Psychiatry and Behavioral Sciences

AF712613

Psychiatry and Behavioral Sciences

An Introduction for Clinical Learners

FIRST EDITION

Written and edited by

Edore Onigu-Otite, Sindhu A. Idicula,

Kammarauche Asuzu, and Asim Shah

cognella®

SAN DIEGO

Bassim Hamadeh, CEO and Publisher
John Remington, Executive Editor
Gem Rabanera, Senior Project Editor
Casey Hands, Production Editor
Jess Estrella, Senior Graphic Designer
Kylie Bartolome, Licensing Associate
Natalie Piccotti, Director of Marketing
Kassie Graves, Vice President of Editorial
Jamie Giganti, Director of Academic Publishing

Copyright © 2022 by Cognella, Inc. All rights reserved. No part of this publication may be reprinted, reproduced, transmitted, or utilized in any form or by any electronic, mechanical, or other means, now known or hereafter invented, including photocopying, microfilming, and recording, or in any information retrieval system without the written permission of Cognella, Inc. For inquiries regarding permissions, translations, foreign rights, audio rights, and any other forms of reproduction, please contact the Cognella Licensing Department at rights@cognella.com.

Trademark Notice: Product or corporate names may be trademarks or registered trademarks and are used only for identification and explanation without intent to infringe.

Cover image: Copyright © 2021 iStockphoto LP/Tinnakorn Jorruang.
Interior design images: Copyright © 2015 Depositphotos/moleks.
Copyright © 2018 Depositphotos/fokas.pokas.
Copyright © 2020 Depositphotos/ylivdesign.
Copyright © 2021 Depositphotos/somen.

Printed in the United States of America.

cognella® ACADEMIC PUBLISHING
3970 Sorrento Valley Blvd., Ste. 500, San Diego, CA 92121

CONTENTS

ACTIVE LEARNING

This book has interactive activities available to complement your reading.

Your instructor may have customized the selection of activities available for your unique course. Please check with your professor to verify whether your class will access this content through the Cognella Active Learning portal (http://active.cognella.com) or through your home learning management system.

cognella® | ACTIVE LEARNING content

ACCESSING WEB-BASED RESOURCES

This book has QR codes available to complement your reading.

The author has selected additional web-based content for further engagement using QR codes, which are intended for those who have purchased print copies of the book. Those who have purchased a digital copy may simply click on the corresponding hyperlinks. Please check with your professor to confirm whether your class will access this content independently or collectively.

Cognella maintains no responsibility for the content nor availability of third-party links. However, Cognella makes every effort to keep texts current. Broken links may be reported to studentreviews@cognella.com. Please include the book's title, author, and 7-digit SKU reference number (found below the barcode on the back cover of the book) in the body of your message.

cognella®
SAN DIEGO

PREFACE

Welcome to the first edition of the *Psychiatry and Behavioral Sciences: An Introduction for Clinical Learners*! This textbook aims to lay a solid foundation in psychiatry and behavioral sciences for medical students and other future medical practitioners. As students go through their training, they invariably encounter patients, not just within psychiatry but in every aspect of medicine, for whom their knowledge of psychiatry and behavioral sciences becomes applicable. Understandably, most medical students will not specialize in psychiatry or any allied mental health field. However, after graduation, given the shortage of psychiatrists nationally and globally, nonpsychiatry providers invariably manage mental health symptoms while waiting to transfer care—when that is even an option.

OUR WRITING TEAM AND GOALS

We put together a team of experienced academic faculty who are active medical educators from reputable medical schools across the United States and a few from Europe and Africa. Our editing team included the main editor, the senior editor, and two contributing editors. Our goal was to simplify the essential psychiatry and behavior concepts and related material as well as possible given the complexities of the field—thereby making it readily accessible and applicable to patient care. Notably, the materials presented in this textbook were vetted by medical students themselves, who provided direct anonymous feedback to the editors on each chapter. We hope that this becomes a go-to resource for medical students and other future medical practitioners seeking a deeper understanding of psychiatric issues relevant to the patients they encounter during their training. This textbook also serves as a medical educators' "ready-to-go resource" for those teaching in psychiatry and behavioral sciences at the medical student level. We aim to improve the medical educators' toolkit for raising awareness among medical students who may not intend to specialize in psychiatry but will invariably encounter or be tasked with managing patients with emotional or behavioral problems, including those related to nonpsychiatry conditions.

TEXTBOOK LAYOUT

The text is comprehensive and covers relevant aspects of psychiatry. The information is presented in simple language and incorporates images, figures, and tables to make the material more visual and facilitate retention and recall. The book is organized into five units, each containing multiple chapters, with each unit building upon the preceding one.

CHAPTER LAYOUT

Each chapter starts with a quote that reflects some profound truth about the topic discussed. The objectives focus the reader on the goals of the chapter. Patient cases are a powerful way of bringing real-world patient and provider experiences to life. Except for a handful of chapters which cover topics that do not lend themselves to patient cases, each chapter contains a case vignette, or vignettes, that showcases patients' journey through their disorder, treatment, and recovery from their symptoms. Special attention is given to highlighting medical symptoms and disorders related to the mental health condition being discussed. The chapters include additional resources for further reading if desired. As much as possible, care was taken to utilize material references in the public domain or accessible to most readers online with or without institutional accounts. Parenthetical citations are included in the text, and full reference lists are provided at the end of each chapter.

Side bars that identify vital concepts, give clinical pointers, and facilitate retention and recall of important material are included in each chapter. They are organized into key points, quick points, clinical tips, and memory tips with corresponding icons. "Key points" appear in the red side bars. They identify essential concepts, including must-know content often tested in exams. "Quick points" are in the orange side bars. They include fast facts relevant to the topic and help put things in larger context. "Clinical tips" are in the green side bars. They are applicable to providers in medical or mental health settings and provide useful pointers for clinical situations. "Memory tips" appear in the blue side bars. They contain analogies and condensed material in the form of useful mnemonics, acronyms, and comparisons and contrasts of related concepts. These all serve as memory hooks to facilitate retention and later recall in clinical, test, or other situations.

UNIT I: INTRODUCTION TO THE PSYCHIATRY PATIENT

The textbook begins by giving learners a global overview of psychiatry and behavioral sciences. Learners are then introduced to the critical tools of a psychiatry assessment with particular focus paid to the psychiatry interview and safety assessment. Detailed attention is given to the mental status examination. The MSE is presented in a unique format to promote knowledge organization, retention, recall, and application. The major components of the MSE are introduced and then systematically developed through the MSE and corresponding terminology. Examples and sample questions to ask the patient are provided to facilitate understanding.

UNIT II: DEVELOPMENT ACROSS A LIFE SPAN

Diagnosis in psychiatry leans on deviation from the norm. In this unit, learners are first given the framework to understand what normal human development is or is considered to be.

The work of notable developmental theorists, who have contributed to our understanding of human development across the life span, is presented. Development occurs progressively along multiple streams. To unify themes, development is discussed along the biopsychosocial domains of development as best as is feasible. Infant and preschool development and mental health is covered in precise detail not elsewhere attainable by the medical student. A comprehensive table that summarizes developmental milestones across multiple domains, including highlights and "red flags" or early signs of problems with development, is presented. The chapter also contains a summary table of evidence-based interventions in infants and toddlers. The school-aged chapter details cognitive development in children. The adolescent chapter discusses pivotal aspects of adolescent development and identity development in detail. The chapter on adulthood contains a case that depicts an adult's life from early through late adulthood. Additional aspects of development, including speech, language, neurocognitive, and psychosexual development, are presented. Attachment, familial influences of development, and the development of defense mechanisms are also discussed in detail.

UNIT III: CLINICAL PRESENTATION OF PSYCHIATRIC DISORDERS

We present psychiatry disorders going by the *DSM-5* and corresponding *ICD-11* diagnostic criteria. For each condition, clinical presentations, diagnosis, and treatment are covered. Common disorders, such as attention-deficit/hyperactivity disorder, autism, anxiety, bipolar disorder, depression, and psychotic symptoms, are discussed. Less commonly discussed, yet problematic, conditions, such as adjustment disorders, grief-related disorders, sleep, and somatoform disorders are discussed. Delirium and dementia are discussed in detail with several useful summary tables. Personality disorders are presented with both categorical and dimensional considerations, simplified for easy assimilation. The chapter on addiction and substance use disorders is comprehensive and particularly difficult to find consolidated in a text written at the medical student level. It provides information in a clinically useful manner, including specific ways of detecting alcohol and other substance use patterns. The subsequent chapter on prescription drug abuse discusses factors related to the opioid epidemic, including the behaviors that may precede the abuse or drug diversion, where clinical intervention can be initiated to interrupt progression to a fatal overdose. A discussion on appropriate prescription practices is presented.

UNIT IV: TREATMENT OF PSYCHIATRIC DISORDERS

This unit covers the different treatment modalities used in psychiatry. The psychotherapy chapter introduces medical students to the core concepts of psychotherapy. Importantly, the chapter discusses empathy and gives a sense of control or structure to the complex emotions that can arise when working with difficult patients in mental health or other medical fields.

Beyond psychiatry, the chapter discusses the evidence-based utility of psychotherapy in medical disease states. Psychopharmacology constitutes a major part of treatment in psychiatry. Medications are presented according to their medication class and disorders treated. Crucially, this chapter presents medical syndromes associated with psychiatry medications, alerting learners to the more subtle clinical signs of known drug-adverse effects, acute and subacute drug–drug interactions, withdrawal and intoxications states, and ways to address these. The neurostimulation chapter covers procedural treatments in psychiatry, including electroconvulsive therapy (ECT), transcranial-magnetic stimulation (TMS), vagus nerve stimulation (VNS), light therapy, and the more-recent ketamine therapies recently approved for treatment-resistant depression. This chapter also highlights the use of electroconvulsive therapy (ECT) in acute medical conditions, such as different catatonic states, regardless of the cause.

UNIT V: SPECIAL TOPICS IN PSYCHIATRY

This unit discusses special topics in psychiatry, including aspects of social medicine, including environmental factors that influence mental health and disability and sociopolitical factors that may be involved. Adverse childhood experiences (ACEs), social determinants of health, diversity, ethnicity, and cultural psychiatry are discussed. Mental health care delivery to particular patient groups, including the young and the old, is presented. Given the shortage of psychiatrists, primary care providers are invariably called on to manage more mental health care disorders than they may have been trained for. For this reason, a pediatrician and a geriatrician were included as authors to provide primary care providers' perspectives. Conversely, the chapter on psychosomatic medicine describes mental health symptoms on the medical floor and ways to address them. The chapter on research contains helpful tips on how to extract relevant information from research articles. It outlines the FDA process of drug and device development and provides tips on categorizing the strength of studies. Finally, the chapter on professional demeanor and boundaries addresses the principles guiding provider–patient relationships and safeguards for both parties.

This text serves as a ready resource for medical students and medical educators to learn and teach psychiatry and behavioral sciences. We hope the goal of introducing medical students to psychiatry and behavioral sciences is an educational as well as a fun process!

ACKNOWLEDGMENTS

We are grateful to Dean of Baylor College of Medicine Jennifer Christner and to our curriculum department faculty, including Nadia Ismail, David Rowley, Clay Goodman, and Cara Foldes, for their support through this process. We are particularly grateful for the encouragement and support of Department Chair Wayne Goodman and Vice-Chair Asim Shah. We are indebted to the medical educators who took on this project during a challenging pandemic year and delivered it in record time! Finally, we are thankful to each medical student and resident who read and provided constructive feedback during this project.

DISCLAIMER

This textbook is designed to complement clinical training. It should not be used as a substitute for sound clinical training, which is essential for learning and mastering the science and art of patient care. This textbook in no way replaces the need to master the current diagnostic criteria set forth by the *DSM* and *ICD*. The mnemonics used are intended to aid memory and may not include all aspects of the conditions discussed.

UNIT I

INTRODUCTION TO THE PSYCHIATRIC PATIENT

This first unit is at the foundation of effective clinical assessment of the psychiatric patient. The science and art of the psychiatry interview, conducting a mental status examination, and using accurate terminology are crucial skills to develop. The unit starts with an overview of psychiatry and behavioral sciences, then it introduces the psychiatry patient. A detailed process of how psychiatry assessments are performed, including interviewing and mental status examinations, is discussed. The terminology used in psychiatry practice is detailed with explanations of how to use each term accurately.

CHAPTER 1

Overview of Psychiatry and Behavioral Sciences

Edore Onigu-Otite, M.D. and Asim Shah, M.D.

> *"Wherever the art of medicine is loved, there is also a love of humanity."*
>
> — Hippocrates

OBJECTIVES

After completing this chapter, students will be able to do the following:

- define psychiatry and behavioral sciences
- recognize the impact of mental health on total health and the general burden of diseases
- provide a general description of psychiatry patient diagnosis and treatment modalities

> **KEY POINT**
>
> A mental illness is a health condition involving changes in emotion, thinking, or behavior (or a combination of these) associated with distress or problems functioning in social, work, or family activities, which are at variance with the individual's culture (APA, 2020, WHO, 2001).

DEFINITIONS AND KEY CONCEPTS

Health is defined as a state of complete physical, mental, and social well-being and not merely the absence of disease or infirmity (World Health Organization, 1946). Without attending to mental health issues, the notion of health remains elusive. Psychiatry is the branch of medicine focused on studying, diagnosing, treating, and preventing mental, emotional, and behavioral disorders, and behavioral science is the scientific study of human and animal behavior. Like two sides of a coin, both are important for understanding normal and aberrant behavior based on an understanding of mental illnesses. A mental illness is a health condition involving changes in emotion, thinking, or behavior (or a combination of these) associated with distress or problems functioning in social, work, or family activities, which are at variance with the individual's culture (American Psychiatric Association [APA], 2020; World Health Organization [WHO], 2001, 2003).

INTRODUCTION

There is no health without mental health (WHO, 2005). The origins of modern medicine can be traced to ancient Greece. Hippocrates, the father of modern medicine, emphasized the need to understand the patient's health and autonomy of mind and the importance of harmony between the individual, social, and natural environment. Thus, the tenet of keeping "a healthy mind in a healthy body" is a significant component of the Hippocratic philosophy, as reflected in the Hippocratic Oath related to the study and practice of medicine (Roger, 2017, Wood, 2016).

Traditionally, an early sign of a medical problem is a change in an individual's behavior. With improved screening and genetic testing, evidence of illness can now be detected before a behavior change manifests. Nevertheless, the response to disease states and treatment still encompasses many behavioral components, such as changes in mood, sleep, appetite, energy, and interests.

With the increasing acknowledgment of the impact of a patient's state of mind on their readiness, willingness, and ability to comply with treatment, psychiatrists are often called on to help manage behavioral problems in patients with medical disorders. For the physician, precise knowledge of psychiatry and behavioral sciences becomes instrumental, regardless of their field of specialty. Such knowledge and attention to the patient's behaviors can significantly impact the treatment journey and affect patient outcomes.

QUICK POINT

Mental health disorders are a significant cause of the global burden of disease (see Table 1.1). About 450 million people currently suffer from mental disorders, making them a leading cause of illness and disability worldwide (WHO, 2001).

EPIDEMIOLOGY

Mental health disorders are a significant cause of the global burden of disease (see Table 1.1). About 450 million people currently suffer from mental disorders, making them a leading cause of illness and disability worldwide (WHO, 2001). Globally, one in four people will suffer a mental or neurological disorder at some point in their life (World Health Organization, 2001).

TABLE 1.1 Global Burden of Disease, 2010

	Proportion of total DALYs (95% UI)	Proportion of total YLDs (95% UI)	Proportion of total YLLs (95% UI)
Cardiovascular and circulatory diseases	11.9% (11.0–12.6)	2.8% (2.4–3.4)	15.9% (15.0–16.8)
Diarrhea, lower respiratory infections, meningitis, and other common infectious diseases	11.4% (10.3–12.7)	2.6% (2.0–3.2)	15.4% (14.0–17.1)
Neonatal disorders	8.1% (7.3–9.0)	1.2% (1.0–1.5)	11.2% (10.2–12.4)
Cancer	7.6% (7.0–8.2)	0.6% (0.5–0.7)	10.7% (10.0–11.4)
Mental and substance use disorders	7.4% (6.2–8.6)	22.9% (18.6–27.2)	0.5% (0.4–0.7)
Musculoskeletal disorders	6.8% (5.4–8.2)	21.3% (17.7–24.9)	0.2% (0.2–0.3)
HIV/AIDS and tuberculosis	5.3% (4.8–5.7)	1.4% (1.0–1.9)	7.0% (6.4–7.5)
Other noncommunicable diseases	5.1% (4.1–6.6)	11.1% (8.2–15.2)	2.4% (2.0–2.8)
Diabetes, urogenital, blood, and endocrine diseases	4.9% (4.4–5.5)	7.3% (6.1–8.7)	3.8% (3.4–4.3)
Unintentional injuries other than transport injuries	4.8% (4.4–5.3)	3.4% (2.5–4.4)	5.5% (4.9–5.9)

Note: DALYs = disability-adjusted life years. YLDs = years lived with disability. YLLs = years of life lost. UI = uncertainty interval (confidence interval). Proportion of YLDs, YLLs, and DALYs explained by the 10 leading causes of total burden in 2010. Adapted from Vos et al., 2012.

More than 50% of individuals will be diagnosed with a mental illness or disorder in the United States at some point in their lifetime (Kessler et al., 2007). Nearly one in five Americans (18.9%) will experience a mental illness each year with fewer than half (42.6%) receiving mental health services. One in 25 Americans lives with a severe mental illness, such as schizophrenia, bipolar disorder, or major depression. One in five children, either currently or at some point during their life, has a seriously debilitating mental illness. Mental health disorders are associated with substantial societal-level impairments. Having a severe mental illness in the preceding 12 months significantly predicts earnings (Kessler et al., 2008). Individual-level socioeconomic characteristics and population-level macroeconomic conditions are associated with behavioral health outcomes (Centers for Disease Control and Prevention [CDC], 2018). The percentage of adults who had mental health outpatient visits increased to 23% from 2014–2015. Increased visits primarily drive the management of mental illness to providers who are not specialized in providing mental health care or services. Adults with less severe psychological distress account for most of the increase, while adults with severe psychological distress experienced a greater relative increase in outpatient mental health service use (Germack et al., 2020; Olfson et al., 2019).

THE PSYCHIATRIC PATIENT

The psychiatric patient is an individual who experiences psychiatric symptoms to the extent that it causes distress or functional impairment in their life. More than 70% of people with mental illness do not seek help from a health professional. Overall, more women with mental health illnesses receive mental health services than men with mental health illnesses. Barriers to accessing care include lack of knowledge and awareness of symptoms, stigma, the expectation of discrimination, and neglect of mental health needs. The psychiatric patient often experiences microaggression from family, friends, and professionals. Such experiences include invalidation, being blamed for their experience, and viewing their needs as excessive or unnecessary (Barber et al., 2019). With acceptance and positive engagement along the treatment journey, psychiatric patients can do exceptionally well and lead successful lives.

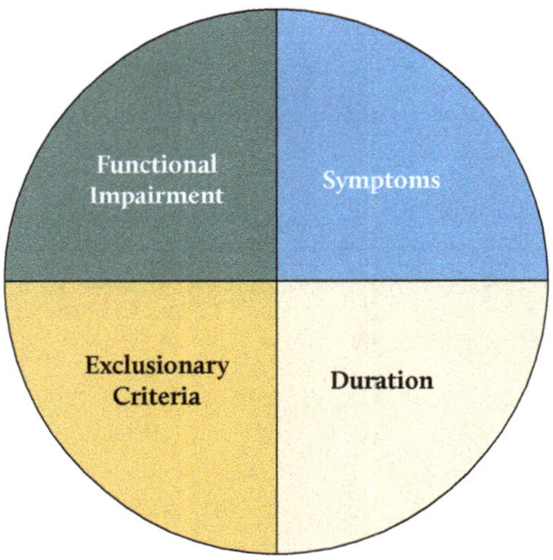

FIGURE 1.1 Essential components in the diagnosis of a mental health disorder.

DIAGNOSIS OF MENTAL HEALTH DISORDERS

Criteria from the *Diagnostic and Statistical Manual of Mental Disorders* (*DSM-5*) (APA, 2013) and the *ICD-11* (WHO, 2018) provide the basis for diagnoses of mental health disorders. In the *DSM-5*, these criteria include symptoms, illness durations, functional impairments, and exclusionary criteria (Figure 1.1). Accurate diagnosis of a psychiatric disorder requires knowledge and skill. While most psychiatric patients are straightforward to manage, others are more challenging. Conducting a proper comprehensive assessment is key for an accurate diagnosis, treatment planning, and, ultimately, patient outcomes.

TREATMENT OF MENTAL HEALTH DISORDERS

Psychiatrists have a variety of effective treatment modalities to reduce symptoms and improve patient functioning. However, patients' and their families' beliefs and attitudes toward mental health significantly impact the initiation and maintenance of treatment. The idea that mentally ill individuals are dangerous is associated with higher use of medications. In contrast, the idea that they never recover, do not want to recover, or have themselves to blame is associated with lower and less regular use of treatment, including medications and psychotherapy (Lewer et al., 2015).

Psychopharmacology is the scientific study of the effects of medications on the mind and behavior. Medications are used in the short term to reduce or resolve symptoms or the long term for maintenance and prevention of relapse. Psychiatrists primarily prescribe psychotropic medications. The use of psychotropic medications in the United States has steeply increased in the past two decades. Data from the National Center for Health Statistics revealed that the rate of antidepressant use in the United States among teens and adults (people ages 12 and older) increased by almost 400% between 1988–1994 and 2005–2008 and does not vary by income status (Pratt et al., 2011). About 75% of retail psychotropic prescriptions in the United States are written by nonpsychiatrists (Mark et al., 2009). Besides, many medications prescribed by nonpsychiatrists have psychopharmacological effects. In general, the greater the number of medications a patient is taking, for either psychiatric or nonpsychiatric symptoms, the higher the risk of drug-to-drug interactions. Therefore, knowledge of psychopharmacological agents is essential for the physician.

Psychotherapy is a form of treatment conducted by talking with a psychiatrist, a psychologist, or an allied mental health provider. Psychotherapy can be short term, lasting weeks to months, or long term, lasting years. Different types of psychotherapy can be used based on the patient's diagnosis and symptoms. Psychotherapy is an effective treatment method that affects psychological and social functioning and neurobiology. In patients treated with psychotherapy, about 75% report some benefit (APA, 2020). Some types of psychotherapy are considered the gold standard for specific disorders, some are used as adjuncts to medications, and others help resolve symptoms and psychosocial stressors even without medications. Other psychosocial interventions are also employed in the treatment of individuals with mental illness.

Neuromodulating treatments include procedures like electroconvulsive therapy (ECT), transcranial magnetic stimulation (TMS), and vagus nerve stimulation (VNS). These treatment modalities result in neurobiological changes via different mechanisms, leading to reduced symptoms and improved functioning.

CLINICAL TIP

- Psychiatrists have a variety of effective treatment modalities to reduce symptoms and improve functioning in patients.
- Psychopharmacology is the scientific study of the effects of medications on the mind and behavior.
- Psychotherapy is a form of treatment conducted by talking with a psychiatrist, a psychologist, or an allied mental health provider.
- Other psychosocial interventions are also employed in the treatment of individuals with mental illness.

QUICK POINT

The use of psychotropic medications in the United States has steeply increased in the past two decades. Data from the National Center for Health Statistics revealed that the rate of antidepressant use in the United States among teens and adults (people ages 12 and older) increased by almost 400% between 1988–1994 and 2005–2008 and does not vary by income status (Pratt et al., 2011). About 75% of retail psychotropic prescriptions in the United States are written by nonpsychiatrists (Mark et al., 2009).

CLINICAL TIP

Understanding psychiatric manifestations of medical illnesses and, conversely, medical symptoms associated with psychiatric illness clarify patients' symptoms and move them to their best possible patient outcome.

MEDICAL CONSIDERATIONS

Understanding psychiatric manifestations of medical illnesses and, conversely, medical symptoms associated with psychiatric illness helps clarify patients' symptoms and move them to their best possible patient outcome. Individuals with medical diseases or conditions are more likely to experience mental illness symptoms. Conversely, the risk of developing medical illnesses is higher in individuals with mental illnesses. The risk of developing medical illnesses is higher in individuals with mental illness. Therefore, in medical training, keen attention to mental health is essential to achieve good patient outcomes and best practices and to optimize health services delivery.

SUMMARY

Psychiatry and behavioral science is the branch of medicine that deals with human behavior in health and disease states. Without mental health, there is no true health. Neuropsychiatric disorders are associated with a high global and national burden of disease. Neuropsychiatric disorders are common. Effective treatments exist and continue to be developed. A good understanding of human behavior is essential for becoming a good clinician and providing effective inpatient and health service management.

RESOURCES

1 World Health Organization, Mental Health
Mental health (who.int)
https://www.who.int/health-topics/mental-health#tab=tab_1

2 US Department of Health & Human Services, Mental Health
Home | MentalHealth.gov
https://www.mentalhealth.gov

3 Centers for Disease Control, Mental Health
Mental Health - Home Page - CDC
https://www.cdc.gov/mentalhealth/index.html

4 National Institute of Mental Health, Transforming the Understanding and Treatment of Mental Health
NIMH » Home (nih.gov)
https://www.nimh.nih.gov

5 American Psychiatry Association
Home | psychiatry.org
https://www.psychiatry.org

REFERENCES

American Psychiatric Association. (2013). *Diagnostic and statistical manual of mental disorders* (5th ed.).

American Psychiatric Association. (2020). *What is mental illness?* https://dictionary.apa.org/mental-health

American Psychological Association. (2020). *Understanding psychotherapy and how it works.* https://www.apa.org/topics/psychotherapy/understanding

Barber, S., Gronholm, P. C., Ahuja, S., Rusch, N., & Thornicroft, G. (2019). Microaggressions towards people affected by mental health problems: A scoping review. *Epidemiology and Psychiatric Sciences, 29*, e82. https://doi.org/10.1017/S2045796019000763

Centers for Disease Control and Prevention. (2018, January 26). *Learn about mental health.* https://www.cdc.gov/mentalhealth/learn/index.htm

Germack, H. D., Drake, C., Donohue, J. M., Golberstein, E., & Busch, S. H. (2020). National trends in outpatient mental health service use among adults between 2008 and 2015. *Psychiatric Services.* https://doi.org/10.1176/appi.ps.201900576

Kessler, R. C., Angermeyer, M., Anthony, J. C., De Graff, R., Demyttenaere, K., Gasquet, I., De Girolamo, G., Gluzman, S., Rureje, O., Haro, J. M., Kawakami, N., Karam, A., Levinson, D., Mora, M. E. M., Oakley Browne, M. A., Posada-Villa, J., Stein, D. J., Tsang, C. H. A, Aguilar-Gaxiola, S., Alonso, J. ... Ustun, T. B. (2007). Lifetime prevalence and age-of-onset distributions of mental disorders in the World Health Organization's World Mental Health Survey Initiative. *World Psychiatry, 6*(3), 168–176.

Kessler, R. C., Heeringa, S., Lakoma, M. D., Petukhova, M., Rupp, A. E., Schoenbaum, M., Wang, P., Zaslavsky, A. M. (2008). Individual and societal effects of mental disorders on earnings in the United States: Results from the National Comorbidity Survey replication. *American Journal of Psychiatry, 165*(6), 703–711. https://doi.org/10.1176/appi.ajp.2008.08010126

Lewer, D., O'Reilly, C., Mojtabai, R., & Evans-Lacko, S. (2015). Antidepressant use in 27 European countries: Associations with sociodemographic, cultural and economic factors. *British Journal of Psychiatry, 207*(3), 221–226. https://doi.org/10.1192/bjp.bp.114.156786

Mark, T. L., Levit, K. R., & Buck, J. A. (2009). Datapoints: Psychotropic drug prescriptions by medical specialty. *Psychiatric Services, 60*(9), 1167. https://doi.org/10.1176/ps.2009.60.9.1167

Olfson, M., Wang, S., Wall, M., Marcus, S. C., & Blanco, C. (2019). Trends in serious psychological distress and outpatient mental health care of US adults. *JAMA Psychiatry, 76*(2), 152–161. https://doi.org/10.1001/jamapsychiatry.2018.3550

Pratt, L. A., Brody, D. J., & Gu, Q. (2011). Antidepressant use in persons aged 12 and over: United States, 2005–2008. *NCHS Data Brief,* (76), 1–8.

Roger, J. (2017). "Mens Sana." *British journal of general practice* 67.663: 435–435.

Vos, T., Flaxman, A. D., Naghavi, M., Lozano, R., Michaud, C., Ezzati, M., S., Kenji, Salomon, J. A, Abdalla, S., Aboyans. V., Abraham J., Ackerman, I., Aggarwal, R., Ahn, S. Y., Ali, M. K, Alvarado, M., Anderson, H. R., Anderson, L. M., Andrews, K. G, . . . Memish, Z. A. (2012). Years lived with disability (YLDs) for 1160 sequelae of 289 diseases and injuries 1990–2010: A systematic analysis for the Global Burden of Disease Study 2010. *Lancet, 380*(9859), 2163–2196. https://doi.org/10.1016/S0140-6736(12)61729-2

Wood, D.F. "Mens Sana in Corpore Sano: Student Well-Being and the Development of Resilience." *Medical education* 50.1 (2016): 20–23.

World Health Organization. (1946). *Constitution.* https://www.who.int/about/who-we-are/constitution

World Health Organization. (2001). *The World Health report: Mental health: New understanding, new hope.* https://www.who.int/whr/2001/en/whr01_en.pdf?ua=1

World Health Organization. (2003). *Invest in mental health.*

World Health Organization. (2018). *International classification of diseases for mortality and morbidity statistics* (11th ed.).

CHAPTER 2

The Psychiatric Patient Interview[1]

Kammarauche Asuzu, M.D., M.H.S.; Zainab Malik, M.D.; and Edore Onigu-Otite, M.D.

> *"A doctor who cannot take a good history and a patient who cannot give one are in danger of giving and receiving bad treatment."*
>
> — Paul Dudley White

OBJECTIVES

After completing this chapter, students will be able to do the following:

- outline the components of a comprehensive psychiatry interview
- describe the process of a comprehensive psychiatry interview
- identify the tasks of the interviewer and clinical skills used while interviewing the psychiatry patient

DEFINITIONS AND KEY CONCEPTS

The psychiatry interview provides an opportunity to begin to learn about the patient, establish a therapeutic rapport that can determine treatment success, gather adequate information for differential diagnoses, assess for safety, and guide treatment planning.

1 Readers may also see "The Psychiatric Patient Interview" (chapter 2) for related material.

INTRODUCTION

Learning about patients, including from their perspective, is critical in psychiatry. It could be the beginning of a long-term doctor–patient relationship. Obtaining a good history is pertinent for any clinical evaluation and is particularly vital for the psychiatry interview. Starting with the psychiatry interview and including the mental status examination, a thorough clinical assessment is often the first, and sometimes the only, diagnostic tool at our disposal. In some cases, after completing the clinical assessment, a provisional diagnosis is made until further collateral information from other parties and results of laboratory investigations are obtained, when indicated.

CLINICAL SKILLS

While talking with the patient, the psychiatric interviewer performs three simultaneous tasks (Sullivan, 1954):

- considers what the patient could mean by what they (the patient) say
- considers how they (the interviewer) can best phrase what they wish to communicate to the patient
- observes the general pattern of the events and experiences shared by the patient. This should include paying attention to events that may be emotionally weighted for the patient.

To do this successfully requires using and progressively improving specific clinical skillsets. Directing the interview process and keenly observing the patient's response are two sides of the coin in the psychiatry interview (see Figure 2.1). Several factors contribute to ensuring that a psychiatric interview is successful. Understanding how people communicate helps our understanding of what is being shared beyond the words used. People communicate in both verbal and nonverbal ways. Paying attention to both aspects of communication provides a more robust awareness of what the patient is imparting.

CLINICAL TIP

While talking with the patient, the psychiatric interviewer performs three simultaneous tasks (Sullivan, 1954):

- considers what the patient could mean by what they (the patient) say
- considers how they (the interviewer) can best phrase what they wish to communicate to the patient
- observes the general pattern of the events and experiences shared by the patient. This should include paying attention to events that may be emotionally weighted for the patient.

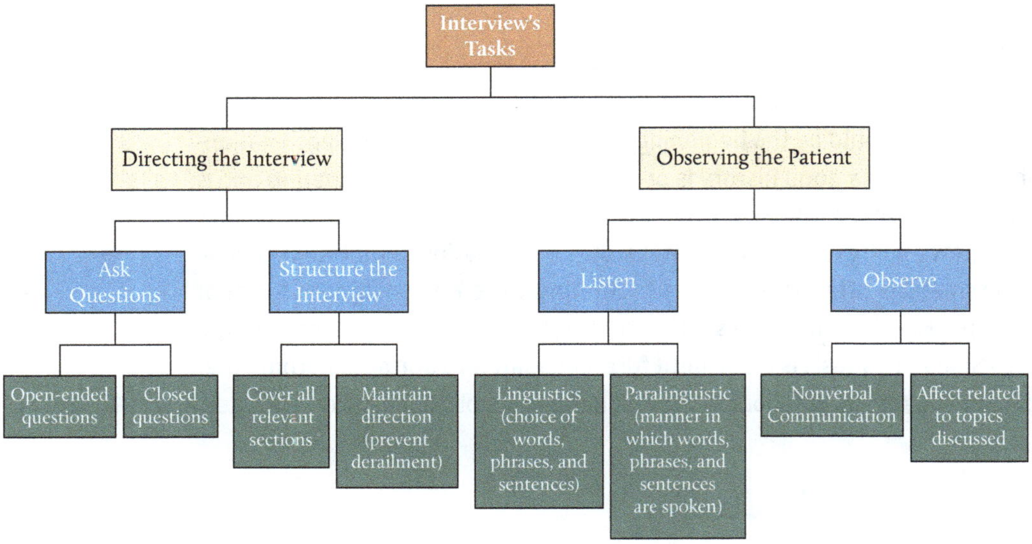

FIGURE 2.1 Breakdown of clinical skills used during the process of a psychiatry interview.

Verbal Communication

Verbal communication consists of both linguistic and paralinguistic communication. Linguistic communication refers to the actual words spoken. This includes the choice of words the patient uses and how they string their sentences together. The paralinguistic elements of communication elements relate to ways people show what they mean apart from the words they use. This includes tone of voice, emphasis on words, changes in volume or rate of speech, length or absence of pauses, muttering under their breath, and so on. What they say and how they say it could reveal their emotions related to the topic. Rapidly escalating tones or volume can indicate a patient is upset or angry about the topic being discussed. Slowing down and lowering voice tones can reveal that a patient struggles emotionally with the subject and may want to avoid speaking about it altogether. It could also indicate that they are emotionally distressed and, in cases of trauma, it could lead to dissociation. Stalling or stuttering over words (in a nonstutterer) could reveal anxiety around the subject matter discussed.

Nonverbal Communication

Nonverbal communication is commonly understood to be body language. For example, tapping or nail biting may indicate anxiety in general or around the subject being discussed at the time. On the other hand, some individuals may habitually engage in tapping at baseline, such as those with attention-deficit/hyperactivity disorder (ADHD). Eye contact is an important aspect of nonverbal communication. Looking away with the head bent down may signal shame around the subject matter. The patient tilting their head down and shaking their head may signal disapproval, including regret related to the issue. On the other hand, individuals with depression can be withdrawn and look down, avoiding eye contact a significant amount of the time. An individual with autism may make avoidant eye contact where they look anywhere but at the interviewer's face while responding to interaction. A patient experiencing psychotic symptoms may look to other parts of the room as if communicating with unseen persons in the room.

Attention to Affect

Affect is the internal experience and external expression of a person's internal emotions. The affect displayed in response to different subject matters discussed during an interview is often key in identifying problem areas.

CLINICAL TIP

Affect is the internal experience and external expression of a person's internal emotions. The affect displayed in response to different subject matters discussed during an interview is often key in identifying problem areas.

A tearful or crying patient is usually easy to spot. However, more subtle cues reveal emotional struggles related to the subject matter being discussed and may be missed if the interviewer is not keenly observing the patient during the interview process. These cues can guide the interviewer's subsequent questions or further evaluation. Upon display of affect by the patient, the interviewer can make a simple observation, then ask a follow-up question. For example, an interviewer might ask, "I noticed that you became tearful when you mentioned your mother. Can you tell me a little more about what makes it difficult to talk about your mother?" On the other hand, if a patient becomes guarded while discussing a particular subject matter, the interviewer may need to tread carefully and respect the patient's need to be reticent on a particular issue—at least for the time being. The interviewer may return to the subject matter later in the course of the interview if this is a critical piece of information to be obtained. How a patient communicates about a specific event or experience should be noted. Paying close attention to changes, fluctuations, or shifts in affect can cue the interviewer to explore further or temporarily avoid certain areas of the conversation that could precipitate intense emotional reactions or derail the interview.

THE INTERVIEWER'S COMMUNICATION STYLE

The interviewer needs to be mindful of their own verbal and nonverbal communication. As best as possible, questions should be worded in simple language and suited to the individual's understanding and developmental stage. The interviewer should be mindful of their own body language and gestures because this is relevant to the process. Leaning slightly in the direction of the patient, making appropriate eye contact (without staring or glaring), and using a calm tone and even pace of voice can help put the patient at ease. It helps to bear in mind that often the patient has never met the interviewer outside a professional capacity. There is a power differential between the clinician and the patient, making the process even more intimidating for some patients.

In the psychiatry interview, we ask the patient to share personal aspects of their life, some of which may be less socially palatable than others. It helps the process if the interviewer puts the patient at an appropriate level of comfort, based on their condition. In general, a calm patient is easier to interview and more likely to volunteer relevant information. On the other hand, an interviewer would not want to put an intoxicated or disoriented patient at a level of too much ease, as this can sometimes be dangerous. There are situations in which firm boundaries are essential to the process. Any interference caused by note-taking, computer use, or electronics use should be minimized. This allows the interviewer to direct the interview while observing the patient, and it communicates respect of the patient's time and person.

Empathic Listening

CLINICAL TIP

Empathic listening is a structured listening and questioning technique that allows the clinician to develop and enhance rapport with the patient based on a stronger understanding of what is being conveyed, both intellectually and emotionally.

Empathic listening is a structured listening and questioning technique that allows the clinician to develop and enhance rapport with the patient based on a stronger understanding of what is being conveyed, both intellectually and emotionally. Patients may be at their most vulnerable as they tell their stories. The use of validating statements, such as, "I can imagine how challenging it must have been for you," can convey empathic understanding. However, being overly sympathetic (e.g., openly crying with the patient while consoling them) can be problematic. This can derail the interview process for both the patient and the provider and confuse the patient. Allowing briefly for the show of affect, expressing empathy, and then leading the patient from that point on to continue or complete the interview as best as possible may be a more efficient use of the often limited interview time.

Question Types

The answer an interviewer gets is only as good as the question they ask. Mastering the skill of question asking makes the interview more efficient and often yields high-quality and specific information. A combination of open-ended and closed-ended questions is often used. Open-ended questions convey curiosity and are typically used at the beginning of the interview or to introduce new subject matters. Open-ended questions usually yield more general information. The information gained from asking open-ended questions can signal which follow-up closed-ended questions to ask. Closed-ended questions provide more specific information that helps clarify diagnosis and differential diagnoses and guides treatment planning. Note that close-ended questions are used at the beginning of the interview to collect specific data, including identifying information such as name, age, marital status, job status, and so on.

Clarifying and Summarizing

The use of clarification and summary communicates to the patient that the interviewer is interested in understanding what the patient is relaying. The interviewer can use repeating, rephrasing, paraphrasing the last few patient statements (now in the interviewer's own words), and checking whether they understood the patient correctly.

Providing Structure

While the interviewer should give the patient the time and space to express their feelings and concerns, it is essential to have a direct and focused interview. Without this, the interview could go on a tangent and get derailed without obtaining enough information and necessary background to arrive at an accurate diagnosis or treatment plan. The patient, or even the interviewer, going on a tangent should be addressed as early as possible. For example, "We were talking about subject A, but we are *now* talking more about subject B. I'm curious to learn more about subject A. Let's go back and talk a bit more about subject A."

THE SETTING OF THE INTERVIEW

The setting of the psychiatric interview can determine how comprehensive the assessment is. The focus in the emergency room (ER) setting is different from the office setting. The interview needs to be modified to attend to the most crucial elements, while being as thorough as the situation necessitates. In the ER, a complete and comprehensive safety assessment is paramount and must be given priority. Under those circumstances, other aspects of the interview (e.g., early developmental history) may not be assessed in great detail, unless they are particularly relevant to the presenting complaint. Regardless of the setting, the clinician should strive to interview the patient in a private environment with optimal environmental stimulation because these can impact the psychiatry interview process. Specifically, overstimulation caused by frequent, loud, or sudden sounds, noises, or movements should be kept at a low level. Other environmental factors, including lighting and temperature, should be kept to an optimal level (i.e., not too bright or dark and not too hot or cold).

ADDRESSING CONFIDENTIALITY

Confidentiality involves the ethical duty of the clinician not to disclose information without the patient's authorization. This should be established at the outset of the interview. The parameters of confidentiality may vary according to the clinical setting or jurisdiction (e.g., military, forensic, or correctional facilities). It should be clarified to the patient that there are

> **KEY POINT**
>
> Confidentiality involves the ethical duty of the clinician not to disclose information without the patient's authorization. This should be established at the outset of the interview. The parameters of confidentiality may vary according to the clinical setting or jurisdiction.

exceptions to the duty of confidentiality. These exceptions are primarily due to safety concerns. A child needs to be informed that confidentiality will be broken if they report abuse or safety concerns. Confidential information may be revealed to comply with state-mandated laws, such as child and elder abuse reporting. If the patient is a minor or an individual with an intellectual disability, consent from a legally authorized surrogate decision-maker (e.g., a parent or a guardian) needs to be obtained. In general, a clinician may disclose confidential information in response to a court order by a judge of competent jurisdiction. In many states, if a patient threatens to harm a third party, the provider has a duty to warn the third party. In all cases, the clinician should stay up-to-date on and follow the confidentiality laws of the state in which they are conducting an interview.

COMPONENTS OF A PSYCHIATRIC INTERVIEW

The psychiatric interview has different parts, each serving a different purpose. The different components are geared toward obtaining a specific category of information with the overarching aim of obtaining a comprehensive, yet specific, view of the patient's current presentation in light of their past and background.

Chief Complaint

The chief complaint is usually captured in the patient's own words. Examples of chief complaints include, "I've been feeling sad lately," "I worry all the time," "I lost my job," "My spouse just left me," "I don't know why I'm here," "I have behavior problems," "My child has trouble focusing," "The police brought me here," "The FBI is after me," "My wife thinks I'm crazy," and several others. Otherwise, the reason the patient is seeking help can be captured, (e.g., depression, anxiety, behavior problems, suicidal ideation, etc.). For individuals with neurodevelopmental conditions, including nonverbal patients unable to communicate by alternative means, such as sign language, patients with intellectual disabilities, and young children, their parents or legal guardians often state or describe the chief complaint.

History of Presenting Illness

The history of presenting illness (HPI) expands on the concern that the patient presents with. HPI includes details related to the following:

- *The onset*—Ask when the symptom(s) started. For example, a question like, "When was the last time you felt happy?" can help indicate the onset of depression. "When did this start?" invites the patient to identify an apparent beginning. "How old were you the first time you noticed you had trouble focusing?" provides information about the developmental stage of the individual. "Did you begin using drugs before or after you felt depressed?" provides information on whether this is a primary depression or possibly a substance-induced depressive state.

- *Occurrence or reoccurrence*—Ask whether this is the first episode or the patient has had similar past experiences?
- *The precipitating event(s)*—Ask for any associated, precipitating, or triggering, events. For example, "What happened before you got depressed?" or "Did anything lead up to your becoming depressed?"
- *The durability of symptoms*—Ask whether the symptoms or concerns have been persistent or intermittent.
- *The progression of symptoms*—Ask if the symptoms are worsening or getting better.
- *The severity*—Ask for a sense of how severe the symptoms are.
- *Functional impairment*—It is imperative to gather information about how the symptoms might be interfering with daily functioning across multiple domains. This includes functioning in individual areas, such as neurovegetative functioning (the acronym MASE [mood, appetite, sleep, energy] is helpful for thinking about neurovegative functioning) and functioning in social settings (e.g., school, work, relationships, etc.).

Past Psychiatric History

The past psychiatric history focuses on gathering information about the patient's history of psychiatry treatment to date. Organizing information obtained on a timeline can help an interviewer understand this information. Examples of timelines include dates (e.g., the month or year), developmental stages (e.g., as a child, teen, or young or middle adult), a period in the patient's life (e.g., while in elementary school, middle school, high school, college, their first or last workplace, after marriage, after divorce), etc. Timelines may also be based on significant events in the patient's life (e.g., before or after they lost a friend or family member or experienced another traumatic event).

KEY POINT

The past psychiatric history focuses on gathering information about the patient's history of psychiatry treatment to date. Organizing information obtained on a timeline can help an interviewer understand this information.

The past psychiatric history includes information on any previous diagnoses, medication trials, and treatment settings, including outpatient providers and treatment facilities attended. Treatment facilities include outpatient mental health clinics, intensive outpatient programs, partial hospitalization programs, residential treatments, drug rehabilitation treatment programs, and inpatient hospitalizations. This also includes ER visits for mental health concerns, treatment received, and the outcome or disposition (e.g., hospitalization, transfer to a different facility, referral to outpatient programs or services, or other discharge from the ER).

The history of hospitalizations should be specifically obtained. Inpatient psychiatry hospitalizations are the most typical way of delivering high-intensity mental health services. However, for many reasons, a patient may receive mental health services while admitted to a nonpsychiatry service. This can occur for medical reasons when being treated for acute medical conditions in a different service. Given the shortage of mental health facilities, this can also occur in situations in which there is limited inpatient psychiatry treatment capacity. Specifically, due to the lack of inpatient psychiatry facilities available to accept patients from the ER, sometimes relatively high-intensity mental health services are delivered during ER stays, and some of which are prolonged for days. For hospitalizations, the number of hospitalizations, involuntary commitments, the reason for each hospitalization, the length of stay, appropriate or precipitated discharge (e.g., discharges against medical advice), and treatment summary for each encounter should be obtained.

Obtaining the past psychiatry history should include treatment modalities, including medications (e.g., pills or monthly shots), psychotherapy, and neurostimulation treatments (e.g., electroconvulsive therapy, trans-magnetic stimulation). Obtaining a history of medication trials is vital, as this helps guide future medication options. Finally, including the patient's perspective on treatment success, including what they perceived as helpful and unhelpful in their past treatment is useful.

KEY POINT

The psychiatric review of systems focuses on gathering information about the patient's history of psychiatry symptoms to date. Organizing information obtained on a timeline can help the clinician understand this information. This includes checking for a history of symptoms in other areas of psychiatry, including major disorders, such as depression, anxiety, bipolar disorder, psychosis, substance use, trauma history, and any other relevant areas.

Review of Systems (ROS)

The review of systems (ROS) encompasses the standard organ systems reviewed in clinical evaluations, such as the cardiovascular, respiratory, gastrointestinal, neurology, and endocrine systems. It includes the psychiatry ROS, which is conducted more meticulously during the psychiatry assessment. The psychiatry ROS is separated and conducted earlier in the interview process, while the rest of the standard clinical ROS is conducted later.

The psychiatric review of systems focuses on gathering information about the patient's history of psychiatry symptoms to date. Organizing information obtained on a timeline can help the clinician understand this information. This includes checking for a history of symptoms in other areas of psychiatry, including major disorders, such as depression, anxiety, bipolar disorder, psychosis, substance use, trauma history, and any other relevant areas. The criteria for each of these disorders in the *Dicgnostic and Statistical Manual* (*DSM*) provides a guide to questions to review for each of these disorders and any subthreshold symptoms (i.e., symptoms being present but not quite meeting full criteria should be noted). Pertinent questions about substance use include age at first use, frequency of use, average and the greatest amount of use, duration of use, tolerance, withdrawal, overdose incidents, and other problems associated with substance use. This is crucial information to obtain from patients reporting substance use.

Past Medical History

Past medical history encompasses all other nonpsychiatric history, including any medical conditions and disorders onset in childhood, such as asthma, allergies, and past surgeries. The patient's current medication history is essential to note, especially to avoid negative drug–drug interactions. Obtaining the contact information of the patient's primary care physician and other providers linked to their care is important for collaborating with other providers involved in the patient's care. Sometimes, this information is prepopulated in electronic medical records.

Family History

Family history includes information about the history of psychiatric and nonpsychiatric illness among relatives on both the paternal and maternal sides of the family. If a family history is present, the individual's relationship to the patient, the diagnosis, and, if available, the treatment found most effective or not effective at all is good information to note. In situations in which a person is adopted, the interviewer needs to ask about the family history of their biological family as well as the adopted family. Family history of suicide is essential, including the details relating to the psychiatric diagnosis and how suicide was completed if that is the case. If a biological family member with a diagnosis of a psychiatric illness has a history of favorable treatment response to a particular medication, this may help with treatment planning. In some cases, the history of violence committed by family members, including homicides, is important to note.

Social History

Social history is focused on gathering important information about current and past social experiences or events. The current social information includes where the patient lives, family and household members, and the general atmosphere in the home.

Developmental history is important to obtain, especially when evaluating children or adolescents. This includes pregnancy and birth history, temperament as a child, separation from parents, and adjustment with transitions (e.g., daycare, elementary, middle, high school, or college). The patient's school history, including academic ability, learning or academic problems and behavior or disciplinary problems, and the highest education level attained by the individual or their parents is also important. To obtain this information in adult patients, the interviewer may want to ask what the patient's experience growing up was like. Drug use history should be inquired about if not already assessed under ROS. History of abuse or trauma, including physical, emotional, and sexual abuse, whether ongoing or in the recent or remote past, should be assessed in an empathic and sensitive manner.

Information about the patient's current and past work experiences and relationships is good to obtain. Information about their work history can give you a window into their relationship with colleagues, work ethic, and any current or past sources of difficulty. In assessing relationship history, you also want to find out about sexual preferences and psychosexual history. Other important information includes their current social support system, including friends and family.

Legal History

Asking about legal history, such as charges related to driving under the influence of alcohol or substances (DUIs), custody cases, and child or adult protective services involvement, can give the clinician important information. This also provides an insight into the patient's life, family dynamics, and functioning and determines the need to obtain further collateral and inform treatment planning and setting.

Religion or Spirituality History

Religion and spiritual history are often neglected in the psychiatric interview but may be significant. In many patients, this is viewed as a protective factor. Conversely, in others, various forms of religion, including hyper-religiosity or even extremism, may signal troubling underlying problems.

Cultural Background

Asking about the patient's cultural background, such as the culture of their family of origin, the culture they were raised in, and the culture they ascribe to, can provide insight into their presentation and perception of their symptoms.

CLINICAL TIP

The clinician should obtain history and information from the patient's family, friends, and caregivers whenever possible or needed. Collateral information is especially important for discharge planning where safety concerns have been raised by the patient's behavior, history, or diagnosis.

OBTAINING COLLATERAL INFORMATION

The clinician should obtain history and information from the patient's family, friends, and caregivers whenever possible or needed. For children, getting additional information from school is often helpful for assessing the child or teen. This may help the clinician understand presentations such as a change in behavior, or atypical behavior, or psychotic symptoms like delusions and hallucinations. Collateral may also be helpful for understanding cultural factors that may be contributing to the clinical presentations. Collateral information is useful in the ER setting to assure safety and disposition planning. Collateral information is especially important for discharge planning where safety concerns have been raised by the patient's behavior, history, or diagnosis.

ASSESSING FOR AGGRESSION AND SAFETY

While most patients with mental health disorders are not aggressive, statistically, individuals with mental health disorders are at an increased risk of violence when compared to the general population. Bearing this in mind, a psychiatric interview is incomplete without an assessment of safety, which includes assessing the patient's potential for inflicting harm to themselves, others, or property. Figure 2.2 shows types of aggression that can be uncovered during a psychiatry interview.

Aggression is a term used to describe several behaviors, including self-injurious behavior, violence, hostility, and crime. Aggression can be defined as behaviors that are intended to hurt or harm oneself, others, or property. Aggression refers to inflicting emotional or physical pain, harm, or destruction to humans (to self or others), animals, or property. Aggression can be verbal or physical. Verbal aggression can range from using ugly words toward a person, cursing angrily at a person, suggesting or warning of an intent to harm (e.g., "You better watch your back") to making outright threats to harm (e.g., "I am going to kill you/them" or "I'm going to burn down the place") that can be considered a terroristic threat. A terroristic threat is a threat to commit a violent crime. This includes a threat to cause bodily injury to another person. Physical aggression can range from inflicting wounds (e.g., cuts, scratches, burns, or punches), fighting, threatening, or using a weapon to attempt to or ultimately end life. *Hostility* is a more loosely defined term that refers to irritability, suspiciousness, uncooperativeness, jealousy, or aggression. *Crime* is more specifically defined as the intentional violation of criminal law.

KEY POINT

Aggression is a term used to describe several behaviors, including self-injurious behavior, violence, hostility, and crime. Aggression can be defined as behaviors that are intended to hurt or harm oneself, others, or property.

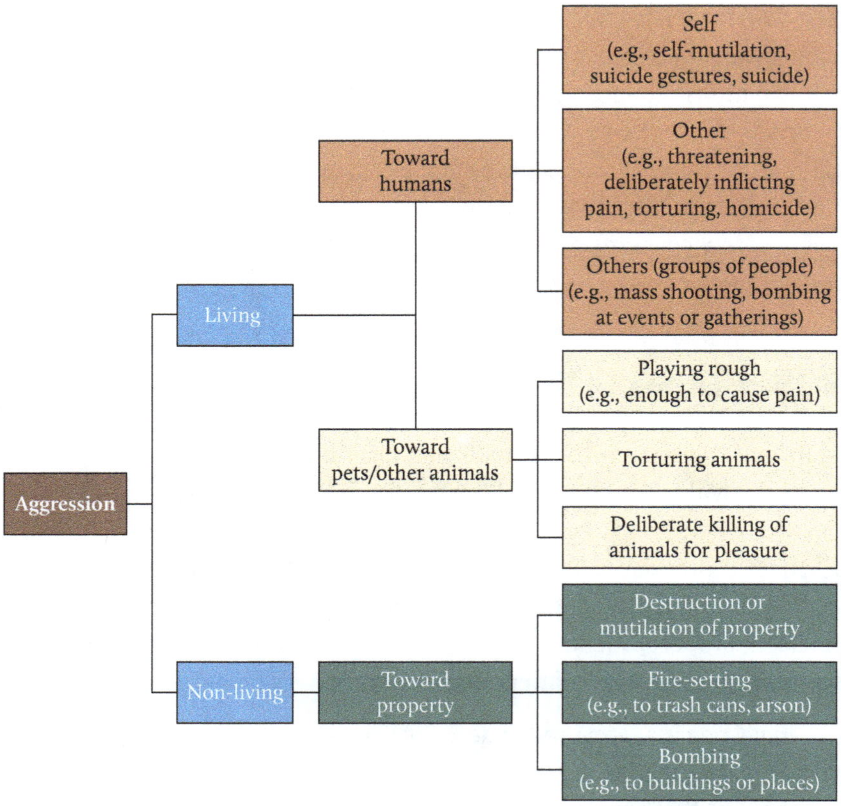

FIGURE 2.2 Types of aggression.

Assessing for safety is a critical function of the psychiatry interview. This means being on the alert for any expression of violent ideations, including suicidal or homicidal thought content, in the interview. More specifically, it includes assessing for suicidal or homicidal ideation, intent, or plan(s). Explicitly asking for a history of suicidal ideation and attempts is essential. When assessing suicidal ideation, we assess the presence of ideation, intent, plan, actual attempt(s), and outcome of the action taken. The means used should be asked for. Note that the intent behind the action makes it a suicide attempt, not the means used. For example, a child who believes they would die if they choked themselves with a pillow and goes through with the action of placing the pillow over their head but can still breathe, and therefore is not successful, may be noted as a suicide attempt. If present, it is important to ask about any preparation for the act (e.g., researching pill types, storing pills, writing notes to loved ones, giving things away). If a patient began the process of attempting, it is crucial to ask if and how the process was intercepted or interrupted. It is vital to ask if the attempt was previously disclosed, the details of what occurred, the severity, and if this medical attention was sought or needed. Asking whether a suicide attempt led to hospitalization indicates the grave severity of the condition.

CLINICAL TIP

Assessing for safety is a critical function of the psychiatry interview. This means being on the alert for any expression of violent ideations, including suicidal or homicidal thought content, in the interview.

The safety assessment includes gathering information about access to means to inflict harm, such as weapons and guns. You should clearly ask if the patient with active mental health symptoms (including adult or minor) has access to a gun or other lethal weapon and document their response. If the patient has guns in the home, additional questions should be asked. These include questions about the storage of firearms and ammunition, including whether they are stored in a secured location; whether there is ammunition; and whether the ammunition is stored separately from the firearm. It may surprise some to know that information pertaining to opening different gun safes may be readily available on the internet—even to minors.

Individuals may become aggressive for different reasons at different times in their life. Assessing the risk of a patient committing a brutal, aggressive act, or set of actions, includes obtaining the history of their level of aggression to themselves or others, which is a critical piece of the psychiatry interview. Certain risk factors increase the likelihood of committing brutal, aggressive acts. These include a prior history of aggression, current substance use, mental health symptoms (e.g., depression or psychotic symptoms), or inadequate response to treatment. Related factors include a lack of insight, poor impulse control, and the presence of specific personality disorders (e.g., antisocial or borderline personality disorders). Social factors, including poor social support, a chaotic home environment, and access to weapons or other means to commit violent acts, are critical risk factors for committing violent acts (Webster et al., 2009). Figure 2.3 shows some useful categories to inquire about during a safety assessment.

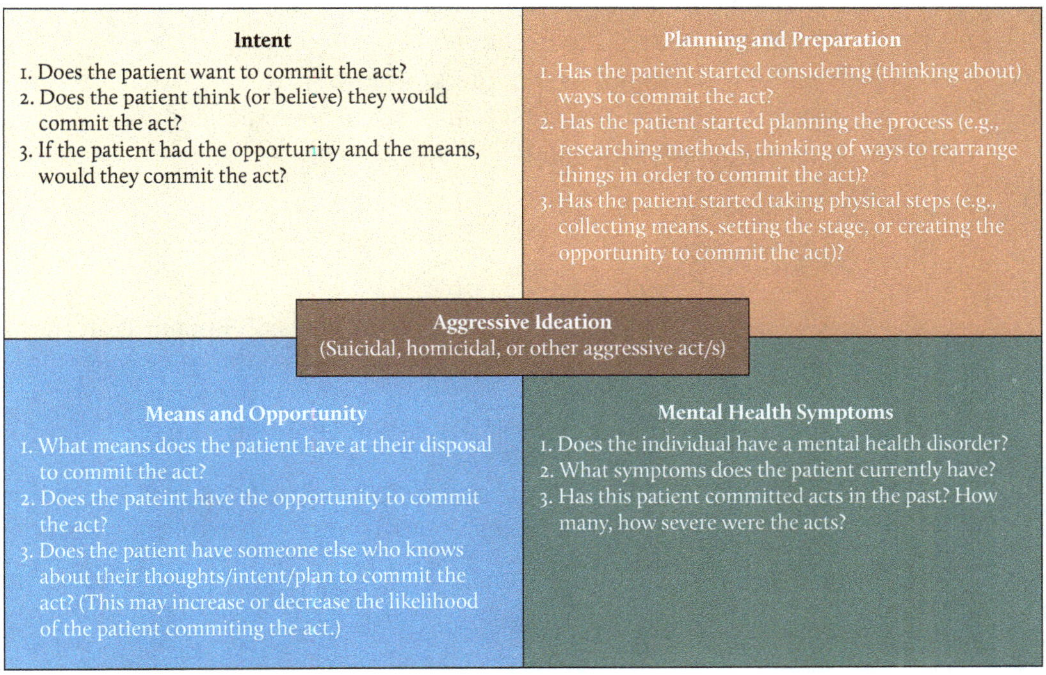

FIGURE 2.3 Assessing for safety and the potential for imminent violence—some questions to think about during the psychiatry interview.

THE DUTY TO WARN (THE TARASOFF LAW)

In some states, providers have a statutory duty to warn potential victims of a patient's violent conduct. Failure to warn the third party may result in the provider being liable for malpractice if the patient follows through with their plan in some states (Gorshkalova & Munakomi, 2020). This is commonly known as the Tarasoff law. In some states, providers may warn medical or law enforcement authorities if the patient is a danger to themselves, to the treating physician, or to others. For the provider, it is advisable to remain aware of the current laws in the states in which they practice that relate to individuals and patients with threats of aggression or safety concerns.

CLINICAL TIP

In psychiatry, a high-quality clinical assessment is often the first and sometimes the only clinical tool to diagnose and inform treatment planning. When done successfully, this fosters the therapeutic alliance with the patient, imbues trust in the psychiatric treatment, reduces the likelihood of incorrect diagnoses, and guides treatment planning.

SUMMARY

The comprehensive assessment of a patient presenting with a psychiatric concern begins with a psychiatry interview that can be adapted to the patient's setting. In psychiatry, a high-quality clinical assessment is often the first, and sometimes the only, clinical tool to diagnose and inform treatment planning. When done successfully, this fosters the therapeutic alliance with the patient, imbues trust in the psychiatric treatment, reduces the likelihood of incorrect diagnoses, and guides treatment planning. As providers, we owe it to our patients to progressively develop this clinical skill set to serve patient engagement, diagnosis, and treatment.

RESOURCES

1. Association of Directors of Medical Student Education in Psychiatry. Clinical Simulation Initiative eModules Description.
   https://www.admsep.org/csi-emodules.php?c=emodules-description
2. American Association of Directors of Psychiatric Residency Training (AADPRT). The Interview Arc Learning the Patient Interview.
   https://umn.qualtrics.com/jfe/form/SV_e9Frr24rKXYqGlT?Q_JFE=qdg
3. How to conduct a psychiatric interview
   https://www.youtube.com/ watch?v=ZGR4Lnn8VCw

REFERENCES

American Psychiatric Association. (2013). *Diagnostic and statistical manual of mental disorders* (5th ed.). https://doi.org/10.1176/appi.books.9780890425596

Gorshkalova, O., & Munakomi, S. (2020). Duty to warn. In: *StatPearls*. StatPearls Publishing. https://www.ncbi.nlm.nih.gov/books/NBK542236

Massachusetts General Hospital and McLean Hospital Residents and Faculties. (2009). *The Massachusetts General Hospital/McLean Hospital residency handbook of psychiatry* (Illustrated edition). Lippincott Williams & Wilkins Company.

Nordgaard, J., Sass, L. A., & Parnas, J. (2013). The psychiatric interview: Validity, structure, and subjectivity. *European Archives of Psychiatry and Clinical Neuroscience, 263*(4), 353–364. https://doi.org/10.1007/s00406-012-0366-z

Sullivan, H. S. (1954). *The psychiatric interview.* W.W. Norton & Company.

Webster, C. D., Bloom, H., & Augimeri, L. (2009). Violence risk assessment in everyday psychiatric practice: Twelve principles to help guide clinicians. *Psychiatric Times, 26*(12), 40.

CHAPTER 3

The Mental Status Examination and Terminology Used in the Practice of Psychiatry[1]

Edore Onigu-Otite, M.D. and Sindhu Idicula, M.D.

"It is alertness to such things as intonation, rate of speech, difficulty in enunciation, rather than by preoccupation with the words spoken, that the psychiatric interview becomes meaningful."

— Harry Stack Sullivan

KEY POINT

The mental status examination (MSE) is the psychological equivalent of a physical examination. The MSE is a structured way of observing, describing, examining, and documenting a patient's cognition and behavior at a given point in time.

OBJECTIVE

Summarize the components of the mental status examination and terminology commonly used in psychiatry.

DEFINITIONS AND KEY CONCEPTS

The mental status examination (MSE) is the psychological equivalent of a physical examination. The MSE is a structured way of observing, describing, examining, and documenting a patient's cognition and behavior at a given point in time.

1 Readers may also see "The Mental Status Examination and Terminology Used in the Practice of Psychiatry" (Chapter 3) for related material.

INTRODUCTION

The practice of psychiatry, much like the practice of medicine, can sometimes feel like speaking a foreign language with a variety of different terms that have specific meanings and that communicate useful information to other clinicians. The vocabulary of psychiatry has significant overlap with neurology, as both have a tremendous focus on the brain.

This chapter serves as an introduction to terms used in psychiatry. This terminology is most useful in the MSE, which serves as the "physical exam" portion of a psychiatrist's work. It includes both subjective experiences described by the patient as well as objective observations of the psychiatrist. It is also applicable to aspects of the psychiatric interview and diagnostic assessments.

THE MENTAL STATUS EXAMINATION

The MSE begins the very minute the clinician encounters the patient. The MSE is conducted by observing the patient, asking pertinent questions, listening for both content and the process by which the story is told, and testing aspects of cognitive functioning. The MSE is documented in each patient encounter, including initial evaluations and follow-up encounters. Careful attention is given to a variety of different aspects of the patient's appearance, emotional states, thoughts, movement, and understanding. To better put the information into context, it is helpful to have background information, such as the patient's level of education, cultural background, and related social factors.

CLINICAL TIP

The MSE begins the very minute the clinician encounters the patient. The MSE is conducted by observing the patient, asking pertinent questions, listening for both content and the process by which the story is told, and testing aspects of cognitive functioning.

Just as physical vital signs may fluctuate, the findings of the examination of the mental status are fluid and may change from moment to moment. The examination represents a "snapshot in time" for the patient, and sometimes, the changes between snapshots may convey useful information about the diagnosis. For example, if a patient is suffering from delirium, a state where a medical issue may present in the brain as confusion, hallucinations, and disorientation, the MSE may change from time to time. A delirious patient may be confused at one patient encounter and lucid at another, which would help the astute clinician recognize as the hallmark of the diagnosis of delirium.

The four main categories of an MSE are appearance, affect, thought, and cognition (Figure 3.1). Tables 3.1a to 3.1d summarize the MSE components by category with the corresponding tasks of observing, listening, and asking.

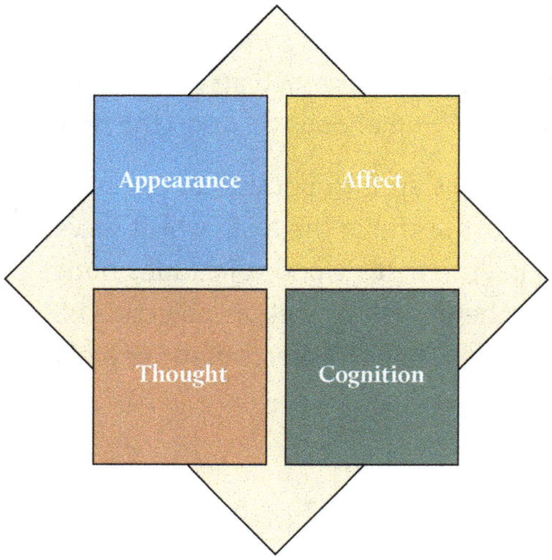

FIGURE 3.1 Major components of a mental status examination.

KEY POINT

Appearance describes how the patient looks, moves, sounds, and interacts within their environment. This includes their general look, physical description, demeanor, and interaction with others present.

Appearance

In the MSE, appearance describes how the patient looks, moves, sounds, and interacts within their environment. This includes their general look, physical description, demeanor, and interaction with others present. It also includes how the patient presents themselves and how they behave in the circumstances, including their interaction with the examiner, their cooperation with the interview, and the appropriateness of their behavior.

TABLE 3.1A MSE Clinician Tasks—Appearance

MSE Clinician Tasks—Appearance

MSE component	Item and description	Interviewer's tasks	Things to note	Examples	Useful tips and questions
Appearance	Physical look	Observe	Age, build, and posture	• Looks stated age, older than stated age, or younger than stated age • Well-developed, thin, cachectic, etc.	• Notice general things about the patient and anything that stands out
			Gender	• Male, female, transgender, or other	
			Dressing and grooming	• Clean and neatly dressed • Disheveled (dirty/odorous) • Casual/formally/overly dressed • If pertinent, may comment on makeup	
			Prominent physical characteristics	• Noticeable physical characteristics (e.g., tattoos, skin piercings, needle marks, bruises, or cuts, etc.)	• Notice things that make your patient stand out in a waiting room
	Movement	Observe	Gait	• Within the normal limit • Limping • Wide-based • Shuffling	• May utilize the walk to your consulting room as an opportunity to get a head start on this
			Rate of movement	• Calm • Restless • Fidgety • Hyperactive • Bradykinetic • Agitated • Posturing	• Notice how they are sitting or if they need to move around while giving history
			Abnormal movements	• Tics • Tremors • Stereotypies	• May take note of the time of these abnormalities taking place, such as during stressful moments in the history
			Unusual postures	• Bizarre posturing or waxy flexibility	• Notice whether unusual postures or movements occur

(continued)

TABLE 3.1A (Continued)

MSE Clinician Tasks—Appearance

MSE component	Item and description	Interviewer's tasks	Things to note	Examples	Useful tips and questions
	Interaction	Observe and listen	Attitude	• Cooperative • Uncooperative • Guarded • Withdrawn • Rapport (friendly/distant) • Hostile/belligerent • Style (unremarkable, worried, dramatic, self-depreciatory, charming, seductive, flattering, entitled, eager-to-please, childish, critical, etc.)	• Notice how they handle questions you ask and their general attitude toward being at the evaluation and toward you as an examiner
			Eye contact	• Good • Poor • Avoidant • Piercing	• Notice how this varies with the history and exam, and moments when shifts happen (e.g., during periods of discussing emotional events)
	Speech	Observe and listen	Volume	• Normal • Loud • Low/soft/gentle tone	• Notice how this varies with the history and exam and moments when shifts happen (e.g., during periods of discussing emotional events)
			Rate	• Normal • Rapid • Pressured • Slow	
			Inflection	• Normal • Increased • Decreased (monotonic)	
			Latency	• Normal • Decreased • Increased (long pauses before answers)	
			Rhythm	• Normal • Decreased • Increased • Unusual (unusual cadence/ intonation)	
			Articulation	• Well-articulated • Poorly articulated • Dysarthric	

Affect

Affect refers to mood and includes the internal experience and external expression of a person's emotions. A patient's emotional state is experienced subjectively and observed objectively. In the MSE, this is further broken down into mood and affect. Mood is the prevailing emotional state as perceived by the patient. Affect is the emotional state as observed by the clinician. In other words, in the MSE, mood is what the patient tells you, while affect is what you observe. Mood is often, but not always, placed as quoted from the patient (see Table 3.1b).

KEY POINT

Affect refers to mood, which is the internal experience and external expression of a person's emotions. A patient's emotional state is experienced subjectively and observed objectively. Mood is the prevailing emotional state as perceived by the patient. Affect is the emotional state as observed by the clinician.

TABLE 3.1B MSE Clinician Tasks—Affect and Mood

MSE Clinician Tasks—Affect and Mood

MSE component	Item and description	Interviewer's tasks	Things to note	Examples	Useful tips and questions
Affect	Affect	Observe and listen	Type	• Tearful • Sad • Angry/irritable/agitated	• Notice how this varies with the history and exam and moments when shifts happen (e.g., during periods of discussing emotional events)
			Range	• Full • Restricted • Blunted • Flat	
			Congruence	• Appropriate/congruent • Inappropriate/incongruent	
			Stability	• Stable • Labile (frequently changing)	
	Mood	Observe, listen, and ask	Normal	• Normal/euthymic • Neutral • Happy • Euphoric/grandiose • Sad/depressed • Angry/irritable • Ashamed/embarrassed • Anxious/worried • Numb	• How are you feeling? • What has your mood been like?

KEY POINT

Thought content refers to the patient's thoughts. It answers the question, "What are they thinking?" Thought process refers to how the patient expresses their thoughts.

Thought

Thoughts are mental acts and a result of the action of thinking. *Thought content* refers to a patient's thoughts. *Thought process* refers to how a patient expresses their thoughts. Thought content refers to the themes that occupy a patient's thoughts and perception. It answers the questions, "What is this patient thinking?", "What is on this patient's mind?", and "Is this patient in a different reality?" Thought process refers to the sequence and logical connection of thoughts. It includes how a patient expresses their thoughts, the rate of their thoughts, how their thoughts flow, how their thoughts are connected, and whether their thoughts get to a final point (see Table 3.1c).

TABLE 3.1C MSE Clinician Tasks—Thought Process and Content

MSE Clinician Tasks—Thought Process and Content					
MSE component	Item and description	Interviewer's tasks	Things to note	Examples	Useful tips and questions
Thought	Thought process	Observe, listen, and ask	Connection	• Logical • Nonlogical • Concrete	• This is how they respond to your questions about various parts of the history. Can you understand their thought process? Do they answer questions in a timely manner? Do they stick with or lose their train of thought?
			Direction	• Linear/goal-directed • Loosening of association • Circumstantial • Tangential • Disorganized	• Do they answer your questions, go off topic, answer with unnecessary detail, give fragmented disjointed answers, or never get to the point?
			Speed and flow	• Flight of ideas • Thought blocking • Thought insertion	• Do you ever feel as if someone has taken an idea out of their brain or put an idea in their head?
			Preoccupations	• Suicidal ideation, intent, plan, means • Urges for nonsuicidal self-injury (self-mutilation, such as cutting) • Homicidal ideation, intent, and plan • Obsessions and Compulsions	• Are there ever times you feel so awful that you start to think about not being around anymore? • Does it get to a point where you think you'd be better off dead? • How long does that thought last? Does it persist or go away? • Do you ever start to think about acting on that thought? If so, what ideas have come to your mind? What pushes you toward acting on it? What keeps you from acting on it? • Do you ever feel like hurting others? (Practicioners can use similar questions for the topic of suicidality.)

MSE Clinician Tasks—Thought Process and Content

MSE component	Item and description	Interviewer's tasks	Things to note	Examples	Useful tips and questions
Thought	Thought content	Observe, listen, and ask			• Do you ever have a particular thought that gets stuck in your head that you think about over and over? Do you have an example? How do you get it out of your head?
			Perceptual disturbances	• Illusions • Hallucinations, including auditory (command, derogatory), visual, tactile, olfactory, and gustatory	• Do you ever perceive (or see, hear, feel, etc.) things that other people don't perceive? • If yes to auditory hallucinations, what kinds of sounds do you hear? Is it a voice or voices? Can you make out what they are saying? Does it feel like a part of you or something outside of you (like my voice)?
			Delusions	• Grandiose, persecutory, religious, nihilistic, etc. • Ideas of reference	• Do you ever have any beliefs that some people consider unusual or odd? • Do you ever start to feel like you have special abilities that are beyond what others can do? Do you start to worry about others coming after you? • Do you ever feel like the TV or radio is sending messages specifically intended for you?

Cognition

Cognition refers to the mental processes involved in thinking, acquiring, comprehending, and utilizing knowledge and experience in decision-making. It includes alertness and orientation; the ability to focus, sustain, and appropriately shift mental attention; and the ability to retain and recall previously learned material. Knowledge acquisition, retention, and utilization are assessed in this section of the MSE. Items assessed include alertness and orientation, attention and concentration, memory (immediate, short-term, and long-term), insight, and judgment. *Attention* and *concentration* are a person's ability to focus, sustain, and appropriately shift mental attention. Insight is awareness of one's own illness and/or situation. Judgment is the ability to anticipate the consequences of one's behavior and make decisions to safeguard one's well-being and that of others. In this process of conducting an MSE on the patient, an estimate of the patient's intellectual functioning is assessed (see Table 3.1d).

KEY POINT

Cognition refers to the mental processes involved in thinking, acquiring, comprehending, and utilizing knowledge and experience in decision-making. It includes alertness and orientation; the ability to focus, sustain, and appropriately shift mental attention; and the ability to retain and recall previously learned material.

TABLE 3.1D MSE Clinician Tasks—Cognition, Insight, and Judgment

MSE Clinician Tasks—Cognition, Insight, and Judgment

MSE component	Item and description	Interviewer's tasks	Things to note	Examples	Useful tips and questions
Cognition	Alertness and orientation	Observe, listen, and ask	Orientation	• Time, person, place, or situation • Sensorium (alert, sleepy, drowsy, or obtunded)	• What is the date? Where are we? About what time of the day is it? • What brings us together right now?
	Attention and concentration	Observe, listen, ask	Immediate recall	Ask patient to: • recall three objects • spell "world" backward • say days of the week backward • Serial sevens (starting at 100, ask the patient to continue subtracting 7 and continue to a total of 5 subtractions. 1 point is given for each correct answer to a maximum of 5 points. • Serial threes (starting at 20, ask the patient to continue subtracting 3 and continue to a total of 5 subtractions. 1 point is given for each correct answer to a maximum of 5 points). • Digit span (Start with a four-digit number and continue until the patient fails to recall the number at a given digit length. The digit span is one digit less than this [the usual is 6 to 7]).	• I'm going to give you three objects to remember, and I will ask you again right away and in about 5 minutes • Please spell the word "world." Please spell it backward. • Please take the number 100 and then subtract 7 and count forward.

MSE Clinician Tasks—Cognition, Insight, and Judgment

MSE component	Item and description	Interviewer's tasks	Things to note	Examples	Useful tips and questions
	Memory	Observe, listen, ask	Recent memory	Ask patient to: • recall recent events in their life	• What did you have for dinner last night?
			Long-term memory	Ask patient to: • name past presidents	• Can you tell me the current president? Who was president before them? • The best estimate of long-term memory is the responses given during the psychiatry interview.
	Estimate of intellectual functioning	Observe Listen Ask	Abstraction	Ask for similarities between objects	• How are apples and oranges alike? (They are both round = more concrete; they are both fruit = more abstract) • What is the similarity between a table and a chair? (They are both made out of wood = more concrete; they are both furniture = more abstract) • How are a watch and a ruler alike? (They both have numbers = more concrete; They are both measurement instruments = more abstract)
				Ask for an interpretation of proverbs	What does it mean when people say? • People in glass houses shouldn't throw stones (so they don't break the glass = more concrete; don't be a hypocrite = more abstract). • Don't cry over spilt milk (crying won't solve the problem because the milk is gone, and you can't drink it anymore = more concrete; what's done is done, and you should move on = more abstract). • Don't put all your eggs in one basket (because they may get broken = more concrete; you've got to diversify = more abstract).

(*continued*)

TABLE 3.1D (Continued)

MSE Clinician Tasks—Cognition, Insight, and Judgment					
MSE component	Item and description	Interviewer's tasks	Things to note	Examples	Useful tips and questions
	Insight	Observe, listen, ask, and assess	From your observation, listening, and asking, assess the extent to which the patient thinks they have a problem	Ask yourself: • How well does this patient understand they are experiencing symptoms? • How well does this patient understand their symptoms as affecting their ability to function or make decisions?	These will depend significantly on the history: • How did you get to this place you are now at in your life? • How did the problems you experience come about? • How do you think about managing the issues that are going on?
	Judgment	Observe, listen, ask, and assess	From your observation, listening, and asking, assess whether the patient is able to take adequate judgment	Ask yourself: • If this patient were to walk out the room now, would I be concerned? • If this patient were to walk out the room now, what would I be concerned about?	• Some will ask questions such as, "If you found an addressed, stamped envelope in front of a mailbox, what would you do?" • May also ask about their plans on managing their illness and to consider how they have managed in the past
	Neuro-cognitive functioning	Observe, listen, ask, and test	Specific screening tools (see Table 3.2): • Folstein's MMSE • ACE-R • Mini-Cog • MOCA	• See Table 3.2	• See Table 3.2

By the end of an MSE, the clinician should have gathered the bulk of necessary information to come to a reasonable assessment of the patient's symptoms and functioning. However, some patients may require additional, more detailed assessments of their cognitive functioning.

COGNITIVE SCREENING TOOLS

Brief cognitive screening tools used in clinical settings can provide physicians with objective data on the cognitive state of the patient at the time. Common screening tools include Addenbrooke's Cognitive Examination—Revised (ACE-R; Mioshi et al., 2006), Mini-Cog, Folstein's

Mini-Mental Status Examination (MMSE; Folstein et al., 1975), and the Montreal Cognitive Assessment (MOCA; Nasreddine et al., 2005; Table 3.2).

TABLE 3.2 Brief Cognitive Status Screening Tools

Name	Utility	Time needed	Accessibility	Links
Addenbrooke's Congitive Examination, Revised (ACE-R)	Neurocognitive functioning and visuospatial proficiency	< 20 mins	Public domain	https://neurovascularmedicine.com/ace.pdf
Mini-Cog	Executive functioning and visuospatial proficiency	< 5 mins	Public domain	http://mini-cog.com/wp-content/uploads/2015/12/Universal-Mini-Cog-Form-011916.pdf
Folstein's Mini-Mental Status Examination (MMSE)	Neurocognitive functioning and visuospatial proficiency	< 10 mins	Copyrighted	https://www.ncbi.nlm.nih.gov/projects/gap/cgi-bin/GetPdf.cgi?id=phd001525.1
Montreal Cognitive Assessment (MOCA)	Neurocognitive functioning	<10 mins	Public domain	https://championsforhealth.org/wp-content/uploads/2018/12/MOCA-8.1.8.2-English.pdf

SAMPLE MSE

Wilson is a 35-year-old male who presents for anxiety.

- *Appearance*—appears younger than stated age, well-groomed, casually dressed male in a fleece shirt and jeans and wearing a baseball cap
- *Movement*—no abnormalities observed in gait, no abnormal involuntary movements, such as tics or tremors
- *Interaction*—calm and cooperative attitude, making good eye contact while sharing his story but looking away when discussing the death of a loved one
- *Speech*—soft-spoken with normal rate and inflection, mildly increased latency with normal rhythm and articulation
- *Affect*—restricted affect with some tearfulness when discussing recent loss but otherwise smiling and euthymic; appropriate to history with overall stability
- *Mood*—"sad"
- *Thought process*—logical, goal-directed with occasional circumstantial thoughts; no evidence of thought blocking or insertion.
- *Thought content*—notes no suicidal or homicidal ideation or urges for self-injury. Notes some thoughts of joining his loved one but also notes no wish for death,

no plans or intention of hurting himself,. No perceptual disturbances or delusions evident in interview.

- *Cognition*—formal testing showed orientation to person, place, time and situation. Patient is alert during interview. Able to spell "world" backward and do serial sevens backward five times. Able to recall three objects immediately, and two thirds objects at five minutes.
- *Insight*—adequate; able to connect difficulty with recent loss
- *Judgment*—adequate; able to seek help and able to function within his life

QUICK POINT

Terms in psychiatry also appear in common language. Learning the accurate use of the term in the psychiatriac field is essential for arriving at an accurate assessment of the patient's condition and communicating symptoms and syndromes to other providers.

TERMINOLOGY

Terms in psychiatry also appear in common language. Learning the accurate use of the term in the psychiatriac field is essential for arriving at an accurate assessment of a patient's condition and communicating symptoms and syndromes to other providers. Table 3.3a contains a list of commonly used terms. Tables 3.3a to 3.3d provide a list of terms applicable to different categories of the MSE. Please note that this list is not exhaustive.

TABLE 3.3A Terminology—Appearance

Appearance		
Terminology component	**Description**	**Applicable terminology**
Motor	Rate and fluidity of patient's movement	• *Catatonia*—abnormality of movement and behavior that can present as a medical or psychiatric emergency. This could include akinetic catatonia (slow movement with the extreme of stupor with mutism), hyperkinetic catatonia (fast movement with the extreme of severe agitation associated with self-harming behavior), or malignant catatonia (hyperthermia, diaphoresis, severe tachycardia and hypertension, and delirium) • *Cataplexy*—temporary loss of muscle tone and weakness precipitated by a variety of emotional states • *Echopraxia*—pathological imitation of movements of one person by another (compare to echolalia) • *Tic*—involuntary, spasmodic motor movement • *Stereotypy*—repetitive fixed pattern of physical action or speech • *Mannerism*—ingrained, habitual involuntary movement • *Chorea*—irregular migrating contraction • *Choreoathetosis*—combination of irregular migrating contractions (chorea) and twisting/writhing (athetosis) • *Dystonia*—twisting/repetitive movement or abnormal fixed posturing • *Tremor*—unintentional, rhythmic, oscillating movement • *Automatism*—spontaneous verbal or motor behavior without patient awareness • *Akathisia*—inner restlessness with an inability to stay still

Appearance		
Terminology component	**Description**	**Applicable terminology**
Speech	Rate, and flow of patient's speech	• *Speech latency*—the time it takes the patient to respond to questions. This is increased (longer) in depression and decreased (shorter) in elevated mood states • *Speech rhythm*—the sense of movement in speech, shown by alternating stressed and unstressed elements and by the timing and quantity of syllables • *Pressured speech*—rapid speech that is increased in amount and difficult to interrupt; the absence of natural pauses in conversation. It is like a water hose pumping out water under pressure without interruption. The words just keep coming at you, and the patient is difficult, and sometimes impossible, to interrupt • *Logorrhea*—copious, coherent, logical speech • *Poverty of speech*—restriction in the amount of speech used; replies may be monosyllabic • *Nonspontaneous speech*—verbal responses given only when asked or spoken to directly; no self-initiation of speech • *Dysarthria*—a mechanical dysfunction of speech • *Stuttering*—speaking with a continued involuntary repetition of sounds

TABLE 3.3B Terminology—Affect and Mood

Affect and Mood		
	Description	**Applicable terminology**
Affect	The observed expression of emotion, possibly inconsistent with the patient's description of the emotion	• *Appropriate affect*—condition in which there is harmony between emotional tone and accompanying idea, thought, or speech; further described as broad or full affect in which a full range of emotions is appropriately expressed • *Inappropriate affect*—disharmony between the emotional tone and accompanying ideas, thoughts, or speech Range of affect: • *Full affect*—normal emotional responsiveness, as usually expressed through facial expressions • *Constricted affect*—limited range of emotional responsiveness, as usually expressed through facial expressions • *Blunted affect*—minimal range of emotional responsiveness, as usually expressed through facial expressions • *Flat affect*—absence of affect or no emotional responsiveness, as usually expressed through facial expressions
Mood	A pervasive and sustained emotion, subjectively experienced and reported by the patient and observed by others; examples include depression, elation, and anger	• *Congruence*—the agreement between two factors (e.g., affect and mood, psychotic symptoms, and mood episode) • *Euthymic mood*—normal range of mood, implying absence of depressed or elevated mood • *Dysphoric mood*—an unpleasant, somewhat sad mood • *Irritable mood*—a state in which a person is easily annoyed and provoked to anger • *Labile mood*—oscillations between mood states (e.g., between euphoria, depression, irritability, or anxiety) • *Expansive mood*—a person's expression of feelings without restraint, frequently with an overestimation of their significance or importance • *Elevated mood*—an air of confidence and enjoyment; a mood more cheerful than usual

TABLE 3.3C Terminology—Thought process and content

Thought Process and Content			
Terminology component	**Description**	**Subcategories**	**Applicable terminology**
Thought process	The flow of expressed ideas, symbols, and associations initiated by a problem or task and leading toward a reality-oriented conclusion	**Logic and connection between thoughts**	• *Coherent*—thoughts expressed are logically connected • *Incoherent*—complete lack of connectedness between thoughts expressed. In this case, it is difficult, and often impossible, to tell what exactly the patient is saying or meaning. • *Loosening of associations*—flow of thought in which ideas shift from one subject to another in a poorly connected or unrelated way; when severe, speech may be incoherent • *Perseveration*—persisting response to a previous stimulus after a new stimulus has been presented; often associated with cognitive disorders • *Neologism*—new word created by a patient, often combining syllables of other words; idiosyncratic and pathological • *Word salad*—incoherent mixture of words and phrases; randomly spoken words • *Clanging or clang association*—speaking with like-sounding words with no connection in meaning; association of words similar in sound but not in meaning; words have no logical connection; may include rhyming and punning • *Verbigeration*—meaningless repetition of specific words or phrases • *Echolalia*—pathological repeating of words or phrases of one person by another; tends to be repetitive and persistent; may be spoken with mocking tone
		Relevance to task or topic	• *Goal-directed*—associations of thought where the speaker gets from desired point to desired goal (i.e., the patient gets to the point) • *Circumstantiality*—indirect speech that is delayed in reaching the point but eventually gets from the original point to the desired goal; characterized by an over inclusion of details and parenthetical remarks (i.e., the patient overly includes circumstances related to, but perhaps not relevant to the point, although they eventually get to the point) • *Tangentiality*—inability to have goal-directed associations of thought; speaker never gets from desired point to desired goal (i.e., the patient goes off on a tangent, talking about unrelated things and is unable to get to the point) • *Derailment*—sudden or gradual deviation in train of thought with thought blocking (i.e., the patient has interruptions in thought, and ends up jumping from one train of thought to another unrelated or indirectly related one)

Thought Process and Content

Terminology component	Description	Subcategories	Applicable terminology
		Speed of thoughts or ideas	• *Racing thoughts*—refers to the speed of thoughts (i.e., fast-paced thoughts) • *Flight of ideas*—rapid, continuous verbalizations or plays on words, producing constant shifting from one idea to another; ideas tend to be connected but too fast for the listener to comprehend. Shifting quickly from one idea to another. In this case, the patient has tons of thought to express. Often due to the rate of their speech, the ideas may initially seem unconnected, but if you examine the ideas, they are logically connected. This often occurs in individuals in elevated mood states, such as mania, but can also occur when patients are anxious or excited. It often goes with pressured speech • *Poverty of thought*—lack of thoughts to express. In this case, the patient has very few thoughts to express • *Thought blocking*—abrupt interruption in train of thinking before a thought or idea is finished; after a brief pause, person indicates no recall of what was being said; sudden stoppage of thoughts—this is like getting to a dead end mid-sentence
Thought content	The reality-drawn conclusions arising in thoughts	**Perception** The process of transferring physical stimulation into psychological information; mental process by which sensory stimuli are brought into awareness	• *Perceptual disturbance*—disruption in perception, causing misinterpretations of the environment • *Illusion*—misperception or misinterpretation of real external sensory stimuli
		Hallucination: A false sensory perception not associated with real external stimuli; there may or may not be a delusional interpretation of the hallucinatory experience	Hallucinations and the five senses: • *Auditory hallucinations*—false perception of sound; usually voices but also other noises, such as music; most common in psychiatric disorders • *Visual hallucinations*—false perception involving sight, consisting of formed images (e.g., people, animals, etc.) and unformed images (e.g, flashes of light); most common in medically related disorders • *Olfactory hallucinations*—false perception of smell; most common in medical disorders, such as the preictus of seizures • *Gustatory hallucination*—false perception of taste, usually unpleasant; most common in medical disorders, such as the preictus of seizures • *Formication* (tactile hallucinations)—false perception of things crawling on one's skin (common in substance intoxication)

(*continued*)

TABLE 3.3C *(Continued)*

Thought Process and Content			
Terminology component	**Description**	**Subcategories**	**Applicable terminology**
			Hallucinations associated with sleep: • *Hypnagogic hallucination*—false sensory perception occurring while falling asleep; generally considered a nonpathological phenomenon • *Hypnopompic hallucination*—false perception occurring while awakening from sleep (getting out of bed); generally considered nonpathological
			Hallucinations and mood: • *Mood congruent hallucination*—hallucination in which the content is consistent with either a manic or depressed mood (e.g., the manic patient could hear voices saying the patient is of inflated worth, power, and knowledge) • *Mood incongruent hallucination*—hallucination in which the content is not consistent with either a depressed or manic mood
			• *Command hallucination*—false perception of orders that a person may feel obliged to obey or unable to resist (often dangerous)
			• *Somatic hallucination*—false sense of things occurring in the body, most often visceral in origin
		Preoccupation: an obsessive theme to one's thought	• *Overvalued idea*—unreasonable, sustained false belief maintained less firmly than a delusion.
			• *Suicidal ideation*—thoughts or a preoccupation about killing oneself
			• *Homicidal ideation*—thoughts or a preoccupation about killing someone else
			• *Assaultive ideation*—thoughts or a preoccupation about hurting someone else without killing them
		Delusion: a fixed false belief, based on incorrect inference about external reality, not consistent with the patient's intelligence and cultural background, cannot be corrected by reasoning	• *Bizarre delusion*—an absurd, totally implausible, strange belief (e.g., invaders from space implanting electrodes in one's brain) • *Nihilistic delusion*—false feeling that self, others, or the world is coming to an end • *Delusion of poverty*—a person's false belief that they are destitute or will be deprived of all material possessions • *Somatic delusion*—false belief involving the functioning of the body (insides are rotting or melting) • *Paranoid delusions*—includes persecutory delusions and delusions of reference, control, and grandeur • *Delusion of persecution*—a person's false belief that they are being harassed, cheated, or persecuted • *Delusion of grandeur*—a person's exaggerated conception of their own importance or power • *Delusion of reference* (sometimes called ideas of reference)—a person's false belief that irrelevant occurrences in the world directly relate to the patient • *Delusions of jealousy*—false belief derived from pathological jealousy about a person's lover being unfaithful • *Erotomanic delusions*—a delusional belief, more common in women than in men, that someone is deeply in love with them from afar

TABLE 3.3C *(Continued)*

Thought Process and Content

Terminology component	Description	Subcategories	Applicable terminology
			Delusions and mood: • *Mood-congruent delusion*—delusion with mood-appropriate content • *Mood-incongruent delusion*—delusions with content that has no association with mood
			Thought delusions: • *Thought withdrawal*—delusions that thoughts are being removed from a person's mind by other people or forces • *Thought insertion*—delusions that thoughts are implanted in a person's mind by other people or forces • *Thought broadcasting*—delusions that a person's thoughts can be heard by others, as though they were being broadcast over the air • *Thought control*—delusions that a person's thoughts are being controlled by other people or forces
		Dissociation: A psychological defense mechanism involving the segregation of any group of mental or behavioral processes from the rest of the person's psychic activity (i.e., a disconnect)	• *Depersonalization*—a person's subjective sense of being unreal, strange, or unfamiliar • *Derealization*—a subjective sense that the environment is strange or unreal; a feeling of changed reality • *Fugue*—taking on a new identity with amnesia for the old identity; often involves travel or wandering to new environments • *Macropsia*—a state in which objects seem larger than they are (can be associated with partial complex seizures) • *Micropsia*—a state in which objects seem smaller than they are (can be associated with partial complex seizures)
		Obsession	• *Obsession*—pathological persistence of an irresistible thought or feeling that cannot be eliminated from consciousness by logical effort (associated with anxiety)
		Compulsion	• *Compulsion*—pathological need to act on an impulse that, if resisted, produces anxiety; repetitive behavior in response to an obsession or performed according to certain rules
		Phobia	• *Phobia*—persistent, irrational, exaggerated, and invariably pathological dread of a specific stimulus or situation, which results in a compelling desire to avoid the feared stimulus

TABLE 3.3D Terminology—Cognition, Insight, and Judgment

Terminology, Cognition, Insight, and Judgment

Terminology component	Description	Subcategories	Applicable terminology
Sensorium	Alertness or level of consciousness	**Disorientation:** Disturbance of orientation in time, place, or person	• *Clouding of consciousness*—incomplete clear mindedness with disturbances in perception and attitude • *Drowsiness*—a state of impaired awareness associated with a desire or inclination to sleep • *Somnolence*—abnormal drowsiness • *Stupor*—lack of reaction to and unawareness of surroundings • *Delirium*—bewildered, restless, confused disoriented reaction; sometimes associated with fear and hallucinations • *Coma*—profound degree of unconsciousness • *Sundowning*—syndrome in elderly individuals that usually occurs at night and is characterized by drowsiness, confusion, ataxia, and falling
Memory	Ability to retrieve previously stored information	**Memory recall**	• *Immediate memory*—reproduction or recall of perceived events within seconds to minutes • *Recent memory*—recall of events over the last few days • *Recent past memory*—recall of events over the past few months • *Remote memory*—recall of events in the distant past
		Amnesia: Partial or total inability to recall past experiences; may be medical or emotional in origin	• *Anterograde amnesia*—amnesia for events occurring after a point in time • *Retrograde amnesia*—amnesia for events occurring before a point in time • *Confabulation*—unconscious filling of gaps in memory by imagined or untrue experiences that a person believes but have no basis in fact
		Memory illusion	• *Déjà vu*—illusion of visual recognition in which a new situation is incorrectly regarded as a repetition of a previous memory
		Memory decline	• *Dementia*—pathological and global deterioration of intellectual functioning • *Pseudodementia*—clinical features resembling dementia not caused by pathological deterioration of the brain; most often caused by depression
Attention	Ability to focus based on internal or external priorities	**Attention**	• *Distractibility*—inability to concentrate attention; a state in which attention is drawn to unimportant or irrelevant stimuli • *Selective inattention*—blocking out only those things that generate anxiety • *Hypervigilance*—excessive attention and focus on all internal and external stimuli; usually secondary to delusional or paranoid states • *Trance*—focused attention and altered consciousness; usually seen in hypnosis and dissociative disorders

Terminology, Cognition, Insight, and Judgment

Terminology component	Description	Subcategories	Applicable terminology
Intelligence	Ability to recall, understand, mobilize, and constructively integrate previous learning into new situations	**Abstract vs. concrete thinking**	• *Abstract thinking*—ability to appreciate nuances of meaning; multidimensional thinking with ability to use metaphors and hypotheses appropriately • *Concrete thinking*—literal thinking; limited use of metaphor without understanding of nuances of meaning, one-dimensional thought
		Intellectual disability: Lower intelligence of such a degree that it interferes with social and vocational performance	• *Mild intellectual disability*—IQ of 50–55 to 70 • *Moderate intellectual disability*—IQ of 35–40 to 50–55 • *Severe intellectual disability*—IQ of 20–25 to 35–40 • *Profound intellectual disability*—IQ below 20–25
Insight and Judgment	The patient's understanding of their mental health and their perspective on their general problem-solving ability within the context of their current mental state	**Insight:** A person's ability to understand the true cause and meaning of a situation (such as a set of symptoms)	• *Impaired insight*—diminished ability to understand the objective reality of a situation
		Judgment: Ability to assess a situation correctly and act appropriately in the situation	• *Impaired judgment*—diminished ability to understand a situation correctly and appropriately; inability to analyze the risk and benefits of decisions

RESOURCES

1 Martin, A., Jacobs, A., Krause, R., & Amsalem, D. (2020). The Mental Status Exam: An Online Teaching Exercise Using Video-Based Depictions by Simulated Patients. MedEdPORTAL: the journal of teaching and learning resources, 16, 10947. https://doi.org/10.15766/mep_2374-8265.10947

2 Mental Status Examination in Neurology, Fourth Edition (2000) by Richard L. Strub, MD, F. William Black, PhD

3 Folstein's MMSE Components https://www.youtube.com/watch?v=st_FaCl-3NCY&feature=youtu.be

4 Snyderman D, Rovner B. Mental status exam in primary care: a review. Am Fam Physician. 2009 Oct 15;80(8):809-14. PMID: 19835342.

5 Montreal cognitive assessment (MoCA) administration: https://www.youtube.com/watch?v=XjrnsIXoSCg

6 Mini-Cog examination: https://www.youtube.com/watch?v=DeCFtuD41WY

REFERENCES

Folstein, M. F., Folstein, S. E., & McHugh, P. R. (1975). Mini-mental state: A practical method for grading the cognitive state of patients for the clinician. *Journal of Psychiatric Research, 12*(3), 189–198. https://doi.org/10.1016/0022-3956(75)90026-6

Mioshi, E., Dawson, K., Mitchell, J., Arnold, R., & Hodges, J. R. (2006). The Addenbrooke's cognitive examination revised (ACE-R): A brief cognitive test battery for dementia screening. *International Journal of Geriatric Psychiatry, 21*(11), 1078–1085. https://doi.org/10.1002/gps.1610

Nasreddine, Z. S., Phillips, N. A., Bédirian, V., Charbonneau, S., Whitehead, V., Collin, I., Cummings, J. L., & Chertkow, H. (2005). The Montreal Cognitive Assessment, MoCA: A brief screening tool for mild cognitive impairment. *Journal of the American Geriatrics Society, 53*(4), 695–699. https://doi.org/10.1111/j.1532-5415.2005.53221.

UNIT II

DEVELOPMENT ACROSS A LIFE SPAN

Unit II provides the background for normal development, upon which psychopathology can then be understood. The contributing work of several developmental theorists, who provide a deeper understanding and conceptualization of human development, are presented. The unit presents development according to different ages or life stages and attempts to cover this by including biological, psychological, and social development at each stage. It includes essential topics, such as attachment, neurocognitive development, language development, and psychosexual development. Defense mechanisms are also presented. Look out for each chapter's case vignette, which depicts a patient's journey through the corresponding developmental stage.

CHAPTER 4

Essentials of Human Development[1]

Edore Onigu-Otite, M.D. and Sindhu Idicula, M.D.

"Until you make the unconscious conscious, it will direct your life, and you will call it fate."

— Carl Gustav Jung

OBJECTIVES

After completing this chapter, students will be able to do the following:

- describe the main concepts proposed by prominent developmental theorists
- summarize the stages of human development in major life domains
- match corresponding theorists' concepts to different ages

CASE VIGNETTE

As a young physician, you begin your day with a new patient who presents with her mother. Her mother discusses how her daughter gets very frustrated when she does not get what she wants. When upset, she stomps her feet, yells, throws things, threatens to hurt herself in some way, and hits out at others who are close—these behaviors last for several minutes until she can calm down. The patient's parents are distressed about this and now avoid taking their daughter to places. One of the tasks is determining whether this is normal for her age or caused by an underlying psychiatric problem. If the patient is 3 years old and typically developing, you may consider this behavior within the normal development scope. Toddlers are novices with language and have trouble expressing what it is they want or how they feel. If the patient is 11 years old, you might think differently about this

(*continued*)

1 Readers may also see "Infant and Preschool Mental Health" (Chapter 5), "School-Aged Children" (Chapter 6), and "Adolescence" (Chapter 7) for related material.

case. Suppose the behavior outbursts are pervasive and interfere with day-to-day life and cause fights with siblings at home. You may want to consider that the patient has trouble managing emotions when frustrated as a younger child would. If the patient is 14 years old and the behavior is new, you may want to consider peer influences, adjustment-related concerns, the onset of mood problems, or substance use in some cases. If this is a 34-year-old adult and this type of behavior has always been present, you may want to consider this to be a stable trait and part of a personality disorder, among other things. If the patient is 85 years old and this behavior is sudden or new, you may need urgent medical work up to exclude medical causes.

DEFINITIONS AND KEY CONCEPTS

Development is the act, process, or result of becoming. In this textbook, we will be exploring development in two different ways. The first is the development of human beings—from birth to older adulthood. This process involves growth, maturation, and individuals' evolution based on a variety of different shifts, both biological and experiential. These changes or shifts can include physical, emotional, intellectual, cognitive, moral, ethical, and social. While these may progress simultaneously, there may also be instances where individuals mature more quickly in one domain than another. For clinicians, having a solid grasp on development helps attune them to the individual they are treating and notice areas where development may not be on track.

Clinicians are also highly interested in development from the standpoint of disease or disorders. How do disorders begin, and how do they continue over time? What is the trajectory of a disorder? At what point do symptoms cease to be expected for an individual's developmental level and become a disorder? The development of disease will be introduced in the chapters discussing the various pathologies.

INTRODUCTION

Psychiatrists face the challenge of evaluating individuals throughout life to discern what may result from a psychiatric disorder and what may not. Some disorders start acutely, and some have a more insidious onset. Disorders vary in their severity, ranging from very mild to floridly severe. To accurately discern the issues with our patients, we need a solid grasp of normal human development. This knowledge helps to distinguish normal from pathological behavior, what disorders are present, and what treatment tools may be helpful, given the patient's developmental stage.

Developmental theories provide a framework for understanding and interpreting human behavior, including emotional, intellectual, cognitive, moral, and other social development aspects through a life span. Several developmental theorists have contributed useful frameworks to help understand human development across the life span. Developmental theorists emphasize the importance of the early childhood and other experiences in influencing human development. In general, individuals who successfully completed the previous stages tend to become more well-adjusted, caring, and secure individuals. However, not all individuals achieve more advanced stages of development. Recognizing this in practice allows for more realistic expectations for the individual when behavior might be at variance with what is expected individually or as part of society.

Developmental theories also exist around specific topics such as sexuality, social identity, race, etc. This chapter introduces developmental theories that propose sequential stages spanning multiple phases of life. Several developmental theorists have influenced the understanding of human development. Sigmund Freud brought to light the development of the conscious and unconscious and an understanding of psychosexual development. Erik Erickson shared a framework on psychosocial developments from birth to older adulthood. Jean Piaget examined cognitive development, while Lawrence Kohlberg investigated moral development. Other developmental theorists whose work focused more on specific developmental stages are discussed in the corresponding chapters. For landmarks of physical development, please refer to the related chapters on infancy through adulthood.

CLINICAL TIP

In psychiatry patients, developmental theories provide a framework for understanding and interpreting human behavior, including emotional, intellectual, cognitive, moral, and other social development aspects through a life span. Several developmental theorists have contributed useful frameworks to help understand human development across the life span.

SIGMUND FREUD

Sigmund Schlomo Freud was an Austrian neurologist who created an entirely new approach to understanding human personality (Oldham, 2006; Cieri & Esposito, 2019). He is the founder of psychoanalysis and famous for providing structure to the individual human subconscious and the psychosexual stages of development. Psychoanalysis is a form of psychotherapy that treats psychopathology through purposeful dialogue between the patient and a psychoanalyst. Freud believed that individuals could be treated by becoming conscious of or gaining insight into their unconscious thoughts and drives. He proposed that the bringing to consciousness and release of repressed emotions and experiences in the subconscious was a treatment that could promote psychopathology.

QUICK POINT

Sigmund Freud created an entirely new approach to understanding human personality. He provided structure to the individual human subconscious, wrote about the psychosexual stages of development, and was the founder of psychoanalysis.

The Human Subconscious

Freud illuminated the unparalleled role of the unconscious in directing and motivating human behavior. In his structural model, Freud recognized three parts of the human mind: the id, the ego, and the superego. The id is the individual mind's drive for pleasure seeking. It seeks out the most basic drives, such as for food or sex, and strives for immediate gratification. The ego is the individual mind's balance-seeking drive. The ego, aware

KEY POINT

Freud proposed that psychological development in childhood and adolescence occurs according to five psychosexual stages: oral, anal, phallic, latency, and genital stages.

that not all personal pleasures can be met simultaneously, creates a balance between seeking personal pleasure and denying oneself personal pleasure based on external considerations. The id and the ego are unconscious, but the ego is in close contact with the outer world. The ego is also referred to as the preconscious because it is the part of the mind that mediates between the unconscious id and the conscious ego. It exerts control on the instinctual demands from the id for self-preservation within the external world. The superego is in the conscious part of the mind, which is thought to develop around age 4 or 5. The superego internalizes societal morals based on caregivers' experiences, placing a sense of right and wrong on acts frowned upon by society. Freud described the Oedipal complex as a boy's desire for sexual involvement with the opposite-sex parent—the mother. This desire is repressed. The child becomes aware of their limitations, followed by anxiety that the parent can destroy him, and resolves this by identifying with the opposite-sex parent. This was suggested within a heteronormative paradigm considered to be the default sexuality of individuals within a society.

The Psychosexual Stages of Development

Freud proposed that psychological development in childhood and adolescence occurs according to five psychosexual stages (Table 4.1). These psychosexual stages revolve around specific physical areas in the individual's body. Each zone (and their related instincts) represents the

TABLE 4.1 Freud's Psychosexual Stages of Development

Stage	Age range	Erogenous zone (area of libido)	Characteristics
Oral	Birth–1 year	Mouth	Pleasure centers on the mouth, including ingesting food and liquids, chewing, sucking, biting, and swallowing. Fixations may be seen in nail-biting, vaping or cigarette smoking, overeating, etc.
Anal	1–3 years	Anus (bowel/ bladder control)	Pleasure centers on the anus, including elimination and withholding elimination until released. This period coincides with toilet training, and the experience of control becomes powerful, including elimination or withholding at will or on command from others. Fixations may be seen in perfectionism or excessive messiness.
Phallic	4–6 years	Genitals (masturbation)	Pleasure centers on the penis/clitoris, including through masturbation, as children become more aware of their genitals. This period coincides with the Oedipal complex (Electra complex with girls).
Latency	6 years–puberty	No clear pleasure focus	During this time, sexual urges become quiet or repressed (go offline). Children direct most of their energy into discovering their world, play, hobbies, and interaction with same-sex peers.
Genital	Puberty–adulthood	Genital (maturing sexual interests)	During this stage, sexual urges resurface (come back online), including through sexual curiosity and exploration. Adolescents direct their sexual desires and urges to others outside of their family.

area of sensitivity and fixation of libido (pleasure, not necessarily overtly sexual) and the corresponding release of tension. Over the years, many of Freud's theories have undergone significant revision (by himself and others after him). Nevertheless, the psychosexual theory is highly referenced and still used psychoanalytically, in whole or in part. Table 4.1 contains a description of Freud's five psychosexual stages.

QUICK POINT

Erik Erikson studied how personality develops in rational, well-ordered individuals and the influence of culture on psychological development. He advanced the notion that personality is shaped through the life span, which allows later experiences to mitigate earlier negative experiences.

ERIK ERIKSON

Erik Homburger Erikson (born Erik Salomonsen) was a German-born American psychoanalyst who practiced child psychoanalysis and studied how the ego operates creatively in rational, well-ordered individuals and the influence of culture on psychological development. Erikson wrote about children being individuals who are aware and developing within their society's expectations, prohibitions, and prejudices. He advanced the notion that personality is shaped through the life span, which allows later experiences to mitigate earlier negative experiences. Erikson wrote on social psychology, the interactions between psychology with history and politics, and cultural effects on psychosocial problems.

KEY POINT

Erickson's psychosocial stages of development span from birth to old age. Each of the eight stages includes a primary psychosocial task, which sparks a crisis that the individual must confront and resolve in preparation for the next developmental stage.

The Psychosocial Stages of Development

Erikson is famous for devising the psychosocial developmental stages that span from birth to old age, each presenting the individual with psychosocial demands (Erikson, 1966). According to Erikson, personal development occurs through a series of crises that the individual must confront and resolve in preparation for the next developmental stage (Erikson, 1953). Erikson's work was further developed by several developmental psychologists, including James Marcia, who formulated the different stages of identity development in adolescence (see Chapter 7, "Adolescence"). Table 4.2 summarizes the eight psychosocial stages of development.

TABLE 4.2 Erickson's Psychosocial Stages of Development

Stage (age range)	Basic conflict	Characteristics	Outcome
Infancy (birth to 1 year)	Trust vs. mistrust	Feeding	Infants develop a sense of trust when they experience consistency in the responsiveness of attentive, reliable, affectionate, and caring caregivers. In the absence of this consistency in care, infants may mistrust that the world is safe.
Early childhood (1 to 3 years)	Autonomy vs. shame and doubt	Toilet training	Toddlers begin to develop physical skills, allowing them a sense of independence and self-reliance. This feeling of autonomy can be overshadowed when failures are followed by feeling ashamed and doubtful, resulting in their genuine selves' inhibition.
Preschool (3 to 6 years)	Initiative vs. guilt	Exploration	Preschoolers begin to develop some sense of control over their environment. They are now able to initiate actions or *projects*. A child who perceives an encouraging environment to do this without fear of being cautioned as *wrong* or *stupid* will develop a stronger sense of initiative. On the contrary, a child who is discouraged from initiating actions or projects may create a sense of guilt ("If I don't try or start anything, I won't be blamed.")
School age (6 to 11 years)	Industry vs. inferiority	School	School-aged children develop skills and a sense of purposeful activity, both individually and with peers. A sense of achievement provides the self-assurance a child needs to resolve this conflict. A sense of failure results in feelings of not being valuable and inferiority.
Adolescence (12 to 18 years)	Identity vs. role confusion	Peer and social relationships	Adolescents need to develop a sense of self and personal identity to function dependably in the world. Success in identity formation results in the ability to be authentic. On the contrary, failure to achieve a strong or consolidated sense of identity leads to inauthentic functioning, where a person cannot see clearly who they are and how they can relate meaningfully in the world.
Young adulthood (19 to 40 years)	Intimacy vs. isolation	Family relationships	Young adults need to establish intimate, loving relationships with other people, including family and marital or mating partners. Failure to achieve these results in isolation and alienation from social experiences.
Middle adulthood (40 to 65 years)	Generativity vs. stagnation	Work and parenthood	Middle-aged adults need to nurture relationships and make changes that will outlast them. This is achieved by selflessly raising children or making positive changes unconditionally that benefit others or the larger world. Adults who do not utilize or create outlets may end up with stagnation, where the individual remains self-absorbed.
Maturity (65 to death)	Ego integrity vs. despair	Reflection on life	This stage coincides with the senior/elderly years and provides an opportunity for reflection over one's life. Seniors who look back and feel a sense of peace with little to no regret within themselves achieve a sense of integrity. The opposite, despair (or disgust), results in regrets from the reflection on perceived wasted opportunities and the wish to turn back to earlier stages to repair this sense of loss.

JEAN PIAGET

Jean William Fritz Piaget was a Swiss psychologist famous for his work on the acquisition of knowledge in children (Piaget, 1970). Piaget described the process of thinking and intellectual development as an extension of the biological functions of adaptation. He described the child as continually creating their version of reality organized as schemas (mental representations of categories of information) and the relationships among them and refining these to progressively achieve mental growth by integrating more straightforward concepts into higher-level concepts. Piaget described cognitive development as the result of two ongoing processes: assimilation (the cognitive process of fitting further information into preexisting schemas) and accommodation (modifying existing schemas to incorporate new information). Of note, Vygotsky, another notable psychologist who studied the acquisition of knowledge in children, viewed the child as a social being with cognitive development that was based on the child's social interactions (see chapter 6, "The School-Aged Child").

KEY POINT

Jean Piaget was a child developmental psychologist who studied how children learn. He described the child as continually creating their version of reality organized as schemas and the relationships between them.

The Cognitive Stages of Development

Piaget proposed that children moved from egocentrism to sociocentrism. Egocentrism is the inability to differentiate self from others. More precisely, it is the inability to disentangle subjective schemas from objective reality, including the inability to see or understand any perspective other than one's own (Piaget & Inhelder, 1971). Sociocentrism is the ability to look at the world from the perspective of one's social group or society. Piaget outlined four stages of cognitive development, as contained in Table 4.3.

KEY POINT

Piaget proposed that, cognitively, children progressively develop from egocentrism to sociocentrism. During this process they make characteristic errors in their thinking. Piaget outlined four stages of cognitive development: the sensorimotor, preoperational, concrete operations, and formal operations stages.

TABLE 4.3 Piaget's Cognitive Stages of Development

Stage	Description (age range)	Characteristics	Outcome, description, and examples
Sensorimotor stage	Infancy (birth–2 years)	*Object permanence*—an understanding that objects exist independently of one's perception of them	Infants coordinate sensory inputs and motor capabilities, forming behavioral schemes that allow them *act on* and *get to know* their environments. Early in the first year, infants treat objects as if they genuinely disappear when they cannot be seen (i.e., out of sight, out of mind). Later, in the first year, when an object is out of sight (e.g., a toy hidden under a blanket), they begin to realize the object is still there, despite not being seen. This is the beginning of object permanence, a cognitive ability that is not fully established until about 12–18 months.
		Symbolism—the ability to use symbols to represent things	Infants begin to talk and gesture, using sounds and actions to represent things. They begin to understand that waving means goodbye.
Preoperational	Preschool–early elementary (2–7 years)	*Egocentrism*—the inability to distinguish one's perspective from another's perspective	The child believes that others see the world precisely as they do. A child may think they're hidden from view because they have a sheet covering their eyes, even though they are in full view of others around them.
		Animism—crediting inanimate objects with lifelike properties, such as feelings	The child ascribes emotions to things, albeit inanimate objects. They may believe a door is hurting because it was slammed shut.
		Centration—a tendency to focus on one salient aspect of a situation, while neglecting other relevant aspects	The child understands reality from one perspective, while leaving out other relevant perspectives. To them, a row of five pennies has more than another row of five pennies if they are spread further apart.
		Appearance as reality—an object's appearance conveys what the object is really like	The child believes an object's appearance is what the object really is. Here, a child may think the milk they are drinking is brown because they are viewing this through tinted sunglasses.
		Irreversibility—the inability to undo mental processes	The child is unable to think back to how an object was before the change (cannot mentally undo an action they have witnessed). Even though the child saw the same liquid poured from a short wide glass to a tall thin glass, they are unable to undo the process mentally and may erroneously believe the tall glass has more liquid.
Concrete operations	Middle and late elementary (7–11 years)	*Conservation/de-centration*—the ability to simultaneously focus on multiple aspects of an object at the same time	The child can see another's perspective. They can now ignore misleading appearances and focus on more than one aspect of a situation. For example, they can now consider the height and area of a liquid's container as important in determining volume.
		Reversibility—the ability to undo mental processes	The child can mentally undo changes they have witnessed (i.e., reversibility).

Stage	Description (age range)	Characteristics	Outcome, description, and examples
		Relational logic—the ability to mentally arrange items along a quantifiable dimension	The child can arrange things by characteristic (e.g., line peers up by height, arrange toys according to color, etc.).
		Transitivity—necessary relations between elements in a series	The child can also solve logical problems involving transitivity, such as if A > B and B > C, then A > C. The child understands the order of numbers and simple mathematic.
Formal operations	Adolescence and adulthood (11 and above)	*Hypothetico-deductive reasoning*—the ability to think hypothetically	The individual can reason systematically and abstractly. They start using hypothetico-deductive reasoning. The individual goes beyond simple to more complex mathematical problem-solving (e.g., the use of variables.) At this stage, an individual can isolate each variable to test their various hypotheses.
		Inductive reasoning—scientific reasoning where hypotheses are generated and then systematically tested in experiments	The individual can use inductive reasoning, which allows for scientific experimentation and prediction. An individual at this stage can predict how fast a pendulum would swing based on different factors, such as weight, length of string, etc.

LAWRENCE KOHLBERG

Lawrence Kohlberg was an American psychologist who expanded on the earlier work of cognitive theorist Jean Piaget to explain children's moral development. He described moral reasoning as a necessary (but not sufficient) condition for ethical behavior. He highlights the distinction between what an individual thinks is the right thing to do and what they do (Kuhn et al., 1977).

KEY POINT

Lawrence Kohlberg described moral reasoning as a necessary (but not sufficient) condition for ethical behavior. He developed three levels, encompassing six stages of moral development.

Stages of Moral Development

Kohlberg believed that moral development follows a series of stages. He defined three levels of moral development: preconventional, conventional, and postconventional, with each level having two stages (Kohlberg, 1994). There is an upward progression within these stages with older individuals achieving higher levels of moral functioning. At the preconventional level, morality is externally controlled with rules imposed by external authority figures. These rules are conformed to avoid punishment or receive rewards. At the conventional level, morality is based on relationships with others, including parents, peers, school authorities, and the government, to win approval or maintain social order. At the postconventional level, morality goes beyond the individual's society and is defined by principles and values applicable to all situations and societies. At this level, individual rights determine behavior,

KEY POINT

Kohlberg defined three levels of moral development: preconventional, conventional, and postconventional with each level having two stages.

and the appropriate action is determined by one's self-chosen ethical principles of conscience, which are abstract and universal in application. This is a more sophisticated level of moral reasoning that incorporates perspectives of every person or group that could potentially be affected by the decision. Kohlberg believed only a few humans achieved the sixth stage or highest level of moral functioning. Table 4.4 summarizes Kohlberg's stages of moral development.

TABLE 4.4 Kohlberg's Stages of Moral Development

Level	Stage	Orientation	Underlying motivation (reason for action)	Example of thought process
Preconventional	Stage 1	The punishment–obedience orientation	Avoid punishment	"It's okay to do it if I don't get caught."
	Stage 2	Instrumental purpose/ naïve hedonism orientation	Gain reward	"It's okay to do it if it makes me happy."
Conventional	Stage 3	"Good boy"/"good girl" orientation	Gain liking or approval	"It's okay to do it if it makes them happy."
	Stage 4	Law and order, maintain social order orientation	Respect authority or keep social order	"It's okay to do it if it keeps things in order."
Postconventional	Stage 5	Social contract orientation	To align with the group's ethics (assumed or proclaimed)	"It's okay to do it if others think I should do it."
	Stage 6	Universal ethics orientation	Alignment with conscience with respect for individual rights	"It's okay to do it if it is the right thing to do."

KEY POINT

Developmental theorists have contributed to understanding normal and pathological development and suggested ways to resolve developmental issues, which often contribute to psychopathology.

SUMMARY

Developmental theorists have contributed to understanding normal and pathological development and suggested ways to resolve developmental issues, which often contribute to psychopathology. Table 4.5 provides a comparison chart between the developmental theories discussed in this chapter. In addition to those discussed in this chapter, several other theorists have contributed to understanding human development and behavior, including Carl Jung, Heinz Kohut, Otto Rank, Alfred Adler, Melanie Klein, Harry Stack Sullivan, and Donald Winnicott to name a few. These theories are often useful when dealing with simple and complex human behavior in psychiatry, forensics, sociology and anthropology, race and diversity, and other sociocultural events and experiences.

TABLE 4.5 Summary and Comparison Chart of Developmental Theories

Life period	Erikson psycho-social			Freud psycho-sexual			Piaget cognitive			Kohlberg moral		
	Age (years)	**Stage**	**Virtue or skill**	**Age (years)**	**Stage**	**Virtue or skill**	**Age (years)**	**Stage**	**Virtue or skill**	**Age (years)**	**Level**	**Stage virtue or skill**
Infancy (0–1)	0–1	Trust vs. mistrust	Hope	0–1	Oral	Weaning	Birth to 2	Sensorimotor Stage	Object permanence			
Toddlerhood (1 – 3)	1–3	Autonomy vs. shame and doubt	Will-power	1–3	Anal	Toilet training	2–7	Preoperational	Causality			
Preschool (3 – 5)	3–5	Initiative vs. guilt	Purpose	3–5	Phallic	Sexual identity				3–10	Preconventional morality	1. Avoid punishment 2. Gain reward
School Age (6 – 11)	6–11	Industry vs. inferiority	Competence	6–11	Latency	Learning and physical skills building	7–11	Concrete Operations	Performance of simple, reversible mental processes	10–13	Conventional morality	3. Gain approval 4. Social order/ respect authority
Adolescence (12 – 18)	12–18	Identity vs. role confusion	Loyalty	12+	Genital	Intercourse	12+	Formal Operations	Abstract thinking			
Young Adulthood (19 – 40)	19–40	Intimacy vs. isolation	Love							13+	Postconventional morality	5. Social contract 6. Universal ethics/ conscience
Middle Adulthood (40 – 65)	40–65	Generativity vs. stagnation	Nurturing									
Maturity (65 and above)	65–death	Ego integrity vs. despair	Wisdom									

RESOURCES

1 Developmental Psychology
https://www.simplypsychology.org/developmental-psychology.html

2 Sigmund Freud
What are the most interesting ideas of Sigmund Freud? (simplypsychology.org)

3 Erik Eriksons Stages of Psychosocial Development
Erik Eriksons Stages of Psychosocial Developmentt (simplypsychology.org)

4 Jean Piagets Theory and Stages of Cognitive Development
Jean Piagets Theory and Stages of Cognitive Development (simplypsychology.org)

5 Kohlberg's Stages of Moral Development
Kohlberg's Stages of Moral Development (simplypsychology.org)

REFERENCES

Cieri, F., & Esposito, R. (2019). Psychoanalysis and neuroscience: The bridge between mind and brain. *Frontiers in Psychology, 10*, 1790. https://doi.org/10.3389/fpsyg.2019.01983

Erikson, E. H. (1953). Growth and crises of the healthy personality, II. *Psyche (Stuttgart), 7*(2), 112–139.

Erikson, E. H. (1966). Eight ages of man. *International Journal of Psychiatry, 2*(3), 281–307.

Kohlberg, L. (1994). *Kohlberg's original study of moral development*. Garland.

Kuhn, D., Langer, J., Kohlberg, L., & Haan, N. S. (1977). The development of formal operations in logical and moral judgment. *Genetic Psychology Monographs, 95*(1), 97–188.

Oldham, J. (2006). Freud's Legacies. *Journal of Psychiatric Practice, 12*(3).

Piaget, J. (1970). *Science of education and the psychology of the child*. (D. Coltman, Trans.). Orion.

Piaget, J., & Inhelder, B. (1971). Mental imagery in the child: A study of the development of imaginal representation. *British Journal of Educational Studies, 19*(3), 343–344.

CHAPTER 5

Infant and Preschool Mental Health[1]

Bishara Bhasi, M.B.B.S. and Joyce Harrison, M.D.

"The first five years have so much to do with how the next eighty turn out."

— Bill Gates, Jr.

OBJECTIVES

After completing this chapter, students will be able to do the following:

- define infant and early childhood mental health
- describe how early childhood psychiatric assessment differs from assessment of older children
- name three common early childhood disorders
- list two common evidence-based interventions for infants and preschoolers

Many ideas presented here have been drawn from *Pre-School Mental Health Disorders: A Review* (Zaim & Harrison, 2020) and *Clinical Guide to Psychiatric Assessment of Infants and Young Children* (Frankel et al., 2019).

CASE VIGNETTE

OVERVIEW:

C. J. is a 2-year and 9-month-old biracial girl with a history of developmental delays who presents to the clinic referred by her pediatrician due to concerns of disruptive behavior, hyperactivity, and impulsivity. C. J.'s mother describes C. J. as an energetic child who is always on the go. At home, she climbs onto furniture, jumps off countertops, hops off stairs, and has run out the home's front door a few times. When outdoors, her mother has to keep

(*continued*)

1 Readers may also see "Essentials of Human Development" (Chapter 4) for related material.

a close watch on her because there have been instances when C. J. has run off in the store with her mother chasing behind. On one occasion, C. J. bolted across the street without looking for oncoming traffic. Luckily, motorists saw her in time and slowed down, so C. J. did not get hurt. C. J. is impatient and quickly gets upset when her needs are not met right away. Several times a day, she has meltdowns, where she cries, screams, throws herself to the ground, bangs her head, throws things, bites, and kicks at her parents. C. J. wants to play with other kids but is aggressive in her play, often snatching their toys or pushing them aside. When meeting strangers, C. J. clings to her mother but also quickly warms up to them. There have been changes in C. J.'s life recently. Four months ago, the family moved to a new home, and a month ago, her mother began a second job. Her mother notes since then, C. J. has trouble falling asleep with worsening behavior.

PREGNANCY AND BIRTH HISTORY:
C. J. was the second pregnancy of two for her mother. She was unplanned, but her parents' reaction to the pregnancy was one of happiness and acceptance. Her mother received prenatal care, and there was no exposure to alcohol or illicit drugs in utero. C. J. was the 6-pound 6-ounce product of a full-term vaginal delivery with no complications after the delivery.

TEMPERAMENT AS AN INFANT:
C. J.'s parents describe her as an "easy baby," but she reacted with high emotional intensity and thrived on sensory stimulation and physical activity.

DEVELOPMENTAL HISTORY:
C. J. had motor developmental delays that became more evident around 12 months old. She sat without support at 7 months, crawled at 10 months, stood with support at 12 months, walked with support at 13 months, and walked unassisted at 15 months. Currently, she can run, climb stairs up and down unassisted, jump, kick, and throw a ball. She can use a fork and spoon, take her clothes off independently, and copy a line. C. J. had language delays, which were evident early on. Although she said her first word around 3–4 months ("doll"), she did not repeat it after that. The first word that she consistently said was "Dad," and this began around 15 months old. Currently, she can meaningfully put two words together like "juice please." Her vocabulary consists of about 10–15 different words, which her mother understands about 90% of the time. Social milestones were met on time. C. J. had a social smile at 1 month. At 12 months she demonstrated a reciprocal smile, looked at things pointed at by her mom, responded to her name, showed objects to her mom, and engaged in two-way communication using vocalization and eye contact. Currently, she engages in parallel play and imitates adults—for example, she imitates speaking on the phone. She has not yet engaged in complex symbolic play. There were no developmental regressions.

PAST MEDICAL HISTORY:
C. J. does not have a history of seizures; heart problems; or thyroid, vision, or hearing problems.

FAMILY HISTORY:
C. J.'s mother has a history of asthma, depression, and anxiety, and she is currently stable on Zoloft. C. J.'s maternal half-brother has a history of ADHD, learning disabilities, and asthma.

There is a history of ADHD, autism spectrum disorder, alcohol abuse, and thyroid dysfunction in the extended maternal family.

PSYCHOSOCIAL HISTORY:

C. J. lives with both parents and her 10-year-old maternal half-brother. C. J.'s mother works two different jobs. Her father is currently unemployed. C. J.'s maternal grandparents assist in caring for C. J. from time to time. The family has had several moves in the past year, including a brief period of homelessness.

Parenting techniques differ in that C. J.'s father has a laid-back approach, allowing C. J. to do whatever she wants most of the time. He, however, also tends to react more angrily when reprimanding her. Her mother, on the contrary, tries to set limits and redirect C. J. frequently.

PAST TREATMENT:

C. J. was evaluated by an early intervention program at 15 months and received physical therapy; occupational therapy; and speech therapy for gross motor, fine motor and speech, and language delays. C. J. has not had any psychiatric interventions or medication trials previously. There is no reported history of exposure to trauma or involvement of child protective services.

MENTAL STATUS EXAM:

C. J. was present at the clinic with her mother. She was thinly built and casually dressed in a gray tank top, pink shorts, and green Crocs. Her hair was braided neatly with pink beads. While C. J. and her mother waited in the playroom for the appointment, C. J. played with several toys strewn on the floor and was constantly on the move. As the provider approached and greeted them, C. J. sought her mother and held on to her mother's hands. As they entered the office, she curiously looked around while still staying by her mother's side. She soon became comfortable enough to venture away from her mother, touching things placed on the provider's desk, picking up the telephone, placing it on her ears, saying "hello," and nudging her mother to do the same by placing the handset to her mother's ears. Soon, her interest moved on to the dollhouse in the corner of the room, but it quickly shifted to other toys. She was constantly on the move, often returning to her mother, wanting to sit on her lap briefly and turning her mother's head toward her as her mother continued to talk with the provider. At one point, C. J. got upset when she couldn't retrieve her mother's car keys from her mother's hand. She struck her mother on her hand a few times but soon got distracted by something else and got engaged in another activity. C. J. did not engage in any self-harming or self-soothing behavior. She was able to label two body parts of a doll in the office. She used a whole hand grasp to hold a pencil and scribbled on the paper provided. She was able to more or less copy a stroke. She was able to stack and make towers of three to four cubes. She was unable to use a key to open a toy chest in the office. She spoke in mostly one- to two-word sentences, such as "hello" and "baby crying." These were difficult to understand most of the time and needed her mother's translation. She struggled to follow through with two-step commands due to her easy distractibility. Her mood was "happy," and her affect was mood congruent, appropriate, and reactive. She had difficulty transitioning and required multiple prompts and redirection to stop playing. As they returned to the waiting area, she demonstrated her skills of walking on her toes, jumping, and running. She was fully alert throughout the visit.

(*continued*)

The following are questions to keep in mind as you read through the chapter:

1. What challenges do you face in diagnosing children as young as C.J.?
2. What would your first line of treatment recommendation be?
3. What additional services does this child require?

DEFINITIONS AND KEY CONCEPTS

Infant and early childhood mental health (IECMH) is synonymous with healthy social and emotional development. Zero to Three is a national nonprofit organization that informs, trains, and supports professionals, policymakers, and parents in the area of IECMH. It defines IECMH as the developing capacity of the child from birth to age five to form close and secure interpersonal relationships; experience, regulate, and express emotions; and explore the environment and learn in the context of family, community, and cultural expectations (Zero to Three, 2017). The World Association of Infant Mental Health (WAIMH) is an international nonprofit organization of scientific and educational professionals with the aim of promoting the mental well-being and healthy development of infants worldwide through the generation and dissemination of scientific knowledge. They define IECMH as an infant or young child's ability to develop physically, cognitively, and socially in a manner that allows them to master the primary emotional tasks of early childhood without serious disruption caused by harmful life events (Osofsky & Fitzgerald, 2000).

KEY POINT

Infant and early childhood mental health refers to an infant or young child's ability to develop physically, cognitively, and socially in a manner that allows them to master the primary emotional tasks of early childhood without serious disruption caused by harmful life events (Osofsky & Fitzgerald, 2000).

INTRODUCTION

They are only babies. For many years, mental health disorders in infants and very young children have been minimized, dismissed, or misunderstood. The field of infant and early childhood mental health (IECMH) has done a great deal since the mid-twentieth century to bring to light the social and emotional life of the infant and the young child, while social sciences and medicine have attempted to recognize, validate, and classify mental health problems in infancy and early childhood.

THEORETICAL AND HISTORICAL BACKGROUND

Infant and early childhood mental health has early roots in psychoanalytic theory but has greatly expanded to incorporate the expanding science of neurodevelopment. Some of the theorists who have contributed to the appreciation of IECMH include:

- *Sigmund Freud* (1856–1939) was among the first to recognize that individuals develop attachment relationships very early and that these relationships have potential to create problems (neuroses) if they are conflictual or do not meet the young child's needs.
- *Anna Freud* (1895–1983) is considered the founder of psychoanalytic child psychology. Her focus was on causes and treatment of behavioral problems in infancy. She was one of the first to make the connection between early childhood behavior and trauma, developmental challenges, and emotional conflict.
- *Jean Piaget's* (1896–1980) major contribution was the understanding of early childhood cognitive processes, which led to the realization that because of their differences in reasoning and understanding the world, young children should be viewed differently from adults (see Chapter 4, "Essentials of Human Development").
- *Donald Winnicott* (1896–1971) was a pediatrician and psychoanalyst who is frequently quoted for, "There is no such thing as a baby," meaning that an infant cannot exist without a caregiver. He stressed the role of parenting in development and supported the idea of the "good enough," as opposed to perfect, parent.
- *Erik Erikson's* (1902–1994) nine stages of development throughout the life cycle include three that describe the foundations of IECMH: trust versus mistrust (0–18 months), autonomy versus shame (1–3 years), and initiative versus guilt (3–5 years).
- *John Bowlby* (1907–1990) is considered the father of attachment theory and was one of the first to describe attachment styles and behaviors. He recognized that the early separation of infants from their mothers had negative effects on children's emotional and intellectual development.
- *Mary Ainsworth* (1913–1999), known as the mother of attachment theory, expanded on Bowlby's work with the development of a procedure entitled the strange situation, which is still widely used as an observational research tool for classifying attachment styles and behaviors.
- *Margaret Mahler's* (1897–1985) theory of separation-individuation described the stages of a young child's acquisition of a sense of identity separate from their mother or caregiver.
- *Selma Fraiberg* (1918–1991) was one of the founding members of Zero to Three and promoted the term social-emotional development. She described the impact of caregivers' early experiences and the concept of transgenerational transmission of trauma in her book *Ghosts in the Nursery*. Her book *The Magic Years* (Fraiberg, 1996) is seminal for students of early childhood development (Stein et al., 2019).

The focus on the caregiver–child relationship and addressing any challenges that arise within the framework of that relationship is at the heart of IECMH (Zeanah et al., 2008). Conversely, a young child's mental health is critical not only to their ability to form relationships but also to regulate a wide range of emotions and explore their environment in a manner that will place the child on an optimal developmental trajectory.

KEY POINT

A young child's mental health is critical not only to their ability to form relationships but also to regulate a wide range of emotions and explore their environment in a manner that will place the child on an optimal developmental trajectory.

The following chapter will provide an overview of the importance of early childhood development in building a foundation for optimal IECMH, approaches to the psychiatric assessment of infants and young children, some common diagnoses, and some evidence-based interventions.

THE DEVELOPING BRAIN

Early childhood is a period of explosive brain development. Brain volume increases from about 36% of the adult volume at 2 to 4 weeks of age to 83% of the adult volume by 2 years of age (Knickmeyer et al., 2008). In the first few years of life, more than one million new neuronal connections are formed every second. After this period, pruning occurs where connections are reduced to make the brain more efficient in its functioning. Sensory pathways, like vision and hearing, develop first followed by early language function and then higher cognitive skills. There are critical periods of impact not only on prenatal brain development but also during infancy and early childhood. For example, language development is greatly impacted by environmental exposure to language in the first two years. A recent fMRI study of 27 brain regions categorized into four functional domains, including vision, motor, language and cognition, identified significantly increased connectivity between 0 and 24 months in the visual and language domains (Yin et al., 2019).

QUICK POINT

The first two years of life are critical for brain development. At birth, the brain is about 25% of its adult size. This rapidly increases in the first month of life to about 36% of the adult brain volume. By age 2, the brain is over 80% the adult volume.

The interactions between genes and environment shape the developing brain. Early childhood experiences impact the foundations of learning, health, and behavior. Stable, caring, and interactive relationships between the parent and child are critical for developing strong foundations. The plasticity of the brain to adapt to changes in environment and interactions is at its maximum during the early childhood years and becomes increasingly difficult to alter over time. Emotional wellbeing and social competence become the foundation for later-emerging cognitive skills and are closely intertwined. Moderate short-lived stress, which is relieved quickly when the child receives support from a caring adult, can promote growth. However, chronic stressors like neglect, extreme poverty, maternal depression, or abuse can alter the development of the brain leading to long term consequences for learning, behavior, and physical and mental health.

STREAMS OF DEVELOPMENT

Developmental milestones are described along five streams of development: gross and fine motor, visual motor problem-solving, language, social skills, and adaptive skills. Developmental disorders arise from:

1. *Delays*—when milestones are attained at a slower rate but are in the proper sequence; they are quantified by the developmental quotient [DQ], which is developmental age/chronological age
2. *Deviances*—when milestones in a single stream develop in an uncustomary sequence
3. *Dissociations*—when the different developmental streams develop at different rates

CLINICAL TIP

Developmental milestones are described along five streams of development: gross and fine motor, visual motor problem-solving, language, social skills, and adaptive skills. Developmental disorders arise from delays, deviances, or dissociations within the different developmental streams.

TABLE 5.1 Developmental Milestones Table

Age	Motor milestones	Language milestones	Social/ emotional milestones	Developmental red flags (if not achieving)
18 months	• Walk upstairs with one hand held • Scribble spontaneously • Stack three blocks	• Knows 10–25 words	• Early symbolic play	• Does not say "mama," "dada," or other names • Unable to follow one-step directions • Does not engage in simple pretend play • Unable to understand spoken language/gesture combinations • Cannot walk independently
24 months	• Run well • Stairs up/ down alone • Imitate stroke • Stack seven blocks	• Can point to 5–6 body parts • Uses over 50 words • Uses pronouns I, you, and me • Uses two-word phrases	• Engages in parallel play but begins to include other children, such as in chase games	• Unable to identify (e.g., by pointing to) body parts when they are named • Points and leads others to items of interest, rather than using names

(continued)

MEMORY TIP

Motor Milestones

Infancy: Using a 3-month timeline as anchors, motor development progresses from head to toe as follows:

- By about 3 months: holds head and shoulders up from prone position
- By about 6 months: sits up without support
- By about 9 months: crawls
- By about 12 months: walks

2-year-old: runs TWO fast
3-year-old: rides TRIcycle
4-year-old: can stand on one foot for two seconds \4/
5-year-old: can do a somersault (imagine a tumbling digit 5)

TABLE 5.1 *(Continued)*

Age	Motor milestones	Language milestones	Social/ emotional milestones	Developmental red flags (if not achieving)
		• Refers to self by name • 50% of speech understood by strangers	• Gets excited when with other children	• Unable to use two-word meaningful phrases (without imitating or repeating)
30 months	• Throws a ball overhand • Washes and dries hands • Brushes teeth with help • Pulls pants up with assistance • Differentiates between vertical and horizontal strokes	• Asks many "What?" and "Where?" questions	• Starts to play with, not just alongside, other kids • Imitates adult activities • Complex symbolic play	• Unable to use two-word unique phrases, including noun–verb combinations • Does not verbally or nonverbally respond or nod/ shake head to questions
3 years	• Rides tricycle • Stack nine blocks • Copy circle	• Three-word sentence • 75% of speech understood by strangers	• Starts to share with/ without prompt • Child can use words to think about what someone else is thinking (Dad thought I was at home)	• Unable to use three-word sentences • Unable to follow two-step directions • Manifests echolalia to questions (repeats questions without answering)

Age	Motor milestones	Language milestones	Social/ emotional milestones	Developmental red flags (if not achieving)
4 years	• Button clothing • Hops and stands on one foot for 2 seconds • Catches a bounced ball most of the time • Copy cross • Copy square	• Name four colors • 100% speech understandable to strangers • Sings songs (e.g., the alphabet song or nursery rhymes)	• Passes Sally and Anne test • Child can be concerned about being deceived or tricked by others • Has a preferred friend	• Ignores or does not respond to other children or to people outside the family • Shows little interest in new or interactive activities. • Does not understand the concepts of *same* and *different*
6 years	• Tie shoes • Copy an arrow or a diamond. • Copy complex shapes (e.g., overlapping circles or a six-sided cube after guidance)	• Asks "Why?" questions • Can follow routines and do daily tasks • Can follow rules and take turns in a game	• Uses the word *because* to explain feelings and actions. • Has best friend, usually of the same sex	• Unable to get dressed without help, brush teeth, wash, or dry hands. • Shows too little or extreme emotions (e.g., withdrawn, worried, angry, or depressed) • Doesn't engage with others • Cannot focus on one activity for more than five minutes

From Misch et al., 2019. Adapted from Gerber, Wilks, and Erdie-Lalena (2010. 2011), Schum (2007).

KEY POINT

Infant and early childhood assessment is a process that may have several goals, including: (1) screening to identify the need for further assessment, (2) diagnosing developmental delay and/or mental health disorders, (3) determining the need for early intervention or special education services, and (4) monitoring the progress of interventions.

ASSESSMENT, DIAGNOSIS, AND FORMULATION

Assessment

Infant and early childhood assessment is a process that may have several goals, including: (1) screening to identify the need for further assessment, (2) diagnosing developmental delay and/or mental health disorders, (3) determining the need for early intervention or special education services, and (4) monitoring the progress of interventions. Screening occurs primarily in primary care offices, while assessment and monitoring in a medical setting typically occur in a specialty clinic (e.g., developmental pediatrics; NICU follow-up; or perinatal, infant, and preschool psychiatric clinics). This section of the chapter will briefly describe the general approach to assessment from a psychiatric perspective. Several tools will be mentioned, but the *DC:0–5: Diagnostic Classification of Mental Health and Developmental Disorders in Infancy and Early Childhood* will be emphasized, as it provides an approach to assessment, diagnosis, and formulation, which is developmentally oriented, multidisciplinary, preventive, and relationship-based.

Before discussing the process and tools for assessment, the distinction between assessment, diagnosis, and formulation should be made. Assessment is the process of gathering data from record reviews, obtaining history and perceptions from interviews, and observations of interactions and behaviors. Diagnosis is the identification and classification of disorders, using a manual, for example *DC:0–5* or *Diagnostic and Statistical Manual of Psychiatric Disorders-5* (*DSM-5*). Formulation is the organization of all the information obtained. It defines the way the very young child is understood in the context of biology, behaviors, relationships, social network, and culture and is central to making decisions about treatment.

The assessment process usually takes more than one session—typically three to five. It requires multiple sources of information, which may be medical records, previous evaluations, or reports from teachers or childcare providers. Interview of the family ideally includes any and all caregivers beyond the primary caregiver. Observation of the child may be both formal and informal, using tools such as the infant and toddler mental status exam (Thomas et al., 1997). Screening tools or standardized instruments may be used, depending on the setting. Diagnostic impression is discussed with the family as well as the formulation of the child. This discussion facilitates joint treatment planning, which often involves recommendations for multidisciplinary referral for further assessment and/or treatment.

Family Interview

The family interview may be conducted with or without the child, depending on the child's age, whether the family can leave the child with other caregivers, whether the clinic has attendants available, or whether the clinician functions as part of a team that can separate the child and caregivers during the visit. Many clinics have parents complete intake forms prior to scheduling an appointment as a way to obtain much of the history.

The interview should begin with a discussion of the practical and administrative considerations and the structure of the day followed by:

- *Reason and source of referral*—The family's expectations of the reasons for the visit should be discussed up front. "What did you hope would happen as a result of today's visit," or "What is your understanding of why you are here today?"
- *Current concerns or difficulties*—"What are you most worried about?" (e.g., timing, setting, and course of concerns)

- *Detailed family history*—Parents and immediate family members' education, learning difficulties, legal difficulties, and medical or mental health illness. The composition of the household is an important part of the family history.
- *Developmental history*—Beginning with conception, "How did you feel when you found out you were pregnant?" Developmental history should include milestones, interventions, and all aspects of development: motor, cognitive, social, and emotional.
- *Physical development and medical history*—Inquire about when the child met their physical developmental milestones, such as when they sat without support, crawled, walked, and so on. Ask about and note any medical concerns, including need for hospitalization or surgeries.
- *Traumatic events*—"Has anything bad or difficult happened to your family or your child recently or in the past?"

Observation

Assessment of the young child in a clinical setting requires flexibility and a range of skills, most importantly observation. There are structured tools that can guide observational assessment, but many of these require specialized training to administer, including the autism diagnostic schedule-2 (Gotham et al., 2007) and the disruptive behavior diagnostic observation schedule (DB-DOS) (Wakschlag, 2002). The infant and toddler mental status exam described by the American Academy of Child and Adolescent Psychiatry's practice parameters for the assessment of infants and toddlers (Thomas et al., 1997) provides a template for systematic observation of a child, the child's interactions with caregivers, and the child's interactions with the clinician. It can be completed through informal observation, play, or cleanup with a parent or play with a clinician and is purely descriptive. It consists of 10 categories: appearance; reaction to situation; self-regulation; motor, speech, and language; thought; affect and mood; play; cognition; and social relatedness. It requires relatively basic general toys that engage young children and may be sensory, aggressive, expressive, pretend, or family-related/nurturing. Some examples include a baby doll and bottle, a playhouse with family figures, puppets, dinosaurs, blocks, bubbles, and squishy toys.

Screening tools, some examples of which follow, can be used to supplement observation. The ages and stages questionnaire is a parent-report developmental screening questionnaire for children ages 1 to 66 months (Goldsmith, 2013). It assesses communication, gross motor, fine motor, problem-solving, and personal/social skills. It can be useful in identifying children with developmental delays that require further assessment. The child behavior checklist 1.5 to 5 is a 100-item parent-teacher self-report that includes DSM-oriented scales of depressive, autism spectrum, attention-deficit/hyperactivity, and oppositional/defiant problems (Achenbach & Rescorla, 2000). The infant-toddler social and emotional assessment (ITSEA) looks at internalizing, externalizing, dysregulation, and competence for ages 12 to 36 months (Carter et al., 2003).

Diagnosis

The purpose of assessment is usually to generate a diagnosis. The basic principles used during assessment and diagnosis of young children include that:

1. The psychological functioning of preschoolers unfolds in the context of relationships/interactions with caregivers.
2. Constitutional characteristics play a major role in how children process life events and emotional experiences.
3. The family's values and parenting beliefs are critical to understanding the child's behavior and developmental course.

The *DSM-5* has now expanded attention to children under 5. Further still, the *DC:0–5: Diagnostic Classification of Mental Health and Developmental Disorders of Infancy and Early Childhood* captures findings relevant to the diagnosis of young children. The DC 0–5 is a multiaxial comprehensive diagnostic system that provides a classification system that is developmentally appropriate, relationship-based, contextually driven, and culturally competent (Frankel, 2018; Zero to Three, 2017).

Formulation and Treatment Planning

Formulation is the way in which the infant or young child's clinical presentation is understood in the context of the young child's relationships, biology, social network, and developmental status. There are many different approaches to formulation, but any comprehensive framework should include biologic and developmental factors intrinsic to the child, psychological factors affecting the caregiver and the child, and social and cultural considerations. The formulation guides treatment planning, which may include additional assessments, educational interventions, family and community support, medical or mental health interventions, social services, or legal involvement, and/or case management referral.

KEY POINT

Psychiatric disorders are present in nearly 10% of preschoolers (Gleason et al., 2016). The most common disorders include externalizing or disruptive behavior disorders, oppositional defiant disorder, anxiety disorders, and mood disorders.

COMMON MENTAL HEALTH DISORDERS IN PRESCHOOL CHILDREN

Psychiatric disorders are present in nearly 10% of preschoolers (Gleason et al., 2016). The most common disorders include externalizing or disruptive behavior disorders, oppositional defiant disorder, anxiety disorders, and mood disorders. In addition to these, trauma and adverse childhood experiences at this age can have a significant impact on future mental health.

Appropriate diagnosis and intervention can help shape healthy social, emotional, and cognitive functioning throughout the life span. For the purposes of this chapter, autism spectrum disorder is not included, even though it commonly presents in early childhood. (Autism spectrum disorders are the subject of another chapter.)

Externalizing/Disruptive Behavior Disorders

Disruptive behaviors include aggression, tantrums, elopement, noncompliance with instructions, and destruction of property. These behaviors, when untreated, can lead to poor academic performance, parent–child relationship problems, and social impairments (Gleason et al., 2016). Preschoolers have the highest rates of school expulsions among all age groups (Gilliam 2005). Tantrums, which are very common in the preschool age group, are distinguished as clinically significant by their quality, intensity, frequency, and context and the degree of dysregulation and impairment (Eisbach et al., 2014). Behavioral problems may be due to a wide range of disorders, including neurodevelopmental disorders like ADHD, medical illness, mood, anxiety, trauma, and attachment-related disorders.

> **CLINICAL TIP**
>
> Disruptive behaviors include aggression, tantrums, elopement, noncompliance with instructions, and destruction of property. Preschoolers have the highest rates of school expulsions among all age groups. Behavioral problems may be due to a wide range of disorders, including neurodevelopmental disorders like ADHD, medical illness, mood, anxiety, trauma, and attachment-related disorders. These behaviors, when untreated, can lead to poor academic performance, parent–child relationship problems, and social impairments.

Attention-Deficit/Hyperactivity Disorder (ADHD)

About 30% of children with ADHD are diagnosed prior to the age of six. ADHD is a neurodevelopmental disorder diagnosed by the presence of inattention or hyperactivity/impulsivity that is developmentally disproportionate and impairing and is present across multiple settings, present beyond 6 months, and is not explained by an alternate diagnosis (American Psychiatric Association, 2013). In the preschool age group, the diagnosis is more difficult to ascertain, as preschoolers may not be engaged in care outside of the home. Many of the standardized screening tools have not been validated in children below the age of 6. The ADHD rating scale-IV preschool version (Alexandre et al., 2018), the child behavior checklist 1.5–5 years (Achenbach & Rescorla, 2000), and the brief early childhood screening assessment (Fallucco et al., 2017) may be used to aid diagnosis, identify comorbid factors, and track symptoms after intervention. The differential diagnosis of ADHD includes comprehension, motor, sensory, medical, and other psychiatric disorders. Treatment of ADHD symptoms includes behavioral interventions, such as parent management training. The American Academy of Pediatrics (AAP) recommends beginning treatment with medications only after age 4, whereas the clinical guidelines from the American Academy of Child and Adolescent Psychiatry recommends a minimum age of 3 years. Stimulants, methylphenidate, and amphetamine preparations are considered first-line medications (Greenhill et al., 2006).

Alpha agonists guanfacine and clonidine and the norepinephrine reuptake inhibitor atomoxetine have some evidence for use in preschoolers as a standalone medication or in combination with the stimulants if the stimulants are ineffective or contraindicated (Harmon & Riggs, 1996; Kratochvil et al., 2011).

Oppositional Defiant Disorder/Conduct Disorder

Oppositional defiant disorder often begins during preschool years and describes symptom patterns of anger, irritability, argumentative, defiant, and/or vindictive behavior lasting more than 6 months and causing impairment in family, school, or social functioning (American Psychiatric Association, 2013). Conduct disorder describes children having symptom clusters, including conflicts with adults and authority figures, serious violations of social norms, and violations of the rights of others. The specifier of childhood onset is used when symptoms occur prior to the age of 10.

Other Disruptive Behavior Disorders

In *DSM-4*, disruptive behavior disorder not otherwise specified was included, which was often the most appropriate diagnosis as underlying developmental etiologies are often not fully developed in preschool children. *DSM-5* no longer includes this diagnosis. The *DC:0–5* defined a disorder of dysregulated anger and aggression (DDAA), which describes young children with dysregulation of mood and behavior. This is considered a precursor to the diagnosis of disruptive mood dysregulation disorder, which can be diagnosed only after 6 years of age (Three, 2016).

Scales for assessment of disruptive behavior include the multidimensional assessment of profile of disruptive behavior (MAP-DP) and the disruptive behavior diagnostic observation schedule (DB-DOS). These can be used to assess preschool disruptive behavior and have been used to accurately diagnose and distinguish clinically significant disruptive behavior from normative early childhood misbehavior (Kaat et al., 2019; Three, 2016; Wakschlag et al., 2008).

Behavioral interventions that address parenting skills and parent–child interaction are the first-line treatment for disruptive behavior disorders. Examples of evidence-based treatment modalities include parent–child interaction therapy, Incredible Years, the Chicago Parent Program, Parent Management Training—The Oregon Model, and Circle of Security (Eyberg et al., 1995; Gross et al., 2009; Hagen et al., 2011; Huber et al., 2015; Webster-Stratton et al., 2011). There is no FDA-approved medication to treat disruptive behavior disorders in young children. There have been studies showing improvement in disruptive behavior with the use of risperidone (Cesena et al., 2002; Ercan et al., 2011) and stimulants (Staller, 2007) in preschool children, but these were small samples or case reports that described side effects, including hyperprolactinemia and weight gain with risperidone.

Anxiety Disorders

Anxiety disorders are among the most common, and yet the most undertreated, mental health disorders in preschool-aged children (Egger & Angold, 2006). The prevalence of preschool anxiety disorders is around 10–20% (Egger & Angold, 2006; Whalen et al., 2017). Most anxiety disorders have an onset in childhood with a waxing and waning course throughout life. Preschool anxiety is associated with an increased risk for anxiety and depression in adulthood (Whalen et al., 2017). Risk factors for development of anxiety disorders include slow to warm temperament, authoritarian parenting style, insecure attachment, maternal anxiety/depression, younger parental age and lower socioeconomic status, and genetic loading (40–65% heritability) (Eley et al., 2003; Whalen et al., 2017). Anxiety disorders are differentiated from normative developmental worries and fears when they persist, are excessive and uncontrollable; impair social, academic, or family function; and occur across multiple settings. Anxiety disorders include specific phobias, generalized anxiety disorder, social phobia, selective mutism, separation anxiety, panic disorder, and agoraphobia (American Psychiatric Association, 2013).

The challenge in diagnosing anxiety disorders in preschool children is that they are often unable to clearly describe their internal experience. Preschoolers may commonly avoid new activities or situations, throw tantrums, cling to their caregivers, ask for reassurance excessively, have difficulty paying attention, have trouble falling asleep, feel irritable and tired, struggle with changes in routine, or endorse somatic complaints like headaches, stomachaches, and chest pain. It is important to rule out medical causes of anxiety-like symptoms, including thyroid dysfunction, medication side effects, asthma, and others. Screening tools like the pediatric symptom checklist, the strengths and difficulties questionnaire, and the preschool anxiety rating scale can be used to aid assessment and treatment progress (Bourdon et al., 2005; Little et al., 1994; Spence et al., 2001).

The treatment of preschool anxiety includes a combination of education, family training and psychotherapy, such as play therapy or cognitive behavioral therapy and parent management (Comer et al., 2012; Connolly et al., 2007; Donovan & March, 2014). There is inadequate evidence for use of medication (Finelli & Gleason, 2019), including SSRIs, which should

QUICK POINT

Anxiety disorders are among the most common, and yet the most undertreated, mental health disorders in preschool-aged children. The prevalence of preschool anxiety disorders is around 10–20%. Preschool anxiety is associated with an increased risk for anxiety and depression in adulthood. Preschool children, due to limited language, are often unable to clearly describe their internal experience. The treatment of preschool anxiety includes a combination of education, family training, and therapy, such as cognitive behavioral therapy and parent management.

CLINICAL TIP

Due to limited language ability, preschool children, are often unable to clearly describe their internal experience. Play therapy is sometimes useful for treatment. The treatment of preschool anxiety includes a combination of education, family training and psychotherapy, such as play therapy or cognitive behavior therapy and parent management.

only be considered if symptoms cause severe impairment or if therapy is ineffective (Gleason et al., 2007).

QUICK POINT

The prevalence of depression in preschool-aged children is 2.1% (Egger & Angold, 2006). Risk factors for early childhood depression include a family history of depression in a parent or sibling, maternal prenatal depression, ACEs, difficulty with peer relationships, low inhibitory control, authoritarian parenting practices, family stress and conflict, low socioeconomic status, and maternal anxiety (Luby et al., 2006).

CLINICAL TIP

In young children, the most common presenting symptoms in this age group include appearing sad (98 %), sleep changes (80%), play themes involving death or killing themselves (74%), and excessive whining or crying (55%). Other symptoms include anhedonia, excessive guilt, and changes in appetite.

Mood Disorders

Depression

The prevalence of depression in preschool-aged children is 2.1% (Egger & Angold, 2006). Risk factors for early childhood depression include a family history of depression in a parent or sibling, maternal prenatal depression, exposure to early adverse events, difficulty with peer relationships, low inhibitory control, authoritarian parenting practices, family stress and conflict, low socioeconomic status, and maternal anxiety (Luby et al., 2006). Though the actual presenting symptoms of depression are not different from older patients, fewer symptoms occur at a given time, and preschool children may have difficulty expressing their symptoms verbally. The most common presenting symptoms in this age group include appearing sad (98%), sleep changes (80%), play themes involving death or killing themselves (74%), and excessive whining or crying (55%). Other symptoms include anhedonia, excessive guilt, and changes in appetite. (Luby et al., 2003). It is important to note that some preschoolers may not have a clear conceptualization of death and its meaning, so suicidal statements may be a general sign of distress rather than related to true suicidal ideations. Preschoolers with depression/suicidal ideations have a better understanding of what it means to die than depressed preschoolers without suicidal ideations or their healthy peers. It is important to consider the context of the suicidal statements and gestures and respond accordingly (Paul & Ortin, 2019).

Screening tools for depression include the pediatric symptom checklist (Jellinek, 2020), the child behavior checklist (Achenbach & Rescorla, 2010), the strengths and difficulties questionnaire (Bourdon et al., 2005), and the preschool feelings checklist (Luby et al., 2004).

Treatment of preschool depression involves psychoeducation, supportive management, school, and family involvement in care (Birmaher et al., 2007). Parent–child interaction therapy—emotional dysregulation has shown efficacy in treating preschool depression (Lenze et al., 2011). Medications are not recommended for first-line treatment, as risks outweigh the benefits (Zuckerman et al., 2007).

Bipolar Disorder

There is controversy about the diagnosis of bipolar disorder in preschool children and whether this diagnosis carries into adulthood (Ghaemi & Martin, 2007; Zuckerman et al., 2007). There is emerging literature that suggests some forms of the disorder may arise as early as 3 years of age (Luby et al., 2009). It is challenging to distinguish irritability in a manic episode from other disruptive disorders. Family history of affective illness is often seen in these children (Luby & Navsaria, 2010). Focus of treatment is on psychoeducation and parent child interactive therapy, and medications are generally not recommended (Finelli & Gleason, 2019).

CLINICAL TIP

Literature suggests some forms of bipolar disorder may arise as early as 3 years of age. However, it is challenging to clearly distinguish irritability in a manic episode from other conditions, such as disruptive disorders (e.g., ADHD), traumatic experiences, or chronic sleep deprivation.

Perceptual Disturbances and Psychotic Symptoms

Seventy-five percent of children aged 3 to 8 have imaginary friends, which is developmentally appropriate. However, the prevalence of childhood onset of schizophrenia is extremely rare (1 in 40,000, or 0.0025%) (Gochman et al., 2011). Young children are more likely to experience psychotic symptoms in the context of mood, anxiety, and trauma-related disorders than schizophrenia (Stevens et al., 2014). Hallucinations may be associated with underlying medical conditions, such as migraine, temporal lobe epilepsy, delirium, encephalitis, and febrile illness. Treatment is focused on the treatment of underlying medical or psychiatric conditions.

CLINICAL TIP

Seventy-five percent of children aged 3 to 8 have imaginary friends, which is developmentally appropriate. Young children are more likely to report psychotic symptoms in the context of mood, anxiety, and trauma-related disorders than schizophrenia.

Trauma

About 12% of preschoolers have at least one type of maltreatment, and 21% have witnessed violence (Saunders & Adams, 2014). Adverse childhood experiences (ACEs) are associated with somatic, mental, and psychosocial problems in adulthood (Felitti et al., 1998). ACEs or trauma during infancy and early childhood can induce changes in hypothalamic pituitary adrenal axis and epigenetics, including shortening of telomere and DNA methylation (Drury et al., 2017; Matosin et al., 2017; Shalev et al., 2013; J. Luby et al., 2013; van Bodegom et al., 2017). Stress and poverty in early childhood are associated with smaller amygdala and hippocampus volumes and decreased connectivity of inferior frontal gyrus in early adolescence (Luby et al., 2013; Luby et al., 2017). Trauma and chronic stress exposure before age three can also increase the risk of developmental delays (Scarborough et al., 2009).

Young children experiencing trauma, commonly present with disturbed sleep, emotional and physical distress, difficulty paying attention, anger, irritability, emotional or social withdrawal, anxious attachment, and exaggerated response to minor stimuli. Children may also show loss of previously acquired developmental skills (e.g., toileting), sleep and eating dysregulation, new onset of aggression or separation anxiety, and new onset of fears.

CLINICAL TIP

Young children with trauma experience, commonly present with sleep disruption, emotional and physical distress, difficulty paying attention, anger, irritability, emotional or social withdrawal, anxious attachment, and exaggerated response to minor stimuli.

TABLE 5.2 Evidence-Based Interventions With Young Children and Families

Name	Age	Length	Target population	Goals/comments
Attachment and biobehavioral catch-up http://www.abcintervention.org	6–24 months	10 sessions	• Children who have experienced abuse, neglect, and/or disruptions in care • Treatment delivered dyadically, focusing on caregiver skills and representation	• Works with parents or other caregivers to help them learn how to (1) behave in nurturing ways when children are distressed; (2) follow their child's lead to behave in delighted ways when children are not distressed; and (3) avoid behaving in frightening or intrusive ways. • Uses videotaped interactions.
Child–parent psychotherapy http://www.cebc4cw.org/program/child-parentpsychoterapy/detailed	Birth–5 years	52 weeks	• Children and primary caregivers who have experienced intimate partner violence and/or trauma • Treatment delivered dyadically through play and psychodynamic interpretation	• Support and strengthen the caregiver–child relationship as a vehicle for restoring and protecting the child's mental health. • Treatment focuses on contextual factors (e.g., culture and socioeconomic and immigration-related stressors).
Circle of Security http://www.cebc4cw.org/program/circle-of-securityparenting/detailed	Birth–5 years	20 sessions	• Dyads with relational and attachment difficulties	• The intervention is organized around the use of the COS graphic, which promotes parental understanding of attachment theory. The intervention includes individualized video clips of caregivers interacting with their young children to increase caregivers' awareness of their children's emotional cues.
Incredible Years http://www.cebc4cw.org/program/the-incredibleyears/detailed	Birth–12 years	10–20 weeks	• Children with disruptive behavior disorders	• Parent program uses videotaped vignettes to demonstrate targeted skills of providing nurturance and reducing harsh discipline. Child program delivered in small groups using dinosaur puppets.
Parent–child interaction therapy http://www.pcit.org	2–8 years	10–20 sessions	• Children with disruptive behavior disorders	• Therapist coaches parents while they interact with their children, teaching caregivers strategies that will promote positive behaviors. • Requires a *bug-in-the-ear* and one-way mirror or video surveillance.
Trauma-focused cognitive behavioral therapy https://tfcbt.org	3–18 years	12–18 sessions	• Children who have experienced traumas, including intimate partner violence, traumatic loss, war, sexual exploitation, and/or multiple complex traumas	• Program integrates cognitive, behavioral, interpersonal, and family therapy sessions as well as trauma interventions. • Provides parallel individual sessions with children and primary caregivers; then joint parent–child sessions.

From Tamkin et al., 2019.

Trauma screening questionnaires include the safe environment for every kid (SEEK) model (Dubowitz, 2014), Centre for Youth Wellness ACE questionnaire (Koita et al., 2018), strength and difficulties questionnaire (SDQ) (Bourdon et al., 2005), survey of well-being of young children (SWYC) (Perrin 2006), and the trauma symptom checklist for children (Briere, 2005).

Evidence-based therapeutic interventions include child–parent psychotherapy and trauma-focused cognitive behavioral therapy, which has been adapted to children as young as 3 (Saunders & Adams, 2014; Scheeringa et al., 2011). There is no evidence for use of medication in this age group for trauma-related disorders, but treating comorbid disorders when appropriate is recommended (Finelli & Gleason, 2019).

INTERVENTIONS

The following chart summarizes some of the most common evidence-based interventions for infants and preschoolers.

SUMMARY

Infancy and early childhood is a period of rapid development that sets the stage for later-life functioning. There are effective tools for assessing and diagnosing infants and preschool children. Early intervention is key in promoting normal development and child mental health, and there are various evidence-based interventions available in this rapidly evolving field.

CASE VIGNETTE COMMENTARY

C. J. was given a preliminary diagnosis of attention-deficit/hyperactivity disorder. Her parents had difficulty accepting this because they hoped she would grow out of it. This delayed the start of services. Eventually, C.J.'s mother began parent–child interaction therapy (PCIT), where she learned to better manage C. J.'s behaviors. C. J. improved in her ability to control her emotions and had fewer outbursts. She was successful at making friends in her preschool and had been invited on some playdates. She still had a short attention span, but with one-on-one help in preschool, she has learned her alphabet and numbers 1 through 10. Now, at age 4, she is anticipated to start kindergarten next year. C. J.'s parents are aware that if their child begins to struggle with her learning or behavior, she may need a reassessment for comorbidities and to determine whether she needs additional services.

RESOURCES

1 https://developingchild.harvard.edu/resources/inbrief-science-of-ecd/

2 https://developingchild.harvard.edu/resources/three-core-concepts-in-early-development/

REFERENCES

Achenbach, T. M., & Rescorla, L. A. (2000). *Child behavior checklist for ages 1 ½–5*. In *Manual for the ASEBA preschool forms & profiles*. Burlington, VT: University of Vermont, Research Center for Children, Youth, and Families.

Achenbach, T. M., & Rescorla, L. A. (2010). *Multicultural supplement to the manual for the ASEBA preschool forms & profiles: Child behavior checklist for ages 1 1/2-5, language development survey, caregiver-teacher report form; an integrated system of multi-informant assessment*. University of Vermont, Research Center for Children, Youth, and Families.

Alexandre, J. L., Lange, A.-M., Bilenberg, N., Gorrissen, A. M., Søbye, N., & Lambek, R. (2018). The ADHD rating scale-IV preschool version: Factor structure, reliability, validity, and standardisation in a Danish community sample. *Research in Developmental Disabilities, 78*, 125–135.

American Psychiatric Association. (2013). *Diagnostic and statistical manual of mental disorders* (5th ed.). https://doi.org/10.1176/appi.books.9780890425596

Birmaher, B., Brent, D., AACAP Work Group on Quality Issues, Bernet, W., Bukstein, O., Walter, H., Benson, R. S., Chrisman, A., Farchione, T., Greenhill, L., Hamilton, J., Keable, H., Kinlan, J., Schoettle, U., Stock, S., Ptakowski, K. K., & Medicus, J. (2007). Practice parameter for the assessment and treatment of children and adolescents with depressive disorders. *Journal of the American Academy of Child and Adolescent Psychiatry, 46*(11), 1503–1526.

Bourdon, K. H., Goodman, R., Rae, D. S., Simpson, G., & Koretz, D. S. (2005). The strengths and difficulties questionnaire: U.S. normative data and psychometric properties. *Journal of the American Academy of Child and Adolescent Psychiatry, 44*(6), 557–564.

Briere, J. (2005). *Trauma Symptom Checklist for Young Children (TSCYC): Professional manual*. Psychological Assessment Resources, Inc. Odessa, FL.

Carter, A. S., Briggs-Gowan, M. J., Jones, S. M., & Little, T. D. (2003). The infant–toddler social and emotional assessment (ITSEA): Factor structure, reliability, and validity. *Journal of Abnormal Child Psychology, 31*(5), 495–514.

Cesena, M., Gonzalez-Heydrich, J., Szigethy, E., Kohlenberg, T. M., & DeMaso, D. R. (2002). A case series of eight aggressive young children treated with risperidone. *Journal of Child and Adolescent Psychopharmacology, 12*(4), 337–345.

Comer, J. S., Puliafico, A. C., Aschenbrand, S. G., McKnight, K., Robin, J. A., Goldfine, M. E., & Albano, A. M. (2012). A pilot feasibility evaluation of the CALM Program for anxiety disorders in early childhood. In *Journal of Anxiety Disorders*, *26*(1), 40–49. https://doi.org/10.1016/j.janxdis.2011.08.011

Connolly, S. D., Bernstein, G. A., & Work Group on Quality Issues. (2007). Practice parameter for the assessment and treatment of children and adolescents with anxiety disorders. *Journal of the American Academy of Child and Adolescent Psychiatry, 46*(2), 267–283.

Donovan, C. L., & March, S. (2014). Online CBT for preschool anxiety disorders: A randomised control trial. *Behaviour Research and Therapy, 58*, 24–35.

Drury, S. S., Howell, B. R., Jones, C., Esteves, K., Morin, E., Schlesinger, R., Meyer, J. S., Baker, K., & Sanchez, M. M. (2017). Shaping long-term primate development: Telomere length trajectory as an indicator of early maternal maltreatment and predictor of future physiologic regulation. *Development and Psychopathology, 29*(5), 1539–1551.

Dubowitz, H. (2014). The safe environment for every kid (SEEK) model: Helping promote children's health, development, and safety: SEEK offers a practical model for enhancing pediatric primary care. *Child Abuse & Neglect, 38*(11), 1725–1733.

Egger, H. L., & Angold, A. (2006). Common emotional and behavioral disorders in preschool children: presentation, nosology, and epidemiology. *Journal of Child Psychology and Psychiatry and Allied Disciplines, 47*(3–4), 313–337.

Eisbach, S. S., Cluxton-Keller, F., Harrison, J., Krall, J. R., Hayat, M., & Gross, D. (2014). Characteristics of temper tantrums in preschoolers with disruptive behavior in a clinical setting. *Journal of Psychosocial Nursing and Mental Health Services, 52*(5), 32–40.

Eley, T. C., Bolton, D., O'Connor, T. G., Perrin, S., Smith, P., & Plomin, R. (2003). A twin study of anxiety-related behaviours in preschool children. *Journal of Child Psychology and Psychiatry, 44*(7), 945–960. https://doi.org/10.1111/1469-7610.00179

Ercan, E. S., Basay, B. K., Basay, O., Durak, S., & Ozbaran, B. (2011). Risperidone in the treatment of conduct disorder in preschool children without intellectual disability. *Child and Adolescent Psychiatry and Mental Health, 5*(1), 10.

Eyberg, S. M., Boggs, S. R., & Algina, J. (1995). Parent–child interaction therapy: A psychosocial model for the treatment of young children with conduct problem behavior and their families. *Psychopharmacology Bulletin, 31*(1), 83–91.

Fallucco, E. M., Wysocki, T., James, L., Kozikowski, C., Williams, A., & Gleason, M. M. (2017). The brief early childhood screening assessment. *Journal of Developmental & Behavioral Pediatrics, 38*(2), 89–98. https://doi.org/10.1097/dbp.0000000000000384

Felitti, V. J., Anda, R. F., Nordenberg, D., Williamson, D. F., Spitz, A. M., Edwards, V., Koss, M. P., & Marks, J. S. (1998). Relationship of childhood abuse and household dysfunction to many of the leading causes of death in adults. *American Journal of Preventive Medicine, 4*, 245–258). https://doi.org/10.1016/s0749-3797(98)00017-8

Finelli, J., & Gleason, M. M. (2019). Psychopharmacologic considerations in early childhood. *Clinical Guide to Psychiatric Assessment of Infants and Young Children*, 285–326. https://doi.org/10.1007/978-3-030-10635-5_9

Fraiberg, S. (1996). *The magic years: Understanding and handling the problems of early childhood.* Simon and Schuster.

Frankel, K. A., Harrison, J., & Njoroge, W. F. M. (2019). *Clinical guide to psychiatric assessment of infants and young children.* Springer.

Frankel, K, Gleason, M., Lieberman, A., Egger, H. L., Zeanah, C. H. (2018). *Diagnostic classification of mental health developmental disorders of infancy and early childhood* (5th ed.). https://doi.org/10.1016/j.jaac.2018.07.843

Ghaemi, S. N., & Martin, A. (2007). Defining the boundaries of childhood bipolar disorder [Review of *Defining the boundaries of childhood bipolar disorder*]. *The American Journal of Psychiatry, 164*(2), 185–188.

Gleason, M. M., Egger, H. L., Emslie, G. J., Greenhill, L. L., Kowatch, R. A., Lieberman, A. F., Luby, J. L., Owens, J., Scahill, L. D., Scheeringa, M. S., Stafford, B., Wise, B., & Zeanah, C. H. (2007). Psychopharmacological treatment for very young children: Contexts and guidelines. *Journal of the American Academy of Child and Adolescent Psychiatry, 46*(12), 1532–1572.

Gleason, M. M., Goldson, E., Yogman, M. W., Council on Early Childhood, Committee on Psychosocial Aspects of Child and Family Health, & Section on Developmental and Behavioral Pediatrics. (2016). Addressing early childhood emotional and behavioral problems. *Pediatrics, 138*(6). https://doi.org/10.1542/peds.2016-3025

Gochman, P., Miller, R., & Rapoport, J. L. (2011). Childhood-onset schizophrenia: The challenge of diagnosis. *Current Psychiatry Reports, 13*(5), 321–322.

Goldsmith, T. R. (2013). Ages and stages questionnaire (2nd ed.). In *Encyclopedia of Autism Spectrum Disorders* (pp. 90–93). https://doi.org/10.1007/978-1-4419-1698-3_283

Gotham, K., Risi, S., Pickles, A., & Lord, C. (2007). The autism diagnostic observation schedule: Revised algorithms for improved diagnostic validity. *Journal of Autism and Developmental Disorders*, 37(4), 613–627. https://doi.org/10.1007/s10803-006-0280-1

Greenhill, L., Kollins, S., Abikoff, H., McCracken, J., Riddle, M., Swanson, J., McGough, J., Wigal, S., Wigal, T., Vitiello, B., Skrobala, A., Posner, K., Ghuman, J., Cunningham, C., Davies, M., Chuang, S., & Cooper, T. (2006). Efficacy and safety of immediate-release methylphenidate treatment for preschoolers with ADHD [Review of *Efficacy and safety of immediate-release methylphenidate treatment for preschoolers with ADHD*]. *Journal of the American Academy of Child and Adolescent Psychiatry, 45*(11), 1284–1293.

Gross, D., Garvey, C., Julion, W., Fogg, L., Tucker, S., & Mokros, H. (2009). Efficacy of the Chicago parent program with low-income African American and Latino parents of young children. *Prevention Science: The Official Journal of the Society for Prevention Research, 10*(1), 54–65.

Hagen, K. A., Ogden, T., & Bjørnebekk, G. (2011). Treatment outcomes and mediators of parent management training: A one-year follow-up of children with conduct problems. *Journal of Clinical Child and Adolescent Psychology, 40*(2), 165–178.

Harmon, R. J., & Riggs, P. D. (1996). Clonidine for posttraumatic stress disorder in preschool children. *Journal of the American Academy of Child and Adolescent Psychiatry, 35*(9), 1247–1249.

Huber, A., McMahon, C., & Sweller, N. (2015). Improved child behavioural and emotional functioning after Circle of Security 20-week intervention. *Attachment & Human Development, 17*(6), 547–569.

Jellinek, M. S. (2020). The pediatric symptom checklist: A bridge to child and adolescent psychiatry from pediatrics. *Journal of the American Academy of Child and Adolescent Psychiatry.* https://doi.org/10.1016/j.jaac.2020.10.020

Kaat, A. J., Blackwell, C. K., Estabrook, R., Burns, J. L., Petitclerc, A., Briggs-Gowan, M. J., Gershon, R. C., Cella, D., Perlman, S. B., & Wakschlag, L. S. (2019). Linking the child behavior checklist (CBCL) with the multidimensional assessment profile of disruptive behavior (MAP-DB): Advancing a dimensional spectrum approach to disruptive behavior. *Journal of Child and Family Studies, 28*(2), 343–353.

Knickmeyer, R. C., Gouttard, S., Kang, C., Evans, D., Wilber, K., Smith, J. K., Hamer, R. M., Lin, W., Gerig, G., & Gilmore, J. H. (2008). A structural MRI study of human brain development from birth to 2 years. *The Journal of Neuroscience, 28*(47), 12176–12182.

Koita, K., Long, D., Hessler, D., Benson, M., Daley, K., Bucci, M., Thakur, N., & Burke Harris, N. (2018). Development and implementation of a pediatric adverse childhood experiences (ACEs) and other determinants of health questionnaire in the pediatric medical home: A pilot study. *PloS One, 13*(12), e0208088.

Kratochvil, C. J., Vaughan, B. S., Stoner, J. A., Daughton, J. M., Lubberstedt, B. D., Murray, D. W., Chrisman, A. K., Faircloth, M. A., Itchon-Ramos, N. B., Kollins, S. H., Maayan, L. A., Greenhill, L. L., Kotler, L. A., Fried, J., & March, J. S. (2011). A double-blind, placebo-controlled study of atomoxetine in young children with ADHD. *Pediatrics, 127*(4), e862–e868.

Lenze, S. N., Pautsch, J., & Luby, J. (2011). Parent–child interaction therapy emotion development: A novel treatment for depression in preschool children. *Depression and Anxiety, 28*(2), 153–159.

Little, M., Michael Murphy, J., Jellinek, M. S., Bishop, S. J., & Arnett, H. L. (1994). Screening 4- and 5-year-old children for psychosocial dysfunction. *Journal of Developmental & Behavioral Pediatrics, 15*(3), 191–197). https://doi.org/10.1097/00004703-199406000-00007

Luby, J., Belden, A., Botteron, K., Marrus, N., Harms, M. P., Babb, C., Nishino, T., & Barch, D. (2013). The effects of poverty on childhood brain development: The mediating effect of caregiving and stressful life events. *JAMA Pediatrics, 167*(12), 1135–1142.

Luby, J. L., Barch, D., Whalen, D., Tillman, R., & Belden, A. (2017). Association between early life adversity and risk for poor emotional and physical health in adolescence: A putative mechanistic neurodevelopmental pathway. *JAMA Pediatrics, 171*(12), 1168–1175.

Luby, J. L., Belden, A. C., & Spitznagel, E. (2006). Risk factors for preschool depression: the mediating role of early stressful life events. *Journal of Child Psychology and Psychiatry, and Allied Disciplines, 47*(12), 1292–1298.

Luby, J. L., Heffelfinger, A. K., Mrakotsky, C., Brown, K. M., Hessler, M. J., Wallis, J. M., & Spitznagel, E. L. (2003). The clinical picture of depression in preschool children. *Journal of the American Academy of Child and Adolescent Psychiatry, 42*(3), 340–348.

Luby, J. L., Heffelfinger, A., Koenig-McNaught, A. L., Brown, K., & Spitznagel, E. (2004). The preschool feelings checklist: A brief and sensitive screening measure for depression in young children. *Journal of the American Academy of Child & Adolescent Psychiatry, 43*(6), 708–717. https://doi.org/10.1097/01.chi.0000121066.29744.08

Luby, J. L., & Navsaria, N. (2010). Pediatric bipolar disorder: Evidence for prodromal states and early markers. *Journal of Child Psychology and Psychiatry and Allied Disciplines, 51*(4), 459–471.

Luby, J. L., Tandon, M., & Belden, A. (2009). Preschool bipolar disorder. *Child and Adolescent Psychiatric Clinics of North America, 18*(2), 391–403, ix.

Matosin, N., Cruceanu, C., & Binder, E. B. (2017). Preclinical and clinical evidence of DNA methylation changes in response to trauma and chronic stress. *Chronic Stress*, 1. https://doi.org/10.1177/2470547017710764

Misch, D., Billings, G., Hong, J. S., & Harrison, J. (2019). Observational Assessment of the young child. In K. A. Frankel, J. Harrison, W. F. M. Njoroge (Eds.), *Clinical guide to psychiatric assessment of infants and young children* (pp. 143–183). https://doi.org/10.1007/978-3-030-10635-5_5

Mulrooney, K., Egger, H., Wagner, S., & Knickerbocker, L. (2019). Diagnosis in young children: The use of the DC:0-5 diagnostic classification of mental health and developmental disorders in infancy and early childhood. In K. A. Frankel, J. Harrison, W. F. M. Njoroge (Eds.), *Clinical guide to psychiatric assessment of infants and young children* (pp. 253–283). https://doi.org/10.1007/978-3-030-10635-5_8

Osofsky, J. D., & Fitzgerald, H. E. (2000). *WAIMH handbook of infant mental health, set.* Wiley.

Paul, E., & Ortin, A. (2019). Correlates of suicidal ideation and self-harm in early childhood in a cohort at risk for child abuse and neglect. *Archives of Suicide Research, 23*(1), 134–150.

Saunders, B. E., & Adams, Z. W. (2014). Epidemiology of traumatic experiences in childhood. *Child and Adolescent Psychiatric Clinics of North America, 23*(2), 167–184. https://doi.org/10.1016/j.chc.2013.12.003

Scarborough, A. A., Lloyd, E. C., & Barth, R. P. (2009). Maltreated infants and toddlers: Predictors of developmental delay. *Journal of Developmental and Behavioral Pediatrics, 30*(6), 489–498.

Scheeringa, M. S., Weems, C. F., Cohen, J. A., Amaya-Jackson, L., & Guthrie, D. (2011). Trauma-focused cognitive-behavioral therapy for posttraumatic stress disorder in three-through six year-old children: A randomized clinical trial. *Journal of Child Psychology and Psychiatry and Allied Disciplines, 52*(8), 853–860.

Shalev, I., Entringer, S., Wadhwa, P. D., Wolkowitz, O. M., Puterman, E., Lin, J., & Epel, E. S. (2013). Stress and telomere biology: A lifespan perspective. *Psychoneuroendocrinology, 38*(9), 1835–1842.

Spence, S. H., Rapee, R., McDonald, C., & Ingram, M. (2001). The structure of anxiety symptoms among preschoolers. *Behaviour Research and Therapy, 39*(11), 1293–1316. https://doi.org/10.1016/s0005-7967(00)00098-x

Staller, J. A. (2007). Psychopharmacologic treatment of aggressive preschoolers: A chart review. *Progress in Neuro-Psychopharmacology & Biological Psychiatry, 31*(1), 131–135.

Stein, R., Njoroge, W. F. M., & Dunn, D. M. (2019). Introduction assessment in early childhood. In K. A. Frankel, J. Harrison, W. F. M. Njoroge (Eds.), *Clinical guide to psychiatric assessment of infants and young children* (pp. 1–20). https://doi.org/10.1007/978-3-030-10635-5_1

Stevens, J. R., Prince, J. B., Prager, L. M., & Stern, T. A. (2014). Psychotic disorders in children and adolescents: A primer on contemporary evaluation and management. *The Primary Care Companion to CNS Disorders, 16*(2). https://doi.org/10.4088/PCC.13f01514

Tamkin, V. L., Dave, B., Whittaker, A. T. N., & Frankel, K. A. (2019). Constructing a joint clinical case formulation and treatment plan with families. In K. A. Frankel, J. Harrison, W. F. M. Njoroge (Eds.), *Clinical Guide to Psychiatric Assessment of Infants and Young Children* (pp. 327–355). https://doi.org/10.1007/978-3-030-10635-5_10

Thomas, J. M., Benham, A. L., Gean, M., Luby, J., Minde, K., Turner, S., & Wright, H. H. (1997). Practice parameters for the psychiatric assessment of infants and toddlers (0–36 months). *Journal of the American Academy of Child & Adolescent Psychiatry, 36*(10), 21S–36S. https://doi.org/10.1097/00004583-199710001-00003

van Bodegom, M., Homberg, J. R., & Henckens, M. J. A. G. (2017). Modulation of the hypothalamic pituitary adrenal axis by early life stress exposure. *Frontiers in Cellular Neuroscience, 11*, 87.

Wakschlag, L. (2002). The disruptive behavior diagnostic observation schedule (DB-DOS): A structured clinical observation tool for the assessment of early conduct problems. *PsycEXTRA Dataset*. https://doi.org/10.1037/e552582012-150

Wakschlag, L. S., Hill, C., Carter, A. S., Danis, B., Egger, H. L., Keenan, K., Leventhal, B. L., Cicchetti, D., Maskowitz, K., Burns, J., & Briggs-Gowan, M. J. (2008). Observational assessment of preschool disruptive behavior, part I: Reliability of the disruptive behavior diagnostic observation schedule (DB-DOS). *Journal of the American Academy of Child & Adolescent Psychiatry, 47*(6), 622–631. https://doi.org/10.1097/chi.0b013e31816c5bdb

Webster-Stratton, C. H., Reid, M. J., & Beauchaine, T. (2011). Combining parent and child training for young children with ADHD. *Journal of Clinical Child and Adolescent Psychology, 40*(2), 191–203.

Whalen, D. J., Sylvester, C. M., & Luby, J. L. (2017). Depression and anxiety in preschoolers: A review of the past 7 years. *Child and Adolescent Psychiatric Clinics of North America, 26*(3), 503–522.

Yin, W., Chen, M.-H., Hung, S.-C., Baluyot, K. R., Li, T., & Lin, W. (2019). Brain functional development separates into three distinct time periods in the first two years of life. *NeuroImage, 189*, 715–726.

Zaim, N., & Harrison, J. (2020). Pre-school mental health disorders: A review. *International Review of Psychiatry, 32*(3), 189–201.

Zeanah, C. H., Stafford, B., Boris, N. W., & Scheeringa, M. (2008). Infant development: The first 3 years of life. In A. Tasman, J. Kay, J. A. Lieberman, M. B. First, M. Maj, *Psychiatry* (pp. 109–134). https://doi.org/10.1002/9780470515167.ch8

Zero to Three. (2017). *DC:0–5: A briefing paper on diagnostic classification of mental health and developmental disorders of infancy and early childhood.* https://www.zerotothree.org/resources/1953-dc-0-5-a-briefing-paper-on-diagnostic-classification-of-mental-health-and-developmental-disorders-of-infancy-and-early-childhood

Zuckerman, M. L., Vaughan, B. L., Whitney, J., Dodds, A., Yakhkind, A., MacMillan, C., Raches, D., Pravdova, I., DeMaso, D. R., Beardslee, W. R., & Gonzalez-Heydrich, J. (2007). Tolerability of selective serotonin reuptake inhibitors in thirty-nine children under age seven: A retrospective chart review. *Journal of Child and Adolescent Psychopharmacology, 17*(2), 165–174.

CHAPTER 6

School-Aged Children[1]

Stephanie Hernandez, D.O. and Edore Onigu-Otite, M.D.

"If children feel safe, they can take risks, ask questions, make mistakes, learn to trust, share their feelings, and grow."

— Alfie Kohn

OBJECTIVES

After completing this chapter, students will be able to do the following:

- review typical development characteristics of school-aged children
- discuss cognitive development and learning theories
- examine types of aggression beginning at school age

CASE VIGNETTE

Zane is a 6-year-old high-strung boy who is prone to arguments. Recently, he got into trouble for punching a kid in school. The kid had accidentally bumped into him on the playground. Instantly, Zane turned around and began bashing the kid with punches, causing him to lose his balance and fall. Zane was sent to the principal's office for in-school detention. After the fact, he was sorry he had hurt the kid, understood it was an accident, and apologized to his classmate. They began talking, and by the end of the week, they were good friends again. At home, his parents gave him a consequence. In addition to his usual chores, he had to do a few extra chores. Zane argued a little about this consequence but did them anyway. To keep up with his high energy level, his parents enrolled him in a local soccer league, which he loved. His parents said he needed to do his homework and keep

(*continued*)

1 Readers may also see "Essentials of Human Development" (Chapter 4), "Neurocognitive Development" (Chapter 11), and "Speech and Language Development" (Chapter 12) for related material.

his grades up to keep going to soccer practice and games. He made excellent grades in school. In soccer, he made many friends he and his family often hang out with outside school and soccer. Zane thrived and enjoyed his childhood experience.

DEFINITIONS AND KEY CONCEPTS

The school-aged child refers to children 6 to 11 years of age. Synonymous with elementary school-aged children, or middle childhood, this developmental stage is when most children begin school-based learning and have increased independence from family. In this chapter, early and late elementary school-aged children refer to 6- to 8-year-olds and 9- to 11-year-olds, respectively. In this developmental period, children experience substantial and rapid physical, psychological, and emotional growth, and development.

INTRODUCTION

School-aged children undergo biological and psychosocial change resulting in increased motor and social skills development and physical and cognitive maturation. For these developments to optimally occur, adequate sleep and physical activity are imperative and often introduced in the home and school environments. School age is also a period in childhood in which many learning and behavioral concerns first present. This chapter focuses on the physical, cognitive, and social development of school-aged children with common presentations of mental health conditions during this developmental period.

KEY POINT

School-aged children undergo biological and psychosocial change, resulting in increased motor and social skills development and physical and cognitive maturation. For these developments to optimally occur, adequate sleep and physical activity are imperative and often introduced in the home and school environments.

BIOLOGICAL DEVELOPMENT

School-aged children undergo physical changes supported by adequate sleep and physical activity. Additionally, the onset of puberty often begins during school age.

Physical Growth

School-aged children undergo periods of slow and rapid growth. On average, they gain about four to seven pounds per year. In early elementary school, the majority of 6- to 8-year-old children are physically in Tanner stage 1, a period without noticeable physical changes in girl or boy bodies; they see the appearance of their first permanent teeth; and they grow slower and more steadily than children in later elementary school (Berk, 2007). By late elementary school, many children begin undergoing growth spurts, and height differences among similarly aged children may range up to six inches. Growth spurts require increased caloric intake, resulting in increased muscle mass and weight gain (Berk, 2007). The onset of pubertal development, or Tanner stage 2, begins, in girls, around age 9 to 11, when they develop the sexual characteristics of areola expansion, breast bud formation, and thin pubic hair on the vaginal lips. Tanner stage 2 in boys begins around age 11, and they develop enlargement of the testicles and scrotum and formation of thin pubic hair at the penile base.

The onset of childhood puberty is associated with genetics, culture, and pediatric obesity. Independent of socioeconomic factors, generally, Black girls enter puberty at earlier ages, followed by Mexican-American and non-Hispanic White girls (Wu et al., 2002). Obese female and male children experience earlier and delayed pubertal onset, respectively (Solorzano & McCartney, 2010). About 12% of American children entering kindergarten are obese, and 17% are overweight. Overweight children in kindergarten are about five times more likely to become obese than same-aged peers of average weight (Cunningham et al., 2014). This is a public health concern because of the association between childhood obesity and future medical complications, such as atherosclerotic vascular disease (e.g., hyperglycemia, hypertension, and dyslipidemia), and insulin resistance (Solorzano & McCartney, 2010).

CLINICAL TIP

School-aged children undergo periods of slow and rapid growth. On average, they gain about four to seven pounds per year. In early elementary school, the majority of 6- to 8-year-old children are physically in Tanner stage 1, a period without noticeable physical changes in girl or boy bodies. By late elementary school, many children begin growth spurts, and height differences among similarly aged children may range up to six inches. The onset of puberty, Tanner stage 2, begins, in girls around age 9 to 11 and in boys begins around age 11.

Motor Development

School-aged children have rapid improvements in gross and fine motor development. By early elementary school (6 to 8 years of age), much of their gross motor skills are well established, and fine motor skills are progressively fine-tuned.

Gross motor skills refer to the use of large muscle groups for movement. Generally, boys have greater motor strength, and girls have better balance. Children in early elementary school have complex muscle coordination, allowing them to use scissors to cut intricate shapes, climb, swim, skate, bicycle ride, skip, gallop, hop, and jump over objects 10 inches high and walk in tandem (Berk, 2007). With these skills, elementary school-aged children have the hand–eye coordination to play organized sports. They are capable of purposeful actions, such as catching and throwing for accuracy and distance and kicking a rolling ball.

Fine motor skills engage the upper extremities and small muscles groups to manipulate objects in the environment. Generally, girls have greater fine motor dexterity than similarly aged boys. Due to improved manual dexterity, school-aged children become increasingly independent with the ability to cut food and manipulate clothing items, such as zippers, buttons, and snaps. They can use blocks to build small structures; solve 16- to 20-piece puzzles; color within lines; connect the dots; legibly print their name; perform rapid finger-to-thumb movements; and draw complex shapes, such as diamonds, asterisks, five-pointed stars, and copy a cube.

Physical Fitness

KEY POINT

Play and physical activity are essential for physical development and psychosocial growth. Structured and unstructured play promotes imagination and creativity and improves memory, attention, and concentration.

Play and physical activity are essential for physical development and psychosocial growth. Structured and unstructured play promotes imagination and creativity and improves memory, attention, and concentration. By promoting prosocial behaviors and social–emotional development through the encouragement of sharing, rule-following, teamwork, and goal setting, play helps build self-esteem and decreases disruptive behaviors.

QUICK POINT

The prevalence of obesity of American school-aged children is 18.5% (Cunningham et al., 2014) with up to 87% of American children exceeding the 1-hour daily media-screen guideline established by the World Health Organization (WHO) (Trinh et al., 2020).

Family culture, teachers, and health care providers have essential roles in encouraging childhood physical activity, which helps counteract childhood obesity and decrease screen technology use. The prevalence of obesity of American school-aged children is 18.5% (Cunningham et al., 2014) with up to 87% of American children exceeding the 1-hour daily media-screen guideline established by the World Health Organization (WHO) (Trinh et al., 2020). It is recommended for school-aged children to have at least 60 minutes of daily moderate to vigorous physical activity. Moderate physical activity includes activities, such as brisk walking or bicycling. Vigorous physical activity is any activity producing large increases in breathing or heart rate. Recommendations also include daily aerobic activity and bone-strengthening exercises at least 3 days per week (e.g., running, jumping, climbing, or doing push-ups). These physical activity guidelines can be met with unstructured play (e.g., open-ended play without a specific learning objective, such as recess) or structured or goal-oriented play (e.g., organized athletics). Organized athletics, however, may be more suitable for older elementary school children, since logic is needed for effective and strategic play (see Table 6.1 for age-appropriate physical activities in school-aged children).

TABLE 6.1 Age-Appropriate Physical Activity in School-Aged Children

Age, years	Developing motor skills	Appropriate physical activities
6- to 8-year-olds	• Dexterity: developing running, skipping, jumping, hopping, throwing, catching, striking, and kicking • Improving balance, movement agility, mind–body coordination • Increasing body awareness • Developing muscle strength, core strength, and stability	• Fun-focused, simple activities focused on motor and cognitive skill development • Activities with flexible rules and little instruction • Examples: recess, playground activity, jumping rope, hula hoop, dribbling a basketball, kicking a soccer ball, beginner push-ups/jumping jacks/hopping/lunging, etc.
9- to 11-year-olds	• Dexterity: throwing for distance and accuracy • Hand-eye coordination is progressing; can make solid contact with a sports ball • Playing more organized team sports requiring logic, strategy, and complex muscle coordination	• Contact, hit, and accurately throw a ball (e.g., baseball, tennis ball, soccer ball, etc.) • More competitive sports with rules are okay • Athletic or sporting events are okay (e.g., short competitive races, distance races, etc.)

CLINICAL TIP

School-aged children are recommended to have *at least 60 minutes of moderate to vigorous physical activity daily*, such as such as brisk walking or bicycling. Vigorous physical activity is any activity producing large increases in breathing or heart rate. Recommendations also include daily aerobic activity and bone-strengthening exercises at least 3 days per week (e.g., running, jumping, climbing, or doing push-ups). These physical activity guidelines can be met with unstructured play (e.g., open-ended play without a specific learning objective, such as recess) or structured or goal-oriented play (e.g., organized athletics).

Sleep

School-aged children are recommended to sleep 9 to 12 hours per 24 hours (Paruthi, 2016). Good sleep hygiene, or habits and practices conducive to sleeping well regularly, is essential for restful sleep, better health, and optimal growth. Examples of healthy sleep hygiene include a good bedtime routine; consistent bedtime and awakening hours; sleeping in a quiet, dark space free of electronic devices and screens; avoiding large meals and liquids before bedtime; and daytime physical activity to decrease nighttime energy. Despite the sleep recommendation, 10% of American children and up to 75% of children with mental health and developmental conditions have sleep problems (Gerber, 2014). Children sleeping less than 10 hours per night have a greater risk of accidental injury and quality of life than older children and adults (Paruthi et al., 2016).

CLINICAL TIP

School-aged children are recommended to sleep 9 to 11 hours per night (National Sleep Foundation, 2015). Good sleep hygiene, or habits and practices conducive to sleeping well regularly, is essential for restful sleep, better health, and optimal growth.

Compared to the late 20th century, children sleep about 1 hour less per night, which may be attributed to increased technology use and familial attitudes regarding sleep. The greatest decline in sleep is for older boys on school days (Matricciani et al., 2012), and *weekend shift* occurs when children stay up later at night and sleep in later on the weekends. This overall decrease in sleep affects neurobiological functioning, mood, and cognitive performance with an IQ decrease of even points on standardized IQ tests (Matricciani et al., 2012). Sleep deprivation may also perpetuate childhood obesity via biologic mechanisms, such as elevated cortisol and decreased growth hormone. It is also associated with increased hunger due to increased levels of ghrelin and decreased leptin levels (Must & Parisi, 2009). Additionally, sleep deprivation in elementary school is associated with poor behavior regulation and impaired executive function and inhibitory control (Sadeh et al., 2002), resulting in behaviors mimicking conduct, mood, or neurologic disorders, such as learning disorders or attention-deficit/hyperactivity disorder (ADHD).

Cognitive Development

In comparison to early childhood, school-aged children are less egocentric, consider different perspectives, and begin understanding concrete information and logic. Though they struggle with planning and future thinking, with improvement in long- and short-term memories, they recall important information and focus on tasks for longer periods of time. Six-year-olds maintain concentration for at least 15 minutes, and 9-year-olds sustain focus for about 1 hour. They can follow three- and five-step commands, respectively. Consequently, school-aged children read longer books, develop, and maintain interest in focused topics, and participate in longer-term projects.

KEY POINT

Jean Piaget's theory of cognitive development uses four sequential stages to explain how children develop in their thinking and understanding about the world around them. At each stage, children have patterns of thinking that manifest characteristic errors in their reasoning. Through the cognitive stages, there is the gradual progression of the child away from egocentrism toward sociocentrism.

Jean Piaget's theory of cognitive development uses four sequential stages to explain how children develop in their thinking and understanding about the world around them. At each stage, children have patterns of thinking that manifest characteristic errors in their reasoning. Through the cognitive stages, there is the gradual progression of the child away from egocentrism toward sociocentrism. This produces a shift from the inability to see any perspective other than one's own to a reality shared with others. While young school-aged children may still be at the preoperational stage, most school-aged children are at the concrete operational stage of cognitive development.

Preoperational Cognitive Stage of Development

The hallmark of the preoperational stage is that children are now able to think symbolically. *Symbolic thinking* is the cognitive ability to use symbols to represent things. It includes the ability to make one thing, such as a word or object, stand for something else. This ability allows children to engage in symbolic, pretend, or role-play. For example, a child may ride on a broomstick, which represents a horse. Preoperational children manifest centration. *Centration* is the tendency to focus on one salient aspect of a situation, while neglecting other relevant aspects. It is the inability to consider multiple factors of a situation simultaneously. This tendency sometimes locks children in this stage into seeing only a single attribute. For example, when given two equal amounts of liquid in two different containers (one narrow and one wide), they will typically think the narrow glass (with taller fluid level) has more liquid even though they saw the water initially measured to be equal then poured into the different containers. *Irreversibility* is the inability to reverse the direction of a sequence of events to their starting point. Children at this stage are unable to undo mental acts. For example, a child is unable to understand that the same water was poured from a tall thin glass into a short wide glass. *Egocentrism* is the inability to distinguish one's perspective from another's perspective. With this, the child assumes what they see, hear, or feel is what everyone else sees, hears, or feels. For example, a 3-year-old talking on the phone to their grandparent may nod their head rather than verbally answer questions.

Magical thinking ascribes a causal link between one's inner or personal experience and the external physical world. It involves the child's belief that their inner wishes or expectations can affect what actually happens in the outer world. For example, a child may assume their cat became seriously ill today because yesterday they were upset at the cat when asked to change the litterbox. Children typically manifest this type of thinking during the preoperational stage of cognitive development. *Animism* is ascribing intentions and feelings to inanimate objects. Children begin to show this type of thinking in the preoperational stage of cognitive development. For example, a child at this stage may think the sun is unhappy on a cloudy day or that a car hurts when it is in an accident. Appearance as reality is the tendency for a child to believe how a thing looks is how it is. For example, a child may become frightened when meeting a costumed animal character in an amusement park.

> **KEY POINT**
>
> Operational thinking is the ability to carry out mental processes and figure out things in one's head. With this, children are able to figure things out in their head about concrete objects. The hallmarks of the concrete operational stage are conservation and transitivity. *Conservation* is the ability to understand that a certain material is the same, despite the adjustment of its appearance (e.g., shape or size). *Transitivity* is the ability to understand how things are related.

Concrete Operations Cognitive Stage of Development

Considered the turning point of cognitive development, the concrete operational stage represents the beginning of logical or operational thought. Operational thinking is the ability to carry out mental processes and figure out things in one's head. Here, thinking becomes more logical, and there is methodical manipulation of symbols (mental representations of objects). The child can now perform mental operations independent of the physical objects or appearances around them. Thinking about objects and experiences becomes more logical.

The hallmarks of the concrete operational stage are conservation and transitivity. *Conservation* is the ability to understand that a certain material is the same, despite the adjustment of its appearance (e.g., shape or size). For example, a child can understand that water poured into a tall, thin glass is the same when poured into a shorter, wider glass, and vice versa. Conservation involves reversibility and decentration. *Reversibility* is the ability to do and undo a process mentally. It is the ability to reverse the direction of a sequence of events from the starting to the endpoint, and vice versa. For example, a child can understand that playdough pushed down into a flat round disc will be the same playdough when rolled into a ball, and vice versa. *Decentration* is the ability to consider multiple aspects of the same situation simultaneously. For example, a child may choose a smaller piece of candy because they prefer the flavor of mint in the smaller piece over the chocolate flavor in the larger piece.

Transitivity is the ability to understand how things are related. It involves the ability to hold two relationships in mind at the same time. Transitivity involves relational logic and seriation. *Relational logic* is the ability to mentally arrange items along a quantifiable dimension, such as arranging people in order of height. (Piaget, 1952). *Seriation* is the ability to sort objects or situations based on a specific characteristic (e.g., size, shape, color, etc.). For example, children who manifest this can line up their friends or toys according to specific parameters (e.g., height). Children begin to understand relationships between things, which allows them to order and classify things during the concrete operational stage of cognitive development.

These cognitive processes move the child toward understanding others' experience the world differently from the child. They begin to recognize that people have feelings, perceptions, and motives different from their own.

QUICK POINT

Jean Piaget (1896–1980) and Lev Vygotsky (1836–1934) have two of the most recognized learning theories. Piaget described learning and cognitive development as occurring in stages dependent on individual experience, while Vygotsky described learning as occurring progressively and being dependent on social and cultural experiences. Both believed learning is what leads to higher-order thinking in the individual.

LEARNING

Jean Piaget (1896–1980) and Lev Vygotsky (1836–1934) have two of the most recognized learning theories. Piaget described learning and cognitive development as occurring in stages dependent on individual experience, while Vygotsky described learning as occurring progressively and being dependent on social and cultural experiences. Both believed learning is what leads to higher-order thinking in the individual. While Piaget described learning as driven by individual hands-on learning, Vygotsky described learning as socially guided or driven. Both theories are significant in understanding how children learn and develop in their understanding of the world around them.

Piaget described the process of acquiring and organizing knowledge, using assimilation, accommodation, and equilibrium to construct and build upon schemas or mental models of the world. Schemas represent the building blocks of knowledge. Schemas are like data file folders where information is stored. When new information is presented, it is either filed into the existing schemas (assimilation), or the current file system is modified to fit in the new knowledge (accommodation; Figure 6.1). Schemas increase in number and complexity throughout development. Piaget's discovery of learning theory asserts that learning is stage-based, universal, and occurs after physiologic and cognitive development. Children are active learners and use independent, discovery-based activities to initiate and refine their learning. Equilibrium is an ongoing process that refines and transforms existing schemas to incorporate new or puzzling information. Further information assimilates into the existing schema, and cognitive equilibrium balances existing schemes and the new information.

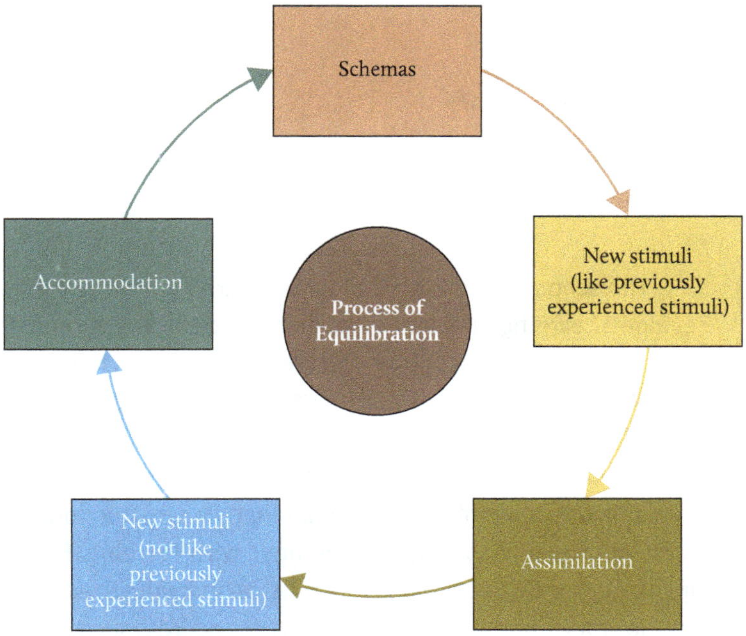

FIGURE 6.1 Piaget's theory of learning: Process of equilibration, schemas, assimilation, and accommodation

Vygotsk's theory of learning asserts that cognition develops through the internalization of language encountered in social and cultural environments. Vygotsky described learning as culturally dependent and based on guidance from a more knowledgeable other (MKO; e.g., a parent, teacher, older sibling, or older peer). In Vygotsky's theory, the MKO's role is to encourage and advance skills learned by providing experiences and opportunities within a child's proximal development zone and facilitating practicing the skill until independence is achieved (Berk & Winsler, 1995). Learning is most efficient when the MKO engages the learner

> **KEY POINT**
>
> Vygotsky described learning as culturally dependent and based on guidance from a more knowledgeable other (MKO). In Vygotsky's theory, the MKO's role is to encourage and advance skills learned by providing experiences and opportunities within a child's proximal development zone and facilitating practicing the skill until independence is achieved.

within the zone of proximal development. Scaffolding is temporary assistance or guidance that enables a child to master a new skill. An example is a parent modeling a skill, such as learning how to tie their shoelaces, which helps their child practice until they can tie a shoe independently. Teaching and learning this skill will likely be more efficient if the child indicates an interest in learning the skill (zone of proximal development; Figure 6.2).

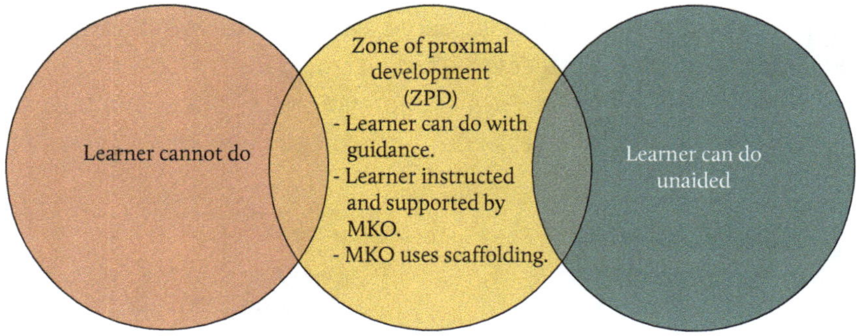

FIGURE 6.2 Vygotsky's theory of learning.

The school age is a time at which learning difficulty may first become evident. Learning difficulties and learning disorders are sometimes responsive to intensive educational intervention. Signs that a child may struggle with learning include difficulty distinguishing right from left or reversing letters, words, or numbers when writing. After first or second grade, difficulty doing tasks with the hands, such as writing, tracing, coloring, cutting, drawing; difficulty remembering or comprehending instructions; or other similar difficulties may also signify challenges with learning. Early interventions including specific attention to deficits, an individualized education plan, or special education services, which can help address such learning difficulties.

> **KEY POINT**
>
> In elementary school age, Erikson's psychosocial stage of development is industry versus inferiority. Here, the child's main psychosocial goal is achieving industry or competency. This stage establishes the foundation for self-concept and feelings of self-worth and is an indicator of future productivity.

PSYCHOSOCIAL DEVELOPMENT

According to Erik Erikson, psychosocial development occurs in eight stages that are often but not necessarily sequential. School-aged children's main psychosocial developmental goal is achieving industry or competency. Children in this stage seek and adhere to rules, peer acceptance, play in small groups, have a best friend, and seek friends of the same sex. Failure to accomplish social and academic goals or successes may result in feeling incompetent, inadequate, and inferior to peers, likely impacting self-esteem. This stage establishes the foundation for self-concept and feelings of self-worth and is an indicator for future productivity.

MENTAL HEALTH IN SCHOOL-AGED AND AGGRESSIVE BEHAVIOR

Mental disorders account for the largest area of aggregate medical spending ($13.8 billion) among all health disorders contributing to overall child health expenses (Soni, 2014). Despite this, mental health care services utilization is relatively low. In the United States, one in six children (17.4%) has a diagnosed mental, behavioral, or developmental disorder (CDC, 2021). Out of this, only 20% to 25% of affected children receive treatment (American Academy of Child and Adolescent Psychiatry, 2009). About half of adults with serious mental health disorders had childhood symptoms by 14 years of age (Kessler, 2005). Children with mental health problems can present with emotional or behavioral symptoms at school age, including anxiety, irritability or anger, and aggression. Parents of school children often worry about their behavioral problems. About 9% of school-aged children are diagnosed with ADHD (Danielson, 2018), about 7% are diagnosed with anxiety, and about 2% are diagnosed with depression (Perou et al., 2013). The prevalence of anxiety and depression increases with age. Learning problems also become more evident during school age. Children with learning difficulties struggle in school for long periods before they are detected. About 8% to 10% of children under age 18 in the United States may have some type of learning disability (National Institute of Neurological Disorders and Stroke, 2021).

CLINICAL TIP

Children in this stage seek and adhere to rules, peer acceptance, play in small groups, have a best friend, and seek friends of the same sex. Failure to accomplish social and academic goals or successes may result in feeling incompetent, inadequate, and inferior to peers, likely impacting self-esteem.

Aggression is one of the most common reasons children are referred for psychiatric evaluation. Aggression is defined as taking actions that are intended to hurt or harm others. Aggression has multiple etiologies, risk factors, and potential sequelae if untreated. It is a common symptom of several childhood mental health conditions, including conduct and oppositional defiant disorders, disruptive mood dysregulation disorder, ADHD, autism spectrum disorder and intellectual disability, anxiety, posttraumatic stress disorder, depressive and bipolar disorders, and may also be a symptom of childhood abuse or substance use. In the school-aged child, aggressive behavior occurs in multiple ways (see Table 6.2). Children with high aggressivity are often belligerent, combative, contentious, and can be outright hostile. Understanding the reason and target of a child's aggression can inform effective interventions. School-aged boys tend to demonstrate more physical or verbal aggression. In contrast, girls generally show more relational aggression, or the act of harming another's social status or relationships through nonphysical actions or exclusion (Kuppens et al., 2008).

QUICK POINT

In the United States, one in six children (17.4%) has a diagnosed mental, behavioral, or developmental disorder. (CDC, 2021) According to the American Academy of Pediatrics, 13% of school-aged children have parents worried about their behavioral problems, and 50% of adults with mental health disorders had childhood symptoms by 14 years of age.

CLINICAL TIP

Aggression is one of the most common reasons children are referred for psychiatric evaluation. Aggression is defined as taking actions that are intended to hurt or harm others. Aggression has multiple etiologies, risk factors, and potential sequelae if untreated. It is a common symptom of several childhood mental health conditions.

CLINICAL TIP

Untreated or suboptimally treated aggression associated with anger and irritability place children at risk for early initiation of substance use, poor social relationships, low academic achievement, and poorer social outcomes. Childhood aggression is a risk factor for suicide-related outcomes, including self-injury and suicidal ideation, attempt, and mortality.

Physiologic correlates of aggression include underarousal or reactivity. Aggressive children (7 to 13 years old) demonstrate elevated heart rate at baseline and lower heart rate reactivity than controls. Male children with early-onset aggression (7 to 12 years old) have low cortisol levels. Children with reactive aggression are associated with reduced sleep quality, reduced central nervous system serotonin levels, and decreased communication between the amygdala and prefrontal cortex (Hernandez et al., 2020).

When associated with anger, childhood aggression predicts poor psychiatric outcomes, increased risk for depression, decreased overall functioning later in development, and increased psychosocial adversity. High levels of outward anger expression are linked to medical illnesses, increased utilization of medical and mental health services, and a worsened health-related quality of life (Hernandez et al., 2020).

Concerning behaviors may range from normal developmental to pathologic and require further workup and intervention by a behavioral health specialist. Since 80% of youth with mental illness do not receive treatment, and the delay between symptom onset and intervention averages 8 to 10 years (American Academy of Pediatrics, 2013), assessing any child demonstrating concerning behaviors is important. Sequelae for unidentified and untreated mental illness are significant, including dropping out of high school, suicide, juvenile delinquency, future impairment, and lost productivity as adults (American Academy of Child and Adolescent Psychiatry, 2013). More specifically, untreated or suboptimally treated aggression in the form of severe anger and irritability place children at risk for early initiation of substance use, poor social relationships, low academic achievement, and poorer social outcomes. It is particularly important to assess children with aggression for associated irritability, anger, and suicidality because anger and irritability is associated with suicide-related outcomes and is a risk factor for suicide-related outcomes, including self-injury and suicidal ideation, attempt, and mortality (Caro-Canizares, 2019; Orri, M. 2018).

The assessment and treatment of childhood aggression include a thorough biopsychosocial clinical evaluation to promote prosocial behaviors and adaptive coping skills. It is important to understand children's reasons for aggressive behaviors and identify the positive and negative consequences of the behavior to help understand factors that reinforce or discourage them. The first-line treatment option is behavioral therapy (e.g., cognitive, individual, family, parent-based behavioral therapy, and school and community-based programs). The second line for treatment of aggression associated with anger and irritability are medications such as selective reuptake inhibitors, alpha-agonists, mood stabilizers, and stimulants (for children diagnosed with ADHD). Noting the baseline number and severity of aggressive behavior and monitoring it through treatment may help indicate the direction of treatment response, particularly in children with elevated symptom levels.

TABLE 6.2 Types of Aggression in Children

	Description	Example
Accidental	Unintentionally hurting another child.	Stepping on another's foot while running playing tag.
Expressive	Committing an aggressive act because the act feels good with no true intent to harm another.	Deliberately destroying another's property (e.g., knocking down another child's blocks of bricks or ripping their papers).
Hostile	Purposeful aggressive act to hurt someone physically or psychologically. Satisfaction from seeing someone hurt.	Taunting, ridiculing, hitting, kicking, shoving, or brushing past with deliberate contact.
Instrumental	Intentional acts intended to obtain a reward (a tangible item or nontangible item, such as recognition or favor).	Shoving another child to attain a certain position (e.g., being the line leader or sitting in a certain spot in class or at the lunch table).
Proactive	Aggressive acts are seen as easy to perform. Acts of aggression are relied upon as a means of solving social problems or as a means of achieving personal objectives.	Commanding, yelling at (verbal), pushing, or shoving (physical) peers to do things. Berating peers when they do not perform as requested .
Reactive	Verbal or physical impulsive retaliation for another person's intentional or accidental actions.	Starting an instant fight after innocently being shoved by a peer during a game.
Relational	Nonphysical acts to hurt the social status or relationships.	Verbal insults, undermining (negative facial expressions or mannerisms, such as rolling eyes), or socially excluding peers (intentionally not talking to, withholding invitation to group activity, or rumor initiation or propagating). Retaliating against one friend to be friends with another. Performing aggressive acts on behalf of a peer (e.g., hitting a peer for telling on a best friend or tattling on a peer to make or keep another as a friend). Common in school-aged children.
Retaliatory	Premeditated and planned aggressive acts elicited by real or imaginary provocations.	Physical (hitting, shoving, or fighting) or verbal (ridiculing or bullying) a peer in response to a perceived hurt or slight.

TABLE 6.3 Summary of Developmental Changes in School-Aged Children

	Biological	Psychological	Social
6- to 8-year-olds	• Tanner stage 1: no obvious physical changes • Physical: Gains 4 to 7 pounds per year, and permanent teeth appear • Dexterity: Developing running, skipping, jumping, hopping, throwing, catching, striking, and kicking • Cognitive: Sustains focus for 15 minutes, and follows three-step commands	• Erikson stage: industry vs. inferiority • Concrete operational stage: Understands conservation. Begins to understand relational logic and transitivity	• Has a best friend • Plays in small groups, usually with same-sex children • Rule following • Children demonstrate more instrumental aggression
9- to 11-year-olds	• Tanner stage 2: areola expansion, breast bud formation, enlargement of scrotum and penis, and thin pubic hair at penis base and on vaginal lips • Physical growth: Gains 4 to 7 pounds per year and begins growth spurt • Dexterity: throwing for distance and accuracy • Playing more organized team sports • Cognitive: sustains focus for one hour and follows five-step commands	• Erikson stage: industry vs. inferiority • Concrete operational stage: understands conservation, relational logic, and transitivity	• Has a best friend, • Plays in small groups, usually with same sex children • May begin showing interest in children of the opposite sex • Boys may demonstrate more reactive aggression. • Girls may demonstrate more relational aggression.

SUMMARY

School-aged childhood development is a time of significant biological, psychological, and social maturation. Such development requires the support of healthy sleep and physical activity. Physically, children fine-tune their gross and fine motor control during this developmental period, and by the end of elementary school, many begin puberty and have observable secondary sexual characteristics. Cognitively, school-aged children acquire an understanding of others' perspectives, develop logical thought, and manipulate abstract concepts by the end of middle childhood. Through the mastery of skills and forming friendships and interests, school-aged children build the foundations of self-esteem and self-concept that they will continue developing as adolescents. Table 6.3 contains a summary chart of the developmental changes in school-aged children.

As health care providers, it is essential to remember that many school-aged children present with symptoms concerning for current or future mental health conditions. Children and their families may not readily ask for help for fear of being teased or looked down upon and instead may try to mask their struggles by objecting to observations or disruptive behaviors. Children who struggle with anxiety or depression may demonstrate somatic symptoms or disruptive behaviors. However, with guidance, support, and thorough evaluation when needed, normal development versus pathologic behavior may be discerned, and school-aged children can optimally develop and prepare for adolescence.

CLINICAL TIP

As health care providers, it is essential to remember that many school-aged children present with symptoms concerning for current or future mental health conditions. Children and their families may not readily ask for help for fear of being teased or looked down upon and instead may try to mask their struggles by objecting to observations or disruptive behaviors.

RESOURCES

1 Piaget's 4 Stages of Cognitive Development
https://www.youtube.com/watch?v=Jt3-PIC2nCs

2 Jean Piaget's Theory of Cognitive Development Explained!
https://www.youtube.com/watch?v=u06yS0t2wyQ&pbjreload=101

3 Vygotsky's Theory of Cognitive Development: How Relationships Increase Learning
www.youtube.com/watch?v=8I2hrSRbmHE

REFERENCES

American Academy of Child and Adolescent Psychiatry Committee on Health Care Access and Economics, Task Force on Mental Health. *Pediatrics, 123*(4) 1248–1251. https://doi.org/10.1542/peds.2009-0048

Berk, L. E. (2007). *Infants and children: Prenatal through middle childhood.* Recording for the Blind & Dyslexic.

Berk, L. E., & Winsler, A. (1995). *Scaffolding children's learning: Vygotsky and early childhood education.* (NAEYC Research into Practice Series, Vol. 7). National Association for the Education of Young Children.

Caro-Canizares, I., García-Nieto, R., Díaz de Neira-Hernando, M., Brandt, S. A., Baca-García, E., & Carballo, J. J. (2019).The SDQ dysregulation profile is associated with self-injurious thoughts and behaviors in adolescents evaluated at a clinical setting. *Revista de psiquiatria y salud mental, 12*(4), 242–250.

Centers for Disease Control and Prevention. (2021). *Child mental health: Data and statistics on children's mental health.* https://www.cdc.gov/childrensmentalhealth/data.html

Cunningham, S. A., Kramer, M. R., & Narayan, K. M. V. (2014). Incidence of childhood obesity in the United States. *New England Journal of Medicine, 370*(5), 403–411. https://doi.org/10.1056/NEJMoa1309753

Danielson M. L., Bitsko R. H., Ghandour R. M., Holbrook J. R., & Blumberg S. J. (2016). Prevalence of parent-reported ADHD diagnosis and associated treatment among U.S. children and adolescerts. *Journal of Clinical Child and Adolescent Psychology.: the official journal for the Society of Clinical Child and Adolescent Psychology, American Psychological Association, Division 53, 47*(2), 199–212. https://doi.org/10.1080/15374416.2017.1417860

Gerber, L. (2014). Sleep deprivation in children: A growing public health concern. *Nursing Management, 45*(8), 22–28. https://doi.org/10.1097/01.NUMA.0000451997.95978.2f

Hernandez, S., Popatia, S., Khan, B., Le, H., Shah, A., & Onigu-Otite, E. (2020). *Pediatric anger management.* Directions in Psychiatry.

Kessler R. C., Berglund P., Demler O., Jin R., Merikangas K. R., Walters E. E. Lifetime prevalence and age-of-onset distributions of DSM-IV disorders in the national comorbidity survey replication [published erratum appears in *Arch Gen Psychiatry, 62*, 768]. *Archives of General Psychiatry*, 2005, *62*, 593–602.

Kuppens, S., Grietens, H., Onghena, P., Michiels, D., & Subramanian, S. V. (2008). Individual and classroom variables associated with relational aggression in elementary-school aged children: A multilevel analysis. *Journal of School Psychology, 46*(6), 639–660. https://doi.org/10.1016/j.jsp.2008.06.005

Matricciani, L., Olds, T., & Petkov, J. (2012). In search of lost sleep: Secular trends in the sleep time of school-aged children and adolescents. *Sleep Medicine Reviews, 16*(3), 203–211. https://doi.org/10.1016/j.smrv.2011.03.005

Must, A., & Parisi, S. (2009). Sedentary behavior and sleep: Paradoxical effects in association with childhood obesity. *International Journal of Obesity, 33*(Suppl 1), S82–S86. https://doi.org/10.1038/ijo.2009.23

National Institute of Neurological Disorders and Stroke. (2021.). *Learning disabilities information page.* https://www.ninds.nih.gov/Disorders/All-Disorders/Learning-Disabilities-Information-Page

Orri, M., Perret, L. C., Turecki, G., & Geoffroy, M. C. Association between irritability and suicide-related outcomes across the life-course. Systematic review of both community and clinical studies. *Journal of Affective Disorders, 239*, 220–233.

Paruthi, S., Brooks, L. J., D'Ambrosio, C., Hall, W. A., Kotagal, S., Lloyd, R. M., Malow, B. A., Maski, K., Nichols, C., Quan, S. F., Rosen, C. L., Troester, M. M., & Wise, M. S. (2016). Consensus statement of the American Academy of Sleep Medicine on the recommended amount of sleep for healthy children: Methodology and discussion. *Journal of Clinical Sleep Medicine, 12*(11), 1549–1561. https://doi.org/10.5664/jcsm.6288

Perou, R., Bitsko, R. H., Blumberg, S. J., Pastor, P., Ghandour, R. M., Gfroerer, J. C., Hedden, S. L., Crosby, A. E., Visser, S. N., Schieve, L. A., Parks, S. E., Hall, J. E., Brody, D., Simile, C. M., Thompson, W. W., Baio, J., Avenevoli, S., Kogan, M. D., Huang, L. N.. Mental health surveillance among children—United States, 2005—2011. *MMWR, 62*(supplement), 1–35.

Sadeh, A., Gruber, R., & Raviv, A. (2002). Sleep, neurobehavioral functioning, and behavior problems in school-age children. *Child Development, 73*(2), 405–417. https://doi.org/10.1111/1467-8624.00414

Solorzano, C. M. B., & McCartney, C. R. (2010). Obesity and the pubertal transition in girls and boys. *Reproduction, 140*(3), 399–410. https://doi.org/10.1530/REP-10-0119

Soni A. The five most costly children's conditions. (2011). Estimates for U.S. civilian noninstitutionalized children, ages 0–17. In: *Statistical Brief (Medical Expenditure Panel Survey).* Agency for Healthcare Research and Quality (U.S.): 2001-. STATISTICAL BRIEF #434. https://www.ncbi.nlm.nih.gov/books/NBK476257/

Trinh, M.-H., Sundaram, R., Robinson, S. L., Lin, T.-C., Bell, E. M., Ghassabian, A., & Yeung, E. H. (2020). Association of trajectory and covariates of children's screen media time. *JAMA Pediatrics, 174*(1), 71–78. https://doi.org/10.1001/jamapediatrics.2019.4488

Wu, T., Mendola, P., & Buck, G. M. (2002). Ethnic differences in the presence of secondary sex characteristics and menarche among U.S. girls: The third national health and nutrition examination survey, 1988–1994. *Pediatrics, 110*(4), 752–757. https://doi.org/10.1542/peds.110.4.752

CHAPTER 7

Adolescence

Edore Onigu-Otite, M.D. and Kammarauche Asuzu, M.D., M.H.S.

> *"Adolescence is a border between childhood and adulthood. Like all borders, it's teeming with energy and fraught with danger."*
>
> — Mary Pipher

OBJECTIVES

After reading this chapter, students will be able to do the following:

- summarize developmental characteristics of adolescents
- understand the development of identity, according to James Marcias
- recognize the emergence of psychiatric disorders during adolescence

CASE VIGNETTE

Ben is biracial. His father, an immigrant, left his birth country when Ben was 2. His mother, a single parent, lived with her parents. His mother worked long hours to provide for him. Ben's grandparents were a stabilizing presence in his life. He excelled in elementary school and was well liked.

In his teens, Ben began to struggle with his identity. He stood out from the other kids in his neighborhood. At age 13, he asked a girl out, but she turned him down rather publicly because her friends thought he was not a good fit for her. Ben suffered his first heartache. He wondered who he was and where he fit in the world. At age 14 he joined a group of friends who prided themselves in having each other's backs. Ben smoked with these friends to numb his emotional pain and his unresolved identity question and to fit in. His grades began to slip, and his mother noticed. She enrolled him in an after-school club, which helped with homework and other fun activities. His mother and grandparents closely monitored him, which Ben resented at first.

(continued)

At age 15, he got depressed and reluctantly admitted to his school counselor that he had considered ending his life. His mother promptly scheduled an appointment with his pediatrician, who treated him for depression. Over the next few months, Ben also saw a therapist regularly. He got better and began reflecting on his past and future life. He began to envision the direction he wanted his life to take. By age 17, Ben had progressively developed his sense of self. Over time, he spent less and less time with his old friends and made new ones. He made good grades, joined his school's basketball team, and became a driving force on the team. By this point, kids wanted to be his friend. By the end of high school, he had a girlfriend he had been steadily dating for a year.

At age 18 he graduated high school with honors and gained admission to a prestigious college. He became a successful professional, built a family, and was always there for his kids. He sometimes looked back and wondered what would have happened if his parents and teachers had not noticed his struggles as a teen and provided the support he needed to navigate the different terrain of his adolescent years.

DEFINITIONS AND KEY CONCEPTS

The word *adolescence* comes from the Latin word *adolescere*, which means to grow up. Adolescence is the transitional period during which a young person develops from a child into an adult. This generally starts with the onset of puberty and continues until the start of adulthood. Puberty is the biological maturation process of a species toward the ability to procreate. Adulthood is the psychological and social state of being able to function independently, including the ability to cater to offspring. While puberty is mostly biologically driven, adulthood is influenced by psychological and social aspects with different cultures expecting different things of the new adult. In most Western societies, legal adulthood begins at age 18 and is meant to signal independence.

INTRODUCTION

Globally, puberty now begins at younger ages compared to the past. The earlier age of puberty onset is attributed to improvements in nutrition, general health, and other social conditions. With this, the onset of adolescence is now earlier than in previous decades. Cultural descriptions and roles of adolescence differ between societies and eras. Some cultures mark the onset of adolescence with cultural ceremonies. Regardless of their cultures, adolescents face different challenges in different societies across different times. Currently, there are 1.2 billion adolescents globally (UNICEF, 2019) and 42 million in the United States, which translates to 12.9% of the U.S. population (U.S. Department of Health and Human Services [HHS]), 2019).

The overarching goal of adolescence is to enable the child to develop the maturity to think and act independently, so they can successfully function as an adult without their parents' supervision. Adolescents have an opportunity to audition or practice adulthood with the benefit of oversight of their parents. As adolescents become more autonomous, they begin to make their own choices about their behavior, who they spend time with, and what direction they choose to pursue in life. They eventually adapt and settle on their identity and role within society. Adolescence is sometimes said to be the second separation individuation with the first being toddlerhood.

KEY POINT

Adolescence is the transitional period during which a young person develops from a child into an adult. This generally starts with the onset of puberty and continues until the start of adulthood. The overarching goal of adolescence is to enable the child to develop the maturity to think and act independently, so they can successfully function as an adult without their parents' oversight.

During this period, adolescents shift their views on themselves, others, and the world. They are now able to think abstractly and consider alternative views. Many adolescents start to think about deeper issues, such as life, beliefs, values, ethics and morality, humanitarian causes, philosophy, spirituality, religion, and politics. Adolescents may consider different ideologies from their parents. Depending on their experiences (e.g., their families' culture and those around them), these shifts may be welcome or may cause conflicts within the family.

Adolescence is a time of significant social shifts with most adolescents venturing out to prioritize relationships with peers over their families. In early adolescence, most associate with the same gender groups. By middle adolescence, teens begin to take interest and make advances toward individuals in other gender peer groups. These relationships are sometimes convoluted with recurrent breaking up and reestablishing romantic partners within both heteronormative and LGBTQ (lesbian, gay, bisexual, transgender, and queer or questioning) relationships. Additionally, some adolescents enter the workforce as a mark of individual responsibility and independence, while others may need to supplement their family income. Adolescents may start to question rules they previously followed without protest or question. While doing this, they sometimes appear to challenge rules based on a developmental desire to acquire and process information and the reasoning behind rules and norms before accepting or rejecting these as such.

Adolescence comes with many pressures and consequences. Many adolescents are faced with peer pressure to use alcohol, nicotine, or other drugs and to initiate sexual relationships, putting themselves at a high risk of unintended pregnancies, sexually transmitted infections (STIs), and intentional and unintentional injuries. Many experience a wide range of psychologically distressing symptoms and mental health problems. Contrary to the common perception of adolescent angst, most adolescents navigate this period without major problems.

ADOLESCENT DEVELOPMENT

The period of adolescence can be divided into three parts: early (ages 10 to 12), middle (ages 13 to 16), and late adolescence (ages 17 to 20). Each stage coincides with different biopsychosocial changes. During adolescence, significant growth occurs, secondary sexual characteristics appear, fertility is achieved, profound psychological changes occur, social connections beyond immediate circles expand, and substantial neurocognitive shifts occur.

Biological Development

Adolescence is a period of rapid physical growth and development. Many biological changes occur with the most obvious being marked increase in height and muscle mass, neurocognitive development, and the development of secondary sexual characteristics.

Puberty

In general, girls' onset of puberty occurs between ages 8 to 14, about 2 years earlier than boys who often begin puberty between ages 9 to 15. Puberty is initiated by a sustained increase in the pulsatile release of the gonadotropin-releasing hormone (GnRH) from the hypothalamus (Abreu & Kaiser, 2016). This leads to surges in the luteinizing hormone (LH) and follicular-stimulating hormone (FSH) from the pituitary gland, both of which stimulate the gonads to release testosterone, estradiol, and progesterone. These hormones promote gametogenesis and the development of secondary sexual characteristics. The process of pubertal maturation is generated primarily by the brain and the hypothalamic–pituitary–gonadal axis, which is influenced by psychosocial environmental influences. There is rapid growth and the development of secondary sexual characteristics during this stage with adolescents becoming physically and sexually mature and now with the capability to procreate. This stage coincides with Freud's genital period. Table 7.1 summarizes the physical changes in adolescence.

QUICK POINT

Adolescence comes with many pressures and consequences. Many adolescents are faced with peer pressures to use alcohol, nicotine, or other drugs and to initiate sexual relationships, putting themselves at a high risk of unintended pregnancies, sexually transmitted infections (STIs), and intentional and unintentional injuries. Many experience a wide range of psychologically distressing symptoms and mental health problems. Contrary to the common perception of adolescent angst, most adolescents navigate this periodwithout major problems.

KEY POINT

The process of pubertal maturation is generated primarily by the brain and the hypothalamic–pituitary–gonadal axis, which is influenced by psychosocial environmental influences. There is rapid growth and the development of secondary sexual characteristics during this stage with adolescents becoming physically and sexually mature and now with the capability to procreate.

TABLE 7.1 Physical (Biological) Changes in Adolescence

General	Girls	Boys
• Weight gain and increases in lean body mass and muscle mass (11–16 years of age) • 95% of adult height (by age 16) • Doubling of heart size and vital lung capacity and an increase in blood pressure and blood volume	• Appearance of breast buds (between 8 and 12 years of age), followed by breast development (13–18) • Development of pubic hair (11–14) • Growth spurt begins (at the average age of 10), which adds inches to height and hip circumference • Menses begins (at the average age of 12 with a normal age range between 9 and 16) • Enlargement of ovaries, uterus, labia, and clitoris; thickening of the endometrium and vaginal mucosa • Appearance of underarm hair (13–16) • Dental changes, which include jaw growth and the development of molars	• Testicular enlargement, beginning as early as 9.5 years of age • Appearance of pubic hair (10–15) • Onset of spermarche, or sperm found in the ejaculate • Lengthening of genitals (11–14) • Rapid enlargement of the larynx, pharynx, and lungs, which can lead to alterations in vocal quality (i.e., voice cracking) • Growth of facial and body hair, which may not be completed until the mid-20s • Dental changes, which include jaw growth and the development of molars • Development of body odor and acne

Neurocognitive Development

Brain development continues through adolescence. Brain maturation allows for faster neural processing and the proliferation of the glial (support) cells, which nourish the neurons. These changes stimulate cognitive growth and development, precipitating qualitative shifts in cognitive ability.

Abstract Thinking

The hallmark of cognitive organization in adolescence is attaining the ability to abstract. This coincides with Piaget's formal operations stage (see Chapter 4). With this ability, adolescents are no longer limited to their own direct experience. With the attainment of abstract thinking, adolescents can engage in hypothetical thinking, including inductive and deductive reasoning, which opens a world of hypothetical possibilities. They can now carry out hypothetical experiments in their minds. With this capability, they can now extend their world beyond their immediate experience and time. They demonstrate a different form of heightened self-focus and may seem more introspective and self-absorbed. They may attribute more power to their thoughts than to the reality around them. In this way, they may perceive the external world through their inner world's lens and strength. For example, a teen may genuinely believe and insist they are performing exceptionally well in school, while the external reality, the objective one, shows their grades are low. Such perceptions may persist and be held firmly until the external realities set in. Piaget believed it was not until adolescents assumed adult roles that they experienced and learned the limits of their thoughts.

> **KEY POINT**
>
> Adolescence is a critical time for brain maturation. Several overlapping processes occur within the brain, sculpting and molding it to its final adult state. Brain maturation generally peaks in late adolescence to young adulthood (18–24 years old). During the adolescent years, the prefrontal cortex's (PFC) relative size decreases and is prominently remodeled. This occurs primarily by two processes: myelination and synaptic pruning. This makes the PFC progressively more efficient in its operations. This promotes the development of the executive functioning system. This higher-order control system regulates the efficiency and accuracy with which information is processed and used to inform goal-directed, future-oriented behaviors (Spear, 2000).

Brain Maturation

Adolescence is a critical time for brain maturation. Several overlapping processes occur within the brain, sculpting and molding it to its final adult state (see Figure 7.1). Brain maturation generally peaks in late adolescence to young adulthood (18–24 years old). During the adolescent years, the prefrontal cortex's (PFC) relative size decreases and is prominently remodeled (Spear, 2000). This occurs primarily by two processes: myelination and synaptic pruning. Myelination is the process of increasing the fatty sheath surrounding neuronal fibers, which increases the efficiency of electrical transmission. Synaptic pruning is the process of elimination of unused synapses. This process begins in childhood through the mid-20s and occurs at different brain sites in corresponding developmental ages. During adolescence, synaptic pruning occurs mainly in the PFC. The connections between the more commonly used neurons are strengthened and become more effective in transmission with these two processes. This makes the PFC progressively more efficient in its operations. Important in this process is the development of the executive functioning system. This higher-order control system regulates the efficiency and accuracy with which information is processed and used to inform goal-directed, future-oriented behaviors (Spear, 2000). Due to this, adolescents can self-manage and organize themselves and their activities with less supervision than in earlier developmental stages.

Executive Functioning and Self-Regulation

Executive functioning and self-regulation are skills that develop in accelerated fashion during adolescence. Executive functioning is "the ability to organize a sequence of actions toward a goal" (Fuster, 2008, p. 191). It includes mental processes and skills that include working memory, mental flexibility, and self-control. These skills enable us direct and focus attention, organize, and plan sometimes multiple overlapping tasks successfully. The PFC controls executive functioning. It directs the prioritization of tasks, filtering distractors and revising previous decisions upon the availability of new data. It is like an air traffic control system that handles multiple streams of information in real time, directing the order of activity to achieve overlapping tasks of airplanes taking off, being in flight, and landing for passenger safety. Successfully achieving goals also involves holding back from taking actions if they are no longer appropriate and controlling impulses to achieve the set goals. Self-regulation is the ability to direct behavior to achieve certain goals or reach certain ideals. It involves monitoring and modulating one's thoughts, emotions, and actions toward goals or ideals. This necessarily includes controlling impulses and persisting in behaviors to reach the goal or ideal. Adolescents develop increased attentional shifting abilities, response inhibition, emotional modulation, discrimination of emotional cues, and behavior modulation. Adolescents become capable of relativistic thinking and develop metacognition and multifactorial decision-making. With this, they become better equipped to handle more complex life decisions.

Sleep

During adolescence, there is a circadian rhythm shift, causing a phase delay in sleep onset. At the same time, the biological need for sleep increases in adolescence. Consequently, adolescents naturally fall asleep and wake up later. Additionally, multiple psychosocial influences impact sleep during adolescence. Adolescents may find their sleep affected by electronic device use, social media, the juggling of academic responsibilities, extracurricular activities, work obligations, and the start time of high school classes. Despite the importance of sleep, there is an "epidemic of sleep deprivation" in adolescence. Chronic sleep deprivation impacts functioning and is associated with feelings of depression, anger, and anxiety (Short & Louca, 2015), reckless driving (Martiniuk et al., 2013), and an increased risk of substance use (Terry-McElrath et al., 2016).

KEY POINT

Executive functioning is "the ability to organize a sequence of actions towards a goal" (Fuster, 2008, p. 191). It includes mental processes and skills that include working memory, mental flexibility, and self-control. These skills enable us direct and focus attention, organize, and plan sometimes multiple overlapping tasks successfully.

CLINICAL TIP

During adolescence, there is a circadian rhythm shift, causing a phase delay in sleep onset. At the same time, the biological need for sleep increases in adolescence. Consequently, adolescents naturally fall asleep and wake up later.

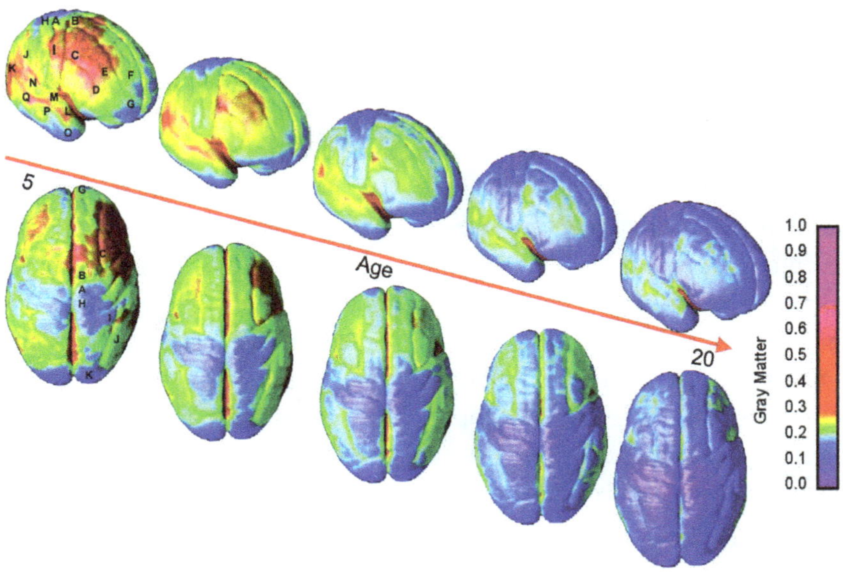

FIGURE 7.1 Maturation of the brain.

Copyright © 2004 by National Academy of Sciences, USA. Reprinted with permission.

Reward-Seeking, Sensation-Seeking, and Impulsivity

Several cognitive processes play an essential role in the adolescent's personal and social functioning. The prefrontal cortex's (PFC) functions, including the cognitive abilities to self-regulate and dampen or inhibit the tendency to act without much prior thought, are not fully developed until late adolescence through early adulthood. In contrast, the reward system matures earlier than the PFC provides a relatively more robust drive toward rewards (strong push forward). The weaker PFC exerts relatively weaker control (weaker pullback). This is the imbalance model, which posits that dynamic neurodevelopmental changes in the adolescent brain result in shifting imbalances in how the brain regulates the individual's behavior around rewards. It takes a dual system perspective similar to the way that both an accelerator and the brakes control a car's movement in the direction of a destination. In adolescence, the accelerator is comparatively more powerful than the weaker brake system. This imbalance is a reason adolescents are reward driven with seemingly less consideration for pausing or slowing down to consider the risks involved. As such, during adolescence through young adulthood, there is a tendency to take risks and seek novel and thrilling experiences, sometimes associated with physical and psychosocial consequences (Figure 7.2).

QUICK POINT

A reward is an event or experience that produces a pleasant or positive emotional experience. Reward-sensitivity is the tendency to detect, pursue, and derive pleasure from positive stimuli. Reward-seeking is the tendency to pursue the desired sensation, feeling, or experience (the reward). Impulsivity is the inability to inhibit behavioral impulses and thoughts. In such instances, the lack of ability to inhibit responses is the problem. Once an idea or urge occurs to the individuals, they are less likely to stop themselves from acting on it.

A *reward* is an event or experience that produces a pleasant or positive affective experience. Reward-sensitivity is the tendency to detect, pursue, learn from, and derive pleasure from positive stimuli. Reward-seeking is the tendency to pursue the desired sensation, feeling, or experience (the reward). Sensation-seeking, also called thrill-seeking or excitement-seeking, is the tendency to seek and pursue new or novel and different sensations, feelings, and experiences. Impulsivity is the inability to inhibit behavioral impulses and thoughts. In such instances, response inhibition is the problem. Once the "go" signal has been registered, the "stop" or "no go" signal is absent, weak, ignored, or overridden, and the thought or action gets carried out. Consequently, without intervention, individuals who are impulse driven lack the ability to adjust their behavior in response to the consequences of their actions. Impulsivity is a trait linked to several mental health conditions, notably ADHD; addictive disorders, including substance use; and other impulse control disorders.

Adolescents have increased reward sensitivity, which contributes to the increased reward-seeking behavior that occurs during this developmental stage. Thus, adolescent risk-taking is not always impulsive but may be planned and undertaken when the reward is pleasing enough. Once the desired reward is in sight for many teens, obstacles in their path become challenges to overcome, sometimes recklessly ignoring the risks. Objectively, with neuromaturation, cognitive control increases linearly. Thus, in essence, from the neurobehavioral standpoint, risk-taking in adolescence is more reward-seeking in origin than impulsive (see Figure 7.2).

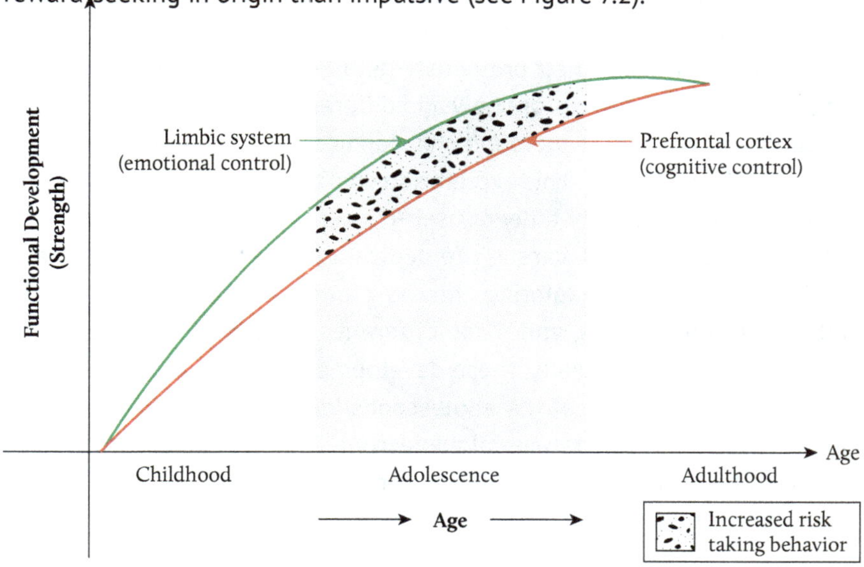

FIGURE 7.2 Reward-seeking and cognitive control in adolescence: Dual-system perspective.

Adapted from Casey BJ et al. Developmental Reviews, 2008; 28:62–77.
Source: https://www.ncbi.nlm.nih.gov/pmc/articles/PMC2500212/pdf/nihms56150.pdf.

Psychological Development

During adolescence, individuals begin to process the existential question of identity. This prompts them to ask themselves the critical question, "Who am I, and where do I fit into this world?" For most adolescents, this is a relatively smooth process. For others, it can bring turbulence into their life and that of their family. Personal identity refers to an individual's sense of self. This includes several substructures of identity, such as ethnicity, sexuality, spirituality, beliefs, values, physical appearance, interpersonal characteristics, and social roles. Identity involves a sense of continuity beneath external changes and the feeling that one is the same person through time, despite physical or other changes.

> **QUICK POINT**
>
> In adolescence, the overarching psychosocial task is to process identity. This often answers the questions, "Who am I?" and "Where do I belong?" A sense of self is an individual's feeling of identity, uniqueness, and self-directedness. Through adolescence, the sense of self evolves. It becomes more organized and coherent and includes various components.

Identity Development

Adolescence coincides with Erickson's psychosocial stage of identity versus role confusion (see Chapter 4). According to Erik Erickson, the primary psychosocial task during adolescence is to achieve a consolidated sense of identity within which one operates in the world. James Marcia, a developmental psychologist, expanded on this concept. Marcia described identity development as a process that evolved through the exploration process by which the adolescent achieves commitment to an identity. Identity development progresses and is catalyzed by experiencing crisis. This crisis, a state of internal angst, creates emotional upheaval and internal conflict. Experiencing such a crisis triggers adolescents to review and question their previously held beliefs and values, shifting them to consider and explore new and different possibilities. The type of exploration is of a more profound philosophical kind, sometimes resulting in physical exploration. This exploration confronts traditional beliefs and often includes facets of a deeper self-concept, such as morality, sexual roles, religious beliefs, career, life dedication, philosophies of life, and political views. While exploring, they may form new and different beliefs, adopt different values, and make different, and sometimes seemingly shocking, decisions. Ideally, these developmental crises lead to the progressive consolidation of the adolescent's identity. Within this process, Marcia described four statuses of adolescent identity development. These can also be viewed as categories, stations, or points along the identity developmental path:

CLINICAL TIP

Adolescents typically explore new and different possibilities. This exploration confronts traditional beliefs and often includes facets of a deeper self-concept, such as morality, sexual roles, religious beliefs, career, life dedication, philosophies of life, and political views. While exploring, they may form new and different beliefs, adopt different values, and make different, and sometimes seemingly shocking, decisions.

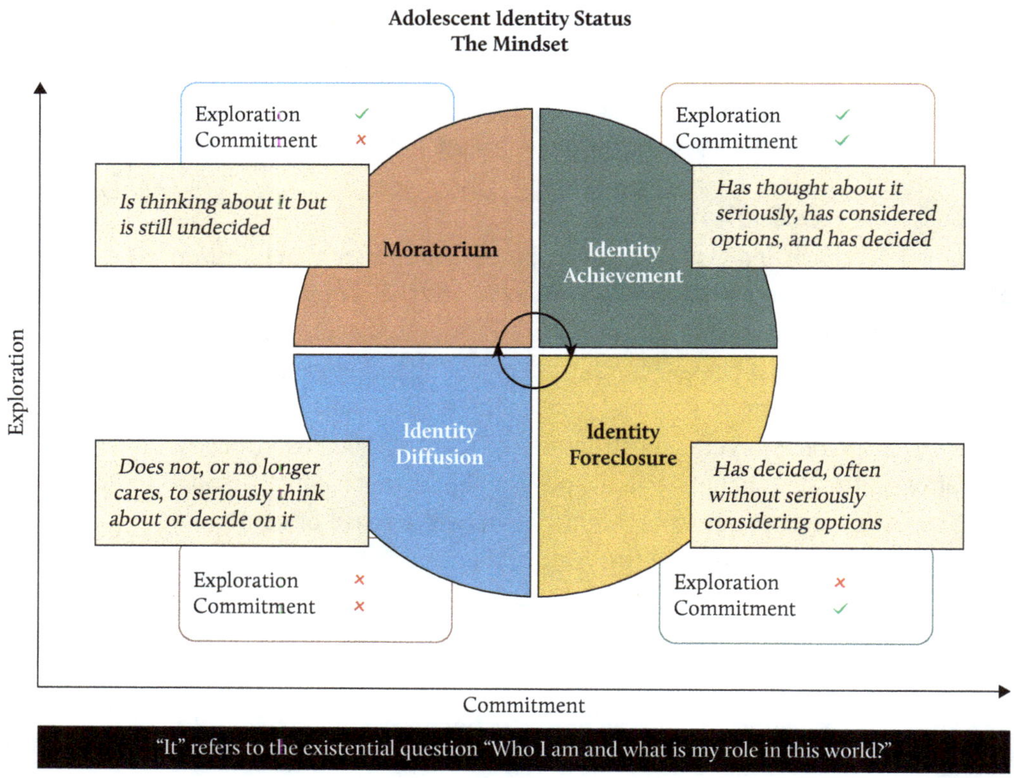

FIGURE 7.3 Adolescent identity status, according to James Marcia.

1. identity diffusion
2. identity foreclosure
3. moratorium
4. identity achievement

> **KEY POINT**
>
> Four adolescent identity statuses were described by Marcia as follows:
>
> 1. identity diffusion
> 2. identity foreclosure
> 3. moratorium
> 4. identity achievement

Identity Diffusion

Identity diffusion involves a low degree of exploration and a low degree of commitment. Here, the adolescent manifests little to no consolidation of their identity. They may no longer experience much internal crisis even when they are yet to settle on their identity. They are like a leaf blowing in the wind, not anchored in specific ideals or identities and seem to be in a state of constant flux. They lack serious consideration or commitment to specific life goals. They tend to assume the identity of persons around them based on momentary factors, including their emotional and other needs at the time. Individuals in this category often change their beliefs or behavior to please others or to succeed.

Identity Foreclosure

Identity foreclosure involves a low degree of exploration and a high degree of commitment. Here, the adolescent consolidates their identity early in the process, often without experiencing much crisis and before much exploration has occurred. This identity type is narrower, prescriptive, precisely defined, and results in a highly specific individual identity. Here, adolescents achieve their identity by accepting preset values and beliefs, usually from their family or culture, without much consideration for alternatives. Individuals in this category decide and settle quickly on their identity and role within their family and community.

Moratorium

Moratorium involves a high degree of exploration and a low degree of commitment. This is a state of crisis and internal conflict, which occurs while the adolescent explores various life facets. Here, the adolescent is in a state of crisis that has yet to be resolved. Nevertheless, in this state, they keep their options open.

Identity Achievement

Identity achievement involves a high degree of exploration and a high degree of commitment. In many ways, this is the ideal status, which results in a secure, consolidated sense of identity. This usually occurs after the active exploration and experience and resolution of the crisis. Individuals in this state manifest a secure sense of self and a strong commitment to a set of values and beliefs, often with a clear life direction.

Although these statuses are points along the developmental path of adolescent identity formation, not all adolescents go through all phases and not to the same degree. While some consolidate their identity early in the process, others never quite consolidate and may continue this way into their adult years. Additionally, adolescents may process their identity based on their individual crisis experience and may be at different identity statuses in different areas (e.g., religion, gender, political views, work, etc.). As such, events occurring during adolescence, particularly major or traumatic ones, could cause some stagnation and significantly impact a teen's sense of self if not adequately managed. Ultimately, identity is multifaceted and includes physical characteristics, habitual traits or patterns of behavior, sexual identity, vocational and academic decisions, relationships, leisure time activities, and life philosophy.

Identity, Sense of Self, Self-Concept, and Self-Esteem

In working through the existential question of identity, several related concepts are sometimes used interchangeably, but each lends a different facet to an individual's identity. A sense of self is an individual's feeling of identity, uniqueness, and self-directedness. Self-esteem is confidence and satisfaction in oneself. Self-concept is one's description and evaluation of oneself. It includes psychological and physical characteristics, qualities, skills, roles, and so on. Self-concepts contribute to the individual's sense of identity over time. Self-concept is partly conscious and includes self-rating, which others sometimes influence, including parental figures and peers.

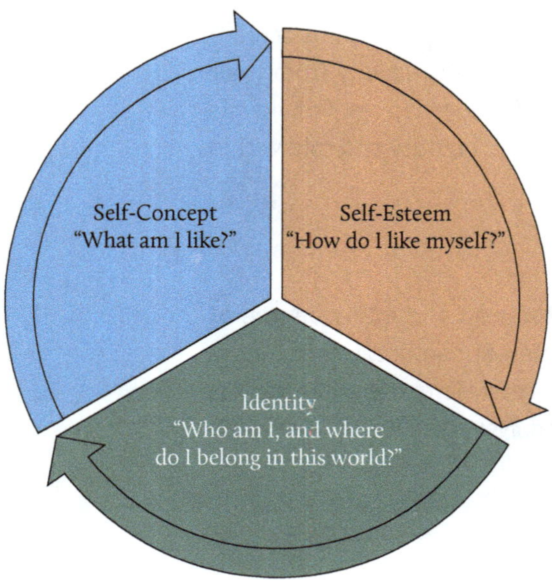

FIGURE 7.4 Various aspects of sense of self.

Through adolescence, the sense of self evolves. It becomes more organized and coherent and includes various components (see Figure 7.4). It often broadens to include both one's assessment and one's perception of others' views of oneself. This is where peers' views become impactful—for better or worse. Adolescents with a weaker sense of self may struggle to do what it takes, including behaving in ways that may be unusual for their personalities, upbringing, and family values, to win their peers' approval. Depending on what type of behaviors are endorsed by peers, adolescents can engage in prosocial or antisocial behaviors. Teens may enter abusive relationships erroneously because the abusive party makes them feel good about themselves. They may also get into drugs as a way of self-medicating to alleviate negative mood states.

Social Development

Social development is a hallmark of adolescent development. During this period, teens expand their relationships with peers, develop intimate relationships, their interaction and relationship with their family of origin changes, and their social circle begins to expand beyond their immediate family.

Peer Relationships

Adolescents go through realigning social ties with members of both the same and the opposite gender. Early adolescents may tend to fall in and out of peer groups, a process that can cause much emotional distress. Adolescents tend to form groups or cliques based on shared norms, interests, and values. A teen's reputation within the group becomes increasingly powerful. These groups provide a sense of belonging. This serves an important social need for adolescents and often facilitates the formation of separate and distinct identities from their families.

Electronic and Social Media

The presence of social media and its use among adolescents has transformed the peer experience. Social media context features change the frequency, immediacy, and duration of peer interaction, which often extends beyond school hours and after usual bedtimes. This increases the demand and supply of peer interaction and its influence on the peer and the peer group. The influence of peer groups can be positive or negative. In the current age, the presence of social media has both positive and negative impacts with an increasing peer social presence and ease of peer victimization.

Separation From Family and Culture of Origin

Adolescents begin to renegotiate roles and balance of power in a quest for autonomy and control. They are sometimes viewed as challenging existing authority. Depending on the prevailing molding social force, this could be viewed as either a positive or an unwelcome development. In individualistic cultures, such as Western cultures, independence is placed over interdependence. In collectivistic cultures, the larger family or community, rather than parents alone, controls the social force. Interdependence, acting with consideration for collective needs, is valued over independence, acting mainly for personal goals. With the globalization of Western culture, social media, immigration, and increasing global travel, increasing numbers of adolescents experience different cultures and subcultures in real life and via social media and develop a more complex understanding of societal and social impact.

Dating, Intimate Relationships, and Sexual Activity

In heteronormative conditions, biological sex, sexuality, and gender identity align. However, the LGBTQ population in adolescence has increased over the years. In early adolescence, relationships and gender interactions change, and dating relationships begin. These dating relationships are more like relationships between close friends from the opposite gender than adult-type romantic relationships, often with more physical than sexual behaviors. This serves as a means of autonomy from parents and peers, providing a sense of "grown-up" status and practicing for intimate relationships later. Dating activities include texting, "Snapchatting," phone calls, and video chats. Breakups may be experienced as devastating for the teen. In the United States, by age 15, about 90% of teens have dated. Double or group dates are common. By middle adolescence, dating relationships become more serious, as adolescents begin to form intimate relationships with other teens. By 15, 33% of U.S. males and 25% of females have had an intimate relationship. This increases through adolescence, and by age 19 86% of males and 80% of females have had intimate relationships. Adolescents also begin to engage in sexual activity. About 7.1% have their first sexual intercourse before 13; more males than females report early sexual intercourse (Cavazos-Rehg, 2009). Some reasons for early sexual activity include peer pressure, curiosity, sexual feelings and desires, and coercions (e.g., date rape), and they sometimes include drugs and alcohol use. In youth aged 15–19, about 42% of females and 44% of males had had their first sexual intercourse (Abma et al, 2017).

Socioeconomic Factors

During adolescence, financial means significantly impact adolescents' development, educational attainment, peer relationships, and socioeconomic potential. Family income is the most critical factor in determining the social settings and experiences within which the adolescent develops. The household environment, housing, neighborhoods, schools, other social opportunities, and experiences are largely controlled by income. The adolescent's socioeconomic status provides, or limits, opportunities for quality and advanced education and training. Family income and employment dictate access to and the quality of health care services, including for mental health. For socioeconomic reasons, some adolescents feel the pressure to enter the workforce prematurely. Others are enticed into illegal dealings, which elevates their risk for involvement with the justice system. For others, work is seen as a mark of independence, and this brings added social experience. Nevertheless, persistent poverty sometimes exerts a high cost on adolescents' development, educational attainment, and socioeconomic potential during this developmental stage. Table 7.2 summarizes the biological, psychological, and social changes in different adolescent age groups.

TABLE 7.2 Summary Chart Showing Biological, Psychological, and Social Changes in Different Adolescent Age Groups

	Biological	Psychological	Social
Early adolescence (ages 10–13)	• Onset of puberty • Increase in acne • Rapid growth spurt • Girls achieve menarche	• Final phase of Erikson's stage of industry vs. inferiority • Questions around self-esteem surface • Begin to seek autonomy • Begin to question value systems • Increasing interest in world issues	• Same-sex peer groups • Decreasing interest in family activities • Increasing interest in peer group activities • Dating interests and behavior develop
Middle adolescence (ages 14–16)	• Lethargy • Increased need for sleep • Girls complete physical development • Girls establish regular menstruation • Boys are still going through the stages of puberty with continued growth in height and muscle, voice cracking, and hair growth • Boys achieve thorarche	• Erikson's stage of identity vs. role confusion • Exploration of various aspects of identity • Increased reward-seeking behaviors • Egocentrism • Oppositionality • Increased abstract thought • Increased interest in morality and social order	• Mixed-sex peer groups • Romantic relationships • Increased desire for privacy • Family conflict • Concerned about body image and personal fashion style
Late adolescence (ages 17–19)	• 95% of adult height • Girls achieve 93% of bone mass • Boys achieve 83% of bone mass	• Identity established • Sense of self is stabilized • Better control of impulsivity • Erikson's stage of identity vs. role confusion • Application of abstract thought to decision-making	• Romantic relationships (more stable) • Establishment of role in society • Establishment of vocational path • Resolving conflict with caregivers

MENTAL HEALTH PROBLEMS IN ADOLESCENCE

Adolescence is a confluence of active brain changes, psychological self-restructuring, and social role construction, all occurring while striving to gain a sense of autonomy and independence. Within this context, adolescence is the time several major mental health disorders are onset. Anxiety occurs in about 32% of 13- to 18-year-olds, depression occurs in approximately 20% of 12- to 17-year-olds, ADHD in 9% of 13- to 18-year-olds, and eating

QUICK POINT

Firearms are the most common mode of suicide in youth, followed by suffocation and poisoning

KEY POINT

Suicide is the second-leading cause of death in adolescents. The majority of children and adolescents who attempt suicide have a significant mental health disorders. Risk factors for youth suicide attempts include depression, feelings of hopelessness or helplessness, aggressive or disruptive behavior, acute loss or rejection, trauma (including bullying), exposure to violence, a family history of suicide attempts, and access to firearms.

CLINICAL TIP

Several mental health disorders, including major depressive disorder, schizophrenia, bipolar disorder, and substance use disorders, often begin in adolescence. Adolescents are at higher risk of substance use initiation due to a combination of reward-seeking behavior with limited control by their relatively weaker PFC and the strength of peer influence.

disorders in about 3% of 13- to 18-year-olds (Merikangas et al., 2010). Adolescents are at increased risk of suicidality, including nonsuicidal suicidal ideation (NSSI), suicide attempts, and completed suicide.

Suicide is the second-leading cause of death in youth (Herron, 2019). Most children and adolescents who attempt suicide have a significant mental health disorder, such as depression, a history of disruptive behavior, or substance use. Risk factors for youth suicide attempts include depression, feelings of hopelessness or helplessness, aggressive or disruptive behavior, acute loss or rejection, trauma (including bullying), exposure to violence, a family history of suicide attempts, and access to firearms. Firearms are the most common mode of suicide in youth, followed by suffocation and poisoning. The initiation of substance use remains a public health problem with different substances waxing and waning in popularity among adolescents, yet all carry significant morbidity and mortality, including alarming rates of opioid overdoses (Levy, 2019; Miech, 2016; Patrick, 2018; Terry-McElrath, 2020a, 2020b).

Several mental health disorders, including major depressive disorder, schizophrenia, bipolar disorder, and substance use disorders, often begin in adolescence. Adolescents are at higher risk of substance use initiation due to a combination of reward-seeking behavior with limited control by their relatively less mature PFC and the strength of peer influence. Not surprisingly, the incidence of substance use initiation peaks between the ages of 14 to 16, coinciding with adolescents' reward-seeking behavior. Substance use in adolescence is often the result of a combination of biological predisposition for substance use, onset, progression, unaddressed, or suboptimally treated mental health problems, and psychosocial factors, such as association with drug-using peers, inadequate parental supervision, community factors, including low school community connectedness.

SUMMARY

Adolescence is an active developmental stage across biological, psychological, and social domains. The biological hallmark of adolescence puberty is initiated by the increase in gonadal hormone secretion, leading to the development of secondary sexual characteristics and the capability to procreate. The cognitive hallmark of adolescence is the capability to think abstractly. The psychological hallmark of adolescence is the development of identity. During adolescence, social and behavioral changes include increases in reward-seeking and risk-taking behaviors and a shift toward peer groups taking on greater importance.

Adolescents worldwide face challenges within the context of their various societies. The successful navigation of the adolescent period results in attaining the overarching goal of independence and the acquisition of skills necessary to function adaptively as an adult. Central to this is the attainment of Erickson's adolescent psychosocial task of achieving identity, as compared to role confusion within society.

Due to the confluence of biopsychosocial factors, adolescence is a tipping point for the onset of multiple mental health disorders, most notably depression and substance use disorders, which are two disorders of significant public health concern. Even with this, the vast majority of adolescents' transition through their adolescent years to begin young adulthood successfully and without major turbulence.

RESOURCES

1 Casey, B. J., Jones, R. M., & Hare, T. A. (2008). The adolescent brain. *Annals of the New York Academy of Sciences*, 1124, 111–126. https://doi.org/10.1196/annals.1440.010

2 Adolescent Development | Youth.gov

3 https://www.apa.org/pi/families/resources/develop.pdf

4 https://www.nimh.nih.gov/health/publications/the-teen-brain-7-things-to-know

REFERENCES

Abma, J. C., & Martinez, G. M. (2017). Sexual activity and contraceptive use among teenagers in the United States, 2011-2015. *National Health Statistics Report*, *104*, 1–23.

Abreu, A. P., & Kaiser, U. B. (2016). Pubertal development and regulation. *The Lancet Diabetes & Endocrinology*, *4*(3), 254–264. https://doi.org/10.1016/s2213-8587(15)00418-0

Casey, B. J., Getz, S., & Galvan, A. (2008). The adolescent brain. *Developmental review*, *28*(1), 62–77. https://doi.org/10.1016/j.dr.2007.08.003

Collins, W. A., Welsh, D. P., & Furman, W. (2009). Adolescent romantic relationships. *Annual Review of Psychology*, *60*, 631–652.

Fuster, J. M. (2008). *The prefrontal cortex*. Elsevier.

Hale, R. E. Y. (2003). *Textbook of clinical psychiatry* (4th ed.). American Psychiatric Association.

Herron, M. (2019). Deaths: Leading causes for 2017. *National Vital Statistics Report*, *68*(6), 1–77. https://www.cdc.gov/nchs/data/nvsr/nvsr68/nvsr68_06-508.pdf

Levy, S. (2019). *Youth and the opioid epidemic*. Pediatrics. 143 (2) e20182752. Retrieved October 16, 2021.

Martiniuk, A. L. C., Senserrick, T., Lo, S., Williamson, A., Du, W., Grunstein, R. R., Woodward, M., Lozier, N., Stevenson, M., Norton, R., & Ivers, R. Q. (2013). Sleep-deprived young drivers and the risk for crash: The DRIVE Prospective Cohort Study. *JAMA Pediatrics, 167*(7), 647–655. https://doi.org/10.1001/jamapediatrics.2013.1429

Merikangas, K. R., He, J.-P., Burstein, M., Swanson, S. A., Avenevoli, S., Cui, L., Benjet, C., Georgiades, K., & Swendsen, J. (2010). Lifetime prevalence of mental disorders in US adolescents: Results from the National Comorbidity Survey Replication–Adolescent Supplement (NCS-A). *Journal of the American Academy of Child and Adolescent Psychiatry, 49*(10), 980–989. https://doi.org/10.1016/j.jaac.2010.05.017

Miech, R. A., O'Malley, P. M., Johnston, L. D., & Patrick, M. E. (2016). E-cigarettes and the drug use patterns of adolescents. *OUP Academic*. https://doi.org/10.1093/ntr/ntv217.

Patrick, M. E., Kloska, D. D., Terry-McElrath, Y. M., Lee, C. M., O'Malley, P. M., & Johnston, L. D. (2018). Patterns of simultaneous and concurrent alcohol and marijuana use among adolescents. *The American Journal of Drug and Alcohol Abuse, 44*(4), 441–451. https://doi.org/10.1080/00952990.2017.1402335

Short, M. A., & Louca, M. (2015). Sleep deprivation leads to mood deficits in healthy adolescents. *Sleep Medicine, 16*(8), 987–993. https://doi.org/10.1016/j.sleep.2015.03.007

Spear, L. P. (2000). The adolescent brain and age-related behavioral manifestations. *Neuroscience & Biobehavorial Reviews, 24*(4), 417–463. https://doi.org/10.1016/s0149-7634(00)00014-2

Terry-McElrath, Y. M., Maslowsky, J., O'Malley, P. M., Schulenberg, J. E., & Johnston, L. D. (2016). Sleep and substance use among US adolescents, 1991–2014. *American Journal of Health Behavior, 40*(1), 77–91. https://doi.org/10.5993/AJHB.40.1.9

U.S. Department of Health and Human Services. (2019). *The Changing Face of America's Adolescents*. Office of Population Affairs. https://www.hhs.gov/ash/oah/facts-and-stats/changing-face-of-americas-adolescents/index.html#:~:text=Today%2C%20there%20are%20almost%2042,12.9%20percent%20of%20the%20population.&text=As%20the%20U.S.%20population%20ages,smaller%20proportion%20of%20the%20total

CHAPTER 8

Adulthood

Kelly Truong, M.D. and Mark Yurewicz, M.D.

> *"Life ultimately means taking responsibility to find the right answer to its problems and to fulfill the tasks which it constantly sets for each individual. These tasks, and therefore the meaning of life, differ from man to man, and from moment to moment."*
>
> — Viktor E. Frankl

OBJECTIVES

After completing this chapter, students will be able to do the following:

- characterize the three phases of development in adulthood, along with their correlated main Eriksonian tasks
- recognize common biological processes that can affect functioning and development in early and late adulthood
- start to interpret how biological, psychological, and social aspects can mutually impact each other

DEFINITIONS AND KEY CONCEPTS

The word *adult* encompasses a surprising range of meanings and interesting intonations when grouped together. First used as an adjective in the 1500s, and later a noun by 1600s, it was likely derived from the Latin and then French words *alere* or *alescere*, meaning "to nourish" or "to be nourished," used in the form of "to be grown up." Biologically, *adult* further indicates an organism is sexually mature and, thus, indicates sexually explicit material. Mixed with historical judgments of different aspects of sexuality, *adult* carries the negative connotation of vulgarity, lewdness, and obscenity. (Surprisingly, *adulterate* or *adultery* arrived earlier in

English, also from Latin's *adultere*. It already had the connotation of both the current English concepts and derived from *ad-*, meaning "to," and *altere*, meaning "alter").

INTRODUCTION

Legal systems stake definitions to adult with the purpose of identifying those who can fully participate in society with all its rights and responsibilities. In the United States, states retain the right to decide this, known as "the age of majority." Still, it is almost universally defined as 18 years old, since the 26th Amendment guaranteed the right to vote by 18 years old in 1971. Legally, adults can be fully independent in making decisions about their health, finances, housing, employment, and marriage. Adults are also responsible for their actions in a court of law, paying taxes, taking care of their children or dependents, and, in many countries, participating in some military or civic registration or active service.

There are more graded steps into full economic adulthood. You likely have personal nostalgia for at least one of these or can think of a number of tropes in movies or TV covering steps into adulthood. It might start with your first summer or after-school job, the first time you could drive by yourself, the first time you or a friend could buy alcohol or nicotine, or, potentially, the first time renting a car. And, if we are lucky, we will all have some experience with retirement, a profound shift in our social lives and daily routines. Later, we may help younger children or loved ones going through the same steps, either by saving, creating wealth, or teaching others.

For the sake of brevity, we will not dive into all the varieties of cultural definitions of adulthood. The age, trials, and celebrations that mark coming of age and adulthood vary incredibly across cultures and subcultures around the world. And, as in the previous stages of development, the transitions within adulthood do have direct and indirect biological correlates. Though there are no distinct biological markers for the beginning of adulthood like there are in earlier stages of development, human life and experience are shaped and funneled through universal biological processes at some point. Almost all of us will have to manage a chronic condition and face a physical limitation, and eventually, all will experience death. Your familiarity with the pathophysiology behind cognitive development, aging, endocrinology, death, and other issues will flesh out your understanding of the psychosocial experiences of your adult patients.

The duration of human maturation is often underestimated. Beyond childhood and adolescence, individuals continue to develop and mature, even as adults. Adult development refers to changes in multiple domains of functioning, including biological, psychological, social, and cognitive, from the end of adolescence until death. Stages are generally split into three: young (20–40), middle (40–65), and late adulthood (65+), each building on the other to allow for more complexity. Changes in multiple domains may occur at different times or simultaneously and influence one another based on environmental contexts. For example, an individual may experience a traumatic event (e.g., war, disease, or assault) that changes the trajectory and direction of their development by impacting their physical health, access, or ability to engage with their external support systems and their own internal coping skills and resilience. Moreover, as the brain undergoes structural changes with age (both constructive and degenerative), cognition and behavior notably shift.

BIOLOGICAL FACTORS INFLUENCING DEVELOPMENT

Physical maturation in weight and height is mostly complete by early adulthood. The reproductive system, central nervous system, and physical or athletic abilities are already at or near their peak. The body begins the aging process at the end of early adulthood (approximately age 30). Based on a longitudinal study on aging that tracked a group of older persons for 50 years, the most important physiological changes relate to disease susceptibility. Nevertheless, patterns associated with aging can be observed in various organ systems, including cardiovascular, respiratory, renal, and endocrine (Gideon, 2008). Table 8.1 contains a summary of biological development that occurs in adulthood.

TABLE 8.1 Biological Development in Adulthood

System	Changes
Cardiovascular	• Decreased maximal heart rate; cannot exercise as intensely • Decreased pliability of pliable left ventricle; susceptible to heart failure and fluid overload • Increased arterial wall rigidity; more likely to have high blood pressure and atherosclerosis • Decreased responsiveness of autonomic mechanisms; more likely to become hypotensive (i.e., dehydration)
Respiratory	• Stiffening of the chest wall and decreased lung capacity; more susceptible to shortness of breath and severe respiratory distress from infections (e.g., flu and pneumonia)
Renal and urinary	• Reduced ability to concentrate urine in response to acute volume losses (i.e., vomiting and blood loss); more likely to experience acute renal failure and electrolyte imbalances • Reduction in dilution and filtration ability (70% of people over 65); prone to fluid overload and decreased clearance of some drugs • Decreased bladder contractility; increased risk of urinary tract infections • Increased production of urine at night due to changes in secretion rhythm of antidiuretic hormone
Gastrointestinal	• Decreased acid secretion; does not appear to affect digestion • Gastric mucosa thinning, decreased absorption of nutrients, and susceptibility to vitamin deficiency (e.g., B12) • Decreased colonic function; susceptible to constipation
Endocrine	• Growth hormone; decline leads to reduction in lean body mass, increased fat, and thinning of skin and bones • Insulin; increased resistance and hyperglycemia with stress • Parathyroid hormone; increase leads to susceptibility to hypercalcemia • Thyroid; no decline in serum total or free thyroxine but increased thyroxine clearance. Those with hypothyroidism often require a lower starting dose of thyroxine
Musculoskeletal	• Decline in muscle mass of 25% by age 70, albeit this can vary depending on exercise • Decreased bone mass, especially during menopause in women

QUICK POINT

The duration of human maturation is often underestimated. Beyond childhood and adolescence, individuals continue to develop and mature, even as adults. Adult development refers to changes in multiple domains of functioning, including biological, psychological, social, and cognitive from the end of adolescence until death.

QUICK POINT

Brain development continues beyond adolescence until age 25, particularly in the prefrontal cortex. Neuroimaging studies show an increase in cortical white matter through myelination. In contrast, there is reduction in gray matter density postadolescence in frontal and striatal regions from dendritic pruning of unused synapses.

NEUROCOGNITIVE DEVELOPMENT

Brain Structural Changes

Brain development continues beyond adolescence until age 25, particularly in the prefrontal cortex. Neuroimaging studies show an increase in cortical white matter through myelination. In contrast, there is a reduction in gray matter density postadolescence in frontal and striatal regions from dendritic pruning of unused synapses (Arain et al., 2013). The combination of myelination and pruning increases speed and efficiency of informational processing (Hochberg & Konner, 2020). While there is limited data on changes that occur during young and middle adulthood, some studies have shown microstructural changes on diffusion tensor imaging (DTI) that suggest greater decline in white matter integrity than previously thought (Lixia & Ma, 2017). A review exploring brain changes during the human life span indicated that after age 35 there is a 0.2% loss in total brain volume annually. After age 60, total volume loss is over 0.5% per year (Hedman et al., 2012).

Changes occur differently in men and women in various stages of the life span. In one study comparing brain changes in men and women between the ages of 34 to 43, women had a greater total volume reduction and reduction on the outer brain surfaces, whereas men had more regional reduction on the inner, midline surfaces (Guo et al., 2016). A large population study of participants between age 65–82 showed greater gray matter atrophy in women than in men, at 0.95% compared to 0.65%, respectively (Crivello et al., 2014). Furthermore, the rate of atrophy does not stay consistent across the life span. Women experience a steep volume reduction at an earlier age in the 50s, then even faster atrophy from 70 to 80. In men, significant volume loss begins at a later age in their 60s, then stays gradual until the 80s (Guo et al., 2016).

Hormonal differences may explain sex differences in brain aging. Reproductive changes are steeper in women than in men during middle age. During perimenopause and menopause, women experience a decline in estrogen levels, which has neuroprotective properties (Bryant et al., 2006).

Cognitive Changes

Cognition is a broad term that encompasses smaller components of intellectual ability, learning, and memory. Intelligence can be further divided into fluid and crystallized intelligence. Fluid intelligence refers to biologically determined abilities, such as spatial orientation, learning, memory, and abstract reasoning. Crystalized intelligence refers to experience and education, which includes verbal comprehension and social judgment. Generally, with age, some components of fluid intelligence decline, whereas crystallized intelligence continues to accumulate. For example, vocabulary, reading, and verbal reasoning may improve with age.

KEY POINT

Fluid intelligence refers to biologically determined abilities, such as spatial orientation, learning, memory, and abstract reasoning. Crystalized intelligence refers to experience and education, which includes verbal comprehension and social judgment. Generally, with age, some components of fluid intelligence decline, whereas crystallized intelligence continues to accumulate.

Executive Functioning and Self-Regulation

Completion of frontal lobe development in the mid-20s allows for the improvement of executive functions in young and middle adulthood. Abstract reasoning—a component of executive functioning—is mostly maintained or may improve with age. A significant decline seems to be associated with a disease process (Gideon, 2008). Working memory (WM), the ability to hold and use information in the moment (i.e., remembering and following a set of instructions), declines in older adults (60+). Working memory requires the combination of attention, short-term memory, processing speed, and problem-solving. Older adults perform more poorly on WM tasks and recruit more brain areas to compensate for deficits (i.e., bilateral versus unilateral activation of the prefrontal cortex [PFC] in older adults; Kirova et al., 2015).

Emotional regulation strengthens in middle adulthood, which can allow for more effective interpersonal interactions and flexibility in use of coping strategies. Older adults perceive themselves as having more control over their emotions and can move out of negative emotional states faster. They may not be as "hot-headed" and may rely less on direct confrontation compared to younger adults (Hay & Diehl, 2011).

Memory

As the brain undergoes structural changes, older adults experience overall decline in informational cognitive processing and memory retrieval. The ability to learn and recall information (declarative memory) worsens with age. Episodic memory involving specific details declines more than semantic memory, which is associated with meaning and conceptual knowledge. For example, older adults may not recall specifics of an event like time and place, but they remember vividly what the event meant to them. Autobiographical memory contains both episodic and semantic components with the latter being more salient to older adults (St. Jacques & Levine, 2007). However, procedural memory, like remembering how to brush one's teeth or riding a bike, largely remains intact.

QUICK POINT

Working memory (WM), the ability to hold and use information in the moment (i.e., remembering and following a set of instructions), declines in older adults (60+). Working memory requires the combination of attention, short-term memory, processing speed, and problem-solving.

Aging and memory are influenced by several factors, such as illness, nutrition, and substance use. Someone with a vitamin B12 or thiamine

> **KEY POINT**
>
> Emotional regulation strengthens in middle adulthood, which can allow for more effective interpersonal interactions and flexibility in use of coping strategies.

> **KEY POINT**
>
> As the brain undergoes structural changes, older adults experience overall decline in informational cognitive processing and memory retrieval. The ability to learn and recall information (declarative memory) worsens with age. Aging and memory are influenced by several factors like illness, nutrition, and substance use.

> **CLINICAL TIP**
>
> Aging and memory are influenced by several factors, such as illness, nutrition, and substance use. Drug and alcohol use can also accelerate memory decline. The presence of psychiatric conditions, such as anxiety and depression, can make effortful memory tasks more difficult.

deficiency will have a significant and faster decline in memory. Many older adults take prescription or over-the-counter medication that can impair memory (e.g., benzodiazepines or anticholinergic medication). Drug and alcohol use can also accelerate memory decline. The presence of psychiatric conditions, such as anxiety and depression can make effortful memory tasks more difficult. Someone with anxiety may find it hard to calm anxious thoughts and focus on the information presented. Furthermore, it is important to differentiate between the normal forgetfulness of aging, mild cognitive impairment (MCI), and dementia—the latter two reflecting a substantial decline in the ability to learn and retain information.

PSYCHOLOGICAL FACTORS INFLUENCING DEVELOPMENT

Multiple psychological factors continue to influence individual development with differing impacts through the various stages of adulthood.

Young Adulthood (Age 20–39)

Young adulthood is when individuals become independent from their caregivers and apply skills they have learned in new social, academic, or professional roles. In most cultures, young adults are perceived as now carrying the full responsibility for their own actions and choices. There are many paths to take for the young adult. Some choose to go directly into the workforce, while others pursue higher education. Some marry and have children quickly, while some wait or perhaps never do either. What they have in common is that they are expected to manage relationships and their own well-being and take on increasing responsibilities for themselves and often others. In this stage, they often worry about their future and how they will support themselves financially and emotionally.

Relationships

This period coincides with Erikson's "intimacy versus isolation" stage of psychosocial development. Young adults face challenges when developing intimate, loving relationships outside of their family members, which may include friendships, work, and romantic relationships. Positive relationships are associated with a sense of well-being, whereas an inability to form close relationships may result in loneliness, low self-esteem, and emotional crises. During this period, people learn how to share a space with a partner, while still developing their identity. As the relationship deepens, conflict will inevitably arise. On one level, two people (either friends or partners) need to compromise when values, goals, or interactional styles differ. Young adults learn a number of strategies to resolve conflicts, while maintaining intimacy. They learn to accept differences with their partners and cope with disappointment.

Additionally, they will hopefully come to forge an identity of a pair or team with different roles and a shared value system. A key ingredient is being able to value the other person more than themselves at times and learning how to maintain self-esteem, while valuing the other person. Successful resolution of this stage allows the person to have a better sense of who they are and what they want in work and love.

KEY POINT

Young, or early, adulthood is when individuals become independent from their caregivers and apply skills they have learned in new social, academic, or professional roles. In most cultures, young adults are perceived as now carrying the full responsibility for their own actions and choices.

Trends in Society

Emerging adulthood is a term defined by the psychologist Jeffrey Jensen Arnett to describe the transition between late adolescence through the 20s. During this period, young adults report uncertainty about their job, identity, and marriage. How the social and psychological processes unfold is influenced by broader social and economic trends (Arnett, 2000). In the 21st century, changes in the economic structure have led to a decreased demand for blue-collar manufacturing jobs. Thus, more people are pursuing higher education to be competitive in the workforce. With a larger number of young adults attending college, the median age for marriage has increased because many want to have stable employment prior to starting a family. In 1950, the median marriage age was 20 for women and 22 for men, and it is 28 and 30, respectively, in 2020 (U.S. Census, 2020). Additionally, women now make up more than half of the college-educated labor force with many preferring to build their career before rearing children.

KEY POINT

Early adulthood coincides with Erikson's "intimacy versus isolation" stage of psychosocial development. Young adults face challenges when developing intimate, loving relationships outside of their family members, which may include friendships, work, and romantic relationships.

Middle Adulthood (Age 40–64)

Midlife is the period that coincides with Erikson's "generativity versus stagnation" stage of psychosocial development. It is the longest period in a person's life and involves a variety of developmental tasks. Individuals begin feeling more stable in work and relationships. They are likely to be in long-term committed relationships and learn how to give and receive love. They become interested in guiding the next generation, often through parenting and mentorship. They put energy into contributions they can make for society.

KEY POINT

Middle adulthood, or midlife, is the period that coincides with Erikson's generativity vs. stagnation stage of psychosocial development. It is the longest period in a person's life and involves a variety of developmental tasks.

As midlife progresses, the individual experiences aging and the loss of their parents. As their children grow up and become their own adults, they may become grandparents. By the end of middle adulthood, many are caring for multiple generations. They learn to cope with grief and other painful aspects of life, while holding to their other commitments. As they near late adulthood, they begin to reevaluate their choices and feel a sense of urgency about meaning in their lives.

As the midlife adult reconciles earlier dreams they had for their life with a potentially disappointing reality, they may feel stagnated and experience emotional turmoil. On the other hand, successful development through this stage of life may confer less depression, higher satisfaction, and overall better global cognitive functioning in late life (Malone et al., 2016).

> **KEY POINT**
>
> Late adulthood, the senior or elderly years, is the stage of life that coincides with the Eriksonian psychosocial development "integrity versus despair." In this period, older adults review their life, reflecting on accomplishments and failures.

Late Adulthood (Age 65+)

This stage of life coincides with Erikson's stage psychosocial development "integrity versus despair." In this period, older adults review their life, reflecting on accomplishments and failures. They find meaning in their choices and who they have been. Many seek to guide younger generations through mentorship or grandparenting. When they accept their lives with their successes and failures and derive meaning from their experiences, they achieve wisdom. They feel gratitude and satisfaction for what they have been able to achieve in relationships and work. Acceptance of inevitable death does not mean they lose all productivity in their waning years. Many older adults continue to work at lower intensity, learn new trades, or even continue their education. If a person struggles to find meaning in their lives so far lived, they are prone to despair and hopelessness. These adults may feel unappreciated and isolated from others, putting them at higher risk for late-life depression and suicide.

CASE VIGNETTE: CASEY

Let's track Casey, a cisgendered, heterosexual female with a Caucasian father and White, Hispanic mother. She is not any one real person or patient but an example for us to explore how biological, psychological, and social factors can interact with each other over adulthood.

THE 20S

Casey's young adult years were busy and exciting. She just finished college at the same school her father attended, the first in his family to graduate college. She had less financial debt than her peers and took a job in a neighboring town to her alma mater. Her parents and younger brother were still home, 100 miles away. However, after one successful year into her career, while driving home, she was rear-ended by an oncoming vehicle. Though she had full health insurance, she developed a concussion with residual inattention and irritability, which impacted her work performance enough to invite constructive criticism from her supervisors. Also, she experienced unwanted attention and some gossip around her appearance at this time. She thought this was partly due to her mixed Hispanic ancestry. She was less confident in herself and her identity, given these two factors. It reminded her of being in high school again. She wanted to establish a core set of friends she trusted, and the group that she grew into led her to more frequent outings on the weekend. She started drinking more heavily than her peers and even drinking at home if her friends were busy. She was able to cut back when she got concerned input from her mother and one of her friends who she started to trust.

COMMENTARY

Casey is struggling with a return of the adolescent phase of ego identity versus role confusion at work after biological factors (a concussion) have affected her work performance, along with social factors of apparent microaggressions related to her cultural minority status. Now in a new role as a young adult in the workforce, she is starting to move into the young adult task of intimacy versus isolation by staying in touch and seeking support and connection with close friends and her mother. As a teen, she had separated and distanced herself from her mother, no longer sharing intimate details. Now, as a young adult, she is beginning to seek support from and trust her mother again. Luckily, due to her friend and mother's intervention (by verbal caution) she did not develop a clear pattern of alcohol use disorder. If she had, this could have made her more vulnerable to impulsivity, especially given her age and concussion history. This may have impacted her ability to build trusting, intimate relationships. And, thankfully, her success at building those kinds of relationships helped her halt a problematic pattern of alcohol use.

THE 30S

Casey started dating a friend, and the two married after a couple of years. Both grew up within a couple hundred miles of each other, shared similar backgrounds and values, and it was easy to decide to have children. After a relatively uneventful pregnancy and the birth of her daughter, Emy, Casey developed moderate to severe postpartum depression, which she did not know ran in her extended family. Though her husband was caring and supportive, she struggled to keep up with her friends. This made her appreciate her hus-

(*continued*)

band's support and dedication even more. They did have some distance and tension in their relationship after her sexual drive decreased following treatment with antidepressants, and the two were worried about their finances.

COMMENTARY

The main task of intimacy versus isolation is playing out for Casey with her husband and friends, as the questions "Who can I love?" and "Who is important enough for me to put them first?" play out. Casey was at risk for postpartum depression, given her family history, which, until after she was diagnosed, was unknown to her, but even other endocrine/gynecological states, such as low estrogen states, could put her at risk. Social isolation can be a cause and effect of depression, and pregnancy and young parenthood are enormous changes in psychological identity and social responsibilities. The developmental task of intimacy was in part challenged by a biological effect of her antidepressant treatment and shaped by a myriad of social factors.

THE 40S

Casey found stability again in her life. She started working and found a work community that she trusted and supported her professional growth. She started making long-term goals for her career and life. Her father became ill unexpectedly and passed away. She found herself caught between growing responsibilities for her preteen daughter and helping her mother, who was starting to go through depression again. While spending more time with her own mother, the two fell into old patterns. Casey's mother commented on Casey's appearance, and Casey found herself expecting her mother's love conditional on "enough" effort or good enough outcomes. Now that she had her husband's support, her wisdom, and occasional individual therapy, she wanted to learn how not to recreate the same dynamics with her own daughter, Emy. Her relationship with her husband is still at times strained due to sexual side effects from her antidepressant. Still, the two maintain a close connection around shared values of parenting and other community projects.

COMMENTARY

Casey is transitioning into middle adulthood, addressing generativity versus stagnation. A main concern is how she can make her life count, especially with work and family members.

THE 50S

After a major restructuring in management at work, Casey found herself under a critical, overcontrolling boss. She was given new assignments, losing opportunities as team leader, and, instead, working alone without any mentoring responsibilities. She again found herself doubting her competence, which was reminiscent of her struggles at work in her 20s. She eventually fell back into a depressed state, almost as significant as the postpartum depression of her 30s. She felt guilty for not being emotionally available for Emy's last year at home before she left for college.

COMMENTARY

Casey continues to address her concern of generativity versus stagnation. At this point she is experiencing a recurrence of depression. This new precipitant—psychosocial factors, primarily at work—highlights the idea of kindling. *Kindling* refers to a process by which an event, especially a neurologic or neuropsychiatric event, is initiated, and its recurrence is made more likely. In Casey's case, the threshold of stress needed to precipitate a depressive episode progressively shrinks with each successive depressive episode.

THE 60S AND 70S

Casey ended her career after one more stable period, making peace with her limited roles but finding meaning in building her financial stability and finding other meaningful volunteer work. She continues to take antidepressants to prevent depression and anxiety. However, the anticholinergic side effects of her antidepressants contributed to a fall. While she still didn't have any serious issues, her fear of a new concussion made Casey hesitant to be physically active with sports and outdoor activities. She had time to spend with her mother in her mother's last two years of life and then was available again to be with her own daughter Emy and supported Emy through a high-risk pregnancy.

COMMENTARY

Casey is starting to be physically more vulnerable to the side effects of medications. While these can directly cause medical complications (which, thankfully, Casey did not experience), the difficulty of managing health conditions and the medications meant to treat them can limit people's social lives, activity levels, and psychological confidence. In terms of Erikson's stages, she is navigating ego integrity, finding acceptance and meaning in her life's work and values at work and beyond.

THE 80S AND 90S

Casey and her husband, well into retirement, continue to spend time with her daughter and now a granddaughter. Casey doesn't have the experience to keep up with the current workforce anymore and is more likely to feel lonely, bored, and anhedonic during the longer stretches between visits from family. Now that Emy is going through motherhood, Casey is more aware of her unresolved frustrations around the time she was depressed in her 50s and emotionally unavailable while Emy was transitioning into adulthood. This conflict doesn't make Casey depressed, but she struggles to make peace with Emy's struggles, which are a reflection that reminds her of her own struggles as a mother.

More significantly, Casey experiences a serious fall for which she is hospitalized. Unfortunately, the doctors were unaware it was actually due to a heart attack until a week later. Casey struggles to remain mentally sharp and physically active with chronic pain medications. Unfortunately, the risk factors underlying her heart attack also led to Casey developing mild vascular dementia. Her family and doctors had a harder time telling whether her inactivity was related to dementia or depression. After her sleep medications were adjusted, she had less sundowning and confusion. And when she entered a memory care living facility, she became more physically active, started eating better, and was less anxious and irritable when her family visited. She was able to spend meaningful time with her extended family.

Sadly, Casey became frailer over time and was unable to travel. When she developed serious pneumonia, Emy took up her role as the medical power of attorney. Casey had made peace with her life and did not want to suffer, so she had requested comfort measures only. A few days later, Casey passed away quietly with her family present.

(*continued*)

COMMENTARY

Casey's cognitive abilities and social life are becoming increasingly shaped by physical aging processes. Being functional and active become less of a given and are usually treatment goals in their own right. Casey demonstrates the additional loss of crystallized intelligence at times, due to dementia or delirium. Also, social factors of gender, and potentially even ethnicity, shaped her health outcomes, highlighting how elder patients, women, and people of color can receive delayed health care, due to their "atypical" signs and symptoms (i.e., ones not classically seen with Caucasian males) or other cultural factors.

SUMMARY

Adulthood hopefully covers the longest developmental period of human life. Thanks to a wide variability in the cultures, social structures, and physical resources available to humanity, it is hard to describe any "right" or "normal" developmental path. Still, there are key core elements; in terms of biological development, adulthood is the completion of cortical development. While loss of biological functioning starts in one's 30s, there are specific types of loss in health and cognitive processes in later life. In terms of psychosocial development, adulthood consists of increasing responsibility for one's actions and choices, along with increasingly complex relationships with oneself and with family and community members. In early adulthood, people seek intimacy, while maintaining self-identity. In middle adulthood, they seek to find meaning and generativity. Lastly, the integrity of their legacy and values is at the core of later adulthood. We then ended with Casey, exploring some possible interactions between biological, psychological, and social factors of development.

RESOURCES

1. https://www.ncbi.nlm.nih.gov/pmc/articles/PMC6970937
2. https://ocw.mit.edu/courses/9-00sc-introduction-to-psychology-fall-2011/pages/adult-development/

REFERENCES

Arain, M., Haque, M., Johal, L., Mathur, P., Nel, W., Rais, A., Sandhu, R., & Sharma, S. (2013). Maturation of the adolescent brain. *Neuropsychiatric Disease and Treatment*, *9*, 449–461. https://doi.org/10.2147/NDT.S39776

Arnett, J. J. (2000). Emerging adulthood: A theory of development from the late teens through the twenties. *American Psychologist*, *55*(5), 469–480.

Bryant, D. N., Sheldahl, L. C., Marriott, L. K., Shapiro, R. A., & Dorsa, D.M. (2006). Multiple pathways transmit neuroprotective effects of gonadal steroids. *Endocrine*, *29*, 199–207.

Crivello, F., Tzourio-Mazoyer, N., Tzourio, C., & Mazoyer, B (2014). Longitudinal assessment of global and regional rate of grey matter atrophy in 1172 healthy older adults: Modulation by sex and age. *PLoS One, 9,* e114478.

Gideon C. A. (2008). Adult development. In S. J. Loue & M. Sajatovic (Eds.), *Encyclopedia of aging and public health.* Springer. https://doi.org/10.1007/978-0-387-33754-8_15

Guo, J. Y., Isohanni, M., Miettunen, J., Jääskeläinen, E., Kiviniemi, V., Nikkinen, J., Remes, J., Huhtaniska, S., Veijola, J., Jones, P. B., & Murray, G. K. (2016). Brain structural changes in women and men during midlife. *Neuroscience letters, 615,* 107–112. https://doi.org/10.1016/j.neulet.2016.01.007

Hay E. L., & Diehl M. (2011). Emotion complexity and emotion regulation across adulthood. *European Journal of Ageing, 8,* 157–168.

Hedman A. M., van Haren N. E., Schnack H. G., Kahn R. S., Hulshoff Pol, H. E. (2012). Human brain changes across the life span: A review of 56 longitudinal magnetic resonance imaging studies. *Human Brain Mapping, 33,* 1987–2002.

Hochberg, Z. E., & Konner, M. (2020). Emerging adulthood, a pre-adult life-history stage. *Frontiers in Endocrinology, 10,* 918. https://doi.org/10.3389/fendo.2019.00918

Kirova, A. M., Bays, R. B., & Lagalwar, S. (2015). Working memory and executive function decline across normal aging, mild cognitive impairment, and Alzheimer's disease. *BioMed Research International, 2015,* 748212. https://doi.org/10.1155/2015/748212

Lixia T., & Ma, L. (2017). Microstructural changes of the human brain from early to mid-adulthood. *Frontiers in Human Neuroscience, 11.* https://doi.org/10.3389/fnhum.2017.00393

Malone, J. C., Liu, S. R., Vaillant, G. E., Rentz, D. M., & Waldinger, R. J. (2016). Midlife Eriksonian psychosocial development: Setting the stage for late-life cognitive and emotional health. *Developmental Psychology, 52*(3), 496–508. https://doi.org/10.1037/a0039875

St. Jacques, P. L., & Levine, B. (2007). Ageing and autobiographical memory for emotional and neutral events. *Memory (Hove, England), 15*(2), 129–144. https://doi.org/10.1080/09658210601119762

U.S. Census Bureau. (2020). *Historical marital status tables, median age at first marriage: 1890 to present.* https://www.census.gov/data/tables/time-series/demo/families/marital.html

CHAPTER 9

Familial Influences on Development

Daniel Vener, M.D. and Sindhu Idicula, M.D.

> *"We are always in a perpetual state of being created and creating ourselves."*
>
> — Daniel J. Siegel

OBJECTIVES

After reading this chapter, students will be able to do the following:

- introduce classical and operant conditioning
- summarize different styles of parenting
- understand the role of parental divorce on development
- discuss sibling relationships and the effect of birth order

CASE VIGNETTE

Alan is a 25-year-old man who comes into your clinic for help with addressing anxiety. Alan first started having feelings of anxiety when he was in high school. He struggles with feelings of inadequacy and insecurity in his relationships. He was raised in a two-parent home with an older sister until he was 10 years old when his parents got divorced. When he was young, his father was a dominating figure who set iron-clad rules about everything from grades to which sports he could play to the clothes he could wear. After his parents' divorce he and his sister lived with his mother, who did her best to be present but struggled to find much time to spend with him because she had to work two jobs. In the 11th grade, Alan started smoking marijuana and drinking alcohol and continues to use both substances regularly to this day. In what ways could the family situation that Alan developed in contribute to his continuing feelings of anxiety?

DEFINITIONS AND KEY CONCEPTS

Family is two or more people related by birth, marriage, or choice, who have strong emotional ties and share responsibilities to each other. *Parenting* refers to the intricacies of raising a child, including the promotion and support of physical, emotional, social, intellectual, and economic wellbeing and development of a child from infancy to adulthood. *Sibling rivalry* is a type of competition or animosity among siblings who may or may not be blood related. *Blended family (also known as a reconstituted family)* refers to a family made up of parents with children from the current and past relationships. *Family disruption* refers to events that cause the rupture of a long-term, committed relationships associated with disruption in the family's structure. These include parental separation, divorce, remarriage, deployment, or death and child removal from the home.

INTRODUCTION

Families serve as a dynamic social system for the continued development of children with impact on later developmental stages. In modern society, the family has taken different forms, including the traditional nuclear family with two adults and at least one child, single-parent families, blended or stepfamilies, grandparent families, childless families, and extended families. Through daily social experiences with parents, siblings, and other family members, the individual acquires beliefs, motives, values, and behavior prioritized by family members.

> **KEY POINT**
>
> *The family* is the first social system for a child. Families serve as a dynamic social system for the continued development of children with impact on later developmental stages.

In childhood, families have a powerful role in shaping how a child experiences and navigates the world through a series of small experiences. The family is often the first social system a child encounters before beginning formal schooling. Children learn from their parents through the rules and demands and by modeling their behavior. Siblings play a significant role by competing for family resources and being peers and mentors. Family disruption can have dramatic effects on children's psyche for years to come.

This chapter highlights essential elements of influence by parents, siblings, and the effect of family disruption. Parents, or the variety of other grown-ups who serve in that role, serve as a powerful model for influencing children as they develop. For brevity, we will refer to all grown-ups who serve in that role (e.g., grandparents, foster parents, other family members, etc.) as parents in this chapter.

THE INFLUENCE OF PARENTING ON DEVELOPMENT

As children start out on their lives, they learn primarily from their parents and families. Much to the chagrin of parents who may want them to do as they say, not as they do, children copy the behaviors of their parents. Through their parents, children also learn what to expect about the world. For example, are days predictable and consistent or unpredictable and chaotic? Do I go to bed at the same time every night, or will it be different day to day? When I am hungry, will I get food, or will I go for several hours being hungry not knowing if or when I will be fed? When I am frustrated, energized, or playful, what are acceptable ways of behaving with family members? The behaviors seen and learned may be appropriate or inappropriate to the larger society. However, what has been modelled in childhood is what is seen as accepted behavior, and the same is repeated through later developmental stages, until alternative behaviors are modelled, taught, or learned to influence change.

Children learn from the adults around them, whether their world and other people are predictable, consistent, and safe. Consistency in a parent's behavior helps a child learn that this parent is predictable. Similarly, consistency in daily aspects of life helps make life more predictable for children. A parent who models consistent and warm behavior teaches that child that the world is predictable and safe and paves the way toward healthy attachment. In the transactional model of development, it is also emphasized that children have a reciprocal effect on parents and that this bidirectional influence shapes the relationship.

Shaping a Child's Behavior Through Parenting

Clinicians in pediatrics, primary care, and psychiatry are often asked about ways to modulate a child's behavior. Some families are proactive and ask questions to help positively influence behavior, some come in after problematic behaviors are a bit more stuck, and some others do not come in at all. This chapter will highlight the theory and clinical practice implications of parenting styles, the use of behavior intervention approaches, and the role of parents in helping children develop skills in emotional regulation and the management of their own behavior.

> **QUICK POINT**
>
> *Parenting* is multidimensional and encompasses several competencies. Parents' awareness, and knowledge, of how to meet their child's physical and emotional needs with adequate synchronicity between parent and child facilitates optimal child development.

Parenting Styles

Parenting is multidimensional and encompasses several competencies. Parents' awareness, and knowledge, of how to meet their child's physical and emotional needs with adequate synchronicity between parent and child facilitates optimal child development. Parenting styles were studied by Baumrind, who noticed two dimensions in various styles. One was of control, or oversight over and expectations of the child's behavior. The other is responsiveness, or warmth of the parent's actions, which includes their cognizance and acceptance of the child's emotional and developmental needs.

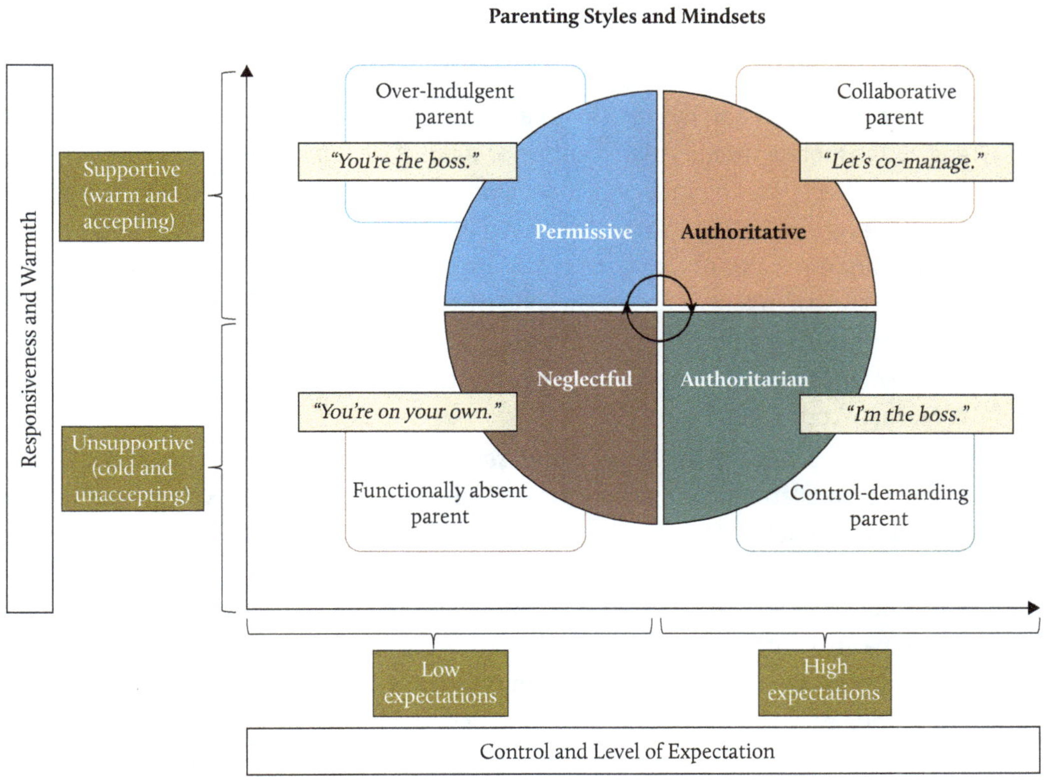

FIGURE 9.1 Parenting styles.

Baumrind found three different parenting styles (Figure 9.1), and a fourth was added by later researchers, as discussed below.

- *Authoritative (high control/high responsiveness)*—An "ideal" parenting strategy, this style encourages development and questioning, while providing a model for how to adjust and conform to societal norms and expectations. They involve their children in decision-making and explain the rationale behind rules, and they are consistent in their enforcement. Authoritative parents accept where a child is at while also setting standards for future conduct. This strategy has the most positive outcomes for children in most metrics, including self-esteem, academic performance, and substance use (Baumrind, 1966).

- *Authoritarian (high control/low responsiveness)*—This style is characterized by a "because I say so" attitude to child rearing. These parents will make rules that they expect their children to follow with a strict obedience. Deviations from parental standards are met with harsh consequences. Unlike authoritative parenting, there is little back-and-forth discussion, which helps children of authoritative parents foster a sense of independence. These strict standards with little heed for children's emotional needs can lead to low self-esteem, average academic performance, and a greater degree of conformity and susceptibility to substance use (Becoña et al., 2012).
- *Permissive (low control/high responsiveness)*—This style of indulgent parenting is an approach in which parents are lax to an extreme, allowing their children free reign and acting more as friends than mentors or support systems. They are involved in their children's lives, but the lack of demands or structure leads their children to become impulsive, poorly self-regulative, and have low self-esteem. To a greater degree than authoritarian and authoritative strategies, children of permissive parents are at risk for substance use as adolescents and beyond (Becoña et al., 2012). In contrast to children of authoritarian parents, those who were raised in a permissive home have a greater feeling of independence, which may be protective against depression (Patock-Peckham & Morgan-Lopez, 2009).
- *Uninvolved or neglectful (low control/low responsiveness)*—This style is characterized by a lack of parental attention to the growth and development of their children. Whether due to being overwhelmed by responsibilities, substance use, or mental illness, parents are unavailable, and there exists an expectation that their children will raise themselves. These parents are often unaware of what their children do, and little effort is made to provide a structure or guidance. Growing up in these homes, children are more likely to be aggressive, they struggle academically, they are more likely to be disciplined (Eckenrode et al., 1993), and are at the highest risk for substance use. These children score the lowest in psychosocial competence and the highest in psychological and behavioral dysfunction (Lamborn et al., 1991).

Behavioral Modification Approaches

When thinking about the behavior of children, behavioral theories are helpful. This includes the ideas of classical and operant conditioning. Classical conditioning is an involuntary and passive process in which the child learns to associate two stimuli together. The typical example was described by Ivan Pavlov. Pavlov rang a bell while feeding his dogs, and over time ringing the bell, even with no food present, led to the salivation response that dogs have with food. Operant conditioning is a voluntary and active learning process in which consequences are used to modulate behavior. These consequences, or *operants*, come in three varieties—neutral, reinforcing, and punishing (Figure 9.2).

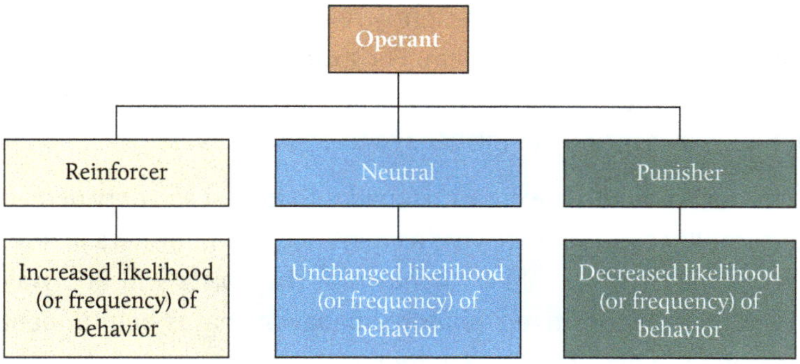

FIGURE 9.2 Operant conditioning.

These operants may be further subdivided into positive and negative types for both reinforcers and punishers. This is further defined with examples in the table below.

TABLE 9.1 Types of Operant Conditioning

Type of operant conditioning	Add/ remove	Stimulus	Effect on behavior	Example
Positive reinforcement	Add	Positive	Enhance Desired	A child receives praise for putting away clothes.
Negative reinforcement	Remove	Aversive	Enhance Desired	A child no longer hears nagging after finishing homework on time.
Positive punishment	Add	Aversive	Deter Undesired	A child gets scolded after hitting a sibling.
Negative punishment	Remove	Positive	Deter Undesired	A child loses screen time after throwing a tantrum when asked to do chores.

MEMORY TIP

Types of Operant Conditioning

- Reinforcements increase behavior *("A plus is a plus; two negatives make a plus.")*
  - Addition of positive reinforcement = ↑ behavior
  - Removal of negative reinforcement = ↑ behavior
- Punishments decrease behavior *("An undesirable thing happens, OR a desirable thing is lost.")*
  - Positive punishment (undesirable thing happens) = ↓behavior
  - Negative punishment (desired thing is lost) = ↓behavior

With this model of shaping behavior, the positive correlates with a stimulus being added, and the negative correlates with a stimulus being taken away. Adding positive stimuli or removing aversive stimuli increases the likelihood of a behavior. Similarly, adding negative stimuli or removing positive stimuli decreases the likelihood of an undesired behavior. Parents often find that they may inadvertently reinforce certain behaviors when they are intending to punish them. For example, a toddler who gets the attention of his father every time he misbehaves, even if that attention is screaming, may continue to misbehave to engage his father.

Behavioral therapists work with families to look at a variety of reactions and to carefully consider their role as reinforcers or punishers in how they shape specific behaviors. Many behavioral therapists will find ways for parents to actively positively reinforce behavior that is helpful behavior, while carefully constructing a plan for tackling problematic behaviors with techniques, such as ignoring, timeouts, losing privileges, etc.

> **CLINICAL TIP**
>
> *Time-ins* can be used to manage problem behaviors. It directs the child to stop the behavior and allows the parent to use the opportunity to facilitate some emotional coaching with the child. The coaching includes understanding where the child is coming from, validating the emotions, and setting firm boundaries around appropriate and inappropriate behavior. Consequences may be employed and are done so in the context of a warm, consistent, and caring relationship. These opportunities throughout childhood allow a child to develop internalized strategies for dealing with emotions and problems in life.

The Role of Parents in Helping Children Learn to Manage Emotions

Time-outs are a strategy that has a behavioral intent—originally being a "time-out from positive reinforcement." Upon misbehaving, the child is removed from the situation and taken away from both fun and the attention of the parent. In studies and in theory, this can be an effective tool when implemented consistently and in the context of a warm and loving parent–child relationship. In real life, it is often used inconsistently without specifying the misbehavior and while the parent is angry. This may lead to a different lesson than intended—that when a child is bad, they will be left alone until the emotion is squashed. Similarly, physical punishment, such as spanking, also has a behavioral intent—adding a painful stimulus should deter the undesired behavior. However, the evidence suggests that corporal punishment is linked to negative outcomes, such as not learning why the behavior was wrong, behaving out of fear in the future, and learning that aggression is an acceptable problem-solving strategy (American Academy of Child and Adolescent Psychiatry Policy Statement on Corporal Punishment, 2017).

> **CLINICAL TIP**
>
> Children can experience intense, and sometimes unexpected, emotions. *Emotion coaching* is a communication strategy that validates emotions, then supports young people to self-regulate and manage their stress responses.

This has led many leaders in mental health to consider the role of parents in helping their children be able to utilize their emotions. A strategy to utilize, instead of walking away from the child, is to join the child in conversation to better understand the situation. This allows the parent to lean into the relationship, understand where their child is coming from, and name and validate the feelings their child is experiencing. While emotions are validated, problematic behaviors are not. For example, a child who hits his brother may hear, "You were really mad at him for taking your toy. It's okay to be mad. It's not okay to hit others. Let's talk about how to handle feeling so mad." This dialogue allows parents to discuss ways of being able to tolerate and manage difficult feelings, helping the child to develop internalized strategies for dealing with emotions and problems in life.

SIBLING RELATIONSHIPS

During childhood, children generally spend more time with siblings than they do with parents. Sibling relationships, or the lack thereof, thus forms a vital part of childhood development. These relationships are highly contextual, based on relative ages of children, parental treatment, childhood experiences, extended family, and their cultures of origin. From as early as the age of 1, children are sensitive to differences in parental treatment. By the age of 3, children understand family rules and can evaluate themselves in relation to their siblings (Dunn, 1988). Children adapt to their circumstances within the family, competing to define who they are as an individual within the family. The psychoanalyst Alfred Adler viewed sibling dynamics and competition over family resources as being central to the developmental process. As children grow, they naturally begin to fill different niches within the family and reduce the sense of competition between one another. Younger children have fewer niches they can fill than their older siblings. Thus, birth order can be highly impactful on determining personalities (Sulloway, 1999). Only children are most like first-born in their temperament; they tend to be ambitious and conform to parental authority. There is no evidence that they are less sociable or experience overindulgence from parents any more than children with siblings do. More recent studies have found no significant differences between birth order, personality scores, or achievement. Thus, it is likely that differences previously attributable to birth order are the sum effect of parenting and the child experiences growing up within their family constellation and not attributable to birth order alone (Lester, 2005; Stannard 2019).

QUICK TIP

Sibling relationships—From as early as the age of 1, children are sensitive to differences in parental treatment. By the age of 3, children understand family rules and can evaluate themselves in relation to their siblings. Sibling rivalry develops naturally, as children compete for resources, toys, and their parent's affection.

Sibling relationships tend to be at their warmest when parents maintain strong relationships with each of their children and when older siblings are encouraged to take on a caretaking role for their younger siblings. Parental conflict, and divorce can have a spillover effect onto children, which can increase emotional distance and hostility (McGuire, 2010).

Sibling rivalry develops naturally, as children compete for resources, toys, and their parent's affection. Sibling rivalries may be exacerbated or ameliorated by several factors, but the role of parent–child relationship is critical. When parents have a more positive relationship with older siblings than with younger, children will rate their sibling relationships more negatively. Generally, as children get older their relationship also tends to sour, as their skill disparities and interests both tend to narrow (Brody, 1994).

FAMILY DISRUPTION

KEY POINT

Family disruption has consequences for all family members, including parents, siblings, and children. Family disruptions include parental separation, divorce, remarriage, deployment, or death and child removal from the home.

Family disruption has consequences for all family members, including parents, siblings, and children. Central to how children perceive and develop through family disruption is how parents introduce the topic to their children and their relationship with and between other family members.

Depending on when in a child's development the time of family disruption is, they may experience different psychological sequelae. Young children may develop separation anxiety, aggression, and sleep problems. Long-term, this can lead to lower self-worth, concerns over their role in causing the disruption, behavior problems, and regression or developmental delays. Middle-schoolers may have conflicted feelings about loyalty, loneliness, and peer-relation difficulties, and in the long-term they may deal with anxiety, unrealistic hopes for reconciliation, and struggle with academics (Mulholland et al., 1991). Adolescents may be angry or depressed. In some cases, family disruption, such as parental divorce, accelerates the adolescent's process of individuation from their parents. In the long term, depending on how the disruption is handled, they are more likely to have substance use issues, relationship problems, and suffer from depression and suicidal ideations (Amato & Keith, 1991; Needle et al., 1990). Families may help children navigate the family disruption, such as divorce, using a few key strategies. Strategies suggested include informing family members, including children, in a timely and developmentally appropriate manner, not discussing faults or blaming any family member(s), clarifying that the disruption is not the fault of any family member(s), and a reassurance that relationships will remain as much as is feasible despite the disruption. Paying attention to children's responses and listening to the questions and concerns that may come up facilitates their processing of the changes headed their way. Sharing that this will be sad and upsetting for everyone and that they can share those feelings with their parents is reassuring to them (American Academy of Child and Adolescent Psychiatry, 2017).

CLINICAL TIP

Strategies to help children navigate family disruption include informing children in a timely and developmentally appropriate manner and not discussing faults or blaming any family member(s). Paying attention to children's responses and listening to the questions and concerns that may come up facilitates their processing of the changes headed their way.

SUMMARY

The family unit is critical for understanding how children begin their life and grow into adulthood. Parent and sibling relationships have a significant impact on the individual's development. Family disruption can influence a child's psychological and behavioral development with sequelae for mental health into their adult years.

COMMENTS ON THE CASE VIGNETTE

Revisiting Alan's case from the beginning of the chapter, we can start to see how the factors discussed may have paved the way for Alan to now be experiencing anxiety and substance use. His father parented with an authoritarian style, leading Alan to conform to the demands of others with a limited capacity to feel he could be an agent of change in his own life. This increases the likelihood of him being anxious about his life and using substances as a way to cope with the distress. The family disruption created a loss of both of his parents. He no longer lives with his father, and now his mother is more occupied at work to help the family survive. These family factors create a perfect storm—a backdrop for Alan to struggle with the issues of anxiety and substance use.

RESOURCES

1 Classical vs Operant Conditioning
https://www.youtube.com/watch?v=PRdCowYEtAg

2 4 Types of Parenting Style
https://www.parentingforbrain.com/4-baumrind-parenting-styles/

REFERENCES

Amato, P. R., & Keith, B. (1991). Parental divorce and the well-being of children: A meta-analysis. *Psychological Bulletin* 110(1).

Amato, P., Loomis, L., & Booth, A. (1995). Parental divorce, marital conflict, and offspring well-being during early adulthood. *Social Forces*, *73*(3), 895-915. https://www.doi.org/10.2307/2580551

American Academy of Child and Adolescent Psychiatry. (2017). *Children and divorce: American academy of child and adolescent psychiatry facts for families*. Retrieved on January 8, 2022, from https://www.aacap.org/AACAP/Families_and_Youth/Facts_for_Families/FFF-Guide/Children-and-Divorce-001.aspx

American Academy of Child and Adolescent Psychiatry. (2012). *Corporal punishment: American academy of child and adolescent psychiatry policy statements*. https://www.aacap.org/aacap/Policy_Statements/2012/Policy_Statement_on_Corporal_Punishment.aspx

Baumrind, D. (1966). Effects of authoritative parental control on child behavior. *Child Development*, *37*(4).

Becoña, E., Martínez, Ú., Calafat, A., Juan, M., Fernández-Hermida, J. R., & Secades-Villa, R. (2012). Parental styles and drug use: A review. *Drugs: Education, Prevention and Policy*, *19*(1), 1–10. https://doi.org/10.3109/09687637.2011.631060

Demo, D. H., & Acock, A. C. (1988). The impact of divorce on children. *Journal of Marriage and Family, 50*(3). http://www.jstor.org/stable/352634

Dunn, J. (1998). *The beginnings of social understanding*. Harvard University Press.

Eckenrode, J., Laird, M., & Doris, J. (1993). School performance and disciplinary problems among abused and neglected children. *Developmental Psychology, 29*(1).

Lamborn, S. D., Mounts, N. S., Steinberg, L., & Dornbusch, S. M. (1991). Patterns of competence and adjustment among adolescents from authoritative, authoritarian, indulgent, and neglectful families. *Child Development*, *62*(5). http://www.jstor.org/stable/1131151http://www.jstor.org/stable/1131151?seq=1&cid=pdf-reference#references_tab_contents

Lester D., & Abdel-Khalek A. (2005). Birth order and personality. *Perceptual and Motor Skills*, *100*(3):882–882. https://www.doi.org/10.2466/pms.100.3.882-882

Mulholland, D. J., Watt, N. F., Philpott, A., & Sarlin, N. (1991). Academic performance in children of divorce: Psychological resilience and vulnerability. *Psychiatry*, *54*(3), 268–280. https://doi.org/10.1080/00332747.1991.11024556

Needle, R. H., Su, S. S., & Doherty, W. J. (1990). Divorce, remarriage, and adolescent substance use: A prospective longitudinal study. *Journal of Marriage and Family*, *52*(1). http://www.jstor.org/stable/352847

Patock-Peckham, J. A., & Morgan-Lopez, A. A. (n.d.). Mediational links among parenting styles, perceptions of parental confidence, self-esteem, and depression on alcohol-related problems in emerging adulthood. *Journal of Studies on Alcohol and Drugs*, *70*(2), 215–226.

Stannard S, Berrington A, Alwan N. (2019). Associations between birth order with mental wellbeing and psychological distress in midlife: Findings from the 1970 British Cohort Study (BCS70). *PLoS One*, *17*; *14*(9): e0222184. https://www.doi.org/10.1371/journal.pone.0222184

Wallerstein, J. S. (1991). The long-term effects of divorce on children: A review. *Journal of the American Academy of Child and Adolescent Psychiatry*, *30*(3), 349–360. https://doi.org/10.1097/00004583-199105000-00001

CHAPTER 10

Attachment[1]

Sohye Kim, Ph.D.; Asna Matin, M.D.; and Sindhu Idicula, M.D.

"The propensity to make strong emotional bonds to particular individuals [is] a basic component of human nature."

— John Bowlby, 1988

OBJECTIVES

At the end of this chapter, students will be able to do the following:

- discuss the historical and scientific advances in the study of attachment
- recognize attachment as the foundation of long-term socioemotional functioning
- discuss factors that contribute to the development of secure attachment and mentalizing
- discuss the concept of intergenerational transmission of attachment and mentalizing and what can break the cycle of insecure attachment and compromised mentalizing

CASE VIGNETTE

Cory is the elder of two children. His parents had a disturbed relationship, which included domestic violence. After his birth, his mother had postpartum depression and was unable to respond to Cory's needs in a consistent manner. His sister was born before he turned 2. Soon after his sister's birth, without any warning, his father abandoned the family. Cory never heard from him again. Corey and his sister were raised by his mom as a single parent. He described his mom as loving and caring. She worked several jobs to make ends meet to provide their needs. It was expected that Cory and his sister were to stay on top of their schoolwork and household chores. Cory made average grades and was active in after-school activities. He felt it did not compare to his sister who made excellent grades.

(*continued*)

1 Readers may also see "Essentials of Human Development" (Chapter 4) and "Infant and Preschool Mental Health" (Chapter 5) for related material.

As a young child, Cory was described as a sensitive child, who would cry easily and took a long time to settle down after a tantrum. Several times his mom had to leave work to pick him up from daycare because he was inconsolable. At school, he was the quiet, shy kid who had a few good friends. He was not prone to fighting or arguing and would often get picked on. As a young adult he felt he got really lucky to be with his girlfriend. He had dated superficially, but this was his first serious girlfriend to whom he felt more deeply emotionally attached. She was different. She was driven to succeed in life. She was a busy college student working to complete her internship, so she would be retained. When apart he would text or call frequently and get upset if she didn't reply right away. He began to question if she was seeing other guys. She wasn't. His incessant calls to his girlfriend became upsetting. She broke off their relationship. Cory was devastated. He cared for his girlfriend and only wanted to be with her. This caused him to decompensate. He became depressed and began therapy. His fears of being abandoned stemmed from his early childhood experiences. He engaged in therapy and has begun the challenging work of uncovering and resolving his attachment problems.

CASE COMMENTARY

Reflecting on attachment is a lot like starting to read a mystery novel in the middle. When a person starts their journey in psychotherapy, they are in the middle of writing their own story. One has to work backward to start to identify attachments with key persons from a young age and make sense of current patterns of attachment. The origin story is also key to writing (or rewriting) a new chapter of earned security. Reflecting on Cory's early childhood, several issues suggest where attachment may have become disrupted. Cory's mother's experience of domestic violence with Cory in utero and onward as well as her struggle with postpartum depression may have compromised her ability to sensitively care for Cory's needs and likely contributed to nonmentalizing interactions with her infant son (see section below on "Intergenerational Transmission of Attachment"). This may have led to an insecure attachment with his mom and possibly even with his sister, whom he felt he did not compare to. Cory's attachment to his father was also disrupted due to the father's departure from the family early in Cory's life. Taken together, these early experiences likely contributed to Cory's "preoccupied" adult attachment that manifested in his anxiety-driving relationship with his girlfriend and his subsequent decompensation after the demise of that relationship. In working with a therapist, Cory can start to reflect, identify, and understand past attachments to take on a more mentalizing stance and practice emotion regulation, while working toward earned security in future attachment relationships. Although Cory cannot change the past, through his work in psychotherapy, he can certainly rewrite the course of his future.

DEFINITIONS AND KEY CONCEPTS

Attachment is the enduring psychological connectedness between human beings. For the infant, attachment refers to the emotional bond between the infant and their caregiver. It is a means by which the infant gets their primary needs for survival and development met. Early attachment goes beyond childhood and becomes the foundation upon which later relationships are built. Like the mooring of a ship by its anchor, emotionally, attachment serves as a stabilizing factor within the turbulence of life. Attachment refers to one's characteristic way of relating to others who are socioemotionally important to them (referred to as *attachment figures*), such as parents, children, and romantic partners. An attachment disorder is a condition that affects an individual's ability to form and maintain stable close relationships, such as with parents, children, and romantic partners.

KEY POINT

Attachment is the enduring psychological connectedness between human beings. Primary attachment occurs during infancy, and this becomes the foundation upon which later relationships are built. Like the mooring of a ship by its anchor, emotionally, attachment serves as a stabilizing factor within the turbulence of life.

INTRODUCTION

Attachment theory offers a life span perspective that highlights the importance of the earliest relational and emotional bond between the child and the caregiver in creating a relational template and strategy for navigating future relationships and the world. The child learns from early relationships how to anticipate and predict how others will respond and how to process difficult emotional experiences. Suppose a young boy had experiences with a caregiver who was consistent, predictable, and kind. He may then expect that others will be consistent, predictable, and kind. On the other hand, if the experiences were erratic, confusing, scary, or even abusive at times, he will come to anticipate that the world is unpredictable, and that he needs to watch out for things that might threaten his safety.

Attachment Theory: Historical Considerations

In developmental psychology, attachment theory is the notion that humans have an inherent need to form close emotional bonds with other humans. This is more evident in infant and caregiver bonds, but also significantly impacts functioning within relationships across a life span.

John Bowlby

John Bowlby, a psychologist, psychiatrist, and psychoanalyst, is considered the father of attachment theory. He noticed that early childhood experiences altered development and postulated that early human connection with attachment figures both facilitated a child's survival and shaped their course of development. He found children seek physical proximity with attachment figures and used signals (crying, clinging, following, smiling, etc.) to elicit a corresponding response from their caregiver. Children used attachment figures as a secure base from which they could explore their environments. Separation, particularly during crucial times, resulted in anxiety and distress (Bowlby, 1969). These attachment behaviors would change over the course of development, and he noticed the pattern below (Gabbard, 2012).

TABLE 10.1 Attachment Behavior Based on Age

Age	Attachment behavior characteristics
0–3 months	Not directed toward specific attachment figures
3–6 months	Directed signals to particular familiar attachment figures
6–12 months	Nuanced and differentiated ways of behaving with different attachment figures, based on previous experience
12+ months	Goal-corrected partnership, where perceived attachment figure's behavior is organized around their goals

Harry Harlow

Harry Harlow was an experimental psychologist whose experiments with macaque monkeys demonstrated that attachment figures (mother monkey) was not only sought for nutritional needs but also for comfort. In one of his experiments, he separated baby monkeys from their mothers and placed them by themselves with only two inanimate mother surrogates. One surrogate was a wire apparatus with milk available. The other was a soft terry cloth monkey with no milk available. Contrary to the popular notion at the time, the baby monkeys spent most of their time on the terry cloth monkey, only briefly visiting the other for food. In frightening situations, the baby monkeys would cling to the terry cloth mother surrogate for comfort, challenging the notion that baby monkeys were only drawn to their mothers for nourishment (Harlow, 1959).

René Spitz

René Spitz was a psychoanalyst in the 1930s, who discovered the effect of maternal deprivation. World War II set the stage for his naturalistic observations, as infants were both orphaned and separated from caregivers due to imprisonment. Spitz noticed that children had significant and patterned reactions to prolonged separation. First, they would grieve and get angry. Over time, they would become progressively more apathetic. If the separation was prolonged for long enough, they would have impacts on their physical development with stunted growth and motor dysfunction, despite having adequate nutrition provided. Some of the children stopped eating and eventually died. He coined the term *anaclitic depression* to describe the social-emotional, physical, and intellectual impairment that can happen when an infant has been separated for a prolonged period from their primary caregiver (Spitz, 1946).

Mary Ainsworth

Mary Ainsworth was a psychologist who devised the "Strange Situation Procedure," a laboratory measure of childhood attachment, which still serves as the gold standard measure in attachment research today. The situation involves children ages 9–18 months, who are present in a simulated laboratory experiment involving their mother, a strange room, a stranger, and a series of three-minute separations and reunions with the mother.

Strange Situation Procedure

1. The mother, baby, and experimenter enter a room unfamiliar to the baby (less than one minute).
2. The experimenter leaves the mother and baby alone.
3. A stranger joins the mother and infant.
4. Separation 1: The mother leaves the baby and stranger alone.
5. Reunion 1: The mother returns, and the stranger leaves.
6. Separation 2: The mother leaves, and the infant is left completely alone.
7. The stranger returns.
8. Reunion 2: The mother returns, and the stranger leaves.

TABLE 10.2 Types of Attachment in the Strange Situation Procedure

	Secure	Resistant	Avoidant
Separation behavior	Distressed when the mother leaves.	Intense distress when the mother leaves.	No sign of distress when the mother leaves.
Behavior with stranger	Avoidant of stranger when alone but friendly when the mother is present.	Avoidant of the stranger—shows fear of the stranger.	The infant is okay with the stranger and plays normally when the stranger is present.
Reunion behavior	Positive and happy when mother returns.	The infant approaches the mother but resists contact and may even push her away.	The infant shows little interest when the mother returns.
Other	Uses the mother as a safe base to explore their environment.	The infant cries more and explores less than the other two types.	The mother and stranger are able to comfort the infant equally well.

Note: Mary Main (described below) later added a fourth category, disorganized, to refer to infants who appear frightened in the presence of their mothers (who were often fear-arousing to their infants) and display a complex array of conflicted behaviors (e.g., crying loudly and suddenly freezing). These infants' "disorganized" behaviors are understood to arise because the caregiver, to whom the infant is hardwired to turn in times of threat, paradoxically also became the source of fear. The disorganized category is strongly associated with later psychopathology.

KEY POINT

The strange situation procedure, developed by Mary Ainsworth, is a measure of childhood attachment, which is often used in attachment research. The original experiment resulted in three categories of attachment—secure, resistant, and avoidant.

QUICK POINT

Attachment is not limited to childhood. Attachment impacts individuals from childhood through adulthood. The adult attachment interview probes lifetime attachment experiences, including potential traumas and losses. Adults manifest secure, preoccupied, dismissive, or unresolved attachment.

The reactions of the baby during the *reunion* with the mother are observed and classified to determine the child's attachment pattern. The following four characteristics were noted: 1) proximity and contact seeking; 2) contact maintenance; 3) proximity and contact avoidance; and 4) resistance to contact and comforting. With these observations, babies were classified into three main categories—secure, resistant, and avoidant (Ainsworth, 1970).

Mary Main

Mary Main, who was a psychology student of Ainsworth, extended this work to adulthood. Main and colleagues developed the adult attachment interview (Main & Goldwyn, 1994; Main, Hesse, & Kaplan, 2005) to systematically assess individual differences in adult attachment. Classifications from the adult attachment interview parallel infant classifications from the strange situation procedure.

Adult Attachment Interview

The adult attachment interview probes lifetime attachment experiences, including potential traumas and losses. It further invites the interviewee to reflect on the meaning and long-term influences of these attachment experiences. Beyond seeking information about the nature of early attachment experiences, the adult attachment interview assesses how the interviewee *currently* thinks and feels about these early experiences and whether they demonstrate *the capacity to freely access, make sense of, and learn from* these important memories. The classifications are determined by the coherence of the interviewee's narrative and quality of their memories and reflections, rather than what happened or did not happen in their life.

TABLE 10.3 Types of Attachment in the Adult Attachment Interview

	Secure-autonomous	Preoccupied	Dismissing	Unresolved
Quality of interview	Coherent, emotionally engaged, and credible	Rambling, overly detailed, and emotionally entangled	Guarded, brief, vague and contradicting memories. Idealization of caregivers is common	Lapses in reasoning during discussion of traumas/losses
Infant attachment classification counterpart	Secure	Ambivalent-resistant	Avoidant	Disorganized

Key Findings in Attachment

Types of Attachment

Adults with *secure* attachment have healthy regard for themselves, can openly share their emotions with others, and are flexible, adaptive, and effective at managing stress. They are comfortable in close relationships and seek out social support when needed. Adults with *preoccupied* attachment tend to vigilantly pursue closeness to others, while also fearing rejection and abandonment. They tend to be easily aroused in times of stress and less able to be soothed. Adults with *dismissing* attachment tend to minimize the importance of close relationships in favor of self-reliance. They tend to dismiss cues of stress and avoid relying on others in times of stress. They may appear calm on the outside, while concurrently showing high physiological arousal. Adults with *unresolved* attachment continue to be influenced by past traumas or losses that have not adequately resolved and carry the highest risk for psychopathology.

CLINICAL TIP

Adults with *secure* attachment have a healthy regard for themselves, can openly share their emotions, and are flexible, adaptive, and effective in managing stress. Adults with *preoccupied* attachment vigilantly pursue closeness to others, while also fearing rejection and abandonment. Adults with *dismissing* attachment tend to minimize close relationships in favor of self-reliance. Adults with *unresolved* attachment continue to be influenced by past traumas or losses that have not adequately resolved and carry the highest risk for psychopathology.

Stability and Change in Attachment

Several longitudinal studies (e.g., *Minnesota Longitudinal Study of Risk and Adaptation* [Sroufe et al., 2005]) have followed infants who completed Ainsworth's strange situation into later childhood, adolescence, and adulthood. These studies demonstrate "impressive continuity and predictable discontinuity" in one's patterns of attachment across the life span (Crowell & Waters, 2005; Main et al., 2005). Studies report positive associations between one's attachment classification in infancy and attachment classification in adulthood. Infants who are securely attached to their primary caregiver (as assessed by the strange situation procedure) are more likely to become adults who are securely attached (as assessed by the adulthood attachment interview), compared to infants who were insecurely attached (Crowell & Waters, 2005; Main et al., 2005). This supports the basic tenets of the attachment theory, suggesting that the earliest attachment relationships serve as some of the most important foundations upon which later relationships are built (Bowlby, 1969/1982).

At the same time, studies observe changes in attachment classifications from infancy to adulthood in the face of significant and meaningful changes in the larger environment (Sroufe et al., 2005), including stressful life events, traumas and losses, social support, and psychotherapy. This demonstrates that attachment patterns are embedded in a broader environmental context and are a result of a cumulative history of interpersonal experiences, which can be modified as one is exposed to new experiences (Allen, 2013).

Intergenerational Transmission of Attachment

A finding that is perhaps as striking as the impressive continuity of attachment from infancy to adulthood is what has been termed the *intergenerational transmission of attachment*. The mother's attachment classification (as assessed by the adult attachment interview) *during pregnancy* predicts her infant's future attachment classification (as assessed by the strange situation procedure) *at age 1* (Fonagy et al., 1991; Iyengar et al., 2014). Simply put, in the absence of intervening factors, attachment patterns can be transmitted from the mother to the infant.

The intergenerational transmission of attachment (Figure 10.1) is mediated by repeated patterns of interactions that mothers provide to their infant during the first year of life. Decades of studies have demonstrated that securely attached mothers are more likely than their insecurely attached counterparts to be sensitive and responsive in their interactions with their infants (Kim et al., 2014). Infants who are consistently exposed to sensitive and responsive social environment are likely to develop confidence that their caregiver will be available and their needs will be met, which is the hallmark of secure attachment in infancy (see Kim, 2015 for a detailed review).

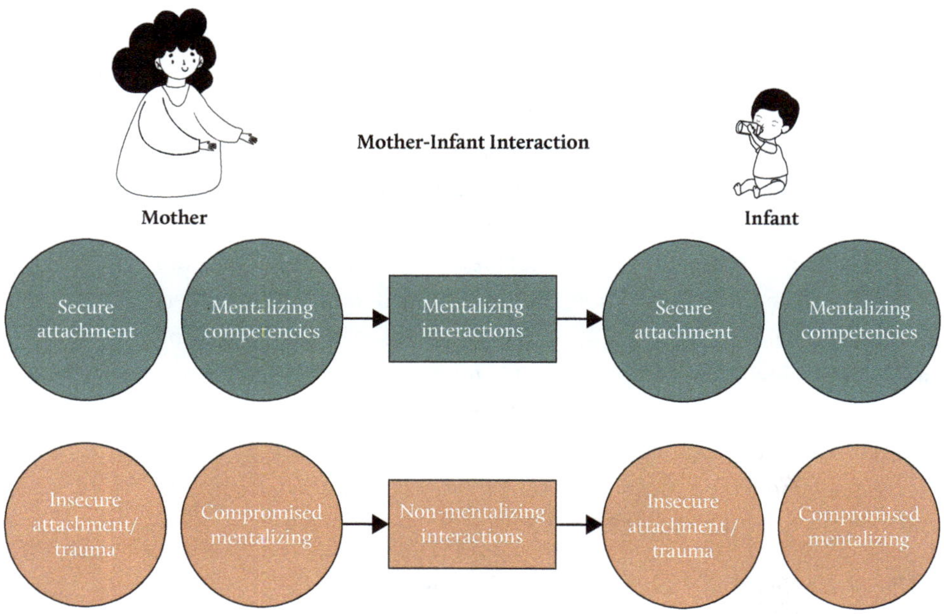

FIGURE 10.1 Intergenerational transmission of attachment and mentalizing. Adapted from Kim, 2015.

Adapted from Sohye Kim, "The Mind in the Making: Developmental and Neurobiological Origins of Mentalizing," Personality Disorders: Theory, Research, and Treatment, vol. 6, no. 4, 2015. Adapted and copyright © by Sohye Kim. Reprinted with permission.
Copyright © 2020 Depositphotos/stockgiu.
Copyright © 2019 Depositphotos/grgroupstock.

CLINICAL IMPLICATIONS

Attachment and Mentalizing

Mentalizing refers to the fundamental human capacity to understand mental states in oneself and others (Allen, 2013). We mentalize when we look beyond a person's behavior and understand mental states (e.g., beliefs, feelings, desires, intentions, and needs) that underlie the behavior. For example, mentalizing occurs when a mother sees her infant frown and recognizes his discomfort or when we speculate about our coworker's heightened stress when witnessing her impatient behaviors. Mentalizing is a distinctly human capacity that allows us to have complex and rich social interactions as part of our daily life. Widespread support exists for the link between attachment security and mentalizing capacity, both in children and adults (Fonagy et al., 1991; Steele et al., 1991). Securely attached individuals are better mentalizers.

KEY POINT

Mentalizing refers to the fundamental human capacity to understand mental states in oneself and others (Allen, 2013). We mentalize when we look beyond a person's behavior and understand mental states (e.g., beliefs, feelings, desires, intentions, and needs) that underlie the behavior.

Mentalizing develops in early attachment relationships. Secure attachment, where the caregiver sensitively recognizes the infant's mental states, is an optimal context for mentalizing to develop. Insecure attachment and attachment trauma, on the other hand, can substantially undermine such development. Note the intergenerational transmission observed here (Kim, 2015). Securely attached mothers are more likely to be capable mentalizers in their interactions with their infants (Kim et al., 2014). These mentalizing interactions they provide foster the development of mentalizing capacity in their children, along with secure attachment.

Attachment and Psychopathology

Secure attachment is a robust protective factor against psychopathology, whereas insecure attachment is a risk factor for overall psychopathology and is over-represented in psychiatric clinical samples. Subtypes of insecure attachment have been differentially associated with different psychiatric diagnoses. Psychiatric diagnoses with internalizing dimensions (e.g., borderline personality disorder) tend to show more associations with preoccupied attachment and/or attachment trauma, whereas diagnoses with externalizing dimensions (e.g., conduct disorder) show an overrepresentation of dismissive attachment (Bakermans-Kranenburg & van IJzendoorn, 2009).

QUICK POINT

Secure attachment is a robust protective factor against psychopathology, whereas insecure attachment is a risk factor for overall psychopathology and is overrepresented in psychiatric clinical samples. Subtypes of insecure attachment have been differentially associated with different psychiatric diagnoses.

The link between attachment and psychopathology is not surprising when considering that individuals first learn to recognize and regulate their emotions in the context of attachment relationships. Children who develop the capacity to skillfully understand mental states in secure attachment relationships are more likely to be capable of adequately managing their emotions. Given this *intricate link between attachment and emotion regulation* (as well as between attachment insecurity and emotion dysregulation), it is important to note that attachment insecurity is associated not only with those clinical presentations in which overt interpersonal dysfunctions are present (e.g., bullying and aggression) but may also play an important role in clinical presentations in which those dysfunctions may seem less obvious (e.g., depression, anxiety, addiction, eating disorders, and perfectionism).

DIAGNOSIS AND TREATMENT

KEY POINT

Reactive attachment disorder (RAD) is a consistent pattern of inhibited and socially withdrawn behavior toward caregivers. It is associated with early social neglect. Children with RAD typically have minimal social responsiveness to others, may not seek or respond to caregiver attempts to comfort them, and often show limited positive affect. They may experience unexplained sadness, fearfulness, and irritability in situations that are nonthreatening.

Impaired attachment results in mental health symptoms, and this manifests across multiple diagnoses in childhood through adulthood. However, the two *DSM-5* diagnoses specific to attachment focus specifically on problems of attachment behaviors in children included within the category of trauma- and stressor-related disorders—reactive attachment disorder (RAD) and disinhibited social engagement disorder (DSED). They both include a diagnostic requirement of social neglect—the absence of adequate caregiving in childhood. While they share a similar cause, RAD expresses itself as an internalizing disorder with depressive symptoms, and DSED brings more disinhibition and externalizing behavior.

RAD consists of an unchanging pattern of inhibited and socially withdrawn behavior toward a caregiver, such as not seeking or responding to comfort. Children with this diagnosis typically have minimal social responsiveness to others, limited positive affect, and may experience unexplained sadness, fearfulness, and irritability in situations that are nonthreatening. The child must have experienced social neglect, which may occur as a result of repeated changes with caregivers or unusual settings (such as an institution) where the child does not get adequate care from caregivers (American Psychiatric Association, 2013). The intervention that has been studied has been the adoption of these children into safe and adequate adoptive families. With consistent caregiving, signs and symptoms of RAD diminish over time (Zeanah & Gleason, 2014).

KEY POINT

Disinhibited social engagement disorder (DSED) is a pattern of disinhibition and overfamiliarity. The child lacks the notion of "stranger danger" and often does not check back with the adult caregiver.

DSED, on the other hand, expresses itself with disinhibition and overfamiliarity. Here, a child may actively approach and interact with unfamiliar adults with little reticence, displaying overly familiar behavior. What is absent is the checking back with the adult caregiver or any qualms about going off with the unfamiliar adult. These behaviors are not the result of impulsivity but the result of social neglect, like RAD (American Psychiatric

Association, 2013). The studied interventions are similar to RAD—providing a safe and adequate adoptive home. The behaviors of DSED may ameliorate with the change in environment; however, some of the symptoms may continue to persist. Further research on interventions may target the continued social cognitive abnormality that may continue in some of these children (Zeanah & Gleason, 2014).

As can be seen in the diagnoses of RAD and DSED, disrupted attachment arises as a critically important factor for children in foster care and adoption. While more research is needed, current understanding is that pre-placement adversity is associated with the child's disrupted attachment, although the development of secure attachment with new caregivers at a stable, long-term placement can facilitate recovery. It is critical that decisions around foster care and adoption are made with the child's attachment in mind.

More broadly, empirically validated attachment-based treatments that focus on parent–child dyads include the Circle of Security (Powell et al., 2014), child–parent psychotherapy (Lieberman et al., 2005), and the Minding the Baby (Sadler et al., 2013). These dyadic interventions have been intensively studied and shown to yield improvements in parent–child attachment relationships.

The most exciting and hopeful finding in the field concerns the capacity for individuals to develop secure attachment later in life (termed *earned security*), regardless of one's early history. Psychotherapy is a well-known predictor of earned security. Although many forms of effective psychotherapy have the potential to yield changes in one's patterns of attachment, specific therapies that have a unique focus on attachment include mentalization-based therapy (Allen, 2013), transference-focused therapy (Kernberg, 1984), or psychodynamic therapy. Much like children who grew up in secure attachment caregiving relationships, adults who later develop secure attachment through psychotherapy learn to skillfully mentalize, grow in their ability to regulate emotions, and capably manage their complex and nuanced socioemotional world.

CLINICAL TIP

Providing a safe and adequate adoptive home with consistent care provided by the caregivers facilitates the relearning of appropriate social interaction and provides the space for successful attachment.

MEMORY TIP

RAD and DSED both occur in children who have experienced early social neglect. However, they are on different ends of the spectrum of social interactivity. While the child with RAD is withdrawn and interacts little, the child with DSED is over interactive.

CLINICAL TIP

Attachment is the enduring psychological connectedness between human beings. The development of secure attachment in childhood is a developmental milestone that is closely associated with the development of mentalizing and emotion regulation.

SUMMARY

Attachment is the enduring psychological connectedness between human beings and is rooted in one's earliest emotional bond with the primary caregiver. The development of secure attachment in infancy is a developmental milestone and is closely associated with the development of mentalizing and emotion regulation. Attachment security provides the foundation upon which one can capably navigate their socioemotional world, while insecure attachment and attachment trauma serve as risk factors for overall psychopathology. Insecure attachment and attachment trauma from early in life (i.e., experiences over which one did not have much control) can be worked through later in life. Psychotherapy is a well-known vehicle for developing secure attachment (i.e., earned security) later in life. For caregivers, this working through is particularly meaningful. Earned security not only allows caregivers to function much more skillfully socioemotionally, but it also enables them to provide the kind of social environment in which their children can develop secure attachment.

RESOURCES

1. Allen, J. G. (2013). *Mentalizing in the development and treatment of attachment trauma*. Karnac Books.
2. Beebe, B., Cohen, P., & Lachmann, F. (2016*). The mother-infant interaction handbook: Origins of attachment*. Norton Professional Books.
3. Cassidy, J. & Shaver, P. (2018). *Handbook of attachment: Theory, research, and clinical applications*. The Guilford Press.
4. Fonagy, P., Gergely, G., Jurist, E., & Target, M. (2005). *Affect regulation, mentalization, and the development of self.* Other Press.
5. Gabbard, G. O., Litowitz, B. E., & Williams, P. (2012). *Textbook of psychoanalysis*. American Psychiatric Publishing.
6. Karen, R. (1998). *Becoming attached: First relationships and how they shape our capacity to love*. Oxford University Press.
7. Kim, S. (2015). The mind in the making: Developmental and neurobiological origins of mentalizing. *Personality Disorders: Theory, Research, and Treatment*, *6*(4), 356–365.
8. Kim, S., & Strathearn, L. (2017). Trauma, mothering, and intergenerational transmission: A synthesis of behavioral and oxytocin research. *The Psychoanalytic Study of the Child*, *70*(1), 200–223.
9. Strathearn, L. (2021). Neurobiology of Attachment. In S. Stahl, M. Lynall, & P. B. Jones (Eds.), *Cambridge textbook of neuroscience for psychiatry*. Cambridge University Press.

REFERENCES

Ainsworth, M. D., & Bell, S. M. (1970). Attachment, exploration, and separation: Illustrated by the behavior of one-year-olds in a strange situation. *Child development*, *41*(1), 49–67.

Allen, J. G. (2013). *Mentalizing in the development and treatment of attachment trauma*. Karnac Books.

Bakermans-Kranenburg, M. J., & van IJzendoorn, M. H. (2009). The first 10,000 adult attachment interviews: Distributions of adult attachment representations in clinical and non-clinical groups. *Attachment and Human Development*, *11*, 223–263.

Bowlby, J. (1969/1982). *Attachment* (2nd ed.). Basic Books.

Bowlby, J. (1969). *Attachment and loss, vol 1: Attachment*. Basic Books.

Crowell, J. A., & Waters E. (2005). Attachment representations, secure-base behavior, and the evolution of adult relationships: The stony brook adult relationship project.

In K. E. Grossman, K. Grossman, & E. Waters (Eds.), *Attachment from infancy to adulthood: The major longitudinal studies*, pp. 223–244. The Guilford Press.

Fonagy, P., Steele, H., & Steele, M. (1991). Maternal representations of attachment during pregnancy predict the organization of infant-mother attachment at one year of age. *Child Development, 62*, 891–905.

Fonagy, P., Steele, M., Steele, H., Moran, G. S., & Higgit, A. C. (1991). The capacity for understanding mental states: The reflective self in parent and child and its significance for security of attachment. *Infant Mental Health Journal, 12*, 201–218.

Gabbard, G. O., Litowitz, B. E., & Williams, P. (2012). *Textbook of psychoanalysis.* American Psychiatric Publishing.

Harlow, Harry F., and Robert R. Zimmermann. (1959). Affectional responses in the infant monkey. *Science, 130*(3373), 421–32. http://www.jstor.org/stable/1758036

Iyengar, U., Kim, S., Martinez, S., Fonagy, P., & Strathearn, L. (2014). Unresolved trauma in mothers: Intergenerational effects and the role of reorganization. *Frontiers in Psychology, 5*(966).

Kernberg, O. F. (1984). *Severe personality disorders: Psychotherapeutic changes.* Yale University Press.

Kim, S. (2015). The mind in the making: Developmental and neurobiological origins of mentalizing. *Personality Disorders: Theory, Research, and Treatment, 6*(4), 356–365.

Kim, S., Fonagy, P., Allen, J., Martinez, S., Iyengar, U., & Strathearn, L. (2014). Mothers who are securely attached in pregnancy show more attuned infant mirroring 7 months postpartum. *Infant Behavior and Development, 37*, 491–504.

Lieberman, A. F., Van Horn, P. J., & Ghosh, I. C. (2005). Toward evidence-based treatment: Child–parent psychotherapy with preschoolers exposed to marital violence. *Journal of the American Academy of Child and Adolescent Psychiatry, 44*, 1241–1248.

Main, M., & Goldwyn, R. (1994). *Adult attachment scoring and classification systems (unpublished scoring manual).* Department of Psychology, University of California, Berkeley.

Main, M., Hesse, E., & Kaplan, N. (2005). Predictability of attachment behavior and representational processes at 1, 6, and 19 years of age. In K. E. Grossman, K. Grossman, & E. Waters (Eds.), *Attachment from infancy to adulthood: The major longitudinal studies* (pp. 245–304). The Guilford Press.

Powell, B., Cooper, G., Hoffman, K., & Marvin, R. (2014). *The Circle of Security intervention. Enhancing attachment in early parent–child relationships*. The Guilford Press.

Slade, A., Holland, M. L., Ordway, M. R., Carlson, E. A., Jeon, S., Close, N., Mayes, L. C., & Sadler, L. S. (2020). Minding the baby: Enhancing parental reflective functioning and infant attachment in an attachment-based interdisciplinary home visiting program. *Development and Psychopathology, 32*, 123–137.

Spitz, R. A. (1946). Anaclitic depression: An inquiry into the genesis of psychiatric conditions in early childhood. *The Psychoanalytic Study of the Child, 2*, 313–342.

Sroufe, L. A., Egeland, B., Carlson, E. A., & Collins, W. A. (2005). *The development of the person: The minnesota study of risk and adaptation from birth to adulthood.* The Guilford Press.

Steele, H., Steele, M., Croft, C., & Fonagy, P. (1999). Infant–mother attachment at one year predicts children's understanding of mixed emotions at six years. *Social Development, 8*, 161–178.

Zeanah, C. H., & Gleason, M. M. (2014). Annual research review: Attachment disorders in early childhood—clinical presentation, causes, correlates, and treatment. *Journal of Child Psychology and Psychiatry, 56*(3), 207–222. https://doi.org/10.1111/jcpp.12347

CHAPTER 11

Neurocognitive Development and Neurodevelopmental Disabilities[1]

Karen D. Evankovich, Ph.D.

> *"From the child of five to myself is but a step. But from the newborn child to the child of five is an appalling distance."*
>
> — Leo Tolstoy

OBJECTIVES

After reading this chapter, students will be able to do the following:

- understand neurocognitive development
- describe intelligence
- discuss intellectual developmental and specific learning disabilities

DEFINITIONS AND KEY CONCEPTS

Neurocognition refers to the processes involved in brain functioning. It involves an understanding of the structure and function of the brain as it relates to thinking, emotions, and behavior. This includes processes such as problem-solving, attention, memory, processing thoughts and emotions, and controlling behavior. These cognitive functions involve various neural pathways that ultimately arise from the brain's substrate at the cellular level.

---

1 Readers may also see "Depression in the Medically Ill" (Chapter 21) and "Adjustment- and Grief-Related Disorders" (Chapter 22) for related material.

INTRODUCTION

It is important for adult and pediatric physicians, from primary care physicians to subspecialists, to acquire a basic understanding of typical brain and cognitive development as well as an appreciation of neurodevelopmental disorders. Approximately 15% of the pediatric population have some form of developmental disability (Boyle et al., 2011), and these children become adults. Depending on the type of developmental disability, patients have increased risk for a wide variety of physical and mental health problems. Thus, as a consequence of neurodevelopmental disabilities, patients may encounter inequities in health care and struggle to adhere to wellness and therapeutic regimens. Moreover, many physicians report feeling as though they are "operating without a road map" when treating patients with neurodevelopmental disorders (Sappok et. al. 2019).

BRAIN DEVELOPMENT

Brain development occurs through a series of complex additive and regressive processes involving both the expression of genes and the impact of environmental experiences (Anderson et al., 2018; Stiles & Jernigan, 2010). Additive growth processes occur in both the gray matter (i.e., neuron proliferation, migration, and differentiation) and white matter (i.e., axonal and dendritic arborization and myelination). Regressive processes in both gray matter (i.e., apoptosis) and white matter (i.e., synaptic pruning) occur later and are modified by environmental influences. These structural changes in the brain continue throughout childhood and adolescence and result in functional differences. Brain regions and functional circuits become specialized for supporting different cognitive, motor, and sensory functions (Stiles & Jernigan, 2010).

KEY POINT

Brain development occurs through a series of complex additive and regressive processes involving both the expression of genes and the impact of environmental experiences.

As depicted in Figure 11.1 (Thompson & Nelson, 2001), the brain begins developing in the third week of gestation and continues throughout much of the life span. The production of neurons begins 42 days after conception and is completed by midgestation (Stiles & Jernigan, 2010). As neurons are produced, they migrate different brain regions, such as the neocortex. Upon reaching the cortex, neurons develop axons and dendrites, forming synapses with other neurons and becoming become committed to specialized functions via this connectivity. Neurons not associated with functional systems may be eliminated by apoptosis—a form of programmed cell death that eliminates cells with unnecessary synaptic connections.

Postnatal brain development appears to follow a set sequence of processes that are largely hierarchical with anterior brain regions being the last to reach maturity (Gogtay et al., 2004). Early development is characterized by rapid synaptogenesis, dendritic development, ongoing myelination, and the development of short cortical-cortical connections and local circuitry. The developing brain becomes more densely packed with the development of axons and arborization of dendrites, so that the surface begins to fold, creating gyri and sulci that serve to increase the surface area of the cortex (Stiles & Jernigan, 2010)

KEY POINT

Rapid dendritic growth and synaptogenesis occur from 8 months to 2 years and reach levels higher than those seen in the adult brain. Synaptogenesis and pruning afford opportunities for environmental experiences to influence brain development.

Rapid dendritic growth and synaptogenesis occur from 8 months to 2 years and reach levels higher than those seen in the adult brain (Walhovd et al., 2014). This period of growth is followed by selective elimination or pruning of synapses. Synaptogenesis and pruning afford opportunities for environmental experiences to influence brain development (Walhvod et al., 2014). Myelination begins about 4 months gestation and peaks in adolescence. Spurts of myelination have been documented at 2 years, 7 to 9 years, and 16 to 19 years (Anderson et al., 2018).

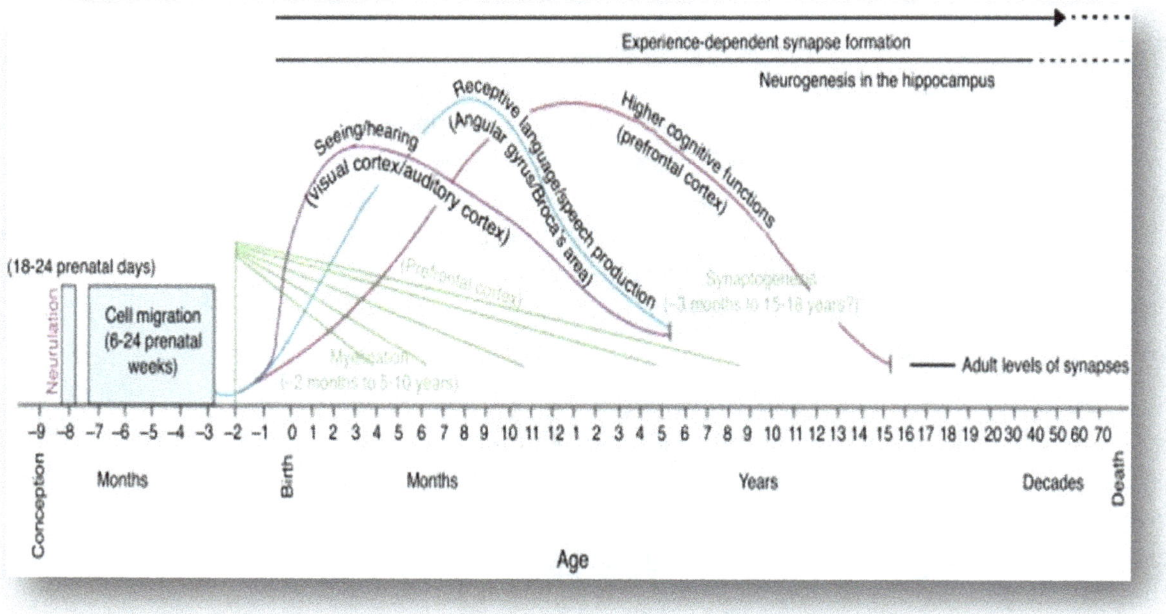

FIGURE 11.1 Early brain development.

R.A. Thompson and C.A. Nelson, "Early Brain Development, from "Developmental science and the media: Early brain development"," American Psychologist, vol. 56, no. 1, p. 8. Copyright © 2001 by American Psychological Association.

COGNITIVE DEVELOPMENT

Associated with the increasing brain maturation, including the ongoing experience-related formation and pruning of synapses and increasing myelination is the parallel development of cognitive skills, as depicted in Figure 11.1 (Thompson & Nelson, 2001; Walhovd et al., 2014). The development of the primary motor and sensory cortex follows vision, hearing, and somatosensory ability as well as fine and gross motor development. The developing senses enable environmental experiences to refine association areas of the brain, which support higher-order cognitive abilities such as receptive and expressive language and visual–spatial ability. Other higher-order cognitive functions reliant on the hippocampus, temporal lobe, and frontal lobe develop simultaneously and persist through the life span. Indeed, the temporal and frontal regions of the brain are last to mature (Gogtay et al., 2004). Higher-order cognitive functions of the temporal lobe, including working and verbal, and visual–spatial memory. Attention and executive functions such as planning and organization, emotional regulation, reasoning, and judgment also begin early in life but are refined with increasing myelination and pruning as a result of interactions with the environment and continue through adolescence and possibly the life span (Baum et al., 2020; Larsen & Luna, 2018; Walhvod et al., 2014). As depicted in Figure 11.2, these higher-order cognitive functions are subserved by localized regions within the different lobes of the brain, including their connections to other brain regions. Sensory and motor functions as well as some higher cortical functions, such as language, verbal and visual spatial memory, and visual–spatial ability are lateralized to the left or right hemisphere.

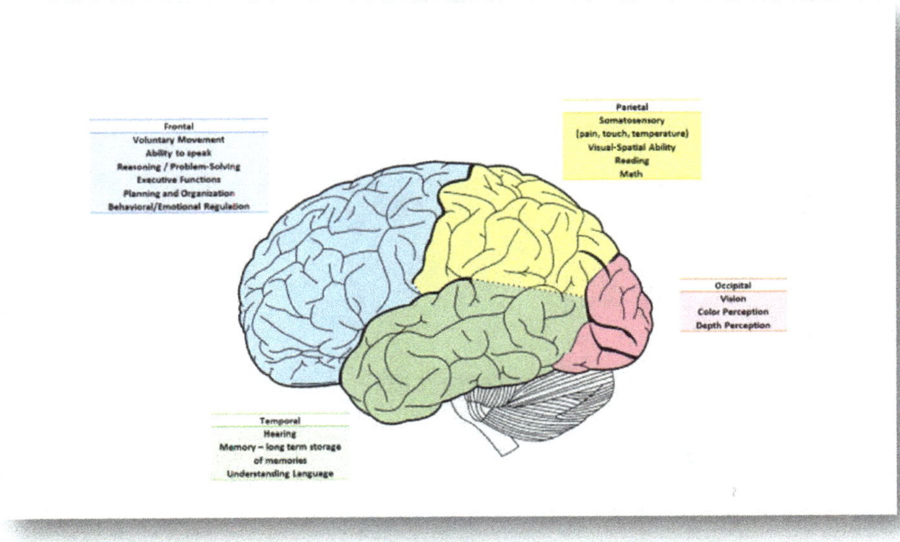

FIGURE 11.2 Brain structure and function

Source: https://commons.wikimedia.org/wiki/File:Lobes_of_the_brain_NL.svg.

MEASUREMENT OF HIGHER-ORDER COGNITIVE FUNCTIONS

Higher-order cognitive functions are measured with individually administered, standardized, norm-referenced tests. Indeed, fields such as neuropsychology, educational psychology, and speech and language pathology are dedicated to the assessment of cognitive functions, as are a variety of test publishing companies. Tests have been developed and standardized to assess discrete cognitive functions, ranging from all aspects of receptive and expressive language to working memory and verbal and visual-spatial memory to processing speed, attention, and executing functions. Arguably, however, the most well-known measure of cognitive functioning is the intelligence or IQ test, which measures a cross section of these skills.

KEY POINT

Intelligence is theorized to be a set of multifaceted, hierarchically organized higher-order cognitive abilities. Intelligence tests are developed to measure these abilities. Discrete cognitive abilities typically include fluid reasoning, verbal comprehension and expression, visual-spatial ability, working memory, and processing speed.

Current views of intelligence, such as the Cattell–Horn–Carrol theory of intelligence depicted in the Figure 11.3, assert that intelligence is not a unitary construct (Schneider & McGrew, 2012, 2018). Rather, intelligence is theorized to be a set of multifaceted, hierarchically organized higher-order cognitive abilities. Intelligence tests are developed to measure these abilities. Discrete cognitive abilities typically include fluid reasoning, verbal comprehension and expression, visual-spatial ability, working memory, and processing speed.

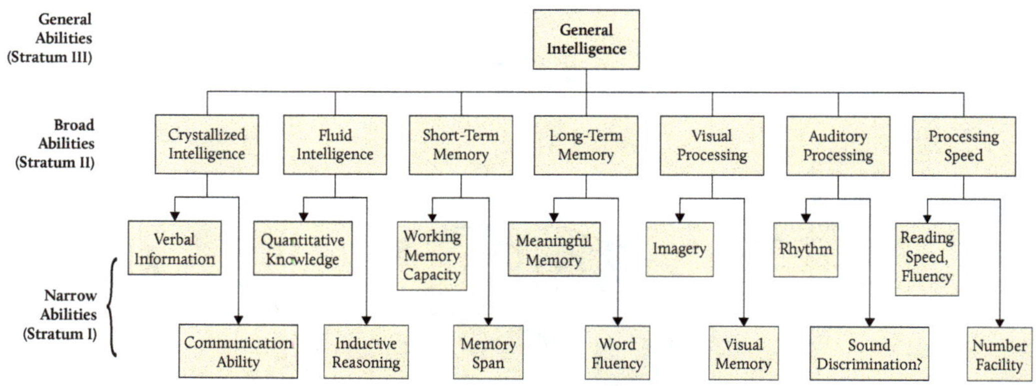

FIGURE 11.3 Cattell–Horn–Carol model of intelligence (as depicted in Scheider & McGrew, 2012).

Adapted from W. Joel Scheider and Kevin S. McGrew, Contemporary Intellectual Assessment: Theories, Tests, and Issues; ed. Dawn P. Flanagan and Erin M. McDonough. Copyright © 2018 by Guilford Press.

Individually administered, standardized, norm-referenced measures of cognitive functions compare an individual's performance on that test to a reference group, typically of other individuals the same age. This comparison is represented by a standard score with a mean of 100 and a standard deviation of 15. Measures of adaptive functioning and academic achievement, discussed later in the chapter, are also individually administered, standardized, norm-referenced tests. The bell curve in Figure 11.4 depicts the ranges of standard scores from the extremely low range to the extremely high range with average scores ranging from 90 to 109 on measures of cognitive, academic, or adaptive functioning.

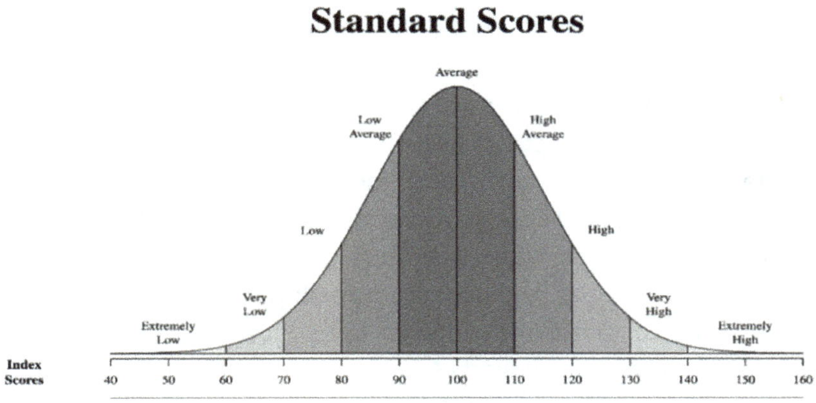

FIGURE 11.4 Standard scores of intelligence quotient.

QUICK POINT

Approximately 15% of the population have some form of developmental disability which, includes intellectual disabilities, specific learning disorders, attention-deficit/hyperactivity disorder, and autism spectrum disorders.

NEURODEVELOPMENTAL DISABILITIES

Neurodevelopmental disabilities result from disruptions in brain and cognitive development due to a multitude of known and yet to be discovered genetic abnormalities, environmental influences, and the convergence of both. Approximately 15% of the population have some form of developmental disability (Boyle et al., 2011), which includes intellectual disabilities, specific learning disorders, attention-deficit/hyperactivity disorder, and autism spectrum disorders. Intellectual disabilities and specific learning disorders will be discussed here, as ADHD and autism are covered in other chapters.

KEY POINT

Neurodevelopmental disabilities result from disruptions in brain and cognitive development due to a multitude of known and yet to be discovered genetic abnormalities, environmental influences, and the convergence of both.

Intellectual Disability

One to 3% of the general population have an intellectual disability (ID). By the fifth edition of *Diagnostic and Statistical Manual* (*DSM-5*; APA, 2013) criteria, these individuals will have deficits in both their intellectual and adaptive functioning. A deficit is defined as two standard deviations below the mean or standard scores less than 70. While the DSM-5 has deemphasized specific IQ scores, an assessment of intellectual functioning remains central to the diagnosis. More important, however, are adaptive skills, which

CLINICAL TIP

Deficits in adaptive functioning necessitate an array of supports for the individual to succeed at school, work, or independent life.

are those skills required to function with age-expected independence in life such as social, communication, and daily living skills. Deficits in adaptive functioning necessitate an array of supports for the individual to succeed at school, work, or independent life. Adaptive functioning is measured using standardized, norm-referenced, culturally appropriate tests.

While people with IDs comprise a small percentage of the population, there is considerable variability in their functioning (APA, 2013; Sappok et al., 2019). As noted in the Table 11.1, the vast majority of individuals will be found to have a mild ID and may be indistinguishable from their peers until elementary school. Individuals with mild ID typically live independently in their communities with supports such as assistance with important decisions and life skills, such as finances, nutrition, shopping, and transportation. Those with moderate ID develop adequate communication skills but need support and supervision. With support and instructions, they can complete most self-care activities and may secure employment in positions requiring limited conceptual ability and social skills. Independent living may be achieved with moderate supports such as those available in group homes. People with severe IDs have very limited communication skills (i.e., words and simple phrases) and require daily assistance for self-care activities and safety supervision. Supported housing is usually necessary. Lastly, those with profound IDs have limited ability to communicate and often have co-occurring sensory or physical limitation. They are dependent on others for all aspects of daily care, typically requiring 24-hour care.

TABLE 11.1 Intellectual Disability: Range of Severity and Associated IQ Scores

Severity	Percent of ID population	Range of IQ scores	Age delays first recognized	Academic skill level
Mild	85	50–55 to 70	5 to 6 years	Fourth to fifth grade
Moderate	10	35 to 55	3 to 5 years	Early elementary
Severe	4	20 to 40	Prior to 3 years	None
Profound	1–2	< 20	Prior to 2 years	None

As depicted in Table 11.2 the most common identified conditions in people with IDs include chromosomal abnormalities (e.g., microdeletions, genetic syndromes), congenital brain malformations, congenital central nervous system infections, inborn errors of metabolism, maternal disease during pregnancy, and in utero exposures to toxins (Karam et al., 2015; Moffat, 2015; Sappok et al. 2019).

TABLE 11.2 Etiologies and Risk Factors for Intellectual Disability

Genetic syndromes	
Large chromosome abnormalities	• Down syndrome
X-linked	• Fragile X
Microdeletions	• Williams syndrome • Prader–Willi Syndrome
Abnormal neuronal migration	• Lissencephaly • Porencephaly
Perinatal factors	• Extreme prematurity • Birth trauma • Breathing problems • Low oxygenation at birth
Childhood CNS infections	• Meningitis • Encephalitis
Infectious diseases (TORCH)	• Toxoplasmosis • Other infections, including syphilis, herpes zoster • Rubella • Cytomegalovirus • Herpes simplex II
Alcohol	• Fetal alcohol syndrome
Toxins	• Lead • Mercury
Degenerative disorders	• Mitochondrial disorders • Inherited metabolic disorders
Trauma	• Severe head injury • Near drowning experience

Relevant to physicians is the finding that individuals with IDs are living longer but experience more age-related health issues. Several reviews from Canada, the United States, Australia, and the United Kingdom have reported that adults with ID are more likely to develop chronic conditions, including congestive heart failure, chronic obstructive pulmonary disease, diabetes, and mental illness than people without ID (Bobbette et al., 2019; Emerson et al., 2012; Havercamp & Scott, 2015; Lunsky et al., 2019). They have increased rates of morbidity and mortality (Sappok et al., 2019). People with ID have expressed dissatisfaction with their health care, particularly communication with their provider and feeling as though their provider does not understand their needs (Brown & Gill, 2009). This, in turn, leads to less frequent primary care visits, increased hospitalizations, and medical errors (Rosenthal, 2008). Even when they do attend to their health, their cognitive limitation may interfere with their ability to understand their diagnosis and treatment plan and interfere with adherence.

Physicians also report difficulty caring for individuals with ID. In a study by Wilkinson et al. (2012), physicians described feeling as though they were "operating without a map," lacked confidence in interacting with patients with IDs, and were unfamiliar with the broad spectrum of patients with ID. They reported being unable to identify potential resources, feeling overwhelmed and out of control about their interactions with their patients, and were anxious about the challenging behaviors patients displayed. Both primary care and ID-focused physicians felt that a curriculum emphasizing how to approach patients would be helpful.

CLINICAL TIP

During well child checkups and pediatric subspecialty visits, parents are asked about their child's development. As early intervention is critical, a history of delayed milestones, learning problems, or the report of a known risk factor warrants a referral.

During well child checkups and pediatric subspecialty visits, parents are asked about their child's development. As early intervention is critical, a history of delayed milestones, learning problems, or the report of a known risk factor warrants a referral, as noted in Table 11.3. Adults with ID often come to medical visits with a family member, who can provide additional history and description of the chief complaint. Nevertheless, to promote communication and a positive patient–physician relationship, the suggestions in Table 11.4 may prove useful.

TABLE 11.3 Sample of Chief Complaints by Age Group

Pediatricians and Pediatric Subspecialists		
Age	**Sign/symptom**	**Next step**
Toddlers and preschool age	• Parent/caregiver report • Delayed milestones • Known risk factor • A sense their child is not developing normally	• Referral to early childhood intervention
School age	• Parent/caregiver report • Child is struggling in school • Social immaturity • Known risk factor • A sense their child is not advancing normally	• Referral for psychoeducational evaluation • Referral for neuropsychological evaluation

TABLE 11.4 Improving Communication With Individuals With Disabilities

	Adult primary care physicians and adult subspecialists
Age	**Steps to improve patient communication**
Adult	• First, speak to the individual with ID and then clarify responses with the family. • Avoid talking to the person as if they are a child. • Use language simple language or a communication aid (e.g., a picture or model). • Ask open questions or change the question to see if the response it the same. • Avoid euphemisms. • Check for understanding by asking them to explain in their own words. • When talking about time, use events the person might understand (e.g., pain began before or after their birthday or what grade they were in). • Do not assume the person will understand the connection between the illness and something they have done or not done or something that has happened to them. Tell them explicitly.

Specific Learning Disorders

According to the *DSM-5*, the prevalence of specific learning disorders, including all academic domains (e.g., reading, reading comprehension, mathematics, and written expression) is approximately 5% to 15% among school-aged children across different languages and cultures (APA, 2013). The prevalence in adults is unknown but is estimated to be approximately 4%. Specific learning disorders are more common in males than females, with ratios ranging from 2:1 to 3:1 and have a high degree of heritability (Elliot & Grigorenko 2014; Shalev et al., 2001). Specific learning disorders are first identified in school but have negative consequences for individuals functioning throughout the life span. These include lower rates of educational attainment, a higher rate of high school dropout, and lower rates of postsecondary education, leading to higher rates of unemployment or underemployment and lower incomes. Thus, it is important to recognize and intervene as early as possible.

KEY POINT

Specific learning disorders are more common in males than females with ratios ranging from 2:1 to 3:1 and have a high degree of heritability. Specific learning disorders are first identified in school but have negative consequences for individuals' functioning throughout the life span.

Specific learning disorders begin during school-aged years but may not become fully manifested until later in life and they persist into adulthood. Specific learning disorders are characterized by difficulty learning or using academic skills in reading (e.g., word level reading, comprehension, and fluency), spelling and written expression, or mathematics (e.g., math calculations and math word problem-solving), despite interventions such as intensive instruction. The affected academic skills are well below age-expected levels and significantly interfere with school functioning

CLINICAL TIP

Specific learning disorders begin during school-aged years but may not become fully manifested until later in life and they persist into adulthood. Specific learning disorders are characterized by difficulty learning or using academic skills in reading (e.g., word-level reading, comprehension, and fluency), spelling and written expression, or mathematics (e.g., math calculations and math word problem-solving), despite interventions, such as intensive instruction.

or occupational performance. The diagnosis is confirmed by individually administered, standardized measures of academic achievement. Diagnostic criteria for a specific learning disorder, however, are met based on the clinical synthesis of assessment data, school reports, and history (e.g., developmental, medical, educational). Neuroimaging and genetic testing are not yet useful for the diagnosis of learning disorders. Of note, the learning disorder cannot be accounted for by an intellectual disability, sensory issue, lack of opportunity, or inadequate instruction.

Knowing when to refer a child or adolescent for a learning disability evaluation is important for the pediatrician and subspecialist. Table 11.5 depicts the typical concerns expressed by parents that may indicate an unrecognized specific learning disability. While adult primary care physicians and subspecialists will not likely need to refer for a learning disability evaluation, learning disabilities persist into adulthood and have the potential to interfere with the individual's ability to understand and adhere to their medical care (Table 11.6).

TABLE 11.5 Supporting Children With Suspected Learning Difficulties

Pediatricians and Pediatric Subspecialists		
Age	**Signs and symptoms**	**Useful step**
School age	• Parent/caregiver report • Inconsistent grades • Memory problems (e.g., knows the information one day and forgets it the next) • Has been retained • Conflict over completing classwork or homework • Family history of learning issues	• Referral for psychoeducational evaluation • Referral for neuropsychological evaluation

TABLE 11.6 Supporting Adults With Suspected Learning Difficulty

Adult Primary Care Physicians and Adult Subspecialists	
Age	**Steps to improve adherence**
Adult	Instruct medical support staff to assist patients and to alert you when patients are observed present with the following: • difficulty or failure to complete pre-visit paperwork • difficulty reading or understanding post-visit summaries • difficulty with adherence to treatment plans • difficulty with treatments requiring complex calculations These are signs the patient may have a learning disability, which could negatively affect their understanding of their medical condition and adherence to your prescribed treatment.

CASE VIGNETTE

A neuropsychological consult was placed for a 15-year-old young woman on an inpatient adolescent medicine unit for eating disorders. She admitted for anorexia but was not following her treatment plan. Her behavior was described as "unusual." She struggled socially on the unit, and the medical team wanted to know if she had an autism spectrum disorder.

The history provided by her mother revealed that the patient was the product of an uncomplicated pregnancy, labor, and delivery. She attained her developmental milestones within the expected timeframes. She was always educated in regular education classes and had just completed the ninth grade. She had a long history of academic problems requiring her to repeat the fourth grade and to attend summer school each year. She had never received special education help or been referred for a psychoeducational evaluation.

During the assessment, the patient was well-mannered, very social, and easily engaged in conversations with the examiner. She displayed a wide range of affect. She was forthright about discussing her difficulties but seemed somewhat less mature for her age. Of note, she was using her personal bedding, which depicted Disney princesses.

The neuropsychologist administered an IQ test, a measure of academic development, and her mother completed a measure of adaptive skills. The scores are depicted in Figure 11.5.

Wechsler Intelligence Scale for Children - V	Standard Score
Full Scale IQ	69
Verbal Comprehension	69
Fluid Reasoning	69
Visual Spatial	71
Working Memory	72
Processing Speed	70

Vineland Adaptive Behavior Scales	Standard Score
Adaptive Behavior Composite	68
Communication	69
Daily Living Skills	65
Socialization	72
Processing Speed	70

(*continued*)

Kaufman Test of Educational Achievement - 3	Standard Score
Reading Composite	72
Letter and Word Recognition	74
Reading Comprehension	69
Math Composite	64
Math Concepts & Applications	66
Math Computation	64
Additional Subtests	
Written Expression	69

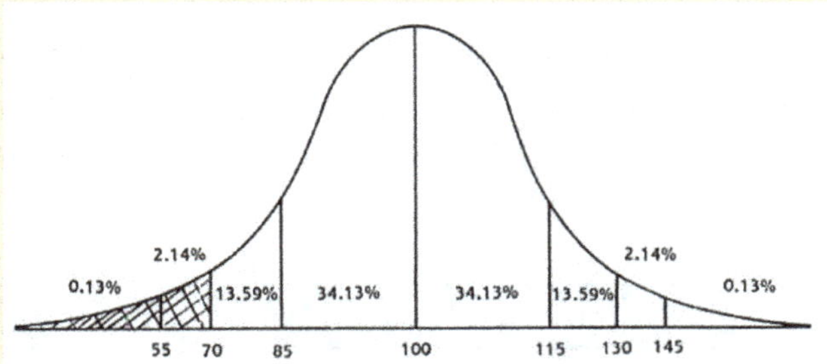

FIGURE 11.5 Patient scores.

The results revealed that she was functioning within the mild range of intellectual ability as both her intelligence (full-scale IQ = 69) and adaptive functioning (adaptive behavior composite = 68) were 2 standard deviations below the mean. Moreover, her reading, math, and written expression were similarly delayed, approximating the fifth-grade level.

As a consequence of her unrecognized mild intellectual disability, she had struggled in school the majority of her life, which had eroded her self-esteem. Because of the ID, she was less mature socially and vulnerable to bullying, which she endured in the eighth and ninth grades. Like many adolescents, she desperately wanted friends and to be accepted. She concluded that her peers would accept her if she were "pretty" and equated beauty with being thin, so she stopped eating. The patient was not following her treatment plan because she simply did not understand why she was in the hospital nor what the unit expected of her with respect to complying with the treatment plan and unit rules.

The neuropsychologist met with her medical team, discussed the findings, and her treatment plan was modified. After the results were discussed with her mother, they were shared with the school district, and she qualified for special education support, which she began to receive her sophomore year.

SUMMARY

Understanding neurodevelopmental disorders is important for pediatric and adult physicians, whether they are primary care practitioners, medical subspecialists, or surgeons. Most, if not all physicians, will be asked to care for a patient with a neurodevelopmental disability at some point in their careers. Depending on the type of developmental disability, patients are at higher risk for chronic physical ailments and mental health problems. The development disability, however, may make it difficult for the patient to understand their health problems and to comprehend and adhere to recommended treatments. Moreover, when physicians do not appreciate neurodevelopmental disabilities and the impact they have on patients' behavior and ability to participate in their care, physicians report feeling overwhelmed and frustrated.

RESOURCES

1 https://www.cdc.gov/ncbddd/developmentaldisabilities/index.html

2 https://www.aacap.org/AACAP/Families_and_Youth/Facts_for_Families/FFF-Guide/Children-with-an-Intellectual-Disability-023.aspx

3 http://www.healthychildren.org/English/health-issues/conditions/developmental-disabilities/Pages/Outlook-for-Children-with-Intellectual-Disabilities.aspx

REFERENCES

American Psychiatric Association. (2013). *Diagnostic and statistical manual of mental disorders* (5th ed.).

Anderson, V., Northam, E., & Wrennall, J. (2018). *Developmental neuropsychology: A clinical approach* (2nd ed.). Routledge.

Baum, G. L., Cui, Z., Roalf, D. R., Rastko, C., Betzel, R. F., Larsen, B., Cieslak, M., Cook, P. A., Xia, C. H., Moore, T. M., Ruparel, K., Oathes, D. J., Alexander-Bloch, A. F., Shinohara, R. T., Raznahan, A., Gur, R. E., Gur, R. C., Bassett, D. S., & Satterthwaite, T. D. Development of structure–function coupling in human brain networks during youth. *bioRxiv*. https://doi.org/10.1101/729004

Bobbette, N., Donnelly, C., Ufholz, L-A., Duggan, J., & Weatherbed, E. (2019). Interprofessional team-based primary health care for adults with intellectual and developmental disabilities: A scoping review protocol. *JBI Database of Systematic Reviews and Implementation Reports*, *17*(12), 2506–2516. https://doi.org/10.11124/JBISRIR-2017-003999

Boyle, C. A., Boulet, S., Schieve, L. A., Cohen, R. A., Blumberg, S. J., Yeargin-Allsopp, M., Visser, S., & Kogan, M. D. (2011). Trends in the prevalence of developmental disabilities in US children, 1997–2008. *Pediatrics*, *127*(6), 1034–1042. https://doi.org/10.1542/peds.2010-2989

Brown, A. A., & Gill, C. J. (2009). New voices in women's health: Perceptions of women with intellectual and developmental disabilities. *Journal of Intellectual and Developmental Disability*, *47*(5), 337–347.

Elliot, J. G., & Grigorenko, E. L. (2014). References. In *The dyslexia debate* (pp. 183–258). Cambridge University Press.

Emerson, E., Baines, S., Allerton, L., & Welch V. (2018). *Health inequalities and people with learning disabilities in the UK.* https://www.basw.co.uk/system/files/resources/basw_14846-4_0.pdf

Gogtay, N., Giedd, J. N., Lusk, L., Hayashi, K. M., Greenstein, D., Vaituzis, A. C., Nugent, T. F., III, Herman, D. H., Clasen, L. S., Toga, A. W., Rapoport, J. L., & Thompson P. M. (2004). Dynamic mapping of human cortical development during childhood through early adulthood. *Proceedings of the National Academy of Sciences, 101*(21), 8174–9. https://doi.org/10.1073/pnas.0402680101

Havercamp, S. M., & Scott, H. M. (2015). National health surveillance of adults with disabilities, adults with intellectual and developmental disabilities, and adults with no disabilities. *Disability and Health Journal, 8*(2), 165–172.

Karam, S. M., Riegel, M., Segal, S. L., Félix, T. M., Barros, A. J. D., Santos, I. S., Matijasevich, A., Giugliani, R., & Black, M.. (2015). Genetic causes of intellectual disability in a birth cohort: A population-based study. *American Journal of Medical Genetics Part A., 167*(6), 1204–1214.

Larsen, B., & Luna, B. (2018). Adolescence as a neurobiological critical period for the development of higher-order cognition. *Neuroscience & Biobehavorial Reviews, 94,* 179–195.

Lunsky, Y., Klein-Geltink, J., & Yates, E. (2019). *Atlas on the primary care of adults with developmental disabilities in Ontario.* https://www.ices.on.ca/Publications/Atlases-and-Reports/2013/Atlas-on-Developmental-Disabilities

Moffat, J. J., Ka, M., Jung, E-M., & Kim, W-Y. (2015). Genes and brain malformations associated with abnormal neuron positioning. *Molecular Brain, 8*(72).

Mürner-Lavanchy, I. M., Koenig, J., Ando, A., Henze, R., Schell, S., Resch, F., Brunner, R., & Kaess, M. (2020). Neuropsychological development in adolescents: Longitudinal associations with white matter microstructure. *Developmental Cognitive Neuroscience, 45,* 100812.

Rosenthal, T. C. (2008). The medical home: Growing evidence to support a new approach to primary care. *Journal of the American Board of Family Medicine, 21*(5), 427–440.

Sappok T., Diefenbacher, A., & Winterholler, M. (2019). The medical care of people with intellectual disability. *Deutsches Ärzteblatt International, 116*(48), 809–816.

Schneider, W. J., & McGrew, K. S. (2012). The Cattell–Horn–Carroll model of intelligence. In D. P. Flanagan & P. L. Harrison (Eds.), *Contemporary intellectual assessment: Theories, tests, and issues* (3rd ed.). Guilford.

Schneider, W. J., & McGrew, K. S. (2018). The Cattel–Horn–Carroll theory of cognitive abilities. In D. P. Flanagan & E. M. McDonough (Eds.), *Contemporary intellectual assessment: Theories, tests, and issues* (4th ed.). Guilford.

Shalev, R. S., Manor, O., Kerem, B., Ayali, M., Badichi, N., Friedlander, Y., & Gross-Tsur, V. (2001). Developmental dyscalculia is a familial learning disability. *Journal of Learning Disabilities, 34*(1), 59–65.

Smith, M. V. A., Adams, D., Carr, C., & Mengoni, S. E. (2019). Do people with intellectual disabilities understand their prescription medication? A scoping review. *Journal of Applied Research in Intellectual Disabilities, 32*(6), 1375–1388.

Stiles, J., & Jernigan, T. L. (2010). The basics of brain development. *Neuropsychology Review, 20*(4), 327–348. https://doi.org/10.1007/s11065-010-9148-4

Thompson, R. A., & Nelson, C. A. (2001). Developmental science and the media: Early brain development. *American Psychologist, 56*(1), 5–15. htttps://doi.org/10.1037/0003-066x.56.1.5

Walhovd, K. B., Tamnes, C. K., & Fjell, A. M. (2014). Brain structural maturation and the foundations of cognitive behavioral development. *Current Opinion in Neurology, 27*(2), 176–184.

Wilkinson, J., Dreyfus, D., Cerreto, M., & Bokhour, B. (2012). "Sometimes I feel overwhelmed": Educational needs of family physicians caring for people with intellectual disability. *Intellectual and Developmental Disabilities, 50*(3), 243–250.

CHAPTER 12

Speech and Language Development[1]

Karol K. Musher, M.A., CCC-SLP and Sindhu Idicula, M.D.

"If you talk to a man in a language he understands, that goes to his head. If you talk to him in his language, that goes to his heart."

— Nelson Mandela

OBJECTIVES

After reading this chapter, students will be able to do the following:

- define components of speech and language
- identify key milestones in the development of speech and language
- recognize early signs of problems with speech and language

CASE VIGNETTE

A 2-and-a-half-year-old boy was brought by his parents for an assessment because of concern about his difficulty speaking. He had recurrent ear infections as a toddler, which had resolved, and his hearing sensitivity, which was recently evaluated, was normal. His father was a late talker, but the family assumed he would start talking by now because of all the conversation and language stimulation in the home and his good comprehension. He was a fairly quiet infant, but he smiled and cooed, played peek-a-boo, waved bye-bye, and appeared to understand general conversation at home and at his Mother's Day Out program. He readily followed one- and two-part commands (e.g., "Get your shoes" or "It's time to go to the park, so get your jacket."). He plays meaningfully with toys and is generally

(continued)

1 Readers may also see "Neurocognitive Development" (Chapter 11) and "Infant and Preschool Mental Health" (Chapter 5) for related material.

good-natured and appropriately interactive with family members and peers but had become increasingly aggressive with siblings and peers (e.g., pulling toys away, biting, and hitting) when trying to "use his words." He used a few words that were fairly well articulated by 14 months, such as "mama" and "dada," and acquired a few others that could be understood by those who know him well if used in context, including "daw"/dog, "baw"/ball "tuhtee"/cookie, "moh"/more, "uh"/up, "doh"/go. A few word combinations were emerging, "doh bye-bye"/go bye-bye and "mama o"/mama home, but were not used consistently and only understood in context. His parents tried getting him to imitate sounds and words, but he was resistant. He liked looking at books and pointed to pictures of animals when named but would not try to imitate names and only sometimes sounds ("oo"/moo, "aaa"/baa). He was not adding words or phrases to his repertoire at any notable rate. He was becoming increasingly frustrated, so his parents sought an evaluation to get help for him. They had been told that the assessment might be traumatic for him, but they were concerned and so proceeded with the appointment.

DEFINITIONS AND KEY CONCEPTS

KEY POINT

Infants quickly learn to differentiate speech from other sound patterns they hear. They pay particular attention to speech and begin to discriminate different rhythms soon after birth.

Speech and language refer to how we say and use words, and both are components of verbal communication (American Speech Language Hearing Association [ASHA], n.d.a.). Speech is the use of articulated sounds to express thoughts and feelings. Articulation is the production of speech sounds using the lips, mouth, and tongue. Fluency is the flow or rhythm of speech production and voice, which involves pitch, loudness, resonance, and vocal quality of utterances. Language refers to the words we use and how we use them. Language involves both comprehension (understanding what others are saying) and expression (expressing our thoughts and feelings). Language is rule governed and generative, meaning that once elements are learned, they are applied to other situations. Components of receptive/expressive language include content (e.g., semantics, vocabulary), form (e.g., syntax or word order, morphology, and grammar), and function (e.g., pragmatics).

It is important to distinguish between speech and language because they are different entities that together facilitate communication. A problem with one or both can interfere with effective communication. Interaction among these components is necessary for effective verbal communication. Verbal communication (speech and language) and nonverbal communication together enable human beings to communicate as we do. The third form of communication—graphic or written language—involves reading, writing, and spelling and will not be included in this discussion.

INTRODUCTION

Speech and language development, a miraculous process we often take for granted, begins immediately after birth. Experts used to teach that a newborn, entirely dependent on caretakers for nourishment and comfort, was not particularly attentive to or was not processing the sounds and visual stimuli around them. We now know they are responding to and learning from these stimuli and that, as early as a few days after birth, infants, especially if appropriately stimulated, begin to develop skills that will enable them to learn to communicate nonverbally, to comprehend and, soon thereafter, to use spoken language.

DEVELOPMENT OF SPEECH AND LANGUAGE

Infants quickly learn to differentiate speech from other sound patterns they hear. They pay particular attention to speech and begin to discriminate different rhythms soon after birth. They not only see and hear, but there is a distinct response to speech from a familiar person or to someone speaking in their native language. They quiet or calm to familiar voices, showing that they have actively been learning from the moment of birth (Vouloumanos & Werker, 2004).

A newborn makes eye contact with their caregiver at close proximity, and by the age of 2–3 months a typically developing child is visibly interacting and communicating nonverbally (ASHA, n.d.b.). Examples include a baby smiling socially, expressing pleasure, and making a conscious effort to connect eyes as a means of engaging.

Other examples of nonverbal communication, such as gesture (e.g., holding out arms to be picked up or shaking head for "no") and facial expressions (e.g., frowns or wide eyes) also begin early; these are used throughout our lives, sometimes to support or supplement oral communication and sometimes stand alone. Considerable refinement will follow, but by 5 months of age, these basic patterns of nonverbal communication are already in place and operating remarkably well.

As a young child communicates nonverbally, their oral communication skills advance rapidly. Infants begin to recognize specific sound patterns (that we call words) and associate these with actions that they then recognize and imitate. Thus, when a parent says and waves "bye-bye," an 8–10-month-old associates that gesture with leaving; the infant may understand so well that she cries, knowing that a loved one is about to disappear. She is likely to wave before she can say "bye-bye" back. By 1 year, she enjoys games, such as peek-a-boo, and recognizes names of common objects. A 2-year-old typically understands the meaning of 1,200 words, points to objects with "show me" questions, and comprehends basic conversation well (ASHA, n.d.c.), and by 3 can follow multipart instructions (ASHA, n.d.d.).

The infant is simultaneously developing expressive language. In just 12 to 24 months, they go from limited expression of discomfort (e.g., crying) and comfort (e.g., cooing) to babbling and producing reflexive sounds that are initially meaningless (e.g., "ma-ma-ma," "ba-ba-ba," and "da-da-da") to combining sounds and syllables into meaningful words (e.g., "mama" and "dada" to refer to "mommy" and "daddy"). Most children say their first meaningful word to communicate feelings and concept by 12 months, and individual words are combined into phrases and sentences using a set of grammatic rules governed by the child's native language by 18 to 24 months. The sounds in words may, at first, not be articulated precisely (e.g., "baw" for ball, "too" for shoe, and "peez" for please), and the grammar or syntax may not be correct (e.g., "daddy car," "go mommy bye-bye," and "mine book"), but in a typically developing child, these aspects of speech sound production and oral language are rapidly refined to conventional forms. At 2, the toddler refers to themself by name, forms some plurals by adding *s* (e.g., "books"), and uses 200 words. They are beginning to ask why questions and enjoy naming objects. Note in the case vignette at the beginning that this child was not meeting expressive language milestones (had fewer than expected words for his age) and was also not articulating in a way that was as clear as was expected at this age.

CLINICAL TIP

Children between the ages of 3 and 5 go through periods of "normal dysfluency" when language is rapidly developing and expanding. It is characterized by tension-free, whole word repetitions (e.g., "I see, I see, I see a bird").

By the age of 4 (ASHA, n.d.e.), a child can talk his way in and out of almost everything with some persisting developmental grammatical errors and vocabulary gaps and comprehends a remarkable amount. Children between the ages of 3 and 5 go through periods of "normal dysfluency" when language is rapidly developing and expanding. It is characterized by tension-free, whole-word repetitions (e.g., "I see, I see, I see a bird"). If these disfluencies develop into struggled or tense repetitions or prolongations and result in word blockages, such as "wh-wh-wh-who is it?" or "Shhhhe's here," that raises a concern for stuttering (Guitar & Conture, 2006).

CLINICAL TIP

By 5 years of age children seem to know and use most correct syntactic structures of their native language and have an extensive vocabulary. They can say all speech sounds in words but may distort sounds, such as *s*, *z*, *r*, *v*, *ch*, *sh*, and *th*.

By 5 years of age (ASHA, n.d.f.), children seem to know and use most correct syntactic structures of their native language and have an extensive vocabulary. They can say all speech sounds in words but may distort sounds such as *s*, *z*, *r*, *v*, *ch*, *sh*, and *th* (Smit et al., 1990) and can relate a short story. They are remarkably good communicators! They continually add new words to their vocabulary to reflect new experiences. They have also learned the social components of language, referred to as pragmatics, which is knowing how to use language to effectively communicate (e.g., saying "please" increases the likelihood of getting ice cream, and "thank you" is greatly rewarded). The richer and more extensive their early experiences, the more vocabulary they are likely to acquire. It is these experiences, background knowledge, and speech-language proficiency that lay the foundation for a child's success in learning graphic or written language (e.g., reading, writing, and spelling)—the next stage of communication. Their increasing interest in and ability to name letters, sounds, and numbers corresponds to starting kindergarten, when formal teaching of reading and writing is accelerated.

REQUIREMENTS FOR NORMAL SPEECH AND LANGUAGE DEVELOPMENT

There is a surprisingly complex array of requirements for normal speech and language development (Figure 12.1; Carter & Musher, 2019a). These include innate or internal characteristics, such as intact hearing sensitivity; motor skills; and integrity of the musculature involved in speech production, perception, memory, attention, cognitive ability, emotional status, ability to relate and interact, and general health.

A favorable environment is also essential, and these factors are subject to a much greater degree of control in the child's learning environment. For children to develop fully to their potential, from a very young age they need to be exposed to rich language and learning experiences that include reading; singing; having life experiences, such as visits to the grocery store, zoo, and park; playing board games; and walking around the neighborhood, looking and talking about things they see and hear. These experiences can readily be provided by parents or caregivers. Shared mealtimes and discussion of daily experiences reinforce all these forms of stimulation. Reading stories and nursery rhymes to young children helps them develop skills required for learning to read, imagine, and reason. By replacing many of these human interactions with screens, technology has eroded these skills essential to language development (Munzer et al., 2019). Exposure to a bilingual environment does not impede language development as long as stimulation in each language is good; recent studies have shown that multilingual exposure enhances rather than detracts from it (Cornell University, 2009).

QUICK POINT

For children to develop fully to their potential, from a very young age they need to be exposed to rich language and learning experiences.

Reinforcement is of greatest importance. Beginning with an infant's early sounds (e.g., cooing and babbling), reinforcing with a smile and imitating their sound combinations help them realize they are communicating and enhances the process. This same need for reinforcement continues throughout childhood. Parents should have realistic expectations about their child's language development; we don't expect a 7-month-old to walk, so why should we expect a 2-year-old to have perfect pronunciation or grammar? Excessive expectations can lead to anxiety about communicating, and if expectations are too low, the child may not reach their potential. Health care professionals should encourage parents to talk, talk, talk and read, read, read to their children.

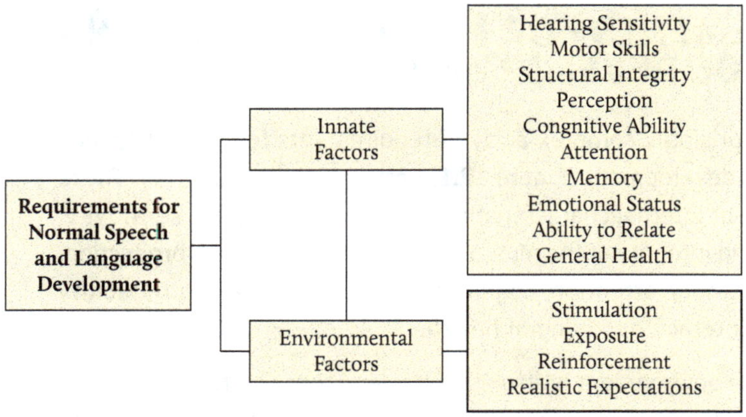

FIGURE 12.1 Requirements for normal speech and language development.

KEY SPEECH AND LANGUAGE MILESTONES

Norms help estimate approximately how a child's skills will develop, and health care professionals need to have some understanding of what is appropriate for children of various ages. It is important to remember that there is a wide range of normal. Part of a clinician's skill is to determine if the child's development falls outside this range. Some key milestones are listed in Table 12.1.

TABLE 12.1 Key Speech and Language Milestones

Age	Nonverbal	Expressive verbal	Receptive verbal
Birth–3 months	• Social smile	• Cooing (pleasure sounds) • Differentiated crying for different needs (e.g., hunger, boredom, or pain)	• Seems to recognize parent's voice and quiets if crying • Quiets or smiles when spoken to
4–6 months		• Chuckles and laughs • Babbles with more consonants	• Responds to changes in tone of voice • Orients and responds to voice • Notices toys that make noise
7–12 months		• Imitates different speech sounds • Uses jargon babbling that sounds like real speech; uses occasional real words with inflection • Uses gesture to communicate (e.g., waves bye-bye)	• May recognize words for common names or objects in environment • Enjoys games like peek-a-boo • Begins to respond to requests, such as "Come here"
10–12 months		• Says "mama" or "dada" and a few other words	• Recognizes names of familiar objects. • Able to respond to simple requests such as, "give it to me," "more juice?"

Age	Nonverbal	Expressive verbal	Receptive verbal
1–2 years		• Combines two words (e.g., "mommy book" and "daddy car") • Uses one- to two-word questions (e.g., "Go bye-bye?") • Vocabulary increases rapidly • Uses expressions (e.g., "oh oh, all gone) • Starts to name pictures in books • Asks what/where/who questions • Uses many different consonant sounds at beginning of words	• Follows simple, one-part directions • Points to pictures in books when named • Points to body parts • Listens to simple stories, songs, and rhymes for a longer time
2 years		• Uses 200+ words	• Comprehends up to 1,200 words • Comprehends basic prepositions (e.g., in, on, or under)
2–3 years		• Understandable to family listeners most of the time • Asks "why" • Has a word for almost everything • Uses two- to three-word sentences • May be dysfluent on words or sounds	• Follows two-part requests
3 years		• Uses up to 900 words	• Up to 3,600 words
3–4 years		• Understandable to strangers most of the time • Talks about what happened during the day; uses four sentences at a time • Can rhyme, use pronouns, plurals, and four-plus word sentences • Uses pronouns like "I," "you," "me," "we," and "they" • Usually talks easily without repeating syllables or words	• Understands words for some colors and shapes • Understands words for family
4–5 years		• Names letters and numbers, tells a short story, and talks in a different way, depending on listener • Keeps a conversation going • Says all speech sounds in words; may misarticulate harder sounds (e.g., *l, s, r, v, z, ch, sh, th)*	• Understands most of what is said at home and school • Understands words for order (e.g., first, next, last) and for time (e.g., yesterday, today, tomorrow) • Follows multipart directions
5–6 years		• Conversation is adult like but still with incorrect formation of irregular past tenses (e.g., "flied"/"flew") and plurals ("mouses"/"mice"). • Subtle development continues, and there is reciprocity between oral and beginning written language skills (e.g., reading and writing) occurs	• Enjoys listening to stories, can hear and understand simple storylines, and can answer simple questions about them.

ABNORMALITIES IN SPEECH AND LANGUAGE

QUICK POINT

The U.S. Centers for Disease Control and Prevention currently estimates that approximately 8% of children have speech–language disorders.

Speech and/or language do not always develop normally. The U.S. Centers for Disease Control and Prevention (CDC) currently estimates that approximately 8% of children have speech–language disorders (Black et al., 2012). Parents often bring their concerns to health care providers who, therefore, must know when to reassure the parent that the child's speech and language is developing normally or when an abnormality may be present and a referral to a speech language pathologist is indicated (Baker & Cantwell, 1987; Feldman, 2019). Having access to developmental norms is helpful for reducing parental anxiety. At the same time, it is important for physicians not to give false reassurance when an abnormality may be present. Children whose speech language development is delayed need to be referred to an appropriate specialist for testing and potential treatment. It cannot be overemphasized that appropriate intervention is the single best predictor of success in managing a speech language disorder, and if one is present, the most common and harmful error is to assure a parent that, "they will just outgrow it."

CLINICAL TIP

Children with significant speech–language disorders may have associated medical or mental health issues and are at high risk for learning disabilities.

Children with significant speech–language disorders may have associated medical or mental health issues and are at high risk for learning disabilities (disorders of written language; Baker & Cantwell, 1987; Langbecker et al., 2020; Lewis et al., 2019). With early intervention, the outcome may be improved and associated frustration, anxiety, and depression, resulting from poor communication be reduced. Table 12.2 lists behaviors that are likely to indicate a need for further evaluation.

TABLE 12.2 Red-Flag Reasons (Causes for Concern) for Referring Young Children for a Speech Language Assessment

Domain	Examples
Changes in pattern of development	Development has slowed down, plateaued, or regressed
Physical abnormalities	Persistent excessive drooling
	Persistent difficulty sucking, chewing, or swallowing
	Child's voice sounds chronically hoarse, nasal, raspy, monotone, or of inappropriate pitch
	Does not react to loud sounds between birth and 3 months (may be a sign of severe hearing impairment)

Domain	Examples
Speech–language abnormalities	Does not respond to name by 12 months
	Does not understand simple instructions by 12–18 months
	Speech consists primarily of vowels
	Does not babble (4–7 months)
	Trouble imitating sounds by 18 months
	No "real" first words by 12–18 months
	No word combinations by 18–24 months
	Parents/caregivers understand less than half a child's speech at 2 years
	Speech difficult for strangers to understand by 3–4 years
	Dysfluencies that are more than tension-free whole word responses (e.g., strained repetitions or prolongations of sounds)
Use of words and language	Child gropes excessively for words; gives associated words or descriptions, such as cutting thing (for knife), it's for your head (for hat)
	Trouble formulating answers, uses vocabulary and sentence structure immature for age, omits word endings, and confuses word order
	Tends to echo or repeat everything they hear with little understanding; may recite TV commercials, read words without comprehension, and lacks give/take of communication
Learning, retention, and memory	Difficulty with rote memory tasks, such as naming basic colors and shapes by 3–3.5 years
	Considerable difficulty learning letter names, sounds, and numbers by the age 5 if they have been exposed
Response to extraneous stimuli	Inconsistent response to sound
	Cannot follow simple directions by 2 years
	Child is excessively distracted by extraneous auditory and visual stimuli and own thoughts; child is impulsive, which adversely affects learning
	Exhibits excessive anxiety with change in routine
	Requires excessive repetition to comprehend simple directions
	Doesn't like being read to
Social concerns	Seems verbally/socially inappropriate even though verbally precocious in some respects; may perseverate on a topic and discuss topic at high level
	Refuses to talk in locations other than home
	Frustrated by communication difficulty; withdraws or acts out (bites, hits, throws toys)
	Teased by peers for "talking funny"
Fine motor concerns	Excessive difficulty with paper/pencil tasks and cutting

Adapted from Carter & Musher, 2019b.

PERNICIOUS MYTHS ABOUT SPEECH OR LANGUAGE DEVELOPMENT

The health care provider must be aware of certain pervasive false myths about speech and language development, some of which are cited. These are rationalizations or explanations that a caregiver may advance as a reason for a child's speech–language delay, but they are *not* valid. For example, common misperceptions of reasons a child does not talk much or clearly are that the child is lazy, older siblings talk for them, they are imitating an older sibling or parent who "talks funny," the parent also did not talk until late, or they are being raised in a bilingual environment. Other examples of improper rationalizations about why a child should not go through testing include they are "too young" or "too old"; testing will make the child self-conscious; or testing is an overreaction, as they will outgrow their speech–language deficits. These rationalizations impede adequate testing and intervention and should be recognized and corrected.

Thinking back through the initial vignette, the boy was evaluated and diagnosed with an expressive language and speech sound (articulation) disorder. He started speech therapy twice weekly for 18 months and made considerable progress. Therapy sessions included direct work with the child and regular interaction with his caregiver, which included recommendations for what should be done at home to reinforce what he did in therapy sessions. He was dismissed when he reached age-appropriate speech and expressive language levels. As his speech and expressive language improved so did his behavior. At dismissal, his speech pathologist recommended that he be reevaluated in one year to check for ongoing progress of speech language development and to monitor his acquisition of early academic skills when he entered kindergarten and elementary school, as children with significant early speech–language disorders are at high risk for having learning disorders.

KEY POINT

Speech and language begin to develop immediately after birth—first with nonverbal communication, followed rapidly by the comprehension of words and use of sounds. Sounds combine to form words, and words combine to express concepts.

SUMMARY

Speech and language begin to develop immediately after birth–first with nonverbal communication, followed rapidly by the comprehension of words and use of sounds. Sounds combine to form words, and words combine to express concepts. Speech is how we say words, and language refers to understanding and using words to express our thoughts and feelings. Subsequently words are expressed by graphic symbols, which includes reading and writing. All this typically occurs over a period of five to six years and continues to develop through life. Strong and ongoing development is dependent on innate and environmental factors. When development does not occur according to norms, the child is best served by referral to an appropriate specialist. Early intervention is of the greatest importance once an abnormality is documented. Communication is a precious gift to be valued and nurtured in our children.

RESOURCES

1. https://www.mayoclinic.org/healthy-lifestyle/infant-and-toddler-health/in-depth/language-development/art-20045163
2. https://www.hopkinsallchildrens.org/Patients-Families/Health-Library/HealthDocNew/Delayed-Speech-or-Language-Development
3. https://www.edc.org/body-work/early-childhood-development-and-learning?gclid=Cj0KCQiA0-6ABhDMARIsAFVdQv-qlQUPLdS5jsUPycc9GGKmbuWqPw_E6W1gExP2XJHdUKv7oC7HJzoaAv4NEALw_wcB

REFERENCES

American Speech Language Hearing Association. (n.d.a.). *What is speech? What is language?* https://www.asha.org/public/speech/development/speech-and-language/

American Speech Language Hearing Association. (n.d.b.). *Developmental milestones: Birth to one year.* https://www.asha.org/public/speech/development/01/

American Speech Language Hearing Association. (n.d.c.). *Developmental milestones: One to two years.* https://www.asha.org/public/speech/development/12/

American Speech Language Hearing Association. (n.d.d.). *Developmental milestones: Two to three years.* https://www.asha.org/public/speech/development/23/

American Speech Language Hearing Association. (n.d.e). *Developmental milestones. Three to four years.* https://www.asha.org/public/speech/development/34/

American Speech Language Hearing Association. (n.d.f). *Developmental milestones. Four to five years.* https://www.asha.org/public/speech/development/45/

Baker, L., & Cantwell, D. P. (1987). A prospective psychiatric follow-up of children with speech/language disorders. *Journal of the American Academy of Child & Adolescent Psychiatry, 26*, 546–553.

Black, L. I., Vahratian, A., & Hoffman, H. J. (2012). Communication disorders and use of intervention services among children aged 3–17 years: United States, 2012. *NCHS Data Brief, 205*, 1–8.

Carter, J., & Musher, K. (2019a). *Etiology of speech and language disorders in children.* Uptodate. https://somepomed.org/articulos/contents/mobipreview.htm?21/11/21695?source=see_link

Carter, J., & Musher, K. (2019b). *Evaluation and treatment of speech and language disorders in children.* Uptodate. https://www.uptodate.com/contents/evaluation-and-treatment-of-speech-and-language-disorders-in-children

Cornell University. (2009). *HD TODAY e-NEWS: Insights from human development's research & outreach.* College of Human Ecology. http://hdtoday.human.cornell.edu/2009/02/12/discovering-child-language-and-cognitive-growth/

Feldman, H. M. (2019). How young children learn language and speech. *Pediatrics in Review, 40*(8), 398–411. https://doi.org/10.1542/pir.2017-0325

Guitar, B., & Conture, E. G. (Eds.). (2006). *The child who stutters: To the pediatrician* (4th ed.). Stuttering Foundation of America.

Langbecker, D., Snoswell, C. L., Smith, A. C., Verboom, J., & Caffery, L. J. (2020). Long-term effects of childhood speech and language disorders: A scoping review. *South African Journal of Childhood Education, 10*(1). http://dx.doi.org/10.4102/sajce.v10i1.801

Lewis, B. A., Freebairn, L., Tag, J., Igo, R. P., Jr., Ciesla, A., Iyengar, S. K., Stein, C. M., & Taylor, H. G. (2019). Differential long-term outcomes for individuals with histories of preschool speech sound disorders. *American Journal of Speech Language Pathology, 28*, 1582–1596.

Munzer, T. G., Miller, A. L., Weeks, H. M., Kaciroti, N., & Radesky J. (2019). Differences in parent–toddler interactions with electronic versus print books. *Pediatrics, 143*(4), e20182012. https://doi.org/10.1542/peds.2018-2012

Smit, A. B., Hand, L., Freilinger, J. J., Bernthal, J. E., & Bird, A. (1990). The Iowa Articulation Norms Project and its Nebraska replication. *Journal of Speech and Hearing Disorders, 55*, 779–798.

Vouloumanos, A., & Werker, J. F. (2004). Tuned to the signal: The privileged status of speech for young infants. *Developmental Science, 7*(3), 270–276. https://doi.org/10.1111/j.1467-7687.2004.00345.x

CHAPTER 13

Psychosexual Development[1]

Josepha Immanuel, M.D.

"The behavior of a human being in sexual matters is often a prototype of the whole of his other modes of reaction in life."

— Sigmund Freud

OBJECTIVES

After completing this chapter, students will be able to do the following:

- define basic terms for gender and psychosexual development
- understand the importance of gender development in healthy sexual development
- explore psychosexual development throughout the life span

CASE VIGNETTE

Tim is a 10-year-old boy, the youngest of three boys. His older brothers are teenagers, play soccer and basketball. Tim often plays basketball and soccer with them and enjoys his time with his brothers. Tim has more girls as friends than boys. At lunch in school, he can invariably be found sitting at the girls' table. His parents are worried. His mother recalls that when Tim was a baby, she had to repeatedly prevent him from pulling at her clothing and touching her upper chest, including while in public. His father recalls that as a toddler, Tim liked to play house with his female cousins whenever they visited. In early elementary school, he got teased because he preferred to play with girls rather than rough and tumble games with boys. He often complimented his female peers' dresses and hairstyles. During a check-up, both parents express concern that at various times, they have seen Tim wearing his mom's heels and some of her jewelry around the home. His parents wonder if his

1 Readers may also see "Essentials of Human Development" (Chapter 4) for related material.

behaviors indicate that Tim is gay. You speak to Tim, who says he is a boy and enjoys playing video games with his friends, basketball, and soccer friends and brothers. Tim tells you that he thinks his mom's clothing is pretty. He finds some girls in his class "cute and fun." How would you handle Tim's parent's question?

At the core of this vignette, Tim's parents are curious if his behaviors are indicators of his sexual orientation and gender identity. It is important to remind his parents that children's sexuality and gender identity is expressed differently based on their developmental stage. Tim's desire to sometimes play with girls or his interest in more stereotypic "feminine" toys is not a signal that he is not masculine or may end up being transgender or gay. Studies have indicated that some begin to question their sexual orientation during adolescence and may engage in same-sex activity. Same-sex activity is also not a clear indicator or homosexuality. Rather than focus on his sexual orientation or gender identity label, advise his parents to redirect their attention to creating a nurturing environment that will allow for healthy sexual and gender development.

DEFINITIONS AND KEY CONCEPTS

The terms used to describe sexual and gender development components have evolved from unidimensional biological fate to a broader paradigm of intersecting factors. In the past, the terms *gender* and *sex* were considered interchangeable. Now, we understand that anatomic sex is based on the medical assessment of genitalia at birth. This assessment tends to be binary, based on the presence of male or female genitalia, with rare cases of individuals with both male and female gonadal tissue. Unlike anatomic sex, gender is a confluence of biology (e.g., chromosomes, hormones, and secondary sexual characteristics) and an individual's sociocultural identity as male, female, or other nonbinary designations. Current gender theory models go beyond binary gender assignments and have introduced the concept of gender diverse, gender queer, gender fluid, and transgender.

QUICK POINT

The terms used to describe sexual and gender development components have evolved from unidimensional biological fate to a broader paradigm of intersecting factors. In the past, the terms ***gender*** and ***sex*** were considered interchangeable. Current gender theory models go beyond binary gender assignments and have introduced the concept of gender diverse, gender queer, gender fluid, and transgender.

INTRODUCTION

Sexual development is a multidimensional construct influenced by genetic, anatomical, physiological, psychological, social, and cultural elements. Healthy sexual development goes beyond sexuality and sexual behavior and includes a recognition of gender, gender identity, gender expression, sexual identity, and sexual orientation. *Gender identity* is an individual's innate

Sexual development is a multidimensional construct influenced by genetic, anatomical, physiological, psychological, social, and cultural elements. Healthy sexual development goes beyond sexuality and sexual behavior and includes recognition of gender, gender identity, gender expression, sexual identity, and sexual orientation.

CLINICAL TIP

The cultural script of "masculinity" and "femininity" is learned in early childhood and manifests in various developmentally age-appropriate behaviors (e.g., play in childhood and sexual roles in adulthood).

awareness of their gender as male, female, nonbinary, or a complete rejection of gender designation. Gender identity should not be confused with sexual identity. *Gender role* is an individual's behaviors, mannerisms and personality traits that are based on their unique social and cultural script of being "masculine" or "feminine." For example, in many cultures, it is considered an appropriate gender role for boys to play roughly and more aggressively than girls. Genotypic males who deviate from the cultural gender "masculine" role are more likely to experience negative social consequences, such as teasing or mockery. Gender role and gender identity often closely correspond. However, in some cases, they diverge (e.g., in the case of dual-role transvestism where an individual who identifies as male adopts a traditionally female gender role through female clothing and behaves effeminately).

The cultural script of "masculinity" and "femininity" is learned in early childhood and manifests in various developmentally age-appropriate behaviors (e.g., play in childhood and sexual roles in adulthood). *Gender expression* is how individuals manifest their internalized and acquired expectations of their gender to the external world. Lastly, *sexual orientation* refers to the direction of an individual's primary attraction (e.g., emotional, physical, romantic arousal) toward a person(s) of the opposite gender (i.e., heterosexual), the same gender (i.e., non-heterosexual), both (i.e., bisexual), neither (i.e., asexual), or an attraction to a person regardless of anatomic sex or gender identity (i.e., omnisexual/pansexual). An individual's *sexual identity* is their assessment of their sexual orientation. Healthy sexual development is not monolithic but a concert of the components above.

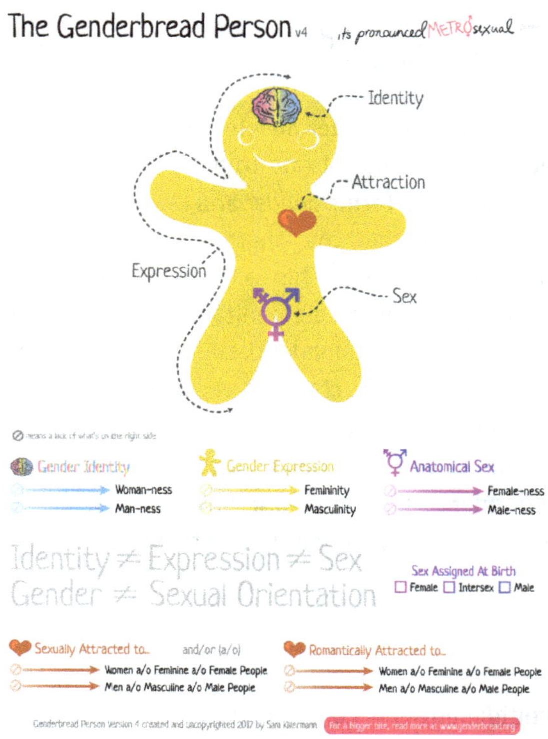

FIGURE 13.1 The genderbread person depiction of different aspects of psychosexual development.

Genderbread Person Version 4. (2017). Created by Sam Killermann. Source: https://www.genderbread.org/resource/genderbread-person-v4-0.

GENDER AND PSYCHOSEXUAL DEVELOPMENT

Human psychosexual development is complex and requires a recognition of what it means to be male, female, or nonbinary and of how this gender discernment is integrated within unfolding sexual identity, behavior, and expression. To explain the workings of gender and sexual development, several theories, including psychoanalytic theory by Freud, cognitive developmental theory, evolutionary theory, gender schema theory, and social cognitive theory, have been proposed (Bussey & Bandura, 1999). From these theories, we have learned there are fundamental gender differences based on evolutionary demands, critical biological events (e.g., chromosomal inheritance, genitalia development, neural, and psychological reaction to hormonal and physical changes), intrapsychic stages that affect self-perception and behavior, cognitive, learned, and sociocultural elements that are negotiated throughout gender and sexual development.

Infancy

Like many aspects of human development, sexual development begins at birth. As early as the first year of life, infants have a rudimentary appreciation of gender features and attributes. Infants as young as 3 months old can distinguish between female and male faces. By 6 months, infants have developed the ability to discriminate faces and voices by gender (Quinn et al., 2002; Rennels & Davis, 2008). Infants have different reactions to female and male faces—with a preference for female faces (Quinn et al., 2002; Rennels & Davis, 2008). The role of male and female is expanded and assimilated into child's gender framework that by age 3, children have reached the self-labeling gender development milestone and can accurately identify their gender (Serbin et al., 2001; Zosuls et al., 2009). As early as 30 months, the awareness of gender roles and gender-type activities is present. In general, boys show more interest than girls in stereotypical "male" objects like cars and tools and engage in rough-and-tumble play, while girls prefer dolls and domestic role-playing activities.

CLINICAL TIP

As early as the first year of life, infants have a rudimentary appreciation of gender features and attributes. Infants as young as 3 months old can distinguish between female and male faces. By 6 months, infants have developed the ability to discriminate faces and voices by gender.

Preschool Age

From age 3 to 5, children's gender stereotyping increases in rigidity and is driven by their awareness of what is expected of their gender group and a strong sense to conform to these expectations (Bussey & Bandura, 1999; Zosuls et al., 2009). Gender segregation, where children will actively reject playmates of the opposite gender, is present as early as 2 years old and

> **KEY POINT**
>
> From age 3 to 5, children's gender stereotyping increases in rigidity and is driven by their awareness of what is expected of their gender group and a strong sense to conform to these expectations.

continues even to age 10, where peers who adhere to gender segregation rules are seen as more socially competent and celebrated (Martin et al., 2013). Girls tends to be more likely to cross gender boundaries, whereas boys are relatively firmer in their boundaries and can be punitive toward other boys who behave effeminately, initiate contact with girls, or sometimes play with cross-sex toys. For example, in some preschool preschool-aged kids, insults such as "Tim is a girl" after seeing Tim play with a dollhouse are common.

The rigidity in the preschool-aged group has been explained by various theories. Kohlberg's cognitive developmental theory indicates that as preschool aged children begin to understand that gender remains constant over time (*gender stability*) and across various situations (*gender constancy*), they begin to act within the expectations of their gender group (Bussey & Bandura, 1999). Social learning theorists have suggested that this emergence of rigid adherence in preschool-aged children is driven by environmental determinants (e.g., peer relations and parental feedback) that punish and reward gender-type behavior, while others suggest that this rigidity is driven by a fear that gender variant behaviors or toys can alter the child's gender (Friedrich et al., 1998). This period of innate pressure to conform to a gender group can be distressing for children, who from an early age, have discomfort with their gender category.

School Age

> **KEY POINT**
>
> By age 7, gender constancy has usually been achieved. At this stage, there is some flexibility in gender stereotypes and increased awareness of gender type and connectedness to the same and sometimes to opposite-gender peers.

By age 7, gender constancy has usually been achieved. At this stage, there is some flexibility in gender stereotypes and an increased awareness of gender type and connectedness to the same and sometimes to opposite opposite-gender peers. By age 8–9 there is some loosening of stereotypic gender role "rules," and this continues as children begin to enter adolescence and sexual drives intensify. Their gender identification at this stage may not entirely signal future sexual or gender orientation.

Freud was one of the first to highlight sexuality as an integral part of human development. Freud believed that sexual energy, or *libido*, was inborn, and to progress to puberty and sexual maturation a person had to progress through and achieve the target in each stage (oral, anal, phallic, latency, and genital; Katz-Wise, 2015). Freud went further to present the *Oedipus complex*, where 3–6-year-old boys (phallic stage) develop a hostile rivalry with their father as a result of their incestuous desire for their mothers. A corresponding complex, the *Electra complex*, was later described in girls by Carl Jung. Freud proposed the idea that *homosexuality* was a result of an arrest in the progression of sexual developmental stages. While some of Freud's theories remain relevant, others have been modified by Freud himself and his followers.

TABLE 13.1 Gender and Psychosexual Milestones

Developmental group	Gender identity milestone	Psychosexual stage	Sexual behavior	Sexual self-concept
Infancy to 1 year	• Awareness of gender differences (in others)	• Oral stage	• May touch genitalia during diaper change or bathing • Male infants may have erections	
Toddler–preschool (2–5 years old)	• Gender self-labeling • Gender segregation • Gender stability	• Phallic stage	• Struggles with boundaries • Taking off clothes sometimes in public • Curiosity about nudity (may watch others disrobe) • May ask questions about genitalia • Self-stimulation in public	• Distinction between self and others
Elementary (5–11 years old)	• Gender constancy • Decreasing rigidity in gender segregation	• Latency stage	• Masturbation continues but increasingly in private • Sex play with same or different gender (e.g., "playing doctor" or "making babies"), typically light-hearted and not aggressive in nature • May explore nudity in person (closer to 5 years old) or via social media or TV (closer to 11 years old)	• Increasing self-awareness of being a sexual being • First crush may happen around 10 years old • Some sexual fantasies present by age 11
Adolescence (12–17 years old)	• Gender identity salience	• Genital stage	• Masturbation (done in private) • May be aware of or question sexual orientation • May or may not engage in sexual acts (may sometimes engage in risky sexual behaviors)	• Increased awareness and importance of sexual self-esteem, self-efficacy, and sexual identity • Exploration of orientation through fantasy or overt sexual acts
Adulthood	• Gender identity secured	• Genital stage	• Continued exploration of sexual desires and fantasy • Sexual experimentation • Sexual technique exploration	• Responsibility for sexual health; ownership of their sexual needs

Adapted from Hillman & Spigarelli, 2009.

Adolescence

In early adolescence, children are usually aware of their sexual orientation, and overt sexual activity is not required for this awareness. There is some experimentation with sexuality through sexual fantasy and masturbation. As children move from early to middle and late adolescence, there is an increased likelihood of overt sexual activity, sometimes with the same gender. It is important to note that same-gender sexual activity or attraction is neither a specific nor sensitive indicator of sexual identity and orientation throughout the individual's life span (Hillman & Spigarelli, 2009). At this stage, both boys and girls continue to assess the physical manifestations of their hormonal changes (e.g., girls wanting to be desired and boys welcoming weight and muscle gain, height, etc.). Girls tend to have a mixed reaction regarding height and breast development, depending on the degree of their physical change. Sometimes girls are teased if they're too tall or have noticeable breast development, whereas boys who mature early enjoy social rewards such as popularity with peers, being socially accepted, and being perceived as confident.

Adulthood

> **KEY POINT**
>
> In adulthood, sexual orientation tends to be clearer, if not solidified, but can remain fluid. With stability in gender identity and sexual orientation, intimacy and relationship with self and others and career development become increasingly important.

As individuals transition from adolescence into adulthood, their gender identity is more stable. Sexual orientation tends to be clearer, if not solidified, at this stage but can remain fluid even in adulthood. With stability in gender identity and sexual orientation, intimacy and relationship with self and others and career development become increasingly important. The developmental process in adulthood is self-regulated and does not have an age-associated end point like in childhood. Experience and social expectations come to the forefront while biological and cognitive milestones take a back seat. Similar to other developmental stages, social expectations are culture dependent (e.g., in the United States, the expectation in adulthood is graduation from school, pursuing higher education or getting a job, having a committed relationship, and having children). Failure to meet these social expectations can be distressing.

SEXUAL BEHAVIOR

Studies have highlighted children's sexual behavior at various age groups (Table 13.1). Prior to 4 years old, children recognize gender categories and the concept of their gender. They become curious about themselves but lack boundaries in their exploration. At this age, children may want to follow their parents to the restroom out of curiosity, disrobe in public, or touch their genitalia or those of other children. Sexual behavior shows an inverse relationship with age with the frequency peaking at about 5 years old for both boys and girls (Katz-Wise, 2015). In the age group of 2–6, mothers reported their children stood too close to people, touched genitalia sometimes in public, or tried to touch their breasts (Hillman & Spigarelli, 2009; Katz-Wise, 2015). From 7–12 years old, mothers reported their children touching genitalia (more often privately) and trying to look at other people when nude or disrobing in person, on the internet, or on television (Katz-Wise, 2015).

Just as social rules are learned in gender development, elementary school–aged children begin to learn understand the social rules for sexual behavior. In childhood, we also see children engaging in sexual play (with the same or opposite gender) that is lighthearted and voluntary, such as "making babies," mimicking adult behavior by kissing or hand hand-holding or playing "doctor." Acts that are aggressive in nature, such as the use of force or coercion or inserting objects into genitalia are concerning and could indicate underlying psychological concerns, including the trauma of abuse or neglect.

As children move into adolescence, sexual self-esteem (an evaluation of one's sense of attractiveness and management of physical changes), sexual self-efficacy (confidence in the ability to navigate sexual situations, including intimacy, closeness, and rejection), sexual identity, and sexual orientation become salient. Cross-culturally, puberty is associated with social status, as it signals a transition into adulthood and the capacity to fulfill the adult potential to reproduce. The metric for the onset of sexual maturation differs for males and females and within each culture (Crockett et al., 2003). For boys, entrance into puberty often marks more independence and freedom. But for girls, in some cultures, it is an end to school, decreased mobility, and sometimes the beginning of marriage preparations.

KEY POINT

Sexuality, sexual identity, sexual expression, and boundaries are influenced by biologic drives, gaining implicit and explicit social knowledge, cultural and religious beliefs, and social experiences. As children develop from early to late adolescence, social media, peers, and societal norms have a broader impact on gender and sexuality than family and sometimes cultural and religious templates.

As children develop from early to late adolescence, social media, peers, and societal norms have a broader impact on gender and sexuality than family and sometimes cultural and religious templates. Middle adolescence is typically the period of a romantic involvement and "first love." Boys and girls tend to place importance on different areas of a relationship. In studies about middle school-aged children, girls emphasized the romantic and emotional aspects of relationships rather than the overt sexual act. The reverse sequence was observed in boys. These divergent gender scripts continue to mold romantic interactions even into adulthood. By late adolescence and adulthood, there is typically increased security in body image, sexual efficacy and sexual self-esteem, gender role, and sexual orientation.

Children learn about sexual behavior and sexuality from observing parents, peers, exposure to social media, and television. The exploration of their knowledge presents differently in each developmental stage. In childhood, sexual behavior, such as self-stimulation (masturbation), is typically driven by curiosity, but in adolescence and adulthood the same sexual behavior can be incentivized by physiological, social, and emotional needs.

CLINICAL TIP

Children learn about sexual behavior and sexuality from observing parents, peers, and exposure to social media and television. The exploration of their knowledge presents differently in each developmental stage. In childhood, sexual behavior, such as self-stimulation (masturbation), is typically driven by curiosity, but in adolescence and adulthood, the same sexual behavior can be incentivized by physiological, social, and emotional needs.

SUMMARY

Biological, cognitive, social, cultural, and religious elements serve as navigation guides throughout gender and sexual development. Sexuality, sexual identity, sexual expression, and boundaries are influenced by biologic drives, gained implicit and explicit social knowledge, cultural and religious beliefs, and implicit and explicit social knowledge, cultural and religious beliefs, and social experiences. The information acquired in childhood about what it means to be male or female is eventually integrated into the understanding of sexuality and behavior as an adolescent and adult. At its core, healthy sexual development involves an understanding and acceptance of one's sense of sexual identity, inclusive of male, female, or nonbinary or a complete rejection of any gender designation.

RESOURCES

1. Clinical Report—The Evaluation of Sexual Behaviors in Children. Nancy D. Kellogg. Pediatrics Sep 2009, 124 (3) 992-998; DOI: 10.1542/peds.2009-1692
2. https://www.youtube.com/watch?v=bFA0pHpR9Ug
3. https://www.youtube.com/watch?v=9Z31bd1ybAs

REFERENCES

Bussey, K., & Bandura, A. (1999). Social cognitive theory of gender development and differentiation. *Psychological Review, 106*(4), 676–713. https://doi.org/10.1037/0033-295x.106.4.676

Crockett, L. J., Raffaelli, M., & Moilanen, K. L. (2003). Adolescent sexuality: Behavior and meaning. In G. R. Adams & M. D. Berzonsky (Eds.), *Blackwell handbook of adolescence* (371–392). Blackwell Publishing.

Friedrich, W. N., Fisher, J., Broughton, D., Houston, M., & Shafran, C. R. (1998). Normative sexual behavior in children: A contemporary sample. *Pediatrics, 101*(4), e9.

Gerlt, T., Blosser, C. G., & Dunn, A. M. (2016, July 24). *Sexuality.* Obgyn Key. https://obgynkey.com/sexuality-3/

Katz-Wise, S. L. (2015). Sexual fluidity in young adult women and men: Associations with sexual orientation and sexual identity development. *Psychology & Sexuality, 6*(2), 189–208.

Hillman, J. B., & Spigarelli, M. G. (2009). Sexuality: Its development and direction. In H. Feldman (Ed.), *Developmental-behavioral pediatrics* (4th ed.; pp. 415–425).

Martin, C. L., Kornienko, O., Schaefer, D. R., Hanish, L. D., Fabes, R. A., & Goble, P. (2013). The role of sex of peers and gender-typed activities in young children's peer affiliative networks: A longitudinal analysis of selection and influence. *Child Development, 84*(3), 921–937. https://doi.org/10.1111/cdev.12032

Quinn, P. C., Yahr, J., Kuhn, A., Slater, A. M., & Pascalis, O. (2002). Representation of the gender of human faces by infants: A preference for female. *Perception, 31*, 1109–1121.

Rennels, J. L., & Davis, R. E. (2008). Facial experience during the first year. *Infant Behavior and Development, 31*(4), 665–678. https://doi.org/10.1016/j.infbeh.2008.04.009

Serbin, L. A., Poulin-Dubois, D., Colburne, K. A., Sen, M. G., & Eichstedt, J. A. (2001). Gender stereotyping in infancy: Visual preferences for and knowledge of gender-stereotyped toys in the second year. *International Journal of Behavioral Development, 25*(1), 7–15. https://doi.org/10.1080/01650250042000078

Zosuls, K. M., Ruble, D. N., Tamis-Lemonda, C. S., Shrout, P. E., Bornstein, M. H., & Greulich, F. K. (2009). The acquisition of gender labels in infancy: Implications for gender-typed play. *Developmental Psychology, 45*(3), 688–701. https://doi.org/10.1037/a0014053

CHAPTER 14

Defense Mechanisms

The Hidden Mental Gymnastics to Protect the Self[1]

Shweta Sharma, Psy.D. and Sindhu Idicula, M.D.

"We don't see things as they are, we see them as we are."

— Anaïs Nin

OBJECTIVES

After reading this chapter, students will be able to do the following:

- define defense mechanisms
- discuss how and why individuals use defense mechanisms
- describe and recognize common defense mechanisms

CASE VIGNETTE[2]

Paul is a 23-year-old cisgender, heterosexual, currently unemployed, single man who was recently diagnosed with celiac disease. For years, he had complained of stomachaches, but his parents passed it off as him making excuses to get out of his soccer practice as a kid. To be fair to his parents, he had been seen by physicians and the nature of the underlying cause of his stomachache was inconclusive. Paul has been playing soccer since elementary school and had always aspired to be a professional soccer player. Now, the diagnosis of celiac disease jeopardized his aspirations. Paul's father, a highly successful business executive, is quite impatient with him and has been verbally and emotionally abusive toward Paul over the years. On the contrary, his mother is overly protective of him, but she also defers to her husband whenever things get tense.

---

1 Readers may also see "Introduction to Psychotherapy for Medical Students" (Chapter 33) for related material.

2 This is a hypothetical case intended to illustrate the potential use of a wide range of defense mechanisms. The case runs through the chapter and is used to provide examples of different defense mechanisms.

DEFINITIONS AND KEY CONCEPTS

Defense mechanisms (or defenses) are mental processes that help protect us against threats, preserve self-esteem, and maintain our psychological equilibrium. The threat is usually some powerful, dangerous, unbearable, or painful emotional experience that exposes an individual to overwhelming anxiety, shame, envy, grief, and the like.

INTRODUCTION

KEY POINT

As humans, we engage in mental processes akin to doing physical gymnastics to protect us from the difficult, or sometimes intolerable, emotions that come with the recognition of our limitations or vulnerabilities. Depending on how they are used, defense mechanisms may impact our functioning positively or negatively.

From the cradle to the grave, we are exposed to frequent reminders of our limitations and vulnerabilities. As humans, we engage in mental processes akin to doing physical gymnastics to protect us from the difficult or sometimes intolerable emotions that come with the recognition of our limitations or vulnerabilities. These mental processes, or defense mechanisms, are hidden and occur across the developmental cycle. They are ubiquitous and essential to everyday life, and none of us would survive without them. They are generally adaptive. However, there can be ways in which the use of defense mechanisms may be problematic and point to the presence of distress or psychological disturbance(s). For example, if their use is excessive, inefficient, or ineffective, it may impair an individual's self-functioning (e.g., self-appraisal, self-esteem regulation, or self-direction) and interpersonal functioning (e.g., empathy, intimacy). The presence or absence of defenses does not define psychological health or distress. Instead, it is the array and type of defenses available to an individual that helps us understand their psychological health with mature and flexible defenses being more adaptive in periods of stress (see Valliant, 2000). Those who have access to sophisticated means of handling complex and disturbing reality and flexible ways of defending against anxiety are likely to be emotionally healthier. This chapter aims to help you understand defense mechanisms and how they operate to protect the self. To achieve this goal, we describe several common defense mechanisms and illustrate how they may operate in clinical work.

UNDERSTANDING DEFENSE MECHANISMS

The concept of defense mechanisms has a long and rich history. Sigmund Freud (1894) introduced the idea of defenses and described them as a mental operation that served to modulate the expression of unacceptable and threatening sexual and aggressive drives and impulses. Although Freud identified defense mechanisms in the context of understanding psychological disturbance, his daughter, Anna Freud, subsequently described them as also occurring as part of normal psychological development (Freud, 1936). Later theorists, like Cooper (1998), described the use and development of defenses to keep unacceptable feelings and needs in check or out of awareness for relational security. Kohut (1977) posited that defense mechanisms protect the self and one's self-esteem from the adverse effects of empathic failures, disappointments, and losses. Below are four crucial points to keep in mind about defenses.

KEY POINT

Defense mechanisms are mental operations we undertake to preserve self-esteem, maintain psychological equilibrium, or feel protected against perceived threats.

Firstly, defense mechanisms are hidden and occur without conscious effort or awareness. In Figure 14.1, for example, Garfield is aggressive but not aware of his aggression. He pushes away from acknowledging or appreciating his aggression toward others by using the defense of projection. Specifically, when he says, "Everybody is against me," Garfield is projecting his aggression onto others. Why would he do this? Perhaps, it allows him to act aggressively without feeling anxious or guilty and responsible for his actions. He laments, "And I don't know why!" Less consciously or defensively, he may not want to know why because, for some reason, he does not want to see himself as aggressive. The hidden mental gymnastics turns the unacceptable experience and act of aggression toward others into justified aggression toward others, and he does not have to take responsibility or change his behavior.

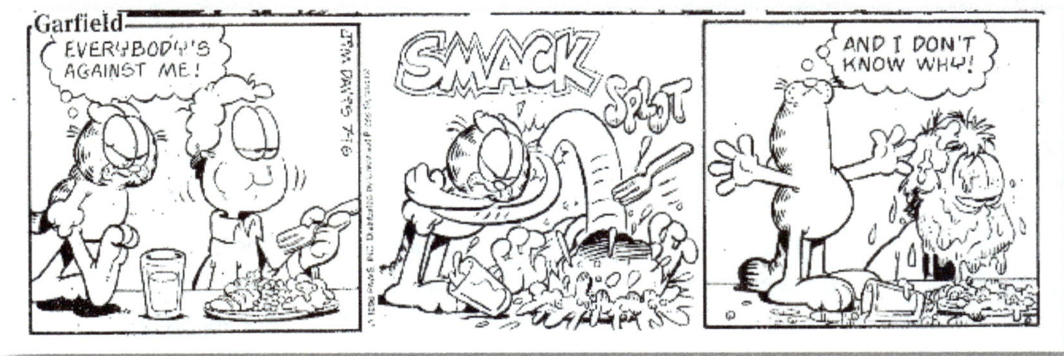

FIGURE 14.1 Illustration showing defense of projection in use.

Copyright © 1996 by Andrews McMeel Universal.

Defense mechanisms primarily operate outside of conscious awareness. Figure 14.1 shows how individuals using defense mechanisms may be internally blind to their own behaviors, which are obvious to external observers. Garfield is aggressive, but not aware of his aggression. He pushes away from acknowledging or appreciating his aggression toward others by using the defense of projection. Specifically, when he says, "Everybody is against me," Garfield is projecting his aggression onto others. The brunt of using defense mechanisms is often borne by other individuals who closely interact with them.

MEMORY TIP

Both defense and coping mechanisms are used to regulate emotions and protect self-esteem. A distinguishing factor between both is that defense mechanisms are mostly unconscious, while coping mechanisms are consciously learned and intentionally used strategies to regulate emotions and protect self-esteem.

Secondly, it is helpful to distinguish between defense mechanisms, coping mechanisms, and defensiveness. Defense mechanisms primarily operate outside of conscious awareness. Unlike defense mechanisms, coping mechanisms are consciously learned and intentionally used strategies to regulate emotions and protect self-esteem. In comparison to defenses that are hidden mental processes, defensiveness refers to interpersonal behaviors or response styles (e.g., counterattack or minimizing) designed to reduce the anxiety that may or may not include the use of defense mechanisms. Both coping mechanisms and defensiveness help deal with "reality." Still, *defense mechanisms change the way we perceive reality.* When using defense mechanisms, our internal reality changes, but our external reality remains the same, leading us to move forward with a distorted perception of our external world.

Thirdly, defenses may be categorized as adaptive or maladaptive and mature or immature (Cramer, 1991; Vaillant et al., 1986). According to empirical studies (e.g., Cramer, 2006), defense mechanisms develop in a predictable sequence as children mature, and their use varies in predominance throughout the life span. For example, denial occurs early, projection develops later, and identification develops still later in life (Cramer, 2006). One way to think about defense maturity or immaturity is within the context of a person's chronological age. The less mature expression generally refers to our natural, adaptive way of experiencing the world as infants. McWilliams (2011) proposed that the immature (lower-order) defenses ignore and distort reality and diffuse the boundary between self and other (including the outer world). In contrast, mature (higher-order) defenses require some appreciation of reality and recognize internal boundaries (e.g., the boundary between our id's primal wishes and our ego's appraisal of what is realistic or responsible). Valliant's (2000) work showed that the use of less adaptive defenses may play a role in understanding why some individuals, when exposed to stress, are at a higher risk of developing psychopathology. In sum, the conceptual distinction between mature and immature defenses is somewhat arbitrary, and most defenses have their less mature and more mature expressions.

CLINICAL TIP

People develop habitual defensive pattern, including a specific defense or a cluster of defenses they typically rely on.

Finally, people develop habitual defensive pattern, including a specific defense or a cluster of defenses they typically rely on. This habitual defense pattern is determined by a complex interaction of several factors, including a person's (a) temperament, (b) nature of childhood stress or adversity, (c) caregiver's temperament and defensive disposition, and (d) positive or negative experiences related with using various defenses (McWilliams, 2011). These patterns can inform our understanding of how a person suffers and manages their distress—such information can aid treatment planning.

COMMON DEFENSE MECHANISMS

While Sigmund Freud identified several distinct defenses, his daughter, Anna Freud, was the first to catalog defense mechanisms using data from children and adults she treated. Defense mechanisms are instructive and helpful in understanding people. In clinical work, understanding defense mechanisms can help you recognize them in your patient, which can aid in your clinical formulation, the development of your differential diagnoses, and planning of thoughtful interventions. Recognizing defense mechanisms in the interview process as well as the content your patient shares (how they talk and interact with you and what they talk about) may cue you in to the hidden and intolerable affect that they are trying to push away or manage. Thinking through the constellation of defenses and whether the pattern is adaptive or disruptive, may assist in the development of a treatment plan that targets the underlying issues at play. Over the course of a century of psychoanalytic thinking clinical theorists have identified and catalogued multitude of defenses (e.g., Blackman, 2004; Freud, 1936; Valliant, 1992; Williams, 2011). We will confine this discussion to the defense mechanisms that we find useful in our clinical practice to help give you an introduction. With each defense, the case of Paul that is discussed above is used in various scenarios to illustrate the defense.

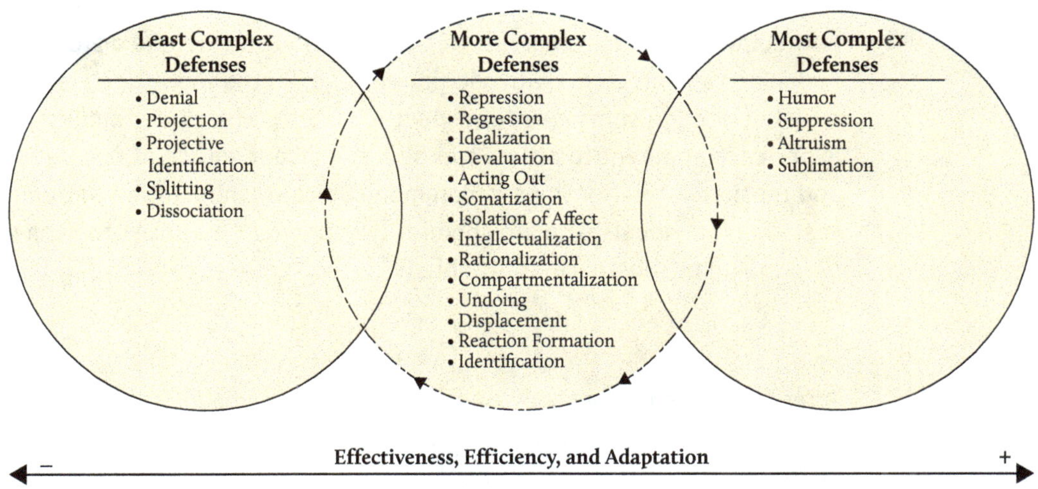

FIGURE 14.2 Common defense mechanisms on a continuum—a visual representation.

Figure 14.2 aims to assist you in thinking about defense mechanisms on a continuum of complexity from earlier and more archaic to later and more sophisticated forms, implying degree of effectiveness, efficiency, and adaptation related to defense use, which is depicted by the shaded arrow. The concept of *complexity* refers to the degree of attunement to reality, maturity of psychological skills involved, and the nature of boundary differentiation involved in defense use. The middle circle depicts how some defense mechanisms have both less mature (i.e., archaic) and more mature (i.e., sophisticated) forms; thus, the open looping arrows. The middle circle also overlaps with the circles on its right and left to underscore how the conceptual division between less mature and more mature defenses is somewhat arbitrary and may depend on how the specific defense is used and the extent of an individual's dependence on the particular defense.

Denial

The operation of most mature defenses involves a component of *denial*, which refers to the refusal to accept unpleasant external reality. Denial involves the mental gymnastics of replacing perceived reality with a distorted version, which then screens out or transforms the unpleasant affect. For instance, Pollyannaish people distort reality in their insistence that everything is fine or for the best. Keep in mind that denial is a misconstrual of reality and is not a conscious deception—that is, it's not a lie. In its adaptive form, denial allows us to function and survive in crises or emergencies by disregarding sensory data that may otherwise overwhelm us. However, beyond its developmentally or situationally appropriate use, persistent use of denial may indicate significant failure of reality testing which is the objective evaluation of an internal emotion or thought against external real life. It may also contribute to distortions in thinking and problems with decision-making. Furthermore, one's refusal to acknowledge some painful aspect of external reality or subjective experience apparent to others can be a significant source of frustration and tension in relationships. A common clinical manifestation of denial is among individuals who are chemically dependent but insist they have no drinking or substance use problem.

KEY POINT

Denial involves replacing perceived reality with a distorted version, which then screens out or transforms the unpleasant emotions.

Paul's Example

After an endoscopy that showed severe intestinal damage, Paul received a diagnosis of celiac disease. However, he reported feeling fine and insisted on resuming his soccer practice right away. He then went online and ordered an expensive pair of soccer cleats to be delivered overnight, despite his physician's recommendation that he abstain from playing soccer during his recovery.

Projection

Projection refers to the mental gymnastics whereby one's unacknowledged or unacceptable feelings, thoughts, or impulses are attributed to others. In its adaptive form, we use the capacity to project our own internal experience to understand other's subjective experiences. Its problematic use involves projecting highly negative aspects of the self onto others in order to get rid of the uncomfortable and unacceptable feelings. Others are then misperceived as judgmental, jealous, envious, distrusting, or dangerous, and significantly misunderstood. Of note, when suspicion of others is realistic or secondary to posttraumatic hypervigilance, it is not considered projection (e.g., healthy cultural suspicion). Individuals with paranoia commonly use the mechanism of projection.

KEY POINT

Projection occurs when a person's unacknowledged or unacceptable feelings, thoughts, impulses are attributed to others. Projection is sometimes used by projecting highly negative aspects of the self onto others to get rid of the uncomfortable and unacceptable feelings.

Paul's Example

Following the endoscopy, Paul develops a slight infection and reacts by expressing anger that his physician was trying to keep him sick and take his parents' money. The physician felt afraid but, using his emotional experience to understand Paul, imagined that underneath his anger Paul may be afraid too. The physician found himself feeling empathic toward Paul, despite being verbally attacked by him.

Projective Identification

Projective identification is a robust and challenging mental process as well as an interpersonal communication that combines projection and introjection. Keep in mind that, in projection, what is inside is misunderstood as coming from outside. On the contrary, in introjection, what is outside is misunderstood as coming from inside. The term projective identification was first introduced by Melanie Klein (1946) and it is used in many ways. Broadly speaking, projective identification is an interpersonal process in which one person's projections influence the other onto whom they are projected to behave, think, and feel in ways that confirm the projections. It is like a self-fulfilling prophecy for the one who projects, making the other identify with what is projected onto them. In its adaptive form, the process of projective identification can involve the contagion of loving, positive feelings in relationships. However, its relentless, intense, and unmodulated use can harm and disrupt interpersonal functioning. The use of projective identification is usually associated with borderline personality organization (Kernberg, 1967).

Paul's Example

Paul projects his angry and resentful feelings toward his physician. The physician feels the hostility in the room and feels an uncharacteristic urge to act aggressively toward Paul. The physician found himself being curt when answering Paul's questions, which surprised him, since he prides himself on being kind and compassionate with his patients. The physician's abrasive behavior, in turn, confirms Paul's projection.

Splitting

> **KEY POINT**
>
> *Splitting* refers to the process of organizing and simplifying the complex life experiences as all good or all bad, especially when they are contradictory, confusing, or threatening.

Splitting refers to the process of organizing and simplifying the complex life experiences as all good or all bad, especially when they are contradictory, confusing, or threatening. We may think of all too familiar split image of good versus evil that pervades all societies. Splitting allows us to organize and make sense of the overwhelming world and find our place in it. It also allows us to avoid internal conflict that may stem from contradictions in our and others' behaviors, thoughts, and feelings—thereby reducing anxiety and maintaining our self-esteem. It's developmentally appropriate to use splitting before developing object constancy (typically set by 1 year of age); still, adults who use splitting struggle with tolerating opposite feelings toward others. The use of splitting is common among individuals with personality disorders.

Paul's Example

Paul describes his physician as the most amazing person and the best in the field, while describing his nurse as angry and incompetent. Similarly, he experiences his father as all good in contrast to his allegedly uncaring and stupid mother.

Dissociation

Dissociation involves the compartmentalization of discrepant ideas, perceptions, feelings, sensations, and behaviors combined with amnesia, which disrupts one's sense of continuity and is manifested as drastic changes in personality. In contemporary theorizing repression is understood as a subset of the dissociative process (see Braun, 1988). Of note, fragmentation of memory involved in trauma (dissociation) also likely involves blocking out of awareness of upsetting wishes and fantasies, and both are different from amnesia due to substance use or brain injury. Dissociation is a common response to trauma but is not limited only to trauma. For instance, consider familiar phenomena like highway hypnosis (Williams, 1963). In its adaptive form, the ability to dissociate or mentally check out allows us to survive life-threatening situations. However, chronic use of dissociation can cause extreme fragmentation of self and dysfunction as evidenced in dissociative identity disorder.

Paul's Example

In addition to verbal and emotional abuse by the father, Paul has a history of sexual abuse by a soccer coach, which he does not recall. Part of his medical evaluation involved a colonoscopy which required a digital rectal exam. Paul became intensely emotionally distressed, started having panic attacks and struggling to exit the room. The distressing and intrusive experience of the examination destabilized him, triggered deep-seated trauma memories, and caused him to feel threatened and unsafe.

Repression

Repression refers to unconscious blocking from awareness of an upsetting idea or impulse, the feeling associated with the idea, or the fantasies and wishes associated with the idea. It is an adaptive way of dealing with disturbing ideas that may otherwise overwhelm us. Its use becomes problematic when it either fails to keep the disturbing thoughts out of awareness or when its excessive use hinders functioning and becomes a source of anxiety. It is important to remember that not all forgetting is due to repression. For instance, substance use or brain injury can cause difficulty remembering. However, the operation of most mature defenses involves a component of repression. Clinically, the use of repression is commonly associated with a hysterical personality style or disorder.

Paul's Example

Paul may have had his follow-up appointment with his physician slip his mind, leading him to arrive late to the appointment. When he arrives, he presents upset and in tears but does not know why. He vaguely speaks about his blood test results that indicated celiac disease, but he can't recall the procedure (endoscopy) he is scheduled for next. His temporary loss of awareness of details that may be typically remembered may function to keep his mind from being completely overwhelmed.

Regression

Regression refers to the unwitting backward slide into habits of a prior developmental phase or functioning. It is a defensive strategy to deal with the internal and external stressors associated with one's present maturational stage by regressing to a relatively helpless and childlike mode of coping with life. For example, somatization, the process of responding to stress by getting sick, would be considered a regression if the person had attained the capacity to put words to feelings before losing them. However, it would not be considered regression if the person is aware of needing extra support or comfort and seeks it out.

Paul's Example

Following the lab tests and endoscopy resulting in the diagnosis of celiac disease, Paul uncharacteristically starts to talk in a childlike manner when visiting with his physician and with his family.

Idealization and Devaluation

Idealization and *devaluation* both represent the psychological process aimed at reassuring oneself of one's power, attractiveness, status, and significance to others. Idealization refers to the tendency to imbue self or others who we depend on with special qualities, values, and power. On the other hand, devaluation refers to the tendency to attribute exaggerated negative quality to self or others. Devaluation is the inevitable downside of idealization. Although unrealistic, to an extent, it is healthy and normal to both idealize and devalue. We all idealize our caregivers and authority figures initially, and with healthy development, (hopefully) de-idealize or devalue them to aid in separation and individuation. These defenses are adaptive when their use is motivating, positively self-fulfilling, and contributes to a feeling of competence and effectiveness in life. However, their use becomes problematic when one cannot tolerate frustration and disappointment related to one's own and others' limitations. The most common clinical manifestation of problematic use of idealization and devaluation is often observed in individuals with narcissistic, psychopathic, sociopathic, or antisocial tendencies.

Paul's Example

Paul describes his soccer performance in glowing terms and contrasts it with the dismal performance of his teammates. When he shifts the focus to his illness and treatment, he describes his physician as the best in the field and his hospital care as perfect. He frequently refers to his previous physicians and makes the point that they were not of the same caliber as his current doctor, and he thinks he should sue them for inadequate care.

KEY POINT

Acting out is avoiding the awareness or experience of painful emotions by acting rather than feeling.

Acting Out

Acting out refers to the mental process of bypassing awareness or experience of painful feelings by putting them into action. By being in action one may unconsciously repeat or enact a conflict or wish that is internally forbidden or traumatic. This may be understood as a hidden effort to master overwhelming feelings. The feeling is unconscious or dissociated, and the action is almost compulsive, impulsive, or automatic. Examples of acting out behaviors may include exhibitionism, counterphobia, masochism, and voyeurism, among others. Acting out is primarily viewed as self-destructive. However, it could be adaptive if it allows for expression of forbidden wishes or conflicts while maintaining one's psychological equilibrium and interpersonal functioning. Clinically, the defense of acting out is seen in many contrasting clinical presentations. For instance, high-risk, self-destructive, and self-sabotaging behaviors are common among individuals with personality disorders.

Paul's Example

Shortly after being diagnosed with celiac disease, Paul gets into several bar fights and wrecks his car twice. Prior to this distressing experience of getting diagnosed with a medical condition, he had no history of reckless or aggressive behaviors.

Somatization

Somatization refers to the mental process of converting emotional stress into physical symptoms. Examples include tension headaches, irritable bowel, or skin rashes. In somatization, emotional states are expressed physically, and the bodily (rather than emotional) concerns are the focus of attention. It is essential to keep in mind that somatic distress is not feigned or all in a person's mind. We may think of the fight–flight–freeze response to stress or blushing in shame. Somatic reactions are hardwired, and part of our maturation is to learn to use language to describe stress-related bodily arousal. Somatization disorders are known to co-occur with most personality disorders (Bornstein & Gold, 2008).

KEY POINT

Somatization is avoiding the awareness or experience of painful emotions or psychological conflict by experiencing medical symptoms.

Paul's Example

Shortly after being diagnosed with celiac disease, Paul becomes preoccupied with vague physical symptoms that do not match his medical condition. He is not reassured despite multiple physical workups that show no cause for concern. All efforts to help him reflect on his emotional concerns and psychological cause or meaning of his physical problems are minimally successful.

Isolation of Affect

Isolation of affect refers to the mental process of separating, denying, or repressing the affect connected with the idea. Isolation does not involve total cut-off from the disturbing experience, but only the feelings associated with it to avoid emotional turmoil. We may think of Sheldon in *The Big Bang Theory*, who is characterized as not being in touch with his feelings. In some extreme situations, it's adaptive to isolate feeling from knowing, as it allows us to function in the moment. But lack of access to feelings and emotional implications of our experiences can be growth-inhibiting. The use of isolation of affect is commonly associated with obsessive compulsive personality disorder.

Paul's Example

Paul talks to his friend about his illness. He shows no emotional response or feelings when discussing his condition, the various procedures he underwent, and the career and life implications of the disease. It is almost as if he is telling a story about someone else's life or someone in a movie he watched.

Intellectualization

Intellectualization refers to the mental process of dealing with emotional overload by excessive use of abstract thinking. For instance, one may report their feelings but in an emotionless manner. By thinking and talking about feelings, one tries to control or minimize the experience of disturbing emotions. Intellectualization is adaptive if one can eventually acknowledge and process the emotional experience. It is problematic when one cannot leave their intellectual position and have no other way to cope with life.

MEMORY TIP

Intellectualization and rationalization both use production of reasons to regulate emotions and protect self-esteem. A distinguishing factor is that intellectualization uses abstract thinking to detach oneself from feelings, while rationalization uses reasons to provide alternative explanations for the facts and motives or rational alternative facts.

Paul's Example

Paul speaks about his anger at being diagnosed with celiac disease and the resultant loss of his career. He expresses himself in a casual and detached manner. He sounds very logical, and it appears he understands it all without any problem. Nothing in his voice or manner reflects any difficulty or struggle with difficult emotions, such as anger, regret, grief, or worry. It is almost as if he is giving a lecture to a virtual audience with no emotions attached.

Rationalization

Rationalization refers to making explanations for or justifying unacceptable attitudes, beliefs, or behaviors after the fact to make them tolerable to oneself. The explanations tend to be reassuring, self-serving, and somewhat incorrect in that they conceal the true motivations for one's thoughts, feelings, or actions. In its adaptive form, rationalization allows one to deal with and learn from a difficult situation with minimal upset. However, it can be used as an unconscious justification for all one's actions or wants.

Paul's Example

Unable to continue to play soccer due to his medical diagnosis, Paul explains the painful outcome as follows, "Well, to tell you the truth I didn't really want to continue to play soccer because I am interested in other things, but playing soccer takes up all of my time."

Compartmentalization

Compartmentalization refers to the rift between two or more incompatible ideas or activities that are all in a person's awareness. The person holds the conflicting ideas, attitudes, or behaviors without feeling confused, guilty, ashamed, or anxious. Adaptively, compartmentalization allows us to tolerate the commonplace discrepancy between our professed beliefs or espoused stance and actual behavior without much emotional discomfort. Less benignly, people deploring abuse can consciously engage in abusive behavior without any sense of guilt and consequent responsibility.

Paul's Example

Paul tends to compartmentalize his anger. One day, he gets upset with his physician and erupts in anger and hurls insults at him. When the physician confronts Paul about his abusive behavior, he is appalled and does not understand why the physician tends to view his behavior as aggressive.

Undoing

Undoing refers to an effort to negate conscious or unconscious guilt or shame related to past behavior, thoughts, or feelings. Think of undoing behavior as actions that symbolically amend or counterbalance past wrongful acts. To atone for actual or imagined wrongdoing, the person may engage in superstitious behavior, compulsive rituals, behavior opposite of the real or imagined wrongful act or behavior that involves self-punishment for the actual or imagined offense. To an extent, remorse can be adaptive and motivate acts of love and care or public service that have the unconscious significance of reparation for a wrong or injury. However, adults are assumed to be healthier if they can take responsibility for their honest mistakes and failures and tolerate the consequent guilt and shame for the unconscious wishes, instead of magically undoing the guilt and shame. Clinically, the use of undoing is commonly associated with obsessional disorders.

Paul's Example

Paul has a longstanding tendency to check the locks on the doors and windows before bed. He insists on rechecking the locks to make sure they are not left open by mistake. Paul is afraid that if he is not careful, his parents' lives could be in danger. He is unaware that by checking and rechecking the locks on the doors and windows, he is trying to symbolically undo and avoid the guilt for his murderous feelings toward his abusive father and passive mother.

Displacement

Displacement refers to redirecting or transferring feelings, preoccupations, or behaviors from their original idea or object to a relatively safe alternative that also resembles the original in some ways to reduce anxiety. We may think of scapegoating. In its adaptive form, displacement may protect an anguished person from the risk of more harm to themselves. More benignly, we may think of channeling anger into a productive activity like cleaning the house or baking. Common clinical manifestation of displacement is found in phobias or perversions.

Paul's Example

Paul gets upset with his physician for double-booking his follow-up appointment but instead yells at his mom when she checks in on him.

Reaction Formation

Reaction formation refers to turning an attitude, wish, or impulse into its polar opposite to make the situation less threatening. We may think of transforming or substituting unacceptable feelings like anger, jealousy, hatred, or envy into their diametrically opposite feelings of love and attraction. This defense is betrayed by the exaggerated or insincere quality of the conscious emotional response. It's adaptive for little kids to have the ego strength to deal with their anger and jealousy toward the newborn by converting it into love and care. But adults are assumed to be healthier if they can acknowledge all their feelings toward any given situation. Reaction formation is generally at play when emotional ambivalence is reduced to one or the other feeling. For instance, obsessive and compulsive individuals inhibit their anger and resentment and are only aware of feelings of respect for the authority figures.

Paul's Example

Paul only feels and expresses positive feelings toward his abusive father, including respect, admiration, and appreciation. He is not aware of negative feelings toward him.

Identification

Identification refers to the mental process by which we identify with important others or with some aspect of important others. This process is defensive when the individual is struggling with identity confusion, fragile self-esteem, or lack of solid sense of self, and is motivated by the need to avoid anxiety, grief, shame, pain or fear, as opposed to wanting to be like those that we admire and value. We may think of young children wanting to be like their caregivers or role models, which can be a healthy emotional basis of motivation to do better. Less benignly, think of bullying victims becoming aggressive to defend against the fear and pain of abuse they themselves have encountered. The mechanism of identification can be partly conscious and partly unconscious. Clinically, this is commonly manifested in patient's propensity to identify with their therapist.

Paul's Example

Paul is afraid of his father's verbal abuse and ruthless criticism of others. At the same time, Paul is often verbally insulting of people around him; however, he is unaware of how much his behaviors reflect his father's.

Humor

Humor refers to the mental process of reducing unpleasant emotion and discomfort by finding funny or ironic elements in challenging situations. This allows for distance from the upsetting situation, creating space for more objectivity and reflection.

Paul's Example

While going through treatment for celiac disease, Paul finds himself sending his close family gluten-free memes to diffuse his stress around having to adapt to the illness-related restrictions on his lifestyle.

Suppression

Suppression refers to a voluntary decision not to attend to a particular feeling, state, or impulse to reduce personal discomfort or unpleasant emotions. We use suppression to delay gratification. Unlike repression, which involves an unconscious process, suppression is a conscious and voluntary action.

Paul's Example

Paul attends a birthday party and feels annoyed looking at the cake that he cannot have due to his dietary restrictions and makes a decision to hang out with friends in the other room away from the cake as a way to not think about it.

Altruism

Altruism refers to the mental process of channeling defensive energy into taking care of the needs of others above and beyond those of one's own as a way of dealing with emotional conflict over one's own needs or dealing with internal or external stressors. An altruistic person commits oneself to the service of others and, in the process, feels gratified, either vicariously or as a response from others. Although altruistic actions are tied to self-interest, vicarious gratification, or direct reward, they are constructive and serve as an avenue for extraordinary achievements and tremendous benefit to society. Altruistic individuals are to some extent aware of their own needs and feelings underlying selfless actions.

Paul's Example

After some months of dealing with his diagnosis, Paul creates a small nonprofit that raises money to help fund support groups for other individuals with celiac disease.

Sublimation

Sublimation involves the mental process of transforming socially or psychologically unacceptable urges, such as destructive impulses, into ones that are considered more productive and socially acceptable. This may involve creative endeavors, such as the arts or channeling aggression through sports. Sublimation is regarded as a hallmark of highest form of ego development.

Paul's Example

Paul channels his anger at the unfairness of his diagnosis into perfecting his moves at the kickboxing gym.

TABLE 14.1 Summary Table of Defense Mechanisms

	Defense mechanism	Description
1.	Denial	Despite overwhelming evidence for its existence, the person refuses to recognize the unpleasant external reality.
2.	Projection	The person attributes their unacknowledged or unacceptable thoughts, feelings, or impulses to others.
3.	Projective identification	This involves a dyad—the projecting person and the identifying person. The identifying person takes on the projecting person's projections and experiences the subtle interpersonal pressure to feel, think, and behave in keeping with the projections, even if it is uncharacteristic of the individual. For the projecting person, the other's identification with their projection becomes a self-fulfilling prophecy.
4.	Splitting	The person sees themselves and others as all good or all bad or vacillates between loving and hating oneself/others.
5.	Dissociation	The person has multiple dispositional states (e.g., traits, skills, and alter identities) hidden from them. In these cases, the individual generally cannot be aware of or access the different mental and physical states simultaneously, despite others perceiving drastic changes in their personality.
6.	Repression	The person unconsciously blocks from the conscious awareness an upsetting idea, impulse, or memory; the feeling associated with it; or the fantasies and wishes associated with it.

	Defense mechanism	Description
7.	**Regression**	The individual unwittingly slides back into habits of a younger maturational stage (e.g., dependency or stubbornness) to escape or avoid the conflicts and tensions associated with their present level of development.
8.	**Idealization**	The person overvalues or exaggerates their positive qualities, or that of others, to bolster their self-esteem or avoid feeling frustrated and disappointed.
9.	**Devaluation**	The person looks down upon others or exaggerates the negative qualities in others to preserve their self-esteem—or the individual exaggerates their negative qualities to avoid experiencing disappointment.
10.	**Acting out**	The person acts on their unpleasant or forbidden wishes or fantasies to avoid or master painful feelings.
11.	**Somatization**	The person redirects their focus to physical symptoms instead of experiencing and expressing their unpleasant emotions. This becomes their primary way of communicating unverbalized emotional distress.
12.	**Isolation of affect**	The person avoids emotional turmoil by cutting off the feelings and meaning associated with a disturbing experience, while still engaging with the experience in a factual or stoic way.
13.	**Intellectualization**	The person excessively thinks and analyzes difficult emotional experiences to gain distance from the associated distressing emotions and avoid feeling them.
14.	**Rationalization**	The person justifies their unacceptable actions or desires by giving reasons that conceal or deny aspects of reality (e.g., true motivations or intentions) to make the actions tolerable.
15.	**Compartmentalization**	The person holds conflicting or incompatible ideas, attitudes, or behaviors without recognizing or acknowledging the contradiction.
16.	**Undoing**	The person engages in superstitious behavior, compulsive rituals, or behaviors involving self-punishment to negate the conscious or unconscious guilt or shame for actual or imagined wrongdoing.
17.	**Displacement**	The person redirects or shifts feelings from their original source to a relatively safer, but similar, alternative to reduce anxiety.
18.	**Reaction formation**	The person feels or acts the opposite of unacceptable wishes or impulses.
19.	**Identification**	The person thinks and acts like a person they admire, a person who abused them, or someone they lost to avoid negative emotions, such as anxiety, shame, pain, fear, or grief.
20.	**Humor**	The person finds funny or ironic elements in a challenging situation to reduce unpleasant feelings.
21.	**Suppression**	The person decides not to attend to a feeling, state, or urge to reduce personal discomfort.
22.	**Altruism**	The person commits to the service of others to deal with emotional conflict over one's own needs.
23.	**Sublimation**	The person channels problematic urges and conflicts into creative and beneficial endeavors.

QUICK POINT

Social experiences are dynamic and have a profound impact on the human psyche. As such, our understanding of defense mechanisms continues to evolve.

ADDITIONAL CONSIDERATIONS

Social experiences are dynamic and have a profound impact on the human psyche. As such, our understanding of defense mechanisms continues to evolve. To this end, Stoute (2021) recently introduced the formulation of "Black Rage" as a necessary adaptive and defensive mental process that allows oppressed people of color who suffer racial trauma and racial degradation to defend against the assault from persecution, demoralization, and self-hate (i.e., internalization of devaluation). Stoute (2021) posits that integrating the concept of Black Rage into psychoanalytic theory validates and allows for the traumatic experiences of the oppressed. She differentiates Black Rage that is mobilized for the purpose of defense and adaptation from the dysfunctional rage that may be suppressed, internalized, or externalized, leading to depression, substance abuse, self-destructive, or other destructive behavior.

CLINICAL APPROACH TO DEFENSE MECHANISMS

CLINICAL TIP

When encountering defense mechanisms in clinical work with patients, it is best to take a nonconfrontational approach.

CLINICAL TIP

By linking problematic or irrational behaviors, symptoms, and attitudes to unpleasurable thoughts and feelings, the patient may start to understand better how their problems developed and perhaps the cost of continuing to function at the status quo.

When encountering defense mechanisms in clinical work with patients, it is best to take a nonconfrontational approach. Confronting the use of defenses is a popular idea in the media, but it has limited clinical utility, depending on the patient's capacity to benefit from this approach. Contrary to what we might hope for, confrontation may cause the patient to dig in rather than give in and this poses the risk of exacerbating their use of defense mechanisms. Figure 14.3 shows how defenses can be maddeningly impervious to influence and how confronting them can backfire. Instead of confrontation, it may be helpful to think of the work as creating a safe interpersonal context in therapy that allows the patient and the therapist to recognize and then challenge the problematic use of defense mechanisms. This work is slow and gradual, involving validation and challenging defenses over time. By linking problematic or irrational behaviors, symptoms, and attitudes to unpleasurable thoughts and feelings, the patient may start to understand better how their problems developed and, perhaps, the cost of continuing to function at the status quo. The linking, over time, can also begin to relieve symptoms and make the use of defense mechanisms less useful as the patient begins to slowly tolerate more and more of the previously unbearable thoughts and feelings. Some patients, however, may struggle with ego functioning (see Busch, 1997; Hartmann, 1939) and may have difficulties with tasks such as perception, reality testing, intelligence, integration, abstraction, executive function, and judgment. For them, becoming aware of previously hidden feelings may not only lack usefulness but may potentially overwhelm or dysregulate them. For these patients, a more helpful strategy in therapy may focus on supporting the patient's functioning instead of exposing or confronting defenses. Schulthesis and Brunstein's (2001) empirical work offers a useful way to approach defense mechanisms. Their research shows that the congruence or incongruence between conscious and unconscious strivings impacts emotional well-being. Simply put, we benefit from increased consistency between our implicit and explicit goals, and increased awareness of unconscious strivings may be used to develop greater consistency. Table 14.1 provides a summary of common defense mechanisms.

Figure 14.3 shows how defenses can be exasperatingly impervious to external evidence. Confronting them can sometimes backfire and result in increased manifestations of the very same defenses. In the figure, the man is labeling the cat's aggressive behavior. He is interpreting fears and conflicts underlying the cat's aggression. His invitation to the cat to think about the meaning of the aggression leads the cat to attack him.

The clinical dilemma of pointing out defense mechanisms is humorously illustrated by the man's continued reading that the cat would likely react with hostility. Timing and delivery are everything in this type of work. Additionally, he seems oblivious to the cat's rising anger and to the evidence of the attack (e.g., the torn clothes, broken glasses, etc.). The work of a good therapist involves careful observation of the patient's mental state and behaviors to

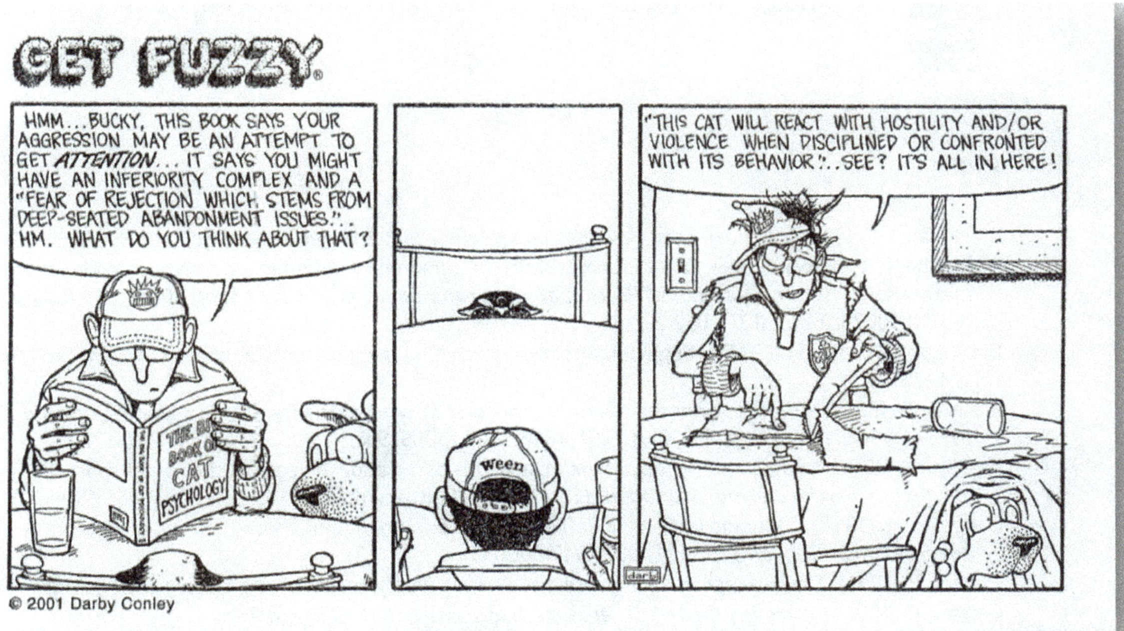

FIGURE 14.3 Illustration showing the risk of confrontation exacerbating the use of defense.

Copyright © 2001 by Andrews McMeel Universal.

inform the movement of the work. Ironically, the dog is more tuned in to the events at hand, noticing the cat's rising anger, and hiding under the table for protection.

SUMMARY

Defense mechanisms are mental processes that allow us to cope with the inescapable vulnerabilities we experience throughout life. While these mental processes may serve us well, there may be patterns in the use of defenses that may be problematic and impair functioning. As clinicians, our ability to recognize these patterns allows us to better understand how our patients function psychologically and emotionally and use that understanding in how we approach the work. With time, patients may begin to tolerate their disavowed experiences more and have more conscious control over how they show up in their lives and the world.

RESOURCES

1 https://www.youtube.com/watch?v=WfeLzjqXemw

2 https://www.youtube.com/watch?v=9bHm8_kq3DA

3 https://www.psychologistworld.com/freud/defence-mechanisms-list

REFERENCES

Blackman, J. S. (2004). *101 defenses: How the mind shields itself.* Brunner-Routledge.

Bornstein, R. F., & Gold, S. H. (2008). Comorbidity of personality disorders and somatization disorder: A meta-analytic review. *Journal of Psychopathology and Behavioral Assessment, 30*(2), 154. https://doi.org/10.1007/s10862-007-9052-2

Braun, B. G. (1988). The BASK (behavior, affect, sensation, knowledge) model of dissociation. *Dissociation, 1*, 4–23.

Brenner, C. (2002). Conflict, compromise formation, and structural theory. *Psychoanalytic Quarterly, 71*(3), 397–418. https://doi.org/10.1002/j.2167-4086.2002.tb00519.x

Busch, F. N. (1997). Understanding the patient's use of free association: An ego psychological approach. *Journal of American Psychoanalytic Association, 45*(2), 407–424. https://doi.org/10.1177/00030651970450020701

Cooper, S. H. (1998). Changing notions of defense within psychoanalytic theory. *Journal of Personality, 66*(6), 947-964. https://doi.org/10.1111/1467-6494.00038

Cramer, P. (1991). *The development of defense mechanism: Theory, research, and assessment.* Springer-Verlag.

Cramer, P. (2006). *Protecting the self: Defense mechanisms in action.* Guilford Press.

Freud, A. (1966). *The ego and mechanism of defense* (revised ed.). International University Press.

Freud, S. (1894). The neuro-psychosis of defense. *Standard Edition, 3*, 45–61. Hogarth Press.

Hartmann, H. (1939). *Ego psychology and the problem of adaptation.* International Universities Press.

Kernberg, O. (1967). Borderline personality organization. *Journal of the American Psychoanalytic Association, 15*(3), 641–684. https://doi.org/10.1177/000306516701500309

Klein, M. (1946). Notes on some schizoid mechanisms. *International Journal of Psycho-Analysis, 27,* 99–110.

Kohut, H. (1977). *The restoration of the self.* International Universities Press.

McWilliams, N. (1994/2011). *Psychoanalytic diagnosis: Understanding personality structure in the clinical process.* Guilford Press

Schulthesis, O. C., & Brunstein, J. C. (2001). Assessment of implicit motives with a research version of the TAT: Picture profiles, gender differences, and relations to other personality measures. *Journal of Personality Assessment, 77*(1), 71–86. https://doi.org/10.1207/S15327752JPA7701_05

Stoute, B. J. (2021). Black rage: The adaptation to the trauma of oppression. *Journal of American Psychoanalytic Association, 69*(2), 259–290. https://doi.org/10.1177/00030651211014207

Valliant, G. E. (1992). *Ego mechanisms of defense: A guide for clinicians and researchers.* American Psychiatric Association.

Valliant, G. E. (2000) Adaptive mental mechanisms. *American Psychologist, 55*(1), 89–98. https://doi.org/10.1037/0003-066X.55.1.89

Vaillant, G. E., Bond, M., & Vaillant, C. O. (1986). An empirically validated hierarchy of defense mechanisms. *Archives of General Psychiatry, 43*(8), 786–794.

Williams, G. W. (1963). Highway hypnosis: An hypothesis. *International Journal of Clinical and Experimental Hypnosis, 11*(3), 143–151.

UNIT III

CLINICAL PRESENTATION OF PSYCHIATRIC DISORDERS

This unit is at the core of psychiatric diagnoses. Each chapter covers a specific set of diagnoses outlined in the fifth edition of the diagnostic and statistical manual of mental disorders, (*DSM-5*; APA, 2013). While comprehensive in content, the authors have created useful figures and tables to understand disease processes and treatment. Check out the case vignettes in each chapter, which illustrate a patient's journey and experience with their disorder and treatment. Key points help identify the main points. Clinical tips give pointers to the busy clinician. Useful mnemonics are included to help facilitate easy retention and recall of important aspects of the diagnoses. Quick points contain fun facts about the conditions.

CHAPTER 15

Autism Spectrum Disorder[1]

M. Frampton Gwynette, M.D. and Emily E. Whisler, D.O.

> *"If you've met one person with autism, you've met one person with autism."*
>
> — Stephen Shore

OBJECTIVES

After reading this chapter, students will be able to do the following:

- obtain a working knowledge of the clinical presentation, diagnosis, and treatment of patients with autism spectrum disorder (ASD)
- describe common comorbid conditions in individuals with ASD
- discuss medical conditions common in patients with ASD

DEFINITIONS AND KEY CONCEPTS

ASD is a condition characterized by deficits in communication and social interaction in addition to patterns of restricted or repetitive interests, behaviors, and activities. This constellation of symptoms results in significant social, educational, and vocational impairment.

INTRODUCTION

ASD is among the most complex conditions in medicine. It impacts the brain in myriad ways, including brain growth, anatomy, connectivity, and information processing, among many others. Autism impacts nearly every organ system and the function in the body, including gross and fine motor coordination, sensory processing, the central nervous system, and

1 Readers may also see "Speech and Language Development" (Chapter 12) for related material.

the GI tract. ASD is often accompanied by other co-occurring psychiatric conditions, most commonly ADHD, mood disorders, anxiety disorder, and insomnia, but also many others.

EPIDEMIOLOGY

ASD impacts one in 54 children in the United States (Maenner et al., 2020). By some counts, it is as many as one in 39 (Zablotsky et al., 2017). ASD prevalence has been rising during the last several decades; the cause for this increase appears to be multifaceted—a combination of genetic and environmental factors. ASD is mostly a lifelong condition, and therefore, the prevalence of adults with ASD is also on the rise with 50,000 individuals with ASD becoming adults each year in the United States. Importantly, there is no evidence that vaccines cause ASD (Flaherty 2011).

QUICK POINT

Nearly one in five individuals with ASD have a known genetic risk factor. Genetic testing is therefore recommended in individuals with ASD. This includes chromosomal microarray testing, as well as testing for fragile X syndrome, to identify genetic mutations that may be contributing to the clinical presentations.

Nearly 20% of individuals with ASD have a known genetic risk factor (Schaefer & Mendelsohn, 2013). It is therefore recommended that all individuals with ASD have chromosomal microarray testing, as well as testing for fragile X syndrome, to identify genetic mutations that may be contributing to the clinical presentations (Muhle et al., 2017). Genetic testing can identify genes that can independently or in combination with other genes cause specific types of ASD (Muhle et al., 2018). Additionally, genetic testing is valuable in clarifying potential treatment pathways for patients according to the underlying genetic origins of their ASD. As an option, please see this brief educational video for a summary of the importance of identifying ASD-associated genes in the advancement of developing customized treatments for patients (Icahn School of Medicine, 2020).

The Benefits of Genetic Testing in Autism

WATCH AT https://www.youtube.com/watch?v=b9nCihlhhk0

Environmental factors can also be associated with ASD. These include advanced parental age (> 40 years for mothers and > 50 years for fathers) and prenatal or perinatal complications, such as maternal metabolic conditions, maternal diabetes or hypertension, infection, umbilical cord accidents, prematurity, low birth weight, hyperbilirubinemia, and numerous others (Lord et al., 2018).

NEUROPATHOLOGY

Numerous differences exist in brain anatomy and connectivity, head size, and other parts of the central nervous system, including nerve connections in the GI tract and nerve connections in the gut. Children with ASD have an abnormal brain growth trajectory, initially characterized by brain overgrowth beginning at approximately 12 months of age until 24 months (Carper & Courchesne, 2005), at which time the growth transitions to a regressive pattern (Hiremath et al., 2021). Further differences exist in the microbiota–gut–brain axis, as compared to typically developing individuals (Srikantha & Mohajeri, 2019).

CLINICAL MANIFESTATIONS

The clinical manifestations of ASD comprise two fundamental areas (American Psychiatric Association [APA], 2013). The first is *impaired social or communication skills*, resulting in difficulty relating to others. For example, individuals may have trouble identifying with peers, hampering their ability to make and keep friends. Social or communication deficits manifest in diverse ways, including poor eye contact, speech delays or being nonverbal, and limited facial expressions or tonality of voice. Deficits can also be more subtle, such as those found in pragmatic speech (i.e., not knowing what to say in a particular social situation). For example, individuals with ASD may have a limited ability to "shift gears" to communicate differently with peers versus teachers.

KEY POINT

The clinical manifestations of ASD comprise two fundamental areas: impaired social/communication skills resulting in difficulty relating to others and restricted or repetitive interests, behaviors, or activities.

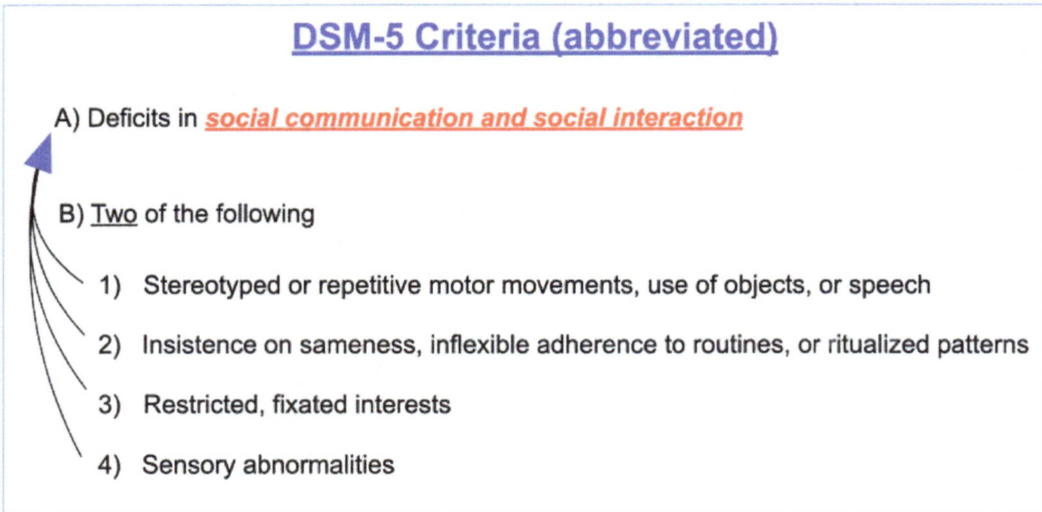

FIGURE 15.1 Abbreviated listing of *DSM-5* criteria with arrows noting the feedback phenomenon whereby criterion B symptoms potentially further impair social communication and social interaction (criterion A).

Adapted from American Psychiatric Association, Diagnostic and Statistical Manual of Mental Disorders. Copyright © 2013 by American Psychiatric Association Publishing. Adapted by M. Frampton Gwynette and Emily E. Whisler.

The second area of clinical manifestations in ASD consists of *restricted or repetitive interests, behaviors, or activities.*

- *Restricted or repetitive interests*—Patients frequently focus on one area of interest. The particular interest or degree of intensity can be unusual when compared to typically developing peers. For example, having a fascination with insects or dinosaurs is developmentally appropriate at age 5; however, increasing intensity of interest may advance from the fascination to extreme perseveration. Unusual topics of interest are also common and may be observed in a child's captivation with weather or train schedules.
- *Restricted or repetitive behaviors*—Order and routine are often important and may be inflexible to a degree that makes changes in the environment intolerable, triggering intense emotional outbursts and/or physical aggression. An individual may require stuffed animals to be organized in a specific order or may engage in ritualistic behaviors, such as a bedtime routine that must be pursued nightly in the same order. A disruption in the procedure can incite anxiety and behavioral disturbances; however, strict pursuance of these desires has the potential to impede other areas of life.
- *Restricted or repetitive activities*—"Stimming," or stereotyped movements, are repetitive movements, such as rocking, hand flapping, and turning lights on and off. One reason patients may do this is to self-sooth. Certain stimming activities are self-injurious in nature and may present with head banging, picking, or biting.

- *Sensory abnormalities*—This is hyper- or hypo-reactivity to sensory input or unusual interest in sensory aspects of the environment, including sensitivity to textures (e.g., food, tooth brushing, or clothing), sounds (e.g., loud noises are problematic), smells, or bright lights.

DIAGNOSIS

Diagnosis of ASD is made by applying the criteria listed in the APA's *Diagnostic and Statistical Manual* and determining whether, in the clinician's judgment, the patient is experiencing significant *impairment* in the areas listed. There are formal tests available to aid in the diagnosis of ASD, including the autism diagnostic observation schedule and the autism diagnostic interview, revised. Both are standardized evaluations designed to have high sensitivity and specificity to be administered by evaluators with specialized training and are normed against standards for reliability. Ultimately, the diagnosis of ASD is made using clinical judgment, rather than psychological tests, lab tests, or brain imaging.

Early diagnosis, with the goal of implementing early intervention, is critical. Parental concerns about ASD in their child should be taken seriously to ensure timely referrals and formal screening for ASD can be made. Screening instruments, such as the M-CHAT, can be reliably predictive of ASD as young as 18 months of age (Havdahl et al., 2017).

TREATMENT

Biological Treatments

There are no evidence-based or FDA-approved biological treatments for core ASD symptoms. Multiple agents are currently being investigated for the treatment of core ASD symptoms, but it remains to be seen whether randomized, double-blind, or placebo-controlled studies will prove efficacy for these potential therapies.

The antipsychotics aripiprazole and risperidone are FDA approved for the treatment of *irritability associated with ASD* in children ages 6 to 17, but irritability is not a core ASD symptom (see *DSM-5* criteria). These two agents, therefore, address a comorbid psychiatric condition, rather than ASD itself. There is emerging evidence that physical activity may be beneficial for social interaction and communication and decrease autism severity in children with ASD (Huang et al., 2020; Toscano et al., 2018). There are no

KEY POINT

The diagnosis of ASD is made by applying the *DSM-V* criteria and determining whether, in the clinician's judgment, the patient is experiencing significant *impairment* in the areas listed. Available standardized tests for aiding the diagnosis of ASD include the autism diagnostic observation schedule (ADOS-2) and the autism diagnostic interview, revised (ADI-R).

MEMORY TIP

Autism, *useful mnemonic*

AUTISTICS

A—Again, and again (repetitive behavior or speech)
U—Unusual (hyper or hypo) reactivity to sensory aspects
T—Toddlers (starts during early development)
I—Insistence on sameness and inflexible adherence to routines; interests are restricted and abnormal in intensity or focus
S—Socioemotional reciprocity deficits
T—To relate with others is a difficulty
I—Impairment in social, occupational, or other functioning
C—Communication (nonverbal) poor for social interaction
S—Social communication below that expected for general development; that is, not due to intellectual disability

(Akunjee, 2009)

evidence-based treatments using nutrition or complementary or alternative medicines for core ASD symptoms. Gluten-free and casein-free diets for children with ASD have been researched extensively, but efficacy data remains insufficient (Alamri, 2020; Piwowarczyk et al., 2018). Brain stimulation, specifically repetitive transcranial magnetic stimulation (rTMS), has emerging data for the treatment of patients with ASD, but treatment protocols and rigorous trials are pending (Cole et al., 2018).

KEY POINT

Applied behavioral analysis (ABA) is a type of therapy that has been adapted for use with success in patients with ASD. ABA therapy involves focused study on the function of behaviors. Patients are rewarded using positive reinforcement for appropriate behaviors, while inappropriate behaviors are not reinforced.

Psychological Treatments

Given the lack of evidence-based biological treatments, behavioral interventions are the bedrock of any successful treatment for patients with ASD. Applied behavioral analysis (ABA) is a type of therapy that has been adapted for use with success in patients with ASD. ABA therapy involves focused study on the functioning of behaviors and intense training on specific skills, such as using speech, making eye contact, and completing academic tasks. Patients are rewarded using positive reinforcement for appropriate behaviors, while inappropriate behaviors are not reinforced.

Antecedent	Behavior	Consequence
Classwork	Aggression	Time on iPad
Classwork	Complete Classwork	Time on iPad

FIGURE 15.2 Summary of applied behavioral analysis (ABA) therapy. In the first example, the patient responds to the antecedent (a request to complete classwork) by becoming aggressive with the goal to escape from classwork and receive time on an iPad. In the second example, the patient responds to the request to complete classwork appropriately, thereby earning time on the iPad. In this case, time on the iPad is used to reinforce the appropriate behavior or completing the classwork as requested.

ABA therapy has been adapted into multiple ABA-based therapy interventions, mostly for very young children. These include early intensive behavioral interventions (EIBI), the early start Denver model (ESDM), and pivotal response treatment (PRT). PRT is among the most studied behavioral interventions for autism with the literature indicating benefit for communication and social function (Mohammadzaheri et al., 2014). Designed as a naturalistic intervention, it focuses on unstructured play and a child's internal motivation and particular set of interests to foster prosocial behaviors. This therapy not only aims to encourage positive behaviors and communication but in so doing also diminish disruptive ones (Mohammadzaheri et al., 2015). Interventionists utilize a child's chosen toy or activity as a source of motivation in eliciting desired behaviors, which are then reinforced with access to the chosen object. For example, if a child wants to play with a ball and verbally requests or attempts with good effort, they are then given the ball as a reward (Koegel et al., 1999).

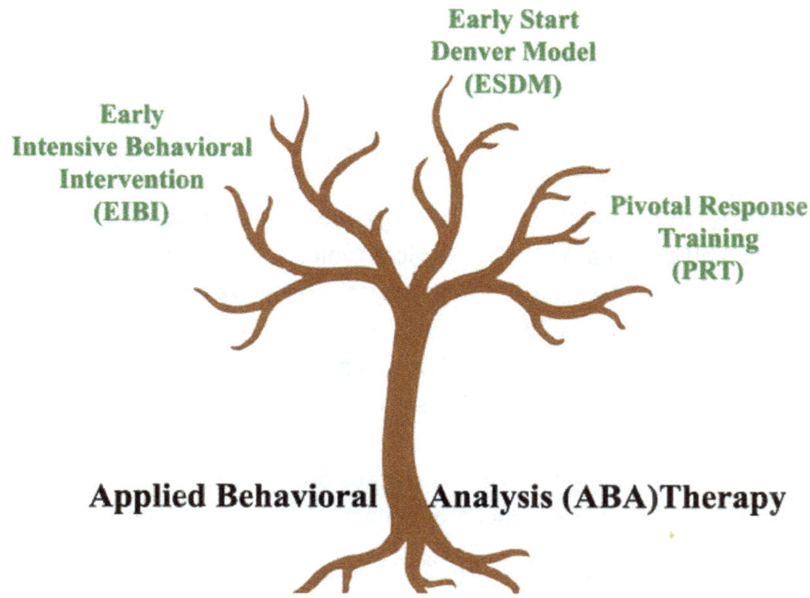

FIGURE 15.3 Diagram showing several offshoots of ABA therapy.

Source: Adapted from https://pixabay.com/vectors/tree-branch-bare-winter-autumn-307047/ by M. Frampton Gwynette and Emily E. Whisler.

Cognitive behavioral therapy (CBT) is evidence-based for the treatment of anxiety disorders for patients with ASD (Sukhodolsky et al., 2013; Wood et al., 2015). The CBT protocol is modified in order to accommodate individuals with ASD.

Social skills training (SST) is a treatment modality, usually delivered in group settings with peers, that aims to help patients with ASD make and keep friends. Parent involvement is an important component, as parent-assisted models of SST have demonstrated significant treatment effects that generalize from the clinic into everyday life and also show long-lasting improvement in social skills (Laugeson et al., 2015; Mandelberg et al., 2014).

Individuals with ASD also frequently receive other therapy services, including speech therapy, physical therapy, and occupational therapy. These services are important components to a successful treatment plan, aiding in language development, gross motor coordination, and fine motor coordination, respectively.

Technology, including tablets, smartphones, wearables, virtual reality, and even humanoid robots, have demonstrated promise in areas such as social skills training, language development, advancing executive skills, and academic achievement for patients with ASD (Gwynette et al., 2018). Technology also has the potential to enhance safety for patients with ASD who either elope or wander—some of the most dangerous behaviors exhibited by these patients. Utilization of technology significantly reduces the likelihood and the emotional toll of elopement or wandering for families (McLaughlin et al., 2020).

Social Interventions

Each individual state in the United States has its own agency or board through which services for patients with ASD are allocated. Clinical interventions, especially for very young children (as young as 12–18 months of age) and case management services typically run through the state's disability board. It is important for clinicians to ensure that the patient's family has made contact with the state's disability board and is working actively with a case manager to establish prompt screening, diagnosis, and delivery of clinical services as early as possible. Notably, the average length of time between the parents' concerns and a diagnosis of ASD is three years (Siklos & Kerns 2007); provider advocacy on behalf of the patient to shorten this wait time can significantly impact long-term outcomes.

Patients with ASD often benefit from school accommodations in the form of academic assistance, behavioral support, speech therapy, bullying prevention, or other focused interventions. An individual education plan (IEP) is the mechanism whereby students with ASD receive school accommodations. Accommodations are essential for two critical areas: behavioral challenges, academic challenges, or both. Due to finite resources within school systems, the child's family and providers often need to play an active role in advocating for accommodations, especially as the child approaches adulthood. IEP meetings routinely occur annually; however, more frequent meetings are available as needed. Importantly, all IEP meetings should be held in the parents' native language or with an interpreter.

QUICK POINT

As a youth with ASD approach legal adulthood, the family needs to carefully consider the child's capacity for medical, legal, and financial decision-making with respect to potential guardianship of the patient.

As a youth with ASD approach 18 years of age, the family needs to carefully consider the child's capacity for medical, legal, and financial decision-making with respect to potential guardianship of the patient. When needed, providers can refer families to a special needs and family attorney to explore options for guardianship, power of attorney, and other legal pathways with the goal of optimizing the welfare and safety of their patients with ASD. Notably, individuals with ASD will by default retain their legal rights upon turning 18, and a significant percentage are capable of making their own decisions and handling their affairs without assistance.

Providers have the opportunity to improve clinical outcomes for patients with ASD by serving foremost in the role of champion for the patient. Leading the coordination of the complexities of the patient's care plan, frequently communicating with other providers, and serving as a navigator for the family will ease their burden as they make their way over the complex landscape of autism services.

CLINICAL TIP

Patients with ASD have a high prevalence of comorbid medical conditions with epilepsy being predominant (occurring in approximately 30% of patients)(Tuchman, 2010,). Other conditions include hypertension, diabetes mellitus, obesity, irritable bowel syndrome, and constipation.

Medical Considerations

Patients with ASD have a high prevalence of comorbid medical conditions with epilepsy being predominant (occurring in approximately 30% of patients) (Tuchman, 2010). Numerous other conditions, including hypertension, diabetes mellitus, obesity, irritable bowel syndrome, and constipation, are commonplace. In fact, gastrointestinal abnormalities have been noted to be four times more likely in patients with ASD (Marler et al., 2017), possibly due to variations in the gut microbiome (Srikantha & Mohajeri, 2019). These higher rates of medical morbidity contribute to more dire consequences, with patients with ASD suffering a decreased life expectancy of on average 16 years shorter than typically developing individuals.

CLINICAL TIP

For individuals with ASD, when it comes to psychiatric illness, comorbidity is the rule, rather than the exception. ADHD, anxiety, mood disorders, insomnia, and multiple others are found in significantly higher rates when compared to typically developing individuals. Patients with ASD are often refractory or have adverse reactions to standard treatments, thus requiring a thoughtful and measured approach on the part of treating clinicians.

Comorbid Psychiatric Conditions

Individuals with ASD have exceedingly high rates of comorbid psychiatric conditions, to the extent that comorbidity is the rule, rather than the exception. ADHD, anxiety, mood disorders, insomnia, and multiple others are found in significantly higher rates when compared to typically developing individuals. Patients with ASD are often refractory or have adverse reactions to standard treatments for the aforementioned conditions, thus requiring a thoughtful and measured approach on the part of treating clinicians. For example, children with ASD are more likely to experience irritability when prescribed stimulant medications for the treatment of ADHD compared to typically developing children. In addition, patients with ASD are more likely to become anxious or activated when prescribed antidepressants for the treatment of depressive or anxiety disorders.

CASE VIGNETTE

Oscar is a 9-year-old male who presents to the child and adolescent psychiatry clinic for evaluation. He is a very bright young boy with normal language skills. He is in all regular classes at school and is performing well academically. He has a history of ADHD, which was treated with long-acting methylphenidate for 1 year. According to pretreatment and posttreatment ADHD rating scales completed by the parent and teacher, Oscar is responding well to the methylphenidate. He does experience some midday decreased appetite and has had mild weight loss since starting the medication. Oscar also has difficulty falling asleep and wakes up one to two times during the night, but this has not changed since the methylphenidate was started.

Oscar struggles socially and has few, if any, friends. When he tries to play with other children in public places, such as parks or playgrounds, Oscar is often excluded by his peers, who say that he is "weird" or "talks too much about random things." Oscar has not been invited to a birthday party or a playdate, aside from family members. At school, Oscar is frequently teased by other children, causing him to become angry and aggressive at times, especially on the school playground. Oscar's peers at school now seem to take pleasure in triggering Oscar to become agitated just so they can laugh at his reaction.

In recent months, Oscar has been telling his mother that he would be better off dead and that he wishes he had sharp teeth and claws, so he could harm the children at school who tease him. This is anxiety-provoking for Oscar's family, since he had previously been a happy child who had never been aggressive.

Oscar is preoccupied with unusual topics for a child his age, such as World War II and UFOs. He enjoys reading and watching videos online about these topics. Given the opportunity, Oscar will turn conversations toward these topics and talk exhaustively about them, not noticing if his conversation partner appears uninterested.

Oscar struggles with changes in his daily routine, becoming frustrated if there is a substitute teacher or if his parents change the family's weekend plans on short notice. At school, Oscar seems especially hyperactive and often requires redirection when transitioning between activities, such as academic classes and recess. Oscar has some sensory abnormalities, including sensitivity to loud noises, various smells and food textures, and an aversion to coarse textures on clothing.

On exam, Oscar mentions that he wants to have friends but that other children just do not seem to like him. He states that he sees no purpose in continuing to live but has no active suicidal or homicidal plans. He has intense interest in fantasy life, wishing he could visit UFOs, but he does not experience psychotic symptoms. Oscar speaks quite clearly, makes minimal eye contact, and seems to have an unusual tone of voice without the normal inflections one might expect.

QUESTIONS ON CASE VIGNETTE

1. Does Oscar meet criteria for ASD?

   In the scenario, a strong case can be made that Oscar does have ASD. He has significant impairment in social skills and his communication with others, while fluid from a language standpoint, is not ideal, given his poor eye contact and unusual intonation while speaking. He also meets multiple criteria for restricted and repetitive interests, behaviors, and activities, given his intense interest in World War II and UFOs, his sensory abnormalities, and his inflexibility with respect to daily routines and schedules. So, according to DSM-5 *criteria, Oscar does have ASD.*

2. How should the social skills deficits be addressed?

   Given his apparently intact cognitive ability, Oscar is a good candidate for social skills training in a group setting. The goals of this treatment would be to help Oscar develop social reciprocity and improve his ability to make and keep friends.

3. As Oscar's psychiatrist, would you want to speak with his teachers or other school staff? If so, what would be the goal for this communication?

   Collaboration with Oscar's school staff would be a very good idea. The goals of this communication would include educating the school about Oscar's diagnosis of ASD, ADHD, depressive symptoms, and suicidal ideation. Additionally, the provider can assist the family in requesting an urgent IEP meeting to address the behavioral challenges Oscar is experiencing. Furthermore, the provider can work to ensure that the school is aware of the bullying toward Oscar, so they can take concrete steps to prevent Oscar from being excluded, teased, or provoked at school. Finally, the provider can recommend that the school consult with the district's autism itinerant in order to develop a comprehensive behavioral plan for Oscar, thereby minimizing his disruptive behaviors during times of transition at school.

4. If Oscar's agitation and aggression worsen to the point that he is hitting peers at school, he may be in danger of getting expelled. What medication(s) might be an option for the treatment of aggression and irritability in the context of ASD?

   Provided that the underlying cause(s) for Oscar's irritability and aggression has been addressed (e.g., bullying), a trial on either risperidone or aripiprazole is reasonable. After detailed discussion with the family regarding potential risks and benefits of medication, starting a low dose of either medication and monitoring closely for side effects, especially increased appetite, weight gain, and abnormal involuntary movements, may be prudent.

SUMMARY

ASD is among the most complex conditions in medicine. It is characterized by deficits in communication and social interaction in addition to patterns of restricted or repetitive interests, behaviors, and activities. The prevalence of ASD has been steadily increasing over the past few decades. ASD is mostly a lifelong condition; therefore, the prevalence of adults with ASD is also on the rise with 50,000 individuals with ASD becoming adults each year in the United States. Currently, for core ASD symptoms, there are no evidence-based or FDA-approved biological treatments. The antipsychotics aripiprazole and risperidone are FDA approved for the treatment of *irritability associated with ASD* in children ages 6 to 17. Applied behavioral analysis (ABA) is a type of psychotherapy that has been adapted for use with success in patients with ASD. Other evidence-based therapies include CBT and SST. Supportive services, including physical therapy and occupational therapy, are important components to a successful treatment plan, aiding in language development, gross motor coordination, and fine motor coordination, respectively. Electronic technology, including tablets, smartphones, wearables, virtual reality, and even humanoid robots, have demonstrated promise in areas such as social skills training, language development, advancing executive skills, and academic achievement for patients with ASD (Gwynette et al., 2018).

RESOURCES

1 For additional resources, please see the Autism/Intellectual Disability resources page on the American Academy of Child and Adolescent Psychiatry (AACAP) website. The page contains teaching videos, practice parameters, and links to articles, texts and other resources curated by the American Academy of Child and Adolescent Psychiatry Autism and Intellectual Committee.

REFERENCES

Akunjee, M., Jalali, S., & Siddiqui, S. (2009). Development assessment, paediatrics. In: *The easy guide to OSCEs for specialties: A step-by-step guide to OSCE success* (pp. 139–140). Radcliffe Publishing Ltd.

Alamri, E. S. (2020). Efficacy of gluten- and casein-free diets on autism spectrum disorders in children. *Saudi Medical Journal, 41*(10), 1041–1046.

American Psychiatric Association. (2013). *Diagnostic and statistical manual of mental disorders* (5th ed.).

Carper, R. A., & Courchesne, E. (2005). Localized enlargement of the frontal cortex in early autism. *Biological Psychiatry, 57*(2), 126–133.

Cole, E. J., Enticott, P. G., Oberman, L. M., Gwynette, M. F. Casanova, M. F., Jackson, S. L. J., Jannati, A., McPartland, J. C., Naples, A. J., & Puts, N. A. J. (2018). The potential of repetitive transcranial magnetic stimulation for autism spectrum disorder: A consensus statement. *Biological Psychiatry, 85*(4), e21–e22.

Flaherty, D. K. (2011). The vaccine–autism connection: A public health crisis caused by unethical medical practices and fraudulent science. *Annals of Pharmacotherapy, 45*(10), 1302–1304.

Gwynette, M. F., Sidhu, S. S., & Ceranoglu, T. A. (2018). Electronic screen media use in youth with autism spectrum disorder. *Child and Adolescent Psychiatric Clinics of North America, 27*(2), 203–219.

Havdahl, K. A., Bishop, S. L., Surén, P., Øyen, A. S., Lord, C., Pickles, A., von Tetzchner, S. Schjølberg, S., Gunnes, N., Hornig, M., Lipkin, W. I., Susser, E., Bresnahan, M., Magnus, P., Stenberg, N., Reichborn-Kjennerud, T., & Stoltenberg, C. (2017). The influence of parental concern on the utility of autism diagnostic instruments. *Autism Research, 10*(10), 1672–1686.

Hiremath, C. S., Sagar, K. J. V., Yamini, B. K., Girimaji, A. S., Kumar, R., Sravanti, S. L., Padmanabha, H., Vykunta Raju, K. N., Kishore, M. T., Jacob, P., Saini, J., Bharath, R. D., Seshadri, S. P., & Kumar, M. (2021). Emerging behavioral and neuroimaging biomarkers for early and accurate characterization of autism spectrum disorders: A systematic review. *Translational Psychiatry, 11*(1), 42.

Huang, J., Du, C., Liu, J., & Tan, C. (2020). Meta-analysis on intervention effects of physical activities on children and adolescents with autism. *International Journal of Environmental Research and Public Health, 17*(6), https://www.doi.org/10.3390/ijerph17061950

Koegel, L. K., Koegel, R. L., Harrower, J. K., & Carter, C. M. (1999). Pivotal response intervention I: Overview of approach. *Journal of the Association for Persons with Severe Handicaps, 24*(3), 174–185. https://doi.org/10.2511/rpsd.24.3.174

Kolevzon, A. (2020, October 7). *The benefits of genetic testing in autism* [Video]. YouTube. https://www.youtube.com/watch?v=b9nCihlhhk0

Laugeson, E. A., Gantman, A., Kapp, S. K., Orenski, K., & Ellingsen, R. (2015). A randomized controlled trial to improve social skills in young adults with autism spectrum disorder: The UCLA PEERS((R)) program. *Journal of Autism and Developmental Disorders, 45*(12), 3978–3989.

Lord, C., Elsabbagh, M., Baird, G., & Veenstra-Vanderweele, J. (2018). Autism spectrum disorder. *Lancet, 392*(10146), 508–520.

Maenner, M. J., Shaw, K. A., Baio, J., Washington, A., Patrick, M., DiRienzo, M., Christensen, D. L., Wiggins, L. D., Pettygrove, S., Andrews, J. G., Lopez, A., Hudson, A., Baroud, T., Schwenk, Y., White, T., Rosenberg, C. R., Lee, L. C., Harrington, R. A., Huston, M., . . . & Dietz, P. M. (2020). Prevalence of autism spectrum disorder among children aged 8 years. *MMWR Surveillance Summaries, 69*(4), 1–12.

Mandelberg, J., Frankel, F., Cunningham, T., Gorospe, C., & Laugeson, E. A. (2014). Long-term outcomes of parent-assisted social skills intervention for high-functioning children with autism spectrum disorders. *Autism, 18*(3), 255–263.

Marler, S., Ferguson, B. J., Lee, E. B., Peters, B., Williams, K. C., McDonnell, E., Macklin, E. A., Levitt, P., Margolis, K. G., Beversdorf, D. Q., & Veenstra-VanderWeele, J. (2017). Association of rigid-compulsive behavior with functional constipation in autism spectrum disorder. *Journal of Autism and Developmental Disorders, 47*(6), 1673–1681.

McLaughlin, L., Rapoport, E., Keim, S. A., & Adesman, A. (2020). Wandering by children with autism spectrum disorders: Impact of electronic tracking devices on elopement behavior and quality of life. *Journal of Developmental and Behavorial Pediatrics, 41*(7), 513–521.

Mohammadzaheri, F., Koegel, L. K., Rezaee, M., & Rafiee, S. M. (2014).. A randomized clinical trial comparison between pivotal response treatment (PRT) and structured applied behavior analysis (ABA) intervention for children with autism. *Journal of Autism and Developmental Disorders. 44*, 2769–2777 (2014). https://doi-org.ezproxy-v.musc.edu/10.1007/s10803-014-2137-3

Mohammadzaheri, F., Koegel, L., Rezaei, M., & Bakhshi, E. (2015). A randomized clinical trial comparison between pivotal response treatment (PRT) and adult-driven applied behavior analysis (ABA) intervention on disruptive behaviors in public school children with autism. *Journal of Autism and Developmental Disorders, 45*(9), 2899–2907. https://doi.org/10.1007/s10803-015-2451-4

Muhle, R. A., Reed, H. E., Stratigos, K. A., & Veenstra-VanderWeele, J. (2018). The emerging clinical neuroscience of autism spectrum disorder: A review. *JAMA Psychiatry, 75*(5), 514–523.

Muhle, R. A., Reed, H. E., Vo, L. C., Mehta, S., McGuire, K., Veenstra-VanderWeele, J., & Pedapati, E. (2017). Clinical diagnostic genetic testing for individuals with developmental disorders. *Journal of the American Academy of Child and Adolescent Psychiatry, 56*(11), 910–913.

Piwowarczyk, A., Horvath, A., Łukasik, J., Pisula, E., & Szajewska, H. (2018). Gluten- and casein-free diet and autism spectrum disorders in children: A systematic review. *European Journal of Nutrition, 57*(2), 433–440.

Schaefer, G. B., & Mendelsohn, N. J. (2013). Clinical genetics evaluation in identifying the etiology of autism spectrum disorders: 2013 guideline revisions. *Genetics in Medicine, 15*(5), 399–407.

Siklos, S., & Kerns, K. A. (2007). Assessing the diagnostic experiences of a small sample of parents of children with autism spectrum disorders. *Research in Developmental Disabilities, 28*(1), 9–22.

Srikantha, P., & Mohajeri, M. H. (2019). The possible role of the microbiota–gut–brain–axis in autism spectrum disorder. *International Journal of Molecular Sciences, 20*(9), 1–29.

Sukhodolsky, D. G., Bloch, M. H., Panza, K. E., & Reichow, B. (2013). Cognitive-behavioral therapy for anxiety in children with high-functioning autism: A meta-analysis. *Pediatrics, 132*(5), e1341–1350.

Toscano, C. V. A., Carvalho, H. M., & Ferreira, J. P. (2018). Exercise effects for children with autism spectrum disorder: Metabolic health, autistic traits, and quality of life. *Perceptual and Motor Skills, 125*(1), 126–146.

Tuchman, R., Cuccaro, M., & Alessandri, M. (2010). Autism and epilepsy: historical perspective. *Brain & development, 32*(9), 709–718. https://doi.org/10.1016/j.braindev.2010.04.008

Wood, J. J., Ehrenreich-May, J., Alessandri, M., Fujii, C., Renno, P., Laugeson, E., Piacentini, J. C., De Nadai, A. S., Arnold, E., Lewin, A. B., Murphy, T. K., & Storch, E. A. (2015). Cognitive behavioral therapy for early adolescents with autism spectrum disorders and clinical anxiety: A randomized, controlled trial. *Behavior Therapy, 46*(1), 7–19.

Zablotsky, B., Black, L. I., & Blumberg, S. J. (2017). Estimated prevalence of children with diagnosed developmental disabilities in the United States, 2014-2016. *NCHS Data Brief, 291*, 1–8.

CHAPTER 16

Attention-Deficit Hyperactivity Disorder (ADHD)[1]

Sindhu Idicula, M.D. and Edore Onigu-Otite, M.D.

> *"Everybody is a genius. But if you judge a fish by its ability to climb a tree, it will live its whole life believing that it is stupid."*
>
> — Albert Einstein

OBJECTIVES

After reading this chapter, students will be able to do the following:

- discuss clinical presentations of ADHD
- review the neurobiology of ADHD
- discuss treatment of ADHD within a biopsychosocial framework

CASE VIGNETTE

Sasha is an 8-year-old presenting with her family for ADHD. Upon diagnosis of ADHD she was started on a longer-acting methylphenidate in the morning. She tolerated the medication, and scales filled out by parents and teachers noted that the medication worked well at controlling her ADHD symptoms while it worked. However, it started working around 8:00 a.m. and would only last until 3:00 p.m., which was when school ended. For the rest of the day, she had worsened symptoms of inattention, hyperactivity, and impulsivity. After school, she had more fights with her little sister, needed frequent reminders to complete her chores, and was argumentative with her parents. The symptoms made it difficult to start and complete homework. Due to this, even though she excelled in her classwork, she had incomplete and missing homework, which brought down her overall

1 Readers may also see "Psychopharmacology" (Chapter 31) for related material.

grades. Upon seeing this information, the physician added a booster dose of a short-acting methylphenidate to be taken around 3:30 p.m. soon after Sarah got home from school. This booster dose added to the duration of the morning methylphenidate, covering Sasha through the rest of the evening. With this, she completed her homework in reasonable time, got along with her siblings, was obedient to her parents, and was a pleasure to deal with in and after school. Sasha's after-school behavior is now more manageable, and her parents have enrolled her in extracurricular activities, including dance and swimming, where she is happy and excelling.

DEFINITIONS AND KEY CONCEPTS

Attention-deficit/hyperactivity disorder (ADHD) is a neuropsychiatric disorder characterized by age-inappropriate problems with attention, impulsivity, and hyperactivity in a pattern that is ongoing and persistent. *Inattention* is the inability to sustain attention on tasks. People with inattention often wander off tasks and avoid, do not complete, or poorly complete tasks that require sustained attention. These problems are *not* due to a lack of understanding or a choice to not participate to defy authority. *Impulsivity* is the inability to inhibit behavioral impulses and thoughts. People with impulsivity have a hard time thinking before they speak or act. Choices they make are poorly thought out and sometimes based on immediate rewards. Individuals may take poorly thought-out decisions and make important decisions, which are sometimes based on immediate rewards without considering the longer-term consequences. *Hyperactivity* is the inability to be still. People with hyperactivity either move constantly or have an inner sense of restlessness or a perception of the need to move. Often, individuals are fidgety, may tap things, or talk a lot.

KEY POINT

ADHD consists of three clusters of symptoms, inattention, hyperactivity, and impulsivity. While hyperactivity is more visible and easier to spot, inattention is more challenging to detect, especially in gifted individuals. Impulsivity often contributes to poorly thought-out decisions and actions, often with social consequences.

INTRODUCTION

ADHD has a long history in medicine and psychiatry. The first publication on ADHD was in 1902 by British pediatrician Sir George Still (1902, 2006), who gave a series of lectures titled Some Abnormal Psychical Conditions in Children, which was later published in the *Lancet*. In this publication, he highlighted a core feature in this subset of children who had an abnormal incapacity for sustained attention without general impairment of intellect. Specifically, he described 43 children who had serious problems with sustained attention and self-regulation; were often aggressive, defiant, excessively emotional, or passionate; and seemed resistant to discipline.

QUICK POINT

In 1902 an article in the Lancet described a group of children who experienced serious problems with sustained attention and self-regulation; were often aggressive, defiant, excessively emotional, or passionate; and seemed resistant to discipline. They showed little inhibitory volition, and though their intellect was normal, they could not learn from the consequences of their actions. These findings could not be accounted for by any fault of environment (Still, 1902, 2006).

They showed little inhibitory volition, and though their intellect was normal, they could not learn from the consequences of their actions. He summarized this as an abnormal defect of moral control in children, which cannot be accounted for by any fault of environment (Still, 1902, 2006).

In 1937, at the Emma Pendleton Bradley Home for children in Rhode Island, psychiatrist Charles Bradley (1950) administered Benzedrine sulfate (a stimulant medication) to children diagnosed with behavioral disorders. After only a week, Bradley observed, a striking change in behavior occurred in the school activities of many of these children. Fifteen of the 30 children responded to Benzedrine by becoming distinctly subdued in their emotional responses—an improvement from the social viewpoint (Bradley, 1950).

In 1955, Ritalin, a stimulant drug, was first approved by the FDA. It was marketed as a "pep pill" stronger than caffeine but not quite as powerful as other stimulants, such as Benzedrine. It was indicated for use in adults with chronic fatigue, lethargy, and depressed states. In 1968, hyperkinetic impulse disorder was included in the *DSM-2*. In the 1980s the disorder evolved to specify that attention was involved, and over time hyperactivity became a subtype of ADHD that was not present for every individual. In the *DSM-3* and *DSM-4*, ADHD was under the category of disruptive behavior disorders. Since 2014, with the current *DSM-5*, ADHD is now categorized as a neurodevelopmental disorder with symptoms manifesting within the first 12 years of life and subtypes varying by the type of presentation (i.e., predominantly inattentive, hyperactive-impulsive, or combined presentations; Table 16.2, Figure 16.1).

Although ADHD symptoms start in childhood, some children are not diagnosed and may continue to have symptoms in adulthood. Children with ADHD may struggle to keep up in school activities or at home with chores. They may also struggle with relationships with other children and with their families. Adults may have consequences at their work and may struggle with romantic relationships, friendships, and with their families. On the other hand, individuals with ADHD can hyper focus on things that interest them. They can grow up to be highly driven adults with outstanding achievements and contributions to society. The life stories of individuals with ADHD highlight the critical importance of parenting, family, and community support in identifying and building on the strengths of the individual with ADHD. As with many disorders, early identification, comprehensive treatment, facilitation of normal developmental activities, the provision of avenues that promote success, and comorbid conditions play a pivotal role in the trajectory and life outcomes for individuals with ADHD (Bernardi et al., 2012; Franke et al., 2018). Although most adults with ADHD remain undiagnosed and untreated, many more are beginning treatment in adulthood with significant improvement in their lives. Attention to this condition, both in children and adults, can mitigate the challenges they face daily due to their condition with significant impact on their life trajectories.

EPIDEMIOLOGY

Population studies show the prevalence of ADHD is 6–9% in youth (i.e., children and adolescents) and 3–5% in adults. Approximately 6.1 million children in the United States had been diagnosed with ADHD. Boys are more likely to be diagnosed with ADHD than girls (12.9% compared to 5.6%), often due to the presence of more disruptive behaviors that are easily noticed by their parents or teachers. The average age of diagnosis is 7 years old, coinciding with the second grade. Boys are diagnosed with all subtypes of ADHD more often than girls. Girls, when diagnosed, are more often diagnosed with an inattentive type of ADHD (commonly called ADD). ADHD symptoms persist over time. At least two thirds of children diagnosed with ADHD continue to experience functionally impairing symptoms as adults. Many children who have ADHD may also have other mental, emotional, or behavioral disorders. Sixty-four percent have some comorbidity, with most having behavioral or conduct problems (52%), followed by anxiety (33%), depression (17%), autism spectrum disorders (14%), and Tourette syndrome (1%). Individuals with ADHD often have sleep problems (Craig et al, 2020; Stein et al., 2012). They are at higher risk of initiating substance use early and of developing substance use disorders (Bierhoff et al., 2019; Howard et al., 2020). Comorbidity studies indicate that neural executive control networks in ADHD may increase susceptibility to developing internet gaming disorders (Vally, 2020; Weinstein & Lejoyeux, 2020; Yen et al., 2017).

ADHD is both over- and underdiagnosed. This means many conditions are misdiagnosed as ADHD, while many individuals with ADHD do not get diagnosed. ADHD is a condition that persists into adulthood. A relative limitation of the diagnostic criteria is that it is more applicable to children than to adults. Clinical studies show that ADHD manifests more subtly in adults than children (Wender, 2001). Population surveys of adults showed full childhood criteria with current symptoms (2.6%), full childhood criteria without current symptoms (4.0%), and subthreshold childhood symptoms (7.5%; Kessler, 2006). Like childhood ADHD, more adult males are diagnosed with ADHD compared to females (OR of 1.6; Biederman, 2004a). Adult ADHD is highly comorbid with many other mental health disorders and associated with substantial role impairment (Kessler, 2006). Adults with ADHD have higher rates of dysthymia (OR of 7.5), bipolar disorder (OR of 7.4),

QUICK POINT

In the general population, the prevalence of ADHD is 6–9% in youth and 3–5% in adults. In children, boys are diagnosed with all subtypes of ADHD more often than girls. Girls, when diagnosed, are more often diagnosed with an inattentive type of ADHD (commonly called ADD). ADHD symptoms persist over time. At least two thirds of children diagnosed with ADHD continue to experience functionally impairing symptoms as adults.

CLINICAL TIP

ADHD is a condition that is both over- and underdiagnosed. This means many conditions are misdiagnosed as ADHD, while many individuals with ADHD do not get diagnosed. About 30% of children with ADHD are diagnosed prior to the age of 6. The average age of diagnosis is 7 years old, coinciding with the second grade. ADHD is a condition that often persists into adulthood but may change the way it manifests.

and major depressive disorder (OR of 2.7). They also have higher rates of anxiety disorders (OR of 1.5–5.5), substance disorders (OR of 1.5–7.9), intermittent explosive disorder (OR of 3.7; Kessler, 2006), and personality disorders, suicide risk, and suicide attempts (Beauchaine, 2020; Biederman, 2004b). Adult ADHD/ADD is associated with poorer social outcomes including higher college dropout rates, poorer job performance, difficulty sustaining employment, lower wages than peers of similar intelligence, poor credit history, and financial stress.

QUICK POINT

ADHD manifests more subtly in adults than children. Population surveys of adults showed full childhood criteria with current symptoms (2.6%), full childhood criteria without current symptoms (4.0%), and subthreshold childhood symptoms (7.5%; Kessler, 2006). Like childhood ADHD, more adult males are diagnosed with ADHD compared to females. Adult ADHD/ADD is associated with poorer social outcomes, including higher college dropout rates, poorer job performance, difficulty sustaining employment, lower wages than peers of similar intelligence, poor credit history, and financial stress.

NEUROPATHOLOGY

ADHD has a complex etiology, and there is not a single pathophysiological entity that is common for all individuals who have it. At the core, ADHD individuals differ in specific region sizes and maturation of the brain. MRI show specific brain areas, including the prefrontal cortex, the striatum, the caudate and putamen in the basal ganglia, and the cerebellum, are smaller in individuals with ADHD when compared to individuals without ADHD. These differences are more prominent in childhood, suggesting delayed brain development (Hoogman et al., 2017). Electroencephalography studies show increased slow-wave activity in the PFC, which is linked to a state of hypoarousal. More evidence is emerging about reduced connectivity in white matter tracts. The science from genetics, pharmacology, imaging, and animal models all point to dopamine dysfunction in the brains of those with ADHD. Current theories are growing to support a model, where multiple genetic and environmental factors interact during early development, creating a susceptibility to the disorder, and a variety of changes in neural networks lead to deficits in neuropsychological functioning, leading to the expression of the disorder. Neurochemically, ADHD reflects a deficit of dopamine in the interneural spaces. Contributing to this, although less impactful, are differences in norepinephrine and serotonin. Figure 16.1 depicts brain areas involved in ADHD and the corresponding symptoms.

KEY POINT

Studies show specific brain areas, including the prefrontal cortex, the striatum, the caudate and putamen in the basal ganglia, and the cerebellum, are smaller in individuals with ADHD when compared to individuals without ADHD. These differences are more prominent in childhood, while some become more comparable by adulthood.

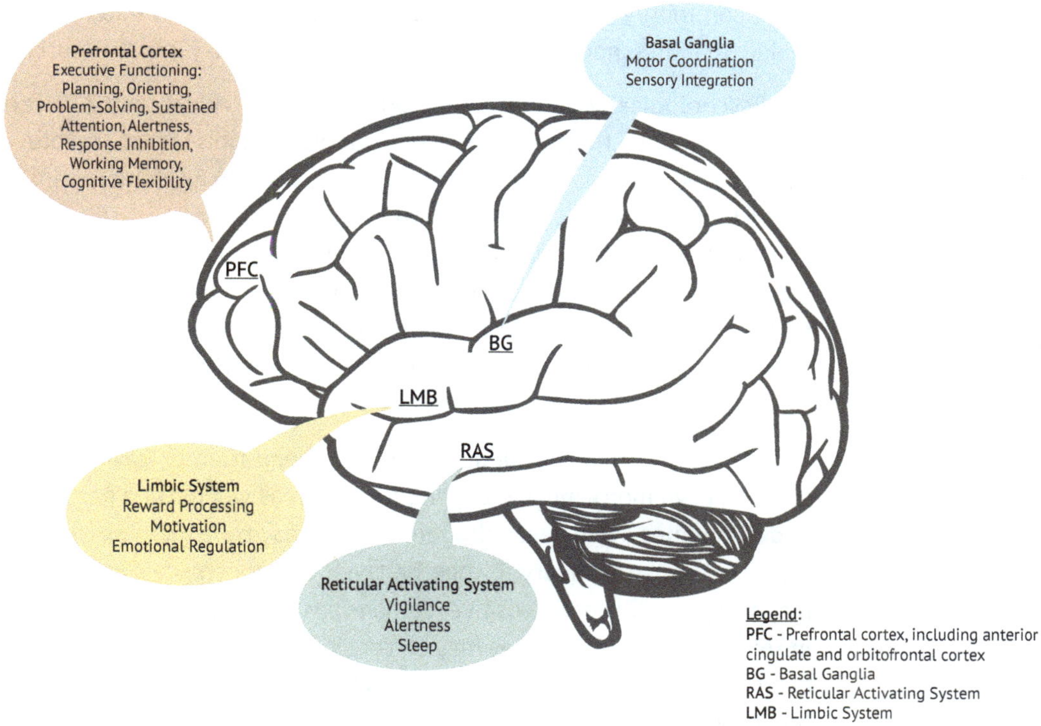

FIGURE 16.1 Brain areas affected and corresponding symptoms in ADHD.

Adapted from Copyright © 2019 Depositphotos/Jolygon.

CLINICAL MANIFESTATIONS

Individuals with ADHD have manifestations that go beyond the core symptoms. These include executive functioning problems, motivational–reward processing problems, motor kinesis control, and emotional dysregulation (Smith et al., 2020). In addition, they often lack response inhibition, which causes them to be seen as impulsive (Lipszyc & Schachar, 2010; Pliszka et al., 2000).

> **KEY POINT**
>
> The brain regions involved in ADHD include the prefrontal cortex, the limbic system, the basal ganglia, and the reticular activating system.

Neurobiologically, in school or work, they may experience learning problems. Their learning deficits may become noticeable early. However, of good note, many individuals with ADHD are of superior intellectual capacity and therefore able to compensate for attentional deficit; as such, they are able to maintain good and even excellent grades, sometimes with significant effort. Precipitous declines in grades and performance occur

> **CLINICAL TIP**
>
> ADHD manifests as core symptoms of hyperactivity, inattention, and impulsivity but also goes beyond this. Individuals with ADHD have other manifestations, including emotional dysregulation, lack of response inhibition (commonly referred to as impulsivity), executive functioning problems, motivational-reward processing problems, and a lack of motor kinesis control.

more commonly with the transition from elementary to middle school, middle to high school, high school to college, and entry into the workforce.

Psychologically, the internal world of the individual with ADHD may include negative themes. They have trouble keeping out of trouble, and what comes relatively easily to others they must put in much more conscious effort to achieve. This may result in a sense of failure or futility of their efforts. Due to this, it is important to intentionally create opportunities for individuals with ADHD to succeed, especially placing them in environments that promote their sense of self. Without this, they resort to defense mechanisms, including denial, minimalization, externalization, or projection. Table 16.2 gives examples of symptoms that may be experienced in ADHD.

Socially, they may struggle to make or keep friends; have more peer conflict; have more bullying experiences, both as victims and perpetrators; and sometimes avoid peers altogether. They may have more disciplinary or legal problems secondary to their behavior or poor choices. At home, they may struggle to maintain positive relationships with their siblings and parents in some cases. At home, they may be considered a "difficult child" or be less liked by their siblings. They may have to live through more school and work failures than individuals without ADHD.

> **KEY POINT**
>
> ADHD remains a clinical diagnosis. A full evaluation, should include additional input from other sources, including school, parents, other relevant adults such as teachers and coaches, or other family members in the case of adults.

DIAGNOSIS

ADHD remains a clinical diagnosis. Specific symptoms of ADHD need to be met to make a diagnosis. Assessing ADHD begins with a full clinical evaluation, which should include additional input from other sources, including school, parents, and other relevant adults, such as teachers and coaches, or other family members in the case of adults. Common forms used in assessing baseline symptoms as well as treatment response include the NICHQ Vanderbilt assessment and follow-up forms, the Conner's teacher and parent rating scales, and the adult ADHD self-report.

Subtypes of ADHD

There are three main domains of symptoms in ADHD: inattention, hyperactivity, and impulsivity. Some individuals may manifest symptoms in one, two, or all three domains. Individuals who manifest only inattention may experience a delay in diagnosis because their symptoms are not as readily noticeable when compared to those with symptoms of hyperactivity or impulsivity. Girls with ADHD are often missed because some may only present with symptoms of inattention, and there is not a problematic

TABLE 16.1 Sample Behaviors of Inattention, Impulsivity, and Hyperactivity in Children, Adolescents, and Adults

Age group	Setting	Inattention	Impulsivity	Hyperactivity
Preschool (2–5 years old)	School	• Plays for short times with random toys • Difficulty cleaning up after play • Wanders off in public places if not closely supervised	• Significant emotional dysregulation (severe tantrums) • Hitting and kicking peers and adults when upset • May have tendency to bite more before language adequately developed	• Unable to sit during story time • Gets up out of seated spot when expected to be seated • High appetite for physical play (does not tire) • Accident prone
	Home	• Wanders off tasks with chores or errands • Forgets parts of multistep tasks (e.g., "Put this dish up, then feed the dog, then clean your room") • Misses details and makes careless errors	• Frequent fights/conflict with siblings • Impatient	• Climbs chairs and tables and furniture • Bounces off the walls; is always on the go
	Social settings	• Wanders off in stores • Difficulty sticking with the group	• Says what they think (has no filters) • Little inhibitory volition; darts across the street	• Difficulty sitting in church/other religious settings • Difficulty waiting
School age (6–11 years old)	School	• Unable to retain newly learned information (forgets lessons learned from one day or week to the next) • Wanders off task with class work • Does not complete classwork • Forgets to turn in assignments in class • Needs frequent reminders to do work	• Interrupts conversations excessively • Blurts out answers before being called on • Difficulty working on group activities	• Gets up out of chair when expected to be seated • Difficulty sitting in group activities
	Home	• Wanders off tasks with chores or errands • Forgets parts of multistep tasks (e.g., "Put this dish up, then feed the dog, then clean your room") • Misses details and makes careless errors	• Frequent fights and conflict with siblings • Impatient	• Climbs chairs and tables and furniture • Bounces off the walls; is always on the go
	Social settings	• Wanders off in stores • Difficulty sticking with the group	• Says what they think (has no filters) • Little inhibitory volition; darts across the street	• May be accident prone • Difficulty remaining still • Difficulty waiting

Age group	Setting	Inattention	Impulsivity	Hyperactivity
Adolescent (12–17 years old)	School	• Easily distracted • Poor task completion • Misses important project and assignment deadlines • Assignments left until the last minute • Disorganized (e.g., school folder and locker have mixed up papers and unorganized items)	• Interrupts often • Off topic in responses or conversations	• Hyperactivity replaced with inner sense of restlessness
	Home	• Procrastinates on chores and family requests • Disorganized (e.g., bedroom is constantly untidy with unorganized items) • May forget or miss important family events	• Says and does things without thinking • Poor decision-making	• May be accident prone • Inner feeling of restlessness • Fidgety behavior • Difficulty remaining still
	Social settings	• Poor planning around activities alone or with peers	• In conversation with peers, contributions may often seem off-topic • Little inhibitory volition; once has an idea, cannot hold back from carrying through • Impulse driven • Higher risk of initiating drug use	• May be accident prone • Inner feeling of restlessness • Fidgety behavior • Difficulty remaining still
Adult (18+ years old)	Work/ college	• Misses important deadlines • Misses details in work assignments • Forgets about appointments • Disorganized and has poor time management	• Poor decision-making • Sudden decision-making	• Inner feeling of restlessness • Fidgety behavior • Difficulty remaining still
	Home	• May forget or miss important family events • Poor home project completion	• Blurts out hurtful comments to family members before (or without) considering the consequence • May make sudden decisions	• Inner feeling of restlessness
	Social settings	• Poor project completion	• Interpersonal conflict • Says what they think (has no filters) • Poor decision-making • May take unnecessary risks	• Inner feeling of restlessness

behavior that teachers and parents notice. They may also keep up their work but with more silent effort.

TABLE 16.2 Subtypes of ADHD Chart

	Inattention symptoms (six out of nine symptoms present)	Hyperactivity-impulsivity symptoms (six out of nine symptoms present)	Diagnosis
Symptoms meeting criteria present?	Yes	No	ADHD: predominantly inattentive presentation
	No	Yes	ADHD: predominantly hyperactive-impulsive presentation
	Yes	Yes	ADHD: combined presentation

TREATMENT

ADHD is considered the most treatable neuropsychiatric condition, and adequate treatment can lead to dramatic improvement in the individual's life. Up to 90% of patients respond to treatment, and with optimum treatment up to 50% normalize. Understanding the significant interactions of biological, psychological, and social factors in ADHD and informing clients of all treatment options, including pharmacological intervention, promote positive treatment outcomes.

The mainstay of treatment for ADHD is biological. This is a departure from many of the disorders treated in psychiatry, where psychosocial interventions are key. The multimodal treatment of ADHD (MTA study) was a multisite randomized clinical trial designed to evaluate efficacy of treatment approaches used in ADHD, including medications, behavior therapy, and a combination of both. The MTA study findings showed that when used as a single modality of treatment, targeted medication management was superior to behavioral therapy. In the study, combined treatment did not yield statistically significant benefits over medication management for the core ADHD symptoms but may have provided benefit for non-ADHD symptoms and positive functioning outcomes (The MTA Cooperative Group, 1999).

Medication treatment provides a robust protective effect, including on academic outcomes, mood disorders, suicidality, criminality, and substance

MEMORY TIP

***ADHD**, useful mnemonic*

CALL FOR FrE d
(six or more inattention symptoms)
C—Careless mistakes
A—Attention difficulty
L—Listening problems
L—Loses things

F—Fails to finish what they start
O—Organizational skills lacking
R—Reluctance to do tasks that need sustained mental effort
FR—Forgetful in routine activities
ED—Easily distracted

RUNS FASTT
(six or more hyperactivity–impulsivity symptoms)
R—Runs or is restless
U—Unable to wait for they turn
N—Not able to play quietly
S—Slow? Oh no! They're on the go!

F—Fidgets with hands or feet
A—Answers blurted out
S—Staying seated is difficult
T—Talks excessively
T—Tends to interrupt

(Stubbe, 2007)

> **CLINICAL TIP**
>
> ADHD is considered the most treatable neuropsychiatric condition. Adequate treatment can lead to dramatic improvement in the individual's life. Medications are effective for the core symptoms, while psychotherapy helps to further improve functional outcomes.

use disorders. Estimates show, when compared to untreated individuals, those who are treated with medications have 31% decreased rate of substance abuse, 43% lower long-term risk of depression at a 3-year follow-up, about 40–58% fewer motor vehicle accidents, and a 32% decrease in the criminality rate for men and 41% for women (Boland et al., 2020; Lichtenstein et al., 2012). Psychosocial treatments delivered without medication treatment provide limited benefits to the individuals who continue to struggle with the core symptoms of ADHD. The different treatments used for ADHD management are discussed below.

PSYCHOPHARMACOLOGY

Medications are effective for all age groups, including preschoolers and newly diagnosed adults with ADHD. Dopaminergic stimulant medications have shown to be the most effective in treating the core ADHD symptoms. Catecholaminergic nonstimulants have shown significant benefit for treating ADHD in adults. Below are the different medications currently used to treat ADHD/ADD.

Stimulant Medications

The first-line treatment for ADHD, regardless of subtype, is the stimulant category of medication. Stimulants have been used as early as 1955 and are, therefore, quite significantly studied. Stimulants are divided into two subcategories: amphetamines and methylphenidates. There are many medications that are modifications of the amphetamine or methylphenidate group. Both categories of stimulants work by increased synaptic availability of dopamine and norepinephrine, including the cortex and the striatum. Amphetamines do so via inhibition of dopamine transporters and norepinephrine transporters. Methylphenidates do so via inhibition of these same receptors and agonistic activity for the 5-HT1A receptors.

The differences between medication often include duration of action (i.e., short-acting versus long-acting) and mode of delivery (i.e., a pill swallowed whole, a capsule that may be opened and sprinkled, a liquid, a patch, etc.). Compared to many psychiatric medications, stimulants work quickly and are metabolized out of the body quickly as well. Given this, a patient may take a stimulant medication in the morning, have it working within an hour of taking it, and find that it wears off hours later. The most common side effects include upset stomach, decreased appetite, difficulty sleeping, and irritability. In addition, more serious issues that are less common include an increase in blood pressure and the potential to decrease the seizure threshold. Thus, monitoring both vital signs as well as symptoms and side effects is key.

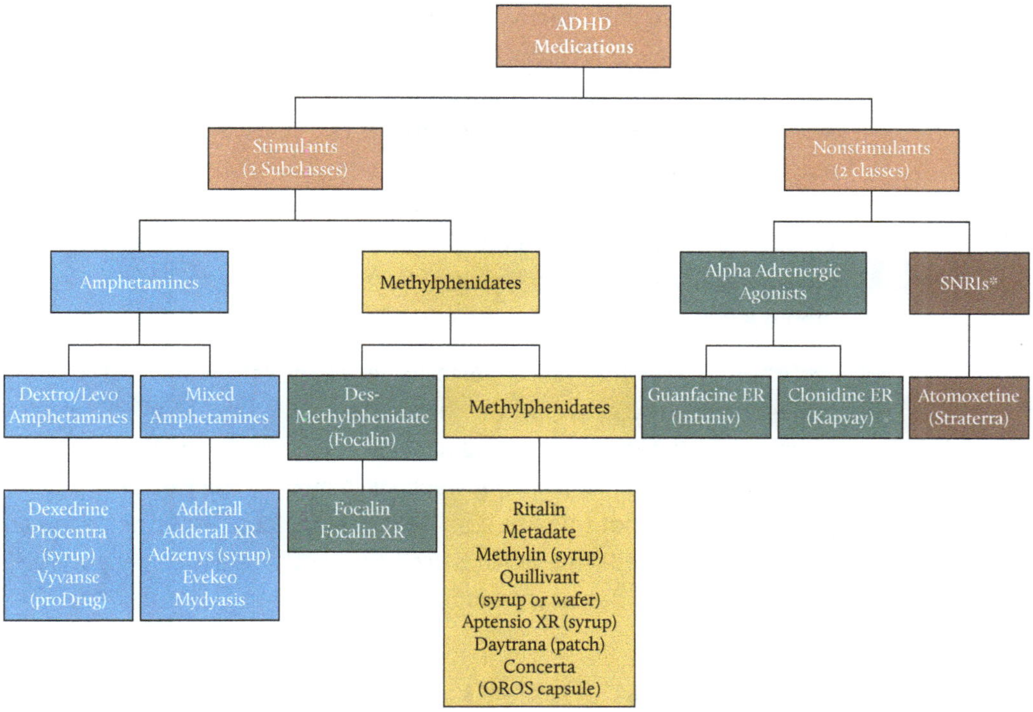

FIGURE 16.2 FDA-approved medications for treating ADHD (this list is not exhaustive). SNRI = Serotonin–norepinephrine reuptake inhibitor.

Methylphenidates and amphetamines generally have similar side effects to each other. There may be some individual differences between the side effects and efficacy of stimulants for a particular patient, but when looking at a whole population, the medications work similarly and have similar side effects. This is true for efficacy, tolerability, adverse effects, treatment discontinuation, and cardiovascular effects, although amphetamines may have some more weight loss and insomnia than methylphenidates.

Typically, stimulant medications are started in the morning (for example, before school), and the effects are monitored throughout the day. With subsequent visits, data from teachers can be collected to monitor, whether the medications are helping with symptoms throughout the day or if there is a premature wearing off of the medications. For individuals for whom a morning dose wears off too quickly, a booster dose of an immediate-acting stimulant may be added. While these medications do not require daily use, as many other medications do, many patients find it helpful to continue their routine of taking it daily, while others may take "holidays" off the medication with no ill effects.

Nonstimulant Medications

Nonstimulant medications that are commonly used include the alpha-adrenergic agonists, such as clonidine and guanfacine. Both are available in their short-acting forms and long-acting forms, and while their mechanism of action for ADHD is poorly understood, they do seem to act on areas that regulate attention and impulse control. They work less effectively than stimulant medications in controlling the symptoms of ADHD, but for some patients, are more tolerable and may be able to help in combination with stimulants as well. As these medications can have an impact on blood pressure, it is important that these medications be scheduled and taken with good compliance to avoid issues with rebound hypertension. Another side effect of sedation may be helpful when employed in the evening to help with sleep.

Another nonstimulant medication is atomoxetine, or Strattera. It is generally more effective on the inattention symptoms of ADHD and less effective on the impulsivity and hyperactivity, with a smaller effect size than stimulants. It, like the alpha-agonists, may be better tolerated by some patients who do not tolerate stimulant medications. Other nonstimulant options include modafinil, which is used off-label for the treatment of ADHD, as well as the antidepressant bupropion (Wellbutrin).

CLINICAL TIP

For children with ADHD, behavior management programs that are rewards-based, such as token economy, are most effective at increasing positive behaviors and reducing negative ones.

PSYCHOTHERAPY

Psychotherapy can be extremely helpful in individuals with ADHD. In preschool children, the focus of therapy is often on supporting and building parental skills to work with the child (e.g., parent management training). Parents are often encouraged to use contingent attention where positive attention is given in response to desired behaviors. Contingent attention could include smiles or nods of approval, positive comments, or showcasing their action as a good example. In school-aged children, behavior management programs are effective when carefully thought out and consistently applied.

The basic principles of behavior management show that the frequency of a behavior increases if it is followed by a reward (i.e., positive/pleasurable consequence) and tends to decrease if not followed by a reward or if followed by a negative consequence. Behavior management programs, which are reward-based, are most effective at increasing positive behaviors and reducing negative ones. A good example is the token economy system, which is like a point system in which the child earns points based on the positive behaviors they perform. These tokens (or points) are then attached to rewards the child earns. Behavior management techniques help improve targeted behaviors (e.g., completing school or homework or keeping the child's hands to themself) but are not usually helpful in reducing core symptoms of inattention, hyperactivity, or impulsivity.

In adolescents, motivational incentives are helpful for promoting and maintaining positive behaviors. Building executive functioning skills is particularly important for the adolescent. In adulthood, executive coaching is helpful. In addition to addressing issues directly stemming for ADHD, patients also benefit from therapy for related conditions, such as CBT for anxiety or depression, mindfulness skills, and therapy for anger management.

SOCIAL AND OTHER INTERVENTIONS

Just as the right environment can promote a child, the wrong environment can limit or even harm a child psychologically in many ways. School is a major part of a child's life. In school, laws, including Section 504, protect individuals against discrimination based on disability. IDEA (Individuals With Disabilities Education Act) relates to children with specific conditions (e.g., intellectual disabilities, emotional disturbances, hearing impairments, speech and language difficulties, and other health impairment [OHI]) if the child is unable to learn in a regular classroom. Students diagnosed with ADHD can request classroom and testing accommodations and have their educational plan individualized to suit their educational needs. Classroom adjustments could include preferential seating; breaking down and presenting work in smaller chunks; keeping instructions written, simple, and clear; monitoring for frustrations; providing frequent breaks; providing the child with the schedule for the day; and so on.

SUMMARY

ADHD is a neurodevelopmental condition with a neurobiological basis. Dopamine deficit is the basic neurochemical dysfunction that causes a low arousal state and motivational problems. ADHD appears to be a stable condition that only changes how it presents through the individual's life. This manifests biologically, psychologically, and socially through the individual's life.

ADHD is the most treatable neuropsychiatric condition. Treatment includes biological (medications), psychological, and social interventions. A robust body of research shows that that ADHD medication treatments are associated with decreases in the risks for a wide range of ADHD-associated functional outcomes. FDA-approved medications include stimulants, alpha-agonists, and a serotonin–norepinephrine reuptake inhibitor. Left inadequately treated, it is associated with the development of a broad range of comorbid conditions; impulsive behaviors; a greater number of traumatic experiences; and a lower quality of life, perceived social support, and social functioning, even after adjusting for additional comorbidities.

The impact of ADHD often begins in childhood and continues through to adulthood. Early diagnosis and adequate treatment of individuals with ADHD in childhood results in fewer secondary problems being carried into adulthood. Effective agents are available for treating this condition. However, especially if left inadequately treatment, ADD/ADHD can exert lifelong impairment.

RESOURCES

1 https://www.youtube.com/watch?v=EpfeWrkV3os

2 https://www.youtube.com/watch?v=Jjf-yHLaXtU

3 https://www.aacap.org/AACAP/Families_and_Youth/Resource_Centers/ADHD_Resource_Center/Home.aspx

4 https://www.mayoclinic.org/diseases-conditions/adult-adhd/symptoms-causes/syc-20350878

5 https://chadd.org

REFERENCES

Beauchaine, T. P., Ben-David, I., & Bos, M. (2020). ADHD, financial distress, and suicide in adulthood: A population study. *Science Advances*, *6*(40): eaba1551.

Bernardi, S., Faraone, S. V., Cortese, S., Kerridge, B. T., Pallanti, S., Wang, S., & Blanco, C. (2012). The lifetime impact of attention deficit hyperactivity disorder: Results from the national epidemiologic survey on alcohol and related conditions (NESARC). *Psychological Medicine*, *42*(4), 875–887.

Biederman J. (2004b). Impact of comorbidity in adults with attention-deficit/hyperactivity disorder. *Journal of Clinical Psychiatry*, *65*(3):3–7.

Biederman, J., Faraone, S. V., Monuteaux, M. C., Bober, M., & Cadogen, E. (2004a). Gender effects on attention-deficit/hyperactivity disorder in adults, revisited. *Biological Psychiatry*, *55*(7):692–700. https://www.doi.org/10.1016/j.biopsych.2003.12.003

Bierhoff, J. Haardörfer R., Windle M., & Berg C. J. (2019). Psychological risk factors for alcohol, cannabis, and various tobacco use among young adults: A longitudinal analysis. *Substance Use & Misuse*, *54*(8), 1365–1375.

Boland H., DiSalvo M., Fried R., Woodworth K. Y., Wilens T., Faraone S. V., & Biederman J. (2020). A literature review and meta-analysis on the effects of ADHD medications on functional outcomes. *Journal of Psychiatric Research*, *123*:21–30.

Bradley, C. (1950). Benzedrine and dexedrine in the treatment of children's behavior disorders. *Pediatrics*, *5*(1), 24–37.

Craig, S. G., Weiss, M. D., & Hudec, K. L., Gibbins, C. (2020). The functional impact of sleep disorders in children with ADHD. *Journal of Attention Disorders*, *24*(4), 499–508.

Franke, B., Michelini, G., Asherson, P., Banaschewski, T., Bilbow, A., Buitelaar, J. K., Cormand, B., Faraone, S. V., Ginsberg, Y., Haavik, J., Kuntsi, J., Larsson, H., Lesch, K. P., Ramos-Quiroga, J. A., Réthelyi, J. M., Ribases, M., & Reif, A. (2018). Live fast, die young? A review on the developmental trajectories of ADHD across the lifespan. *European Neuropsychopharmacology*, *28*(10), 1059–1088.

Hoogman, M., Bralten, J., Hibar, D. P., Mennes, M., Zwiers, M. P., Schweren, L. S. J., van Hulzen, K. J. E., Medland, S. E., Shumskaya, E., Jahanshad, N., Zeeuw, P., Szekely, E., Sudre ,G., Wolfers, T., Onnink, A. M. H., Dammers, J. T., Mostert J. C., Vives-Gilabert, Y., Kohls, G., ... Franke, B. (2017). Subcortical brain volume differences in participants with attention deficit hyperactivity disorder in children and adults: A cross-sectional mega-analysis. *Lancet Psychiatry*, *4*(4), 310–319.

Howard, A. L., Kennedy, T. M., Mitchell, J. T., Sibley, M. H., Hinshaw, S. P., Arnold, L. E., Roy, A., Stehli, A., Swanson, J. M., & Molina, B. S. G. (2020). Early substance use in the pathway from childhood attention-deficit/hyperactivity disorder (ADHD) to young adult substance use: Evidence of statistical mediation and substance specificity. *Psychology of Addictive Behaviors*, *34*(2), 281–292.

Kessler, R. C., Adler, L., Barkley, R., Biederman, J., Conners, C. K., Demler, O., Faraone, S. V., Greenhill, L. L., Howes, M. J., Secnik, K., Spencer, T., Ustun, T. B., Walters, E. E., & Zaslavsky, A. M. *The prevalence and correlates of adult ADHD in the United States: Results from the National Comorbidity Survey Replication. The American Journal of Psychiatry*, *163*(4):716–23.

Lichtenstein, P., Halldner L., Zetterqvist J., Sjölander A., Serlachius E., Fazel S., Långström N., & Larsson H. (2012). Medication for attention deficit-hyperactivity disorder and criminality. *New England Journal of Medicine*, *367*(21), 2006–2014.

Lipszyc, J., & Schachar, R. (2010). Inhibitory control and psychopathology: A meta-analysis of studies using the stop signal task. *Journal of the International Neuropsychological Society*, *16*(6), 1064–1076.

The MTA Cooperative Group (1999). A 14-month randomized clinical trial of treatment strategies for attention-deficit/hyperactivity disorder. Multimodal Treatment Study of Children with ADHD. *JAMA Psychiatry*. 1999 Dec;56(12):1073-86. doi: 10.1001/archpsyc.56.12.1073. PMID: 10591283.].

Pliszka, S. R., Liotti, M., & Woldorff, M. G. (2000). Inhibitory control in children with attention-deficit/hyperactivity disorder: Event-related potentials identify the processing component and timing of an impaired right-frontal response-inhibition mechanism. *Biological Psychiatry*, *48*(3), 238–246.

Smith, Z. R., Langberg J. M., Cusick, C. N., Green, C. D., & Becker, S. P. (2020). Academic motivation deficits in adolescents with ADHD and associations with academic functioning. *Journal of Abnormal Child Psychology*, *48*(2), 237–249.

Stein, M. A., Weiss, M., & Hlavaty, L. (2012). ADHD treatments, sleep, and sleep problems: Complex associations. *Neurotherapeutics*, *9*(3), 509–517.

Still, G.F. (1902). Some abnormal psychical conditions in children. *Lancet*, (1), 1008–1012, 1077–1082.

Still, G.F. (2006). Some abnormal psychical conditions in children: Excerpts from three lectures. *Journal of Attention Disorders*, *10*(2):126-136.

Stubbe, D. (2007). *Child and adolescent psychiatry: a practical guide* (1st. ed.). Lippincott Williams & Wilkins,

Vally, Z. (2020). Symptoms of internet gaming disorder, inattention, and impulsivity: A cross-sectional study conducted in the United Arab Emirates. *Psychiatric Quarterly*, *92*, 301–310. https://doi.org/10.1007/s11126-020-09799-2

Weinstein, A., & Lejoyeux, M. (2020). Neurobiological mechanisms underlying internet gaming disorder. *Dialogues in Clinical Neuroscience*, *22*(2), 113–126.

Wender, P. H., Wolf, L. E., & Wasserstein J. Adults with ADHD. An overview. *Annals of the New York Academy of Sciences*, *931*, 1–16.

Yen, J. Y., Liu, T. L., Wang, P. W., Chen, C. S., Yen, C. F., & Ko, C. H. (2017) Association between internet gaming disorder and adult attention deficit and hyperactivity disorder and their correlates: Impulsivity and hostility. *Addictive Behaviors*, *64*, 308–313.

CHAPTER 17

Anxiety Disorders and Obsessive-Compulsive Disorders[1]

Julie Williams, M.D. and Kim-Lan Czelusta, M.D.

"The only way out is through."

— Robert Frost

OBJECTIVES

After reading this chapter, students will be able to do the following:

- describe the epidemiology, neuropathology, and comorbidity of common anxiety disorders and obsessive-compulsive disorder
- recognize the differences between the different anxiety disorders and obsessive-compulsive disorder using the *DSM-5* criteria, including recognizing where symptoms may be caused by substances or a general medical condition
- outline a biopsychosocial treatment plan for anxiety disorders and obsessive-compulsive disorder

1 Readers may also see "Depression in the Medically Ill" (Chapter 21) and "Adjustment- and Grief-Related Disorders" (Chapter 22) for related material.

CASE VIGNETTE

Eric is a 24-year-old man who presents to your office due to feeling restless, worried, and keyed up all the time. He shares his history that he had difficulty as a young child going to school because he would worry something might happen to himself or his parents. Once at school, he often would enjoy himself and hanging out with his friends. While this improved, Eric notes he has been a "worrier" for most of his life. Now, as a young adult working in a new firm, Eric ruminates on whether he is doing a good job at work, whether his family is okay, and various other responsibilities like caring for his home or his car. He notes it is difficult to relax. Eric is diagnosed with generalized anxiety disorder; treating it with sertraline significantly reduces his symptoms. His anxiety symptoms are not completely gone, but at least he is now able to relax and can begin to enjoy life as it unfolds daily.

DEFINITIONS AND KEY CONCEPTS

Fear is defined as an uncomfortable response to a known threat. *Anxiety* is defined as an uncomfortable response to a threat that is unknown, internal, or vague (Sadock & Sadock, 2007).

INTRODUCTION

Anxiety is present throughout our world and is noted throughout our history. It can be a useful emotion, helping our ancestors avoid predators or helping new parents protect their newborns to ensure their survival. It motivates eager medical students to study long into the night, day after day, for many years! While not everyone will have anxiety symptoms to the degree of a diagnosable disorder, people everywhere will experience worry. This chapter will discuss the varying forms of anxiety and discuss what is considered "appropriate anxiety" versus what a disorder. One of the first historical observances of disordered anxiety comes from ancient Greece. The term *agoraphobia* stems from the Greek words *agora* and *phobos*, meaning fear of the marketplace. Later, soldiers in the Civil War were diagnosed with "irritable heart syndrome," which included some of the first diagnostic criteria of panic disorder. And in 1895, Sigmond Freud introduced the concept of "anxiety neurosis," which included clusters of mental and physical symptoms (Sadock & Sadock, 2007). While no longer categorized under anxiety disorders in the current *DSM-5*, obsessive compulsive disorder shares a similar neurobiological basis, centering on symptoms of uncontrolled

KEY POINT

Anxiety is a part of life. However, high or distressing, levels of anxiety can result in anxiety disorders. The diagnosis of the different anxiety disorders is based on specific criteria.

QUICK POINT

Anxiety affects women twice as commonly as men. Nearly 38% of women and 26% of men will be diagnosed with an anxiety disorder at some point in their lives. Among adults, about 22.8% have had serious impairment and 33.7% have had moderate impairment. Among adolescents, about 31.9% have experienced any anxiety disorder, with a higher prevalence for females than males.

repetitive thoughts. As such, this unique diagnosis will be discussed in this chapter as well.

EPIDEMIOLOGY

As one of the most prevalent disorders, anxiety affects many individuals, both adults and children. Nearly 38% of women and 26% of men will be diagnosed with an anxiety disorder at some point in their lives (Kessler et al., 2012). Among adults, an estimated 22.8% have had serious impairment and 33.7% have had moderate impairment. Anxiety affects women twice as commonly as men. Among adolescents, about 31.9% have experienced any anxiety disorder with a higher prevalence for females than males (Degenhardt, 2007). While anxious thoughts or feelings may be adaptive and allow us to avoid unpleasant sensations, such as pain, punishment, or failure, anxiety disorders disrupt functioning among individuals who have them, keeping them from taking care of themselves and their responsibilities. Figure 17.1 shows past year anxiety disorders among U.S. adults.

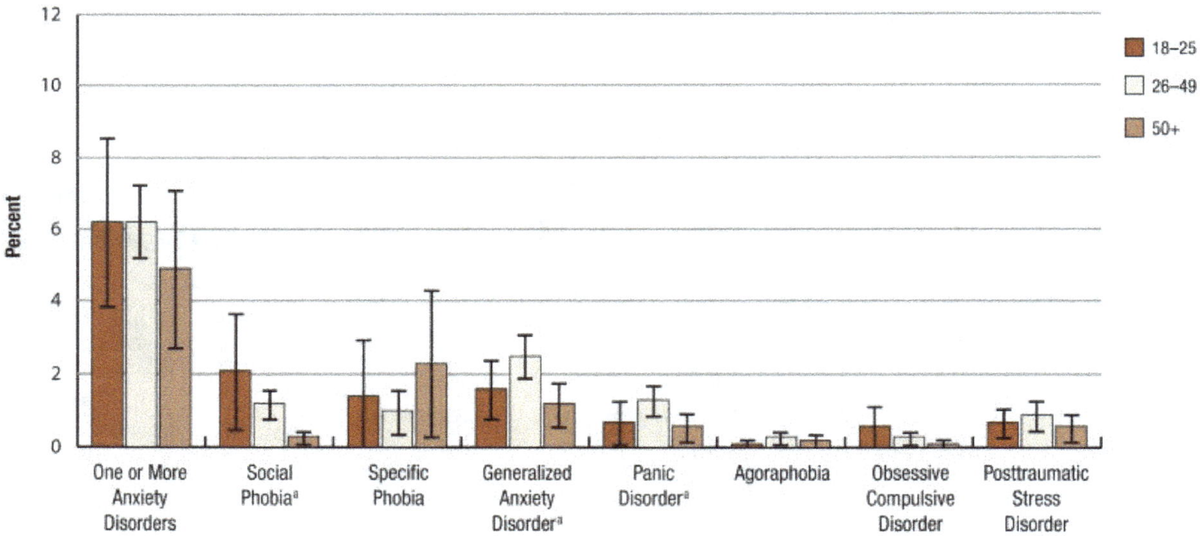

FIGURE 17.1 Past year anxiety disorders among adults aged 18 or older by age group: percentages and 95% confidence intervals. MHSS Clinical Study, 2008–2012. Adapted from Karg et al., 2014.

Rhonda S. Karg, et al., "Past Year Mental Disorders among Adults in the United States: Results from the 2008–2012 Mental Health Surveillance Study," CBHSQ Data Review, p. 13, 2014.

NEUROPATHOLOGY

Anxiety is commonly known to be mediated by the effects of serotonin, norepinephrine, and GABA (gamma-aminobutyric acid). While these neurochemicals may affect other parts of the brain, serotonin, norepinephrine, and GABA have known effects on the amygdala, or the fear center of the brain. The amygdala is an almond-shaped body located in the medial temporal lobe, just anterior to the hippocampus. It is involved in the processing of emotions and memories associated with fear and plays an extensive role in regulating the fear response in humans. Fearful stimuli, such as threatening facial expressions, fear inducing images, and fear conditioned cues, activate the amygdala. On the contrary, when neuronal synaptic transmission is inhibited in the amygdala, glutamate output and the fear response (i.e., panic and phobia) is reduced (see Figure 17.2). In addition to the amygdala, the anterior cingulate cortex and orbitofrontal cortex are also key areas that regulate emotions. Their reciprocal connections to the amygdala help to regulate the fear response (Sadock & Sadock, 2007; Stahl, 2013). Worry (i.e., anxious misery, apprehension, and obsessions) is mediated by the cortico–striato–thalamo–cortical circuit, which is also impacted by serotonin, norepinephrine, and GABA (Stahl, 2013). PET studies have also found that patients with generalized anxiety disorder have reduced metabolic rates in the basal ganglia and white matter of the brain, which correlates with the involvement the cortico–striato–thalamo–cortical circuit (see Figure 17.2, relating to fear and fear conditioning to see the connections between these areas of the brain). These feedback loops are theorized to regulate symptoms of ruminations, obsessions, and other types of recurrent thoughts but are not completely understood.

> **KEY POINT**
>
> The amygdala is an almond-shaped body located in the medial temporal lobe, just anterior to the hippocampus. It is involved in the processing of emotions and memories associated with fear and plays an extensive role in regulating the fear response in humans. Fearful stimuli, such as threatening facial expressions, fear inducing images, and fear conditioned cues, activate the amygdala.

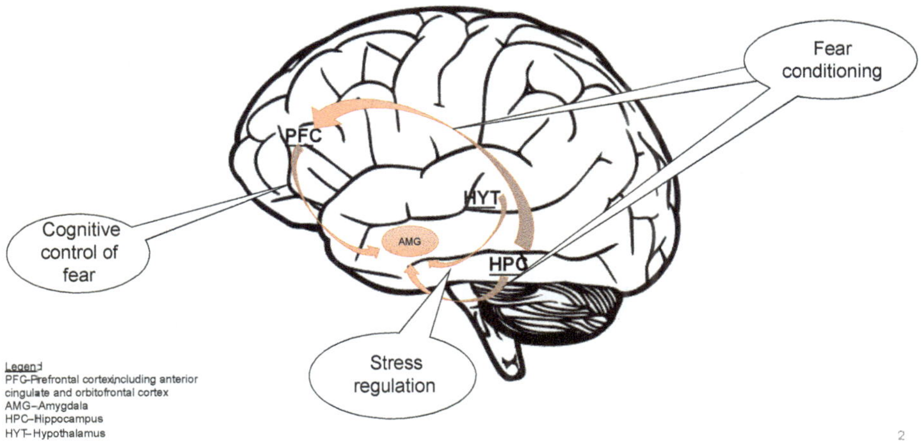

FIGURE 17.2 Fear and fear conditioning

Adapted from Copyright © 2019 Depositphotos/Jolygon.

CLINICAL MANIFESTATIONS

Anxiety presents in a variety of ways—some physical and some mental. For example, patients often first seek help from their primary care physicians for physical symptoms of back pain, headaches, and palpitations. They may also go to the emergency room concerned that they are experiencing a myocardial infarction. Upon careful history and physical examination, an astute physician may find that the back pain and headaches are caused by muscle tension, or the palpitations and diaphoresis may be related to an autonomic response to a stressful trigger. Seeing a negative workup (such as negative EKG and troponin values) along with the context of a stressful event may make the clinician think more closely about an anxiety disorder.

Introspective patients may be aware of their internal distress and present with ruminations and sleeplessness. In children, the fear or anxiety may be expressed by crying, tantrums, shrinking, or failing to speak in social situations. Some of these symptoms are transient and are the mind's way of bringing awareness to a possible threat. However, if the symptoms persist and are severe enough to cause dysfunction in one or more areas of the patient's life, an anxiety disorder should be considered. In the next section, specific criteria of a variety of anxiety disorders will be discussed (APA, 2013).

DIAGNOSIS OF ANXIETY DISORDERS AND OBSESSIVE-COMPULSIVE DISORDER

The diagnosis of an anxiety disorder requires careful assessment and investigation during an interview. When approaching a new patient with complaints of anxiety, the first step in making an accurate diagnosis is to ensure that medical comorbidities and substances are not causing the patient's symptoms. Once medical and substance-related interference is ruled out, the next step in assessing the patient is to determine precisely what the patient is worrying about. Are they particularly triggered by fears of abandonment? Snakes or other perceived threats? Going outside? Being around other people? Everything? Or do their symptoms come without a known trigger, seemingly out of the blue? Answering these key questions will help narrow the diagnoses. It is also important to note that patients can have more than one anxiety diagnoses at any time. If they have symptoms of anxiety related to multiple fears, and each of these fear clusters cause difficulties in their functioning, they will meet criteria for more than one disorder. Also, while any anxiety disorder may be experienced in any age group, certain disorders, such as separation anxiety disorder and selective mutism, are most commonly seen in children and should be considered more strongly for those age groups. General characteristics of anxiety disorders are shown in Table 17.1.

Separation Anxiety Disorder

Separation anxiety disorder is most commonly seen in children. It can be seen in up to 10% of girls and 6% of boys under the age of 17 (Kessler et al., 2012). Like most anxiety disorders, separation anxiety disorder is more commonly seen in females than males. Most children go through "stranger danger" phases when young (generally between 8 and 14 months old). Fear of being separated from one's parents (or primary attachment figure) is common, even in older children. Even college students experience some mild angst when moving out of their parents' home for the first time. However, if the child is older, the significant fear is developmentally inappropriate, and the fear or anxiety is excessive, this disorder may be considered.

The patient must also have at least three of the following symptoms: recurrent excessive distress when anticipating or experiencing separation; worry about losing their parents or something harming them, such as a natural disaster, illness, or accidents; worry about experiencing an untoward event that would cause separation such as getting lost or having an accident; reluctance or refusal to go out of the home due to fear of separation; fear or reluctance to be alone without the attachment figure; reluctance or refusal to sleep away from home or to sleep without the attachment figure nearby; repeated nightmares about separation; and complaints of physical symptoms (e.g., headaches or GI upset) when separated or anticipating separation from their attachment figure. In children, these symptoms must be present at least 4 weeks before the diagnosis can be made. In adults, the symptoms must be present at least 6 months. This diagnosis should be differentiated from other disorders, such as autism, in which the child may react negatively toward change in general, refusal to go outside as in agoraphobia, or worries about illness as in illness anxiety disorder.

When treating this disorder, it is often recommended that patients are kept in a routine as best as possible. For example, if the child is reluctant to go to school due to fear of separation, it is important to continue to take the child to school to habituate to the learning environment. It is also important for parents to avoid unnecessary changes in plans, such as being late for pickup, as this is likely to exacerbate symptoms. Rewards can be used to motivate children to engage in more age-appropriate separation behaviors. Additionally, sometimes parents may themselves be anxious about separation, so involving a component to help parents may also be helpful in improving the outcome for the child.

MEMORY TIP

Separation Anxiety Disorder, *useful mnemonic*

HUG PANDaS

Three of eight for one month in children and adolescents or 6 months in adults; A child will **HUG PANDaS** when they fear or anticipate separation from a major attachment figure. Fear of:

H—Harm or of loss of an attachment figure
U—Untoward event that causes separation or loss of an attachment figure
G—Going out of home avoided due to fear of separation or loss of an attachment figure
P—Physical symptoms with anticipated separation
A—Alone is a big fear
N—Nightmares involving the theme of separation
D—Distress of separation
aS —Sleeping without an attachment figure is distressful

(Kadiyala, 2020)

Selective Mutism

This disorder is also most notable in children but can occur across the life span. Selective mutism is considered relatively rare with a point prevalence of between 0.03–1%, depending on the sample setting. It is often seen upon the child starting school, either kindergarten or some other daycare or preschool setting. This diagnosis can only be applied to children who are previously known to be comfortable speaking in other areas of their lives. Often the teacher will reach out to parents and express concern about the child's language development, completely surprising the parents who have been having daily conversations with their children at home. The diagnosis is hallmarked by a consistent failure to speak in a specific social situation where speaking is expected. The lack of speech interferes with function within that setting and must last at least 1 month (not just occurring in the first month of school). This diagnosis is different from other communication disorders, such as autism or another communication disorder for which knowledge or ability is the limiting factor. Mutism seen in psychotic disorders also excludes this diagnosis.

The treatment for this illness often includes behavioral strategies for both the parents and the child. The parents should be coached to limit speaking for their children, allowing them to order for themselves at restaurants and so on. In addition, children are progressively habituated by talking to others—first, by whispering aloud in the presence of their parents and another person, then by speaking to others in front of their parents, and finally by speaking to others without parents present.

MEMORY TIP

Phobia, *useful mnemonic*

PHOBIA

P—Persistent (> 6 months)
H—Handicapping (restricted lifestyle)
O—Out of proportion
B—Beginning immediately and almost always
I—Intense fear or anxiety about a specific object or situation leading to
A—Avoidance

(Kadiyala, 2020)

Specific Phobia

This disorder is the most common of anxiety disorders with a lifetime prevalence of up to 18% of females and 13% of males. It is characterized by a marked fear or anxiety about a specific object or situation (e.g., flying, heights, needles, and animals). Most everyone can relate to this diagnosis as most everyone is afraid of something in their lives. However, the disorder is present when the fear is out of proportion to the actual danger posed by the objects and to the sociocultural context. For example, most people experience some angst when confronted with a painful medical procedure, but if the fear prevents you from engaging in needed medical care, then a diagnosis of a specific phobia may be considered. Another hallmark of the diagnosis is that the response must be consistent and immediate. People who are only sometimes afraid of a situation or only experience fear after the situation has passed do not meet criteria. The person must experience this significant phobic response at least 6 months or more. It is important to understand the cause of the patient's phobia before making the diagnosis. Patients with posttraumatic stress disorder (PTSD) often have great phobias related to their trauma, but their phobia is better explained by a PTSD diagnosis than a specific phobia as it often occurs in conjunction with other symptom clusters within that diagnosis. Similarly, agoraphobia and social anxiety disorders are given their own diagnoses in the *DSM-5* and are considered separately from specific phobia.

> **MEMORY TIP**
>
> ***Agoraphobia***, *useful mnemonic*
>
> **(FADS)**^{2}
>
> **F—F**eeling **F**earful in open, closed spaces, outside home alone, crowds, and public transport
> **A—A**voidance **A**nxiety attacks that are
> **D—D**isproportionate **D**istressful
> **S—S**ymptoms for **S**ix months
>
> *(Created by Edore Onigu-Otite, 2022)*

Social Anxiety Disorder (Social Phobia)

Social anxiety disorder affects up to 12% of females and 9% of males over the lifetime. As with most anxiety disorders, females are more affected than males. The peak of this gender difference is seen primarily in the adolescent and young adult population. This disorder is characterized by a specific fear about social situations, where one might be scrutinized by others. Performance anxiety falls under this diagnosis, but the diagnosis also includes patients who fear having to talk to unfamiliar people in social situations or being observed eating or drinking. The patient may fear that they will embarrass themselves in some way, but they also may fear that their anxiety related to the situation will also cause them embarrassment. The fear is out of proportion to the actual social situation (e.g., most people feel some level of anxiety when about to give a speech but do not necessarily have a disorder). The fear often causes significant avoidance of the situation or otherwise endured with significant distress, and the fear is consistent—the patient *always* fears meeting new people, not just sometimes. The fear must be present for 6 months or greater.

Other diagnoses that are often confused with this diagnosis are body dysmorphic disorder or schizoid personality disorder. In body dysmorphic disorder, the patient's symptoms primarily relate to their own judgment of themselves rather than anxiety about judgment from others, though this can be a part of the diagnosis. Patients with schizoid personality disorder often have limited social interactions, but these patients prefer to be alone and do not fear judgement from others.

Agoraphobia

Agoraphobia is a rarer disorder, affecting 3% of females and 1.8% of males over the lifetime (Kessler et al., 2012). Incidence peaks in late adolescence and early adulthood. This disorder is a specific fear about two (or more) of the following situations: using public transportation, being in open spaces, being in enclosed spaces, standing in line or being in a crowd, or being outside of the home alone. If the patient has only one of these, consider a specific phobia instead of agoraphobia. Like other phobias, the patient's symptoms are consistent (do not wax and wane when presented with the same threat), the level of fear or anxiety is out of proportion to the actual threat, and the symptoms last 6 months or more. Avoidance continues to be hallmark. Often, the patient has a fear that escape might be difficult, that help may not be available, or that they will experience other incapacitating or embarrassing symptoms (e.g., panic attacks or incontinence). The patient may also require the assistance of a companion to feel comfortable leaving their home.

> **MEMORY TIP**
>
> ***Panic Disorder***, *useful mnemonic*
>
> **STUDENTS Fear 3 Cs**
>
> **S**—Sweating
> **T**—Trembling or shaking
> **U**—Unsteadiness, dizziness, lightheadedness, or fainting
> **D**—Depersonalization or derealization
> **E**—Excessive heart rate or palpitations
> **N**—Nausea or abdominal distress
> **T**—Tingling (numbness or paresthesia's)
> **S**—Shortness of breath or smothering
> **F**—Fear of dying, losing control, or going crazy
> **3 C's**—chest pain, chills, choking
>
> *(Beck, 2011)*

Panic Disorder

Panic disorder affects approximately 5% of women and 2.5% of men over the lifetime (Kessler et al., 2012). The hallmark of this disorder is the presence of panic attacks. Panic attacks are defined as an abrupt surge or intense fear or discomfort, peaking within minutes, including four or more of the following: heart changes (e.g., palpitations, pounding heart, or accelerated heart rate), sweating, trembling/shaking, sensations of shortness of breath, feelings of choking, chest pain or discomfort, nausea or abdominal distress, feeling dizzy/faint/unsteady, chills or heat sensations, paresthesia, derealization or depersonalization, fear of losing control or "going crazy," or fear of dying. The second necessary component to this diagnosis is the presence of either significant worry about having another panic attack or a maladaptive change in behavior to avoid having another panic attack (e.g., avoiding places where panic attacks have occurred in the past) lasting at least a month. Often panic attacks seem out of the blue with unclear triggers. Consider a patient who has panic attacks when faced with socializing with others due to their social anxiety disorder. Their panic attacks are a symptom of their underlying anxiety disorder. However, if they also fear additional panic attacks for 1 month or more, they may also have a comorbid panic disorder.

> **CLINICAL TIP**
>
> Not every incident of intense anxiety is a panic attack. Panic attacks are defined as an abrupt surge or intense fear or discomfort, peaking within minutes, including four or more specified symptoms accompanied with the fear of having another panic attack or avoidance of places where a panic attack may occur.

Generalized Anxiety Disorder

Up to 9% of adults will experience generalized anxiety disorder at some point in their life. The diagnosis peaks in middle age and declines across later years or life. Generalized anxiety disorder is characterized by excessive anxiety and worry about a variety of events. This disorder is often chronic, and symptoms must be present for more days than not for 6 months or greater to meet criteria. The worry is difficult to control and causes dysfunction. The anxiety must be associated with three or more of the following symptoms: restlessness or feeling on edge, fatigue, poor concentration, irritability, muscle tension, and sleep disturbance. Patients with this disorder are sometimes hesitant to treat their underlying disorder due to anxiety about the consequences of treating it. For example, they may express concerns about the side effects of the medications or the financial cost of therapy. They may also worry that if they stop worrying so much, they may fail to complete one or more tasks that their anxiety would otherwise prompt them to address. However, often the dysfunction caused by the disorder (e.g., chronically poor sleep due to worrying about the next day's events) outweighs the potential concerns over treatment.

It is important to note that criteria must be met strictly, or the clinician can consider diagnoses such as other specified anxiety disorder or unspecified anxiety disorder. An overarching requirement when making any anxiety disorder diagnosis is the necessary presence of some form of dysfunction. This could mean poor performance at work or school, restricted social activities, or changes in any other area of functioning important to the patient. After better understanding the patient's symptoms, asking how these symptoms are impacting their day-to-day life is necessary before formally diagnosing a patient with a disorder.

MEMORY TIP

Generalized Anxiety Disorder, *useful mnemonic*

WATCHERS
W—Worry
A—Anxiety
T—Tension in muscles
C—Concentration difficulty
H—Hyperarousal (or irritability)
E—Energy loss
R—Restlessness
S—Sleep disturbance

(Berber, 2000)

Other Specified Anxiety Disorder

This category applies to presentations in which symptoms characteristic of an anxiety disorder that cause clinically significant distress or impairment predominate but do not meet the full criteria for any of the disorders in the anxiety disorders diagnostic class. This diagnosis is used in situations in which the clinician chooses to communicate the specific reason that the presentation does not meet the criteria for any specific anxiety disorder. This is done by recording "other specified anxiety disorder" followed by the specific reason (e.g., "generalized anxiety not occurring more days than not").

Unspecified Anxiety Disorder

The category applies to presentations in which symptoms characteristic of an anxiety disorder that cause clinically significant distress predominate but do not meet the full criteria for any of the disorders in the anxiety disorder diagnostic class. The unspecified anxiety disorder category is used in situations in which the clinician chooses *not* to specify the reason the criteria are not met for a specific anxiety disorder and includes presentations in which there is insufficient information to make a more specific diagnosis (e.g., in emergency room settings).

Anxiety Disorder Due to Another Medical Condition

Many patients first present to their primary care physician for physical manifestations of their anxiety. However, many medical conditions can also cause symptoms of anxiety. For example, hyperthyroidism is well known to cause anxiety symptoms. In addition, air hunger related to chronic obstructive pulmonary disease (COPD), congestive heart failure (CHF), or other respiratory illnesses causing hypoxia can induce symptoms of anxiety. If panic attacks or anxiety is predominant in the clinical picture, a diagnosis of anxiety disorder due to another medical condition can be considered. Importantly, the anxiety must be a direct pathophysiological consequence of the condition. If the anxiety or distress is resultant of the medical condition, but it is not a pathophysiological consequence, diagnoses such as adjustment disorder, somatic symptom disorder, or illness anxiety disorder may be considered. These are discussed elsewhere in the book. Anxiety in the context of delirium is also excluded from this diagnosis. Anxiety symptoms are expected to improve with the resolution of the medical illness.

CLINICAL TIP

Adult patients presenting with no family history, previous personal history or concern for anxiety, and no identifiable psychosocial precipitants for anxiety symptoms should increase the suspicion of substance use or underlying medical condition(s).

Substance- or Medication-Induced Anxiety Disorder

Another factor to consider in the diagnosis of an anxiety disorder is to rule out medications or substances that may be causing anxiety. This may be complicated as some patients struggling with anxiety may turn to substances to help them cope. These include alcohol and cannabis, both known for causing sedation. However, substances and medications (prescribed or over the counter [OTC]) themselves may also cause anxiety. For example, a patient who is prescribed corticosteroids and albuterol for asthma may be at risk for anxiety secondary to the corticosteroids and albuterol.

Establishing a timeline of symptom onset and substance or medication use is particularly helpful when making this diagnosis. If predominant panic attacks and anxiety are developed soon after or during the use of the substance, and the substance is capable of producing such symptoms, a substance- or medication-induced anxiety disorder may be considered. If the patient's symptoms precede the onset of use, the symptoms last more than a month after the cessation of use, or if the patient has had similar symptoms previously without the involvement of the substance of question, an alternative diagnosis should be considered. Substances that are commonly known to cause a substance-induced anxiety disorder are "uppers," such as amphetamines, cocaine, or even caffeine. The diagnoses can also be seen when in acute withdrawal from "downers," such as alcohol, benzodiazepines, or opiates.

TABLE 17.1 General Characteristics of Different Anxiety Disorders

Disorder	General characteristics
Separation anxiety disorder	Often develops in childhood; involves excessive fear or anxiety about separation from attachment figures
Selective mutism	Consistent failure to speak in social situations where there is an expectation to speak
Specific phobia	Anxiety, fear, and avoidance of specific situations or objects
Social phobia	Anxiety, fear and avoidance of social interactions, often with the cognitive basis that others are negatively judging them
Agoraphobia	Fear or anxiety around being in open spaces, crowds, or places where escape or retreat is difficult.
Panic disorder	Recurrent unexpected attacks of acute anxiety with somatic symptoms, often associated with avoidance of triggers and fear of recurrence
Generalized anxiety disorder	Persistent and excessive worry about a variety of activities and events that includes some physical symptoms
Anxiety disorder due to general medical condition	Anxiety symptoms that are biologically caused by another medical condition
Anxiety disorder due to substances	Anxiety symptoms that are biologically caused by a substance (which include prescribed, OTC, and substances that may be misused)

Obsessive-Compulsive Disorder

In the *DSM-5*, obsessive–compulsive disorder (OCD) moved out of the anxiety disorders category into a separate category for obsessive-compulsive and related disorders. OCD affects up to 3% of females and 1.5% of males over the lifetime. While females are diagnosed with this illness more often in adulthood, the illness affects males more commonly in childhood. Interestingly, up to 30% of patients with OCD have a lifetime prevalence of a tic disorder. Patients with OCD struggle with the presence of obsession, compulsions, or both. Obsessions are defined as recurrent and persistent thoughts, urges, or images that are considered intrusive and unwanted and often cause marked anxiety or distress. The patient must also attempt to ignore or suppress the thoughts in some way, often by attempting to neutralize them through performing a compulsion. A compulsion is defined as a repetitive behavior (e.g., hand washing, checking, counting, praying) that the patient feels driven to perform in response to an obsession or in accordance to rigid rules. Additionally, the acts must be aimed at reducing anxiety or distress or preventing some dreaded situation. However, the acts are generally not realistically connected to that which they are designed to neutralize or are excessive.

To meet criteria for OCD, the obsessions or compulsions must take more than one hour or day or cause significant dysfunction. The Yale–Brown obsessive compulsive scale (Y-BOCS) can be used to better characterize the patient's illness. A commonly mistaken diagnosis is obsessive compulsive personality disorder. While patients with both of these disorders may experience preoccupation with orderliness, the patient with obsessive compulsive disorder will experience the obsessions and compulsions as ego-dystonic (or intrusive in some way), whereas the patient with obsessive compulsive personality disorder will experience their symptoms as ego-syntonic (brings them comfort in some way).

> **MEMORY TIP**
>
> ***Obsessive Compulsive Disorder (OCD)****, useful mnemonic*
>
> **Thoughts RIDE TIME; Acts Reduce TIME**
>
> **A.** Presence of obsessions, compulsions, or both
>
> **Obsessions: Thoughts RIDE**
> Thoughts, urges or images that are:
> - **R**ecurrent and persistent
> - **I**ntrusive and unwanted
> - **D**istress (anxiety) provoking
> - **E**ffaced by ignoring or suppressing or neutralizing with other thought or compulsion.
>
> **Compulsions: Acts Reduce**
> - **Acts,** mental or behavioral, repetitively performed in response to an obsession or according to rigid rules
> - **Reduce** or prevent anxiety or distress; prevent a dreaded event
>
> **TIME**
> **B.** **T**ime-consuming or **IM**pair socio-occupational functioning
>
> **C.** **E**xclude being induced by a substance or another medical, or mental health condition
>
> *(Kadiyala, 2020)*

TREATMENT OF ANXIETY DISORDERS

The Biopsychosocial Model

When considering a choice of treatment, it is important to consider the biopsychosocial model of illness. Are there particular biological factors to consider? Comorbid medical conditions that may be contributing to the patient's anxiety level should always be treated as a priority, such as hyperthyroidism, asthma or other respiratory diseases that cause air hunger, and multiple sclerosis. Substance use may also play a role and is discussed later in this chapter. If the patient is at risk for arrhythmia, you would want to avoid medications that would increase that risk, such as citalopram. On the other hand, if the patient struggles with tachycardia, particularly when having to perform in front of others, propranolol might be a good option.

Psychological factors also play a role. What is the patient's primary method of coping? Some common positive coping strategies used to address anxiety include mindfulness meditations, controlled breathing, distraction (e.g., taking a walk, engaging in a pleasurable activity, etc.), or seeking comfort from close family or friends. Sometimes, patients have less healthy means of coping, such as avoiding uncomfortable emotions through the use of substance use, overeating, or even nonsuicidal self-harm behaviors, such as cutting or burning. A patient's psychological function also relates to their chosen defense mechanisms. Patients who primarily use primitive defense mechanisms tend to have a decreased ability to cope with unpleasant emotions. Primitive defense mechanisms include acting out, denial, regression, and projection. For example, if a patient struggles to cope with their anxiety and has immature defense mechanisms, they may cope by regressing to their childhood state (e.g., failing to go to work, moving back in with parents, talking in baby language, or seeking solace in childhood attachment objects such as stuffed animals or blankets). On the other hand, patients who tend to be more resilient to their anxiety generally use mature defense mechanisms, such as altruism, humor, sublimation, and suppression. For example, when a physician is faced with an emergently deteriorating patient, they may take a quick breath in and out before putting aside their anxiety about the situation (suppression) to perform necessary CPR. After the event, in either a good or bad outcome, they then allow themselves time to debrief, breathe deeply, and cope with the doubts and anxiety that generally follow emergent events.

When selecting a therapeutic choice for your patient, it is also important to consider if they have enough insight to allow for introspective psychotherapy, or should you focus on self-soothing techniques? If effective coping is not intact, challenging disordered thoughts in either cognitive behavioral therapy or in psychodynamic therapy may result in further decompensation and engagement in more primitive defense mechanisms. Most patients can benefit from increasing coping strategies. Cognitive behavioral therapy and psychodynamic psychotherapy are discussed later in this chapter.

Finally, understanding the patient's social background is imperative to treatment success. Does the patient have an adequate support system? Do they have the finances and structure needed to adhere to a treatment plan? Are they struggling with a very real threat to which their symptoms are *not* out of proportion? All of these factors must be considered when diagnosing a disorder and selecting a treatment plan.

Psychopharmacology

Medications are used in the treatment of anxiety disorders. This is especially when symptoms are severe, psychotherapy alone is insufficient, or when additional medical or substance use conditions complicate the clinical picture. Common medications used include SSRIs, SNRIs, Benzodiazepines, and other medications.

SSRIs

Selective serotonin reuptake inhibitors (SSRIs) work by stopping the reuptake of serotonin into the presynaptic cell, increasing the amount of serotonin available in the synaptic cleft and increasing the interaction between serotonin and postsynaptic cell receptors. Because much of the effect of the medication requires downstream downregulation, it typically takes 6–8 weeks for patients to see effects. While certain SSRIs carry specific indications for particular anxiety disorders, in general, SSRIs may be used interchangeably as a first-line treatment for anxiety disorders. All SSRIs carry the main side effects of headache, GI upset, and sexual dysfunction. Other notable qualities of specific SSRIs are discussed next. Medications are listed in the order they became available, not by frequency of use. Medication choice is dependent on a variety of factors, including side effect profile, what has worked for the patient or a family member in the past, and cost. For individuals under 24 years of age, SSRIs carry a black box warning about increased risk of suicidality (see Chapter 31, "Psychopharmacology," for additional details.)

Fluoxetine

This medication can sometimes be activating due to its additional activity at 5HT-2C. Some patients with anxiety find this worsens restlessness. Fluoxetine has the *longest* half-life among

SSRIs and can be dosed weekly if the patient struggles with daily medication compliance. It is FDA approved for OCD and panic disorder.

Paroxetine

This medication has some mild muscarinic activity, making it more sedating than other SSRIs. This calming side effect makes it a particularly good choice for anxiety disorders. However, as it has a short half-life, be on the lookout for uncomfortable side effects upon discontinuation. Paroxetine is FDA approved for GAD, social anxiety disorder, panic disorder, and OCD.

Sertraline

This medication is FDA approved for OCD, panic disorder, and social anxiety disorder. It can be somewhat activating like fluoxetine, but it also has anxiolytic activity at sigma 1 like fluvoxamine, making it a respectable choice for anxiety disorders.

Citalopram

This medication is notable to contain *both* the S and R enantiomers of the molecule. The R enantiomer is particularly problematic as it can cause QTc prolongation at high doses. Be cautious with patients at risk for arrhythmia or on other medications that prolong QTc. This medication is only FDA approved for major depressive disorder but is commonly used off-label for the treatment of anxiety disorders, due to its shared mechanism of action with other SSRIs.

Fluvoxamine

This medication is considered first-line for OCD and carries a specific FDA indication for this illness. It is also approved for use in social anxiety disorder. The medication is particularly effective for OCD, as it has additional activity at sigma 1 receptor; this has some anxiolytic properties and may also help with some psychotic processes, such as delusions. While OCD is not a psychotic disorder, some of the obsessions may have a psychotic quality to them that may make the illness particularly susceptible to treatment with this medication.

Escitalopram

This medication is the purest of the SSRIs in that it targets no other receptor (unlike paroxetine) outside of serotonin reuptake. It also has low protein binding, which reduces the likelihood of causing interactions with highly protein-bound drugs. This reduces the risk of unwanted side effects and drug interactions. It is a derivative of citalopram containing *only* the S enantiomer. Hence, there is significantly less risk regarding QTc prolongation. Escitalopram is FDA approved for GAD.

SNRIs

SNRIs work by blocking the reuptake of *both* serotonin and norepinephrine, therefore, increasing the concentrations of these chemicals in the synaptic cleft and allowing for greater attachment to postsynaptic cell receptors. Like the SSRIs, the SNRIs carry varying FDA approvals but are generally considered interchangeable due to their similar mechanism of action. Also, like with SSRIs, it may take 6–8 weeks for clinical impact to be noted by patients. They also have a similar side effect profile with common side effects including headache, GI upset, and sexual side effects. However, SNRIs also may increase the risk for hypertension and hyperhidrosis, due to the increase in extracellular norepinephrine.

Venlafaxine

This medication carries FDA approvals for GAD, social anxiety disorder, and panic disorder. This medication is known to increase blood pressure due to a preferential blocking of norepinephrine reuptake over serotonin reuptake as the dose increases. Be careful with patients already struggling with poorly controlled hypertension or underlying heart conditions.

Desvenlafaxine

This medication is the active metabolite of venlafaxine. It is thought to have fewer side effects and can be titrated quicker than venlafaxine. While desvenlafaxine is only FDA approved for major depressive disorder, it is commonly used to treat anxiety disorders due to its shared mechanism of action with the other SNRIs.

Duloxetine

This medication carries an FDA approval for GAD. It also carries FDA approvals for certain pain conditions, such as fibromyalgia, so it is particularly helpful for patients with anxiety and comorbid pain conditions or those with anxiety related to their painful medical conditions. Unlike venlafaxine, this medication inhibits serotonergic and noradrenergic reuptake equally as the dose increases.

Benzodiazepines

Benzodiazepines are some of the oldest medications approved for the treatment of anxiety. They rose to popularity in the 1960s and by the 1970s were the number one prescribed medication class in the world. The medication works by binding to the GABA-A receptor, increasing the frequency of the channel opening. This is contrasted with barbiturates, which bind to the same receptor but increase the duration of channel opening. This allows an influx of chloride, inhibiting synaptic response of the cell. When this occurs in the amygdala, the release of glutamate and the fear response are reduced. These medications are *highly* effective in treating anxiety acutely, though they are less commonly used now due to a negative side effect profile.

Benzodiazepines are well known to be addictive, allowing patients to build a rapid tolerance, requiring greater and greater doses. If abruptly stopped, the medications can cause a withdrawal phenomenon, which can mimic that of alcohol withdrawal. Patients initially become more anxious (known as a rebound effect), tremulous, and diaphoretic. The symptoms may then progress to increased heart rate and blood pressure and may eventually progress to delirium, seizure, and death.

In addition to addictive potential, benzodiazepines also have other negative effects such as sedation, increased risk of falls, cognitive decline, and increased risk of motor vehicle accidents. Benzodiazepines may be prescribed as a scheduled medication or "as needed" in times of panic or anxious distress.

There are two benzodiazepines that are FDA approved specifically for panic disorder: alprazolam and clonazepam. Selection is typically based on the desired duration of action (see Table 17.2; Shah & Borrensen, 2011). The patient's liver profile also plays into the selection of a benzodiazepine. *LOT* medications (e.g., lorazepam, oxazepam, and temazepam) are metabolized through conjugation rather than oxidation in the liver; therefore, no active metabolites are formed, and they are considered safer for those patients with underlying liver dysfunction. This is particularly useful when treating patients with liver dysfunction related to alcohol use.

TABLE 17.2 Common Benzodiazepines Used in Anxiety Disorders and Duration of Action

Medication name	Onset of action for oral route (hours)	Clinical duration of action (hours)	Half-life of parent drug	Half-life of metabolite	Duration of action
Alprazolam (Xanax)	0.5	3-4	6-12	-	Short-acting
Chlordiazepoxide (Librium)	1	4-6	6-25	3-100	Long-acting
Clonazepam	0.5-1	6-8	18-60	-	Long-acting
Diazepam (Valium)	0.5	4-6	20-70	3-100	Long-acting
Lorazepam (Ativan)	0.5-1	8	10-20	-	Intermediate-acting

Hydroxyzine

Hydroxyzine is an antihistamine, acting on the H1 receptor, similarly to diphenhydramine. However, unlike diphenhydramine, it also has some impact on the 5HT2A receptor and is less anticholinergic than diphenhydramine, making the medication useful for treating anxiety. The goal of the medication is to move the patient from an overactivated, restless, and anxious state to a calmer state by use of the sedating action of the H1 receptor (see Figure 17.3). If the patient is in the midst of burnout, hydroxyzine can help move them toward "optimum stress." However, if the dose is too high, the patient may move into an "inactive" state. A good rule of thumb is to start low and go slow with this and any potentially sedating medication. Hydroxyzine has anticholinergic side effects (e.g., dry mouth, urinary retention, etc.).

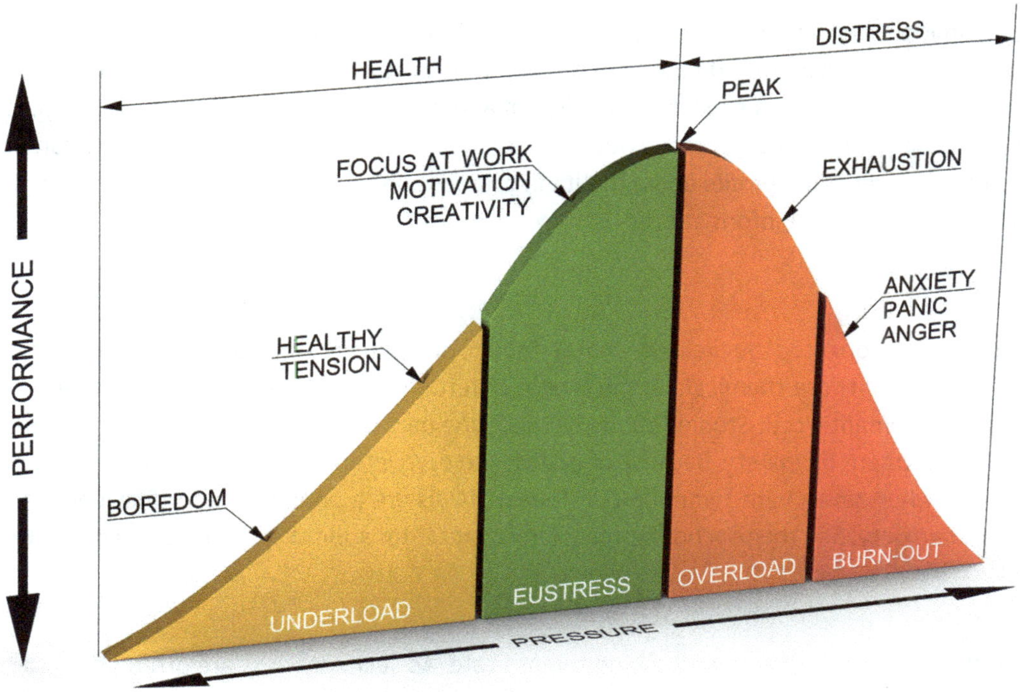

FIGURE 17.3 The stress performance spectrum.

Copyright © 2017 Depositphotos/Olivier26.

Buspirone

Buspirone has a unique mechanism of action—a 5HT-1A partial agonist. As opposed to SSRIs, which increase the amount of serotonin in the synaptic cleft, buspirone targets the postsynaptic receptor itself. This medication is generally prescribed as an augmenting agent due to its less robust efficacy than some other first-line anxiety medications. The most common side effect of the medication is dizziness. Also, the medication is recommended to be prescribed two to three times daily, which is sometimes inconvenient for the patient's schedule.

Propranolol

Propranolol is used to control autonomic symptoms of anxiety, mostly associated with panic attacks or performance anxiety. The medication blocks beta 1 and 2 receptors, thereby reducing heart rate and blood pressure, aiding with symptoms such as palpitations and sweating. As it also acts on beta 2 receptors, it should be used in caution with patients who have underlying asthma or other respiratory conditions that may be sensitive to bronchospasm. The main side effect is dizziness, and patients should be cautioned about delayed hypotension if used chronically.

Tricyclic Antidepressants (TCAs)

Doxepin is the one tricyclic antidepressant that is FDA approved for use in generalized anxiety disorder and is more sedating than the other TCAs. However, many TCAs are often used interchangeably due to a similar mechanism of action. As discussed in Chapter 31, "Psychopharmacology," TCAs are generally not considered first-line for treatment of many disorders due to their side effect profile and lethality in overdose. Please see the psychopharmacology chapter for additional information.

Monoamine Oxidase Inhibitors (MAOIs)

These medications stop the breakdown of serotonin, norepinephrine, and dopamine, increasing the amounts of these chemicals in the synaptic cleft and, therefore, increasing their effects on the postsynaptic cell. Studies do not suggest one particular MAOI over others in its class for the treatment of anxiety. Because of issues with drug interactions as well as the tyramine reaction when taken with tyramine-rich foods, MAOIs are a poor choice for first-line treatment of anxiety. See the psychopharmacology chapter for additional information on MAOIs.

Psychotherapy

Anxiety is a chronic illness with a high relapse rate. As such, patients are often opposed to the prospect of taking medications for years to decades of their life. Psychotherapy offers patients the benefit of reducing anxiety during the acute phase of their illness, while also learning skills to potentially prevent relapse should medications no longer be needed in the future. In addition, therapy can often be useful for anxiety-provoking situations where the threshold for a diagnosis of a disorder is not met. There are two main psychotherapeutic techniques used to treat anxiety: cognitive behavioral therapy (CBT) and psychodynamic therapy.

Cognitive Behavioral Therapy (CBT)

CBT helps patients explore the relationship between their thoughts, emotions, and actions. For example, let's explore the case of a medical student who is anxious about an upcoming examination. The therapist would help the student explore their specific emotions and the reasons behind them: Have they failed a test before? Are the stakes particularly high for this test? The therapist would then help the student explore some of the thoughts that trigger the emotions, such as: "I always do poorly on tests" or "If I don't do well, I will *never* reach my dreams." The next step is to challenge these thoughts. For example, just because tests haven't gone well in the past, it does not automatically predict performance in the future. The patient is asked to think of countering arguments to their own thoughts, similarly to if they had to disprove or prove the statement in a courtroom. By challenging and dispelling erroneous thoughts, the emotions (anxiety) behind them often improve. The patient is also asked to explore their behaviors: Is there anything they are doing or not doing that impacts their anxiety? For example, improper sleep is often linked with worsening anxiety. In addition, new behavioral techniques such as distraction, grounding, and respiratory training are introduced to help cope with anxiety and other negative emotions.

Systematic Desensitization

This technique is a form of behavioral therapy that is most commonly used for specific phobias. The patient is asked to tolerate increasingly triggering stimuli with the goal of desensitizing their autonomic response and therefore reducing their anxiety. For example, if a patient was afraid of snakes, they might be asked to look at a picture of a snake, then hold a toy snake, then tolerate being in a room with a snake in a cage, then in a room with a snake freely exploring the room, then, finally, holding a snake.

Psychodynamic Psychotherapy

Psychodynamic psychotherapy helps the patient gain insight into the development of their anxiety as well as how this anxiety relates to other areas in their life. For example, if a medical student is anxious about upcoming exams, the therapist might help the student explore their relationship between self-worth and external performance measures, whether their parents instilled an overvaluation of external performance in their core values and so on.

TREATMENT OF OBSESSIVE-COMPULSIVE DISORDER (OCD)

Psychopharmacology

The treatment of OCD is similar to that of other anxiety disorders in that the first-line treatment is often SSRIs. There are four SSRIs that have specific FDA indications for OCD (fluvoxamine, fluoxetine, paroxetine, and sertraline). Fluvoxamine is often considered the most effective SSRI for this disorder. Often, SSRI doses higher than the recommended FDA maximum are needed to achieve symptom remission. Second-line agents include TCAs with high serotonergic properties, namely clomipramine, which is often considered the gold standard treatment for OCD. Second-generation antipsychotics are occasionally used in conjunction with SSRIs as an augmenting agent.

Psychotherapy

Psychotherapy plays a large role in the recovery of the highly motivated patient. Studies have shown that cognitive behavioral therapy has similar efficacy in treating OCD as medications but can often have longer lasting effects on the patient's overall functioning and well-being (Sadock & Sadock, 2007). The principle techniques used are exposure and response prevention. For example, if the patient had obsessions related to germs, they might be exposed to a less than sanitary environment but not allowed to wash their hands unless they touched something unsanitary. Alternative coping behaviors and thought challenges may be introduced as well.

SUMMARY

Anxiety is the most common mental illness seen across the life span. The diversity of symptoms and clinical presentations makes this family of disorders one of the most complex and interesting in medicine. Everyone, at some point, will experience worry or fear. However, when symptoms become difficult to control, are long lasting, and cause dysfunction, medications and/or therapy can help reduce the mind's overactivated response.

RESOURCES

1 https://www.nimh.nih.gov/get-involved/digital-shareables/shareable-resources-on-anxiety-disorders

2 https://www.psychiatry.org/patients-families/anxiety-disorders/what-are-anxiety-disorders

3 https://www.aacap.org/AACAP/Families_and_Youth/Resource_Centers/Anxiety_Disorder_Resource_Center/Home.aspx

REFERENCES

American Psychiatric Association. (2013). *Diagnostic and statistical manual of mental disorders* (5th ed.).

Balt, S. (2013). Antipsychotics and anticonvulsants for anxiety disorders. *The Carlat Psychiatry Report, 11*, 1–5. Retrieved January 15, 2022, from https://www.thecarlatreport.com/the-carlat-psychiatry-report/antipsychotics-and-anticonvulsants-anxiety-disorders/

Beck RW. (2011). *Psychoneurological aspects: Functional neurology for practitioners of manual medicine e-book* (2nd ed.). Churchill Livingstone Elsevier Ltd.

Berber MJ. (2000). WATCHERS: Recognizing generalized anxiety disorder. *The Journal of Clinical Psychiatry, 61*(6):447.

Degenhardt, L., Chiu, W. T., Sampson, N., Kessler, R. C., & Anthony, J. C. (2007). Epidemiological patterns of extra-medical drug use in the United States: Evidence from the National Comorbidity Survey Replication, 2001–2003. *Drug and Alcohol Dependence, 90*(2–3), 210–223. https://doi.org/10.1016/j.drugalcdep.2007.03.007

Kadiyala, P. K. (2020). Mnemonics for diagnostic criteria of DSM V mental disorders: A scoping review. *General Psychiatry, 33*(3), e100109. https://doi.org/10.1136/gpsych-2019-100109

Karg R. S., Bose J., Batts K. R., Forman-Hoffman, V. L., Liao, D., Hirsch, E., Pemberton, M. R., Colpe, L. J., & Hedden, S. L. (2014). Past year mental disorders among adults in the united states: Results from the 2008–2012 mental health surveillance study. *CBHSQ Data Review*. https://www.ncbi.nlm.nih.gov/books/NBK379142/figure/Data-Review_N2.f3.5/

Kessler, R. C., Petukhova, M., Sampson, N. A., Zaslavsky, A. M., & Wittchen, H. (2012). Twelve-month and lifetime prevalence and lifetime morbid risk of anxiety and mood disorders in the United States. *International Journal of Methods in Psychiatric Research, 21*(3), 169–184.

Sadock, B. J., & Sadock, V. A. (2007). *Kaplan and Sadock's synopsis of psychiatry: Behavioral sciences/clinical psychiatry*. Wolters Kluwer.

Shah, D., & Borrensen, D. (August). Benzodiazepines: A guide to safe prescribing. *The Carlat Report, 9*, 1–4.

Stahl, S. M. (2013). *Stahl's essential psychopharmacology*. Cambridge University Press.

Yerkes R. M., & Dodson J. D. (1908). The relation of strength of stimulus to rapidity of habit-formation. *Journal of Comparative Neurology and Psychology, 18*(5): 459–482. https://www.doi.org/10.1002/cne.920180503

CHAPTER 18

Trauma- and Stressor-Related Disorders[1]

Kammarauche Asuzu, M.D., M.H.S.; Sophia Banu, M.D.; and Edore Onigu-Otite, M.D.

"There are wounds that never show on the body that are deeper and more hurtful than anything that bleeds."

— Laurell K. Hamilton, Mistral's Kiss

OBJECTIVES

At the end of this chapter, students will be able to do the following:

- describe different trauma- and stressor-related disorders
- understand the pathophysiology of trauma
- discuss common treatment approaches for trauma- and stressor-related disorders

CASE VIGNETTE

Miguel is a 12-year-old male who has been otherwise healthy and has had regular primary care appointments. His vaccinations are up to date. Over the last 6 months, he has had multiple complaints of abdominal pain, which has led to several visits with his primary care provider (PCP), but no abnormalities have been found. After he presented in the emergency room (ER) with severe abdominal pain and vomiting, a consult to the gastrointestinal specialist was placed. A medical work up showed normal physical findings. Following his ER visit, he saw his PCP who screened him using the patient health questionnaire for

(*continued*)

1 Readers may also see "Adverse Childhood Experiences (ACE) and Resilience" (Chapter 36) and "Diversity and Cultural Psychiatry" (Chapter 42) for related material.

adolescents (PHQ-A) and generalized anxiety disorder (GAD7), which found that he was very anxious and depressed. He was referred to psychiatry for further evaluation.

The psychiatrist conducted a psychiatric interview. Miguel lives with his father, mother, and 15-year-old sister. His parents say Miguel jumps at every little sound or sudden movement. He always wants to know his parents are close by. He often checks to ensure the doors at home are locked. Miguel and his sister were close, but recently he seems to be starting up arguments with her daily. Miguel's parents do not understand what the problem is and think this is the "beginning of adolescence." His parents have also become increasingly frustrated with Miguel who gets upset when they try to comfort him with hugs. Miguel was always a good sleeper, but recently, he worries about going to sleep, resists going to sleep, and frequently wakes up in the middle of the night panicked. He often asks to sleep with his parents, which is also a source of concern to the parents. He recently began wetting the bed at night, something he had not done in years. In school, Miguel, previously a good student, now struggles to focus and has started doing poorly. He says he has friends in school. He also mentions that he gets scared, sad, and angry when he sees older boys. Follow-up questions revealed he had been sexually assaulted about 7 months ago by an older teen in his neighborhood. At times memories of this experience flash through his mind and he gets angry and feels like punching things for no reason. When he remembers the assault, Miguel says he sometimes wishes he would disappear, so he doesn't have to remember. He denies wanting to die or hurt himself in any way. He eats well and says he is looking forward to his 13th birthday.

Miguel was diagnosed with posttraumatic stress disorder (PTSD). The psychiatrist met with his parents to explain what Miguel has been going through and how his problematic symptoms are as a result of PTSD. His parents found this helpful and validating. They asked how they could support him. Parents learned that responding in a frustrated manner to Miguel when he is frustrated could be retraumatizing and unsupportive. Miguel and his parents also learned that evidence-based treatment exists and can help Miguel return to functioning well at home and school. Miguel and his family were referred for trauma-focused cognitive behavior therapy (TF-CBT). This involved both parents and child. In a safe environment provided by therapy, Miguel first learned relaxation exercises to manage the strong negative emotions triggered by the memory of the assault. Through the family involvement in treatment, Miguel learned to talk to his parents about his feelings when upset. His parents learned to support Miguel, specifically related to the traumatic event by noticing when Miguel is distressed, helping Miguel put his distress into words, and helping him use his coping strategies. Over the next few months, Miguel began to feel better, and his peri-traumatic symptoms gradually improved. Over the next year, he completed his trauma narrative, which helped him resolve his conflicted emotions around his experience. It also helped him identify experiences that triggered the symptoms of PTSD. His problems with focus in school resolved and his sleep improved. He became happy again and only occasionally now does he have nightmares.

DEFINITIONS AND KEY CONCEPTS

Psychological trauma is a response to an event, a series of events, or a set of circumstances experienced by an individual as physically or emotionally harmful or threatening. This experience often involves terrifying, dangerous, or violent events that threaten the bodily integrity or life of a person or others. The threat of harm occurs when there is an expression of an intention, including using words, gestures, or weapons, to communicate the likelihood of inflicting damage on the individual. The threat of harm can be explicit, such as pointing/waving a weapon at someone, or implicit, such as verbal statements like, "you better watch your back" (signaling to an individual to be on alert because harm is coming their way). Traumatic experiences may occur directly or indirectly through witnessing or learning about the traumatic event. Traumatic experiences can have lasting adverse effects on the individual's functioning and physical, social, emotional, or spiritual well-being (Substance Abuse and Mental Health Services Administration [SAMHSA], 2019).

Various types of trauma can occur on the individual, family, or community levels. Adverse childhood experiences (ACEs) and maltreatment, including abuse and neglect at any age, can have lasting consequences. *Transgenerational* or *intergenerational trauma* refers to the transmission of the experience of trauma to offspring via complex mechanisms. *Historical trauma* refers to the collective emotional harm suffered, due to the traumatic experiences encountered by an individual, group, or generation. *Medical trauma* refers to trauma experienced due to medical illness or treatment, including pain, injury, procedures, or frightening treatment experiences. *Vicarious trauma* refers to a profound shift in world view in providers due to working with clients with trauma. *Complex trauma* describes a profound neuropsychological response to multiple and diverse traumatic experiences that are often invasive and intrapersonal in nature and often recurrent over time. *Race-based trauma* describes cumulative response to witnessing or experiencing racism. These events may include witnessing or experiencing threats of harm or other humiliating experience due to race. *Trauma-informed care* (TIC) is a treatment approach that facilitates engagement and effective health delivery for patients with trauma, including ACEs.

INTRODUCTION

The psychological impact and nature of trauma first came to be understood in the late 19th century by Jean Martin-Charcot. Charcot first observed that hysteria, which was diagnosed among women who had suffered different kinds of violence, was psychological in nature. Before then, hysteria was thought to be due to a disease of the uterus, and women with hysteria underwent hysterectomies. Charcot, along with his student Pierre Janet, also noticed that when women spoke about their traumatic experiences under hypnosis, they got better. Since then, our understanding of traumatic experiences and the effects on physical and mental health has continued to improve. The effect of trauma occurs due to biological, psychological, and social factors, which increase the likelihood of a person developing a mental health disorder. Notably, individual factors increase resilience (the ability to cope despite adversity) and decrease the likelihood of developing poor health outcomes (see Chapter 38, "Psychiatric Emergencies"). Posttraumatic growth refers to developing a new understanding of self, how to relate to others, views of the world, and how to live life following trauma (Tedeschi & Calhoun, 1996).

Trauma threatens a person's sense of safety, and the body's response to this threat is referred to as stress. *Traumatic stress reactions are neuropsychological symptoms and signs that occur in response to a traumatic experience or reminder.* Symptoms may be physical (e.g., muscle tension, palpitations), emotional (e.g., anxiety, anger), or behavioral (e.g., isolation, physical aggression). A person may be aware or unaware of these symptoms, and because of these symptoms, they may struggle with carrying out daily responsibilities at home or work.

TABLE 18.1 Traumatic Events

	Category	Examples
Individual events	Emotional (psychological) abuse	Intentionally causing a state of fright or terror, controlling, demeaning, threatening to hurt or harm, etc.
	Physical abuse	Punching, beating, hitting with objects, etc.
	Sexual abuse	Actual, or threatened, sexual violence, such as rape, sex trafficking, noncontact sexual exploitation (e.g., having a minor engage in acts for another's sexual gratification such as dancing, watching porn, etc.)
	Neglect	Emotional or physical
	Abandonment	Unannounced disappearance of a caregiver
	Accidental injury	Actual or witnessed vehicle accident (e.g., motor, plane, boat, train, etc.)
	Medical trauma	Actual or witnessed experience of a painful, prolonged, or frightening medical treatment
	Physical violence	Being beaten, mugging, kidnapping, torture, or shooting
	Intimate partner violence	Occurs in married, nonmarried, and dating couples, including teens; can include multiple categories of trauma, including emotional, physical, sexual, neglect, etc.
Household events	Household members	Sudden or traumatic death of a household member
	Home environment	Domestic violence, living with household members with substance use problems or mental health disorders, house robberies, house fires, etc.
Community violence	Home community	Home break-ins, robberies, or murders
	School community	Actual or attempted school shootings
	Other community	Mass killings or shootings, wars, genocide
Natural disasters		Earthquakes, tornadoes, floods, forest fires, avalanches, mudslides

Traumatic events may occur at the individual (such as Miguel experienced), household, or community level (see Table 18.1). These events may occur directly to an individual, be witnessed, or indirectly occur when a person learns of an event that happened to a close friend or relative. Trauma- and stressor-related disorders describe disorders that arise in the setting of exposure to these types of events. In the *DSM-5*, trauma- and stressor-related disorders include adjustment disorder, acute stress disorder, posttraumatic stress disorder, reactive attachment disorder, and disinhibited social engagement disorder (APA, 2013).

EPIDEMIOLOGY

Exposure to potentially traumatic experiences (PTE) is common. Traumatic experiences increase the risk of developing subsequent mental health problems, including depression, anxiety, substance use disorders, and PTSD, particularly if left untreated (Lloyd, 2020). Exposure to a traumatic event does not always result in the development of PTSD. However, the higher the number of PTE, the higher the likelihood of experiencing significant psychiatric and physical symptoms as a sequela of the trauma. Multiple abusive experiences, often described as cumulative abuse, increases the risk of physical, mental, and economic problems compared to people without a history of abuse or exposure to a single event (Mcnutt et al., 2002; Sundermann et al., 2013). Exposure to traumatic experiences and PTSD is associated with suicidal ideation and attempts (Afifi et al., 2016; Ryan et al., 2020). Exposure to traumatic events and PTSD may result in significant functional impairment with physical disability, absenteeism, job loss, and lower income.

Children and Adolescents

The younger the age of exposure, the higher the risk of developing psychiatric comorbidities (Dunn et al., 2017). Globally and in the United States, over 50% of children and adolescents aged 2–17 years have been exposed to violence (Finkelhor et al., 2005; Hillis et al., 2016). According to the Centers for Disease Control and Prevention, 686,000 children were victims of maltreatment in 2012, of which 1,646 children died (CDC, 2014). Boys died at a higher rate (2.5/100,000) than girls (1.9/100,000). The most common traumatic event experienced by children and adolescents is the unexpected death of a loved one, followed by exposure to natural or human-made disasters (Martin et al., 2017). There was a racial disparity in death rates with 4.7/100,000 African American children dying compared to 1.6/100,000 for non-Hispanic White children. Children younger than 3 are at the greatest risk of dying following maltreatment, and parents were the most likely perpetrators (80% of cases).

The prevalence of reactive attachment disorder (RAD) and disinhibited social engagement disorder (DSED) are unknown in the general pediatric population, but in children exposed to neglect, RAD occurs in less than 10%, while DSED occurs in about 20% (Gleason et al., 2011). A recent study among institutionalized adolescents found the rates of RAD and DSED to be 9% and 8%, respectively (Seim et al., 2020).

Adjustment disorder is as high as 9–11% in outpatient psychiatric populations (Sundquist et al., 2017; Yaseen, 2017), and the prevalence of PTSD among children and adolescents is 4.7% with a higher prevalence among females (7.3%) compared to males (2.2%; McLaughlin et al., 2013). Although not entirely clear, sex disparity in the development of PTSD may be related to the effect of hormonal changes during puberty on the developing brain and differences in physiologic and limbic responses to stress (Garza & Jovanovic, 2017; McLaughlin et al., 2013). High estrogen levels at puberty are associated with increases in amygdala volumes, which is associated with heightened fear-based responses (Garza & Jovanovic, 2017). In addition, females are more likely to experience sexual trauma, which carries a higher risk of developing PTSD (Garza & Jovanovic, 2017). The risk of developing PTSD varies by the type of traumatic event exposure (Martin et al., 2017). Fortunately, children and adolescents are less likely to develop PTSD from the most common PTEs, such as the unexpected death of a loved one (Martin et al., 2017).

Adults

In a global sample of adults, 70.4% reported exposure to at least one traumatic event (Benjet et al., 2016). In a national sample of U.S. adults, 89.7% reported exposure to at least one traumatic event (Kilpatrick et al., 2013). Accidents or injuries and the unexpected death of a loved one were the two most common types of traumatic events. Intimate partner violence (IPV) refers to physical, sexual, or emotional abuse or the threat of physical or sexual violence inflicted on a person by an intimate partner (Saltzman et al., 1999). Globally, females were more likely to experience intimate partner/sexual violence (32%), although IPV also occurs among males (28%) (Breiding et al., 2014). IPV can occur across various life stages and is associated with chronic health conditions and depression (Sanz-Barbero et al., 2019), and it can result in homicide (Smith et al., 2014). Sex trafficking, a form of human trafficking, involves force, fraud, or coercion to make a child or adult engage in commercial sex acts. Sex trafficking increases the risk of sexually transmitted infections, pregnancy, infertility, chronic pain, substance use, mental disorders, and other physical conditions such as diabetes (CDC, 2020; Dovydaitis, 2010).

Individuals who have experienced childhood trauma are at increased risk of developing personality disorders, including borderline personality disorder and antisocial personality disorder. It is not entirely clear if exposure to the trauma directly leads to the development of these personality disorders or if personality disorders and trauma disorder share similar predisposing factors such as growing up in harsh family environments (Berenz et al., 2013). The prevalence of adjustment disorder in the general adult population ranges from 1%–2% (Casey et al., 2006; Maercker et al., 2012), and the lifetime prevalence of PTSD among adults ranges from 6.8%–8.6% (Kessler et al., 1995; Kilpatrick et al., 2013).

Elderly

Elder abuse remains significantly underrecognized and underreported. Up to 10% of the elderly experience abuse (Dong, 2015). The elderly may experience all forms of abuse, neglect, psychological, and financial abuse being the most common forms of abuse. Elder abuse increases the likelihood of mortality (Bond & Butler, 2013). Perpetrators are usually household members or caretakers. Elders who experience abuse often do not report this for fear of retaliation, fear of being placed in a nursing home, and feeling like they are a burden anyway. Risk factors for elder abuse include having a chronic health condition with impairments in activities of daily living, dementia, increased age, or a caregiver with mental health disorders (Berkowsky, 2020; Bond & Butler, 2013).

Military Trauma

Military personnel are highly trained, skilled, and resilient human beings. Conditions associated with military service can expose persons in the military to life-threatening incidents. Combat trauma refers to traumatic experiences that occur during war. These include bomb explosions with resultant concussions, traumatic brain injuries, loss of body parts, or death. Witnessing individual or mass violence can result in trauma. About 15.7% of military members (3.9% among men and 38.4% among women) report military sexual trauma (MST; Wilson, 2018). MST is grossly underreported for a number of reasons, including fear of retaliation and jeopardizing military careers as well as concern that nothing will be done (Wolff & Mills, 2016). Military trauma is associated with depression, PTSD, substance use disorders, suicidal behavior, eating disorders, and chronic pain disorders (Blais et al., 2017; O'Brien & Sher, 2013).

NEUROPATHOLOGY AND PATHOPHYSIOLOGY

Stress is a part of daily life. In response to encountering stress certain biological changes occur. Under normal circumstances, the body's stress response resolves when the stressor is gone. However, with toxic, chronic, or traumatic stress, the body's stress response can become dysregulated resulting in psychological and physiological symptoms.

Normal Stress Response

Following exposure to a stressful event, the body responds by activating the hypothalamo–pituitary–adrenal (HPA) axis (Chu et al., 2020; Tsigos et al., 2000). In response to signals from the sensory organs (e.g., eyes, ears, skin, and nose), signals are sent to the amygdala, which deciphers the information as stressful and activates the hypothalamus (Figure 18.1). The hypothalamus responds by releasing the corticotropin-releasing hormone, which stimulates the pituitary gland to secrete the adrenocorticotropic hormone (ACTH; Chu et al., 2020; Tsigos et al., 2000). ACTH stimulates the adrenal glands to secrete cortisol and epinephrine responsible for the fight, flight, or freeze response. Cortisol and epinephrine affect multiple systems to enable a person to adequately respond to the perceived threat, including cardiovascular (increased HR), respiratory (increased lung volumes), neuromuscular (to flee if needed), and endocrine (to produce more glucose) responses. Once the threat has passed, cortisol acts in a negative feedback fashion to stop CRH release from the hypothalamus.

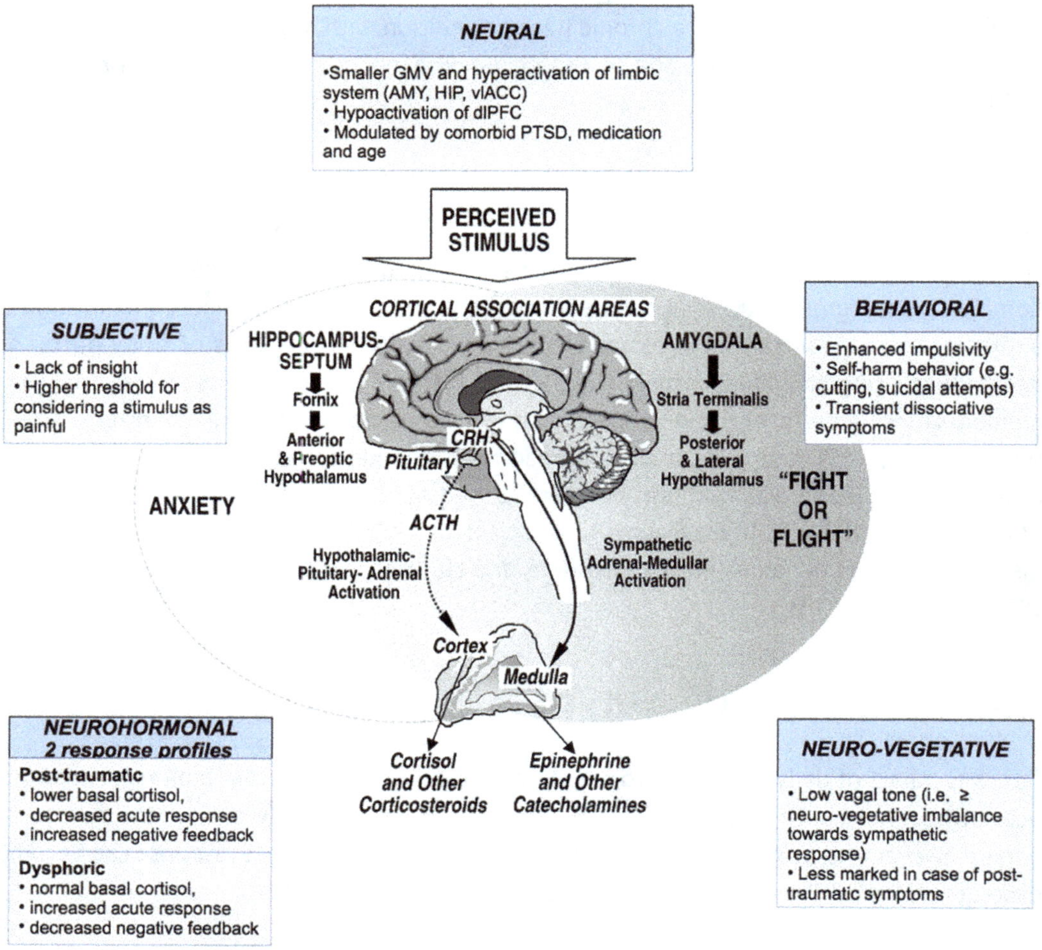

FIGURE 18.1 The stress system.

Copyright © by Nadège Bourvis, et al. (CC by 4.0) at https://www.frontiersin.org/articles/10.3389/fpsyg.2017.02054/full.

TABLE 18.2 Summary of Neurobiological Features With Identified Abnormalities and Functional Implications in Patients With Posttraumatic Stress Disorder

Feature	Change	Effect
A. Neuroendocrine		
Hypothalamic–pituitary–adrenal axis	Hypocortisolism	Disinhibits CRH/NE and upregulates response to stress
		Drives abnormal stress encoding and fear processing
	Sustained, increased level of CRH	Blunts ACTH response to CRH stimulation
		Promotes hippocampal atrophy
Hypothalamic–pituitary–thyroid axis	Abnormal T3: T4 ratio	Increases subjective anxiety
B. Neurochemical		
Catecholamines	Increased dopamine levels	Interferes with fear conditioning by mesolimbic system
	Increased norepinephrine levels/activity	Increases arousal, startle response, and encoding of fear memories
		Increases pulse, blood pressure, and response to memories
Serotonin	Decreased concentrations of 5 HT in dorsal raphe, median raphé, and dorsal/median raphé.	Disturbs dynamic between amygdala and hippocampus
		Compromises anxiolytic effects
		Increases vigilance, startle, impulsivity, and memory intrusions
Amino acids	Decreased GABA activity	Compromises anxiolytic effects
	Increased glutamate	Fosters derealization and dissociation
Peptides	Decreased plasma NPY concentrations	Leaves CRH/NE unopposed and upregulates response to stress
	Increased CSF b-endorphin levels	Fosters numbing, stress-induced analgesia, and dissociation
C. Neuroanatomic		
Hippocampus	Reduced volume and activity	Alters stress responses and extinction
Amygdala	Increased activity	Promotes hypervigilance and impairs discrimination of threat
Cortex	Reduced prefrontal volume	Dysregulates executive functions
	Reduced anterior cingulate volume	Impairs the extinction of fear responses
	Decreased medial prefrontal activation	Unclear

CRH: corticotropin-releasing hormone; 5HT: serotonin; GABA: y-aminobutyric acid; NPY: neuropeptide Y; ACTH: adrenocorticotropin; NE: norepinephrine; CSF: cerebrospinal fluid

QUICK POINT

At a neural level, trauma-related symptoms are associated with disordered neural pathways. Images of the brain show abnormalities in the prefrontal cortex (PFC), the amygdala, and the hippocampus in patients with PTSD (Sherin & Nemeroff, 2011).

Disordered Stress Response

In some patients with trauma exposure, this normal response to stress becomes dysregulated. The state of heightened arousal persists beyond the acute stressful event and is easily activated in situations where there is no actual threat, also called fear conditioning. As a result, there is a feeling of a loss of control. Attempts at regaining control usually manifest in trauma-related symptomatology. At a neural level, trauma-related symptoms are associated with disordered neural pathways. Images of the brain show abnormalities in the prefrontal cortex (PFC), the amygdala, and the hippocampus in patients with PTSD (Sherin & Nemeroff, 2011).

The amygdala is important in emotion processing and fear conditioning. Along with the hippocampus, which is also involved in memory storage and retrieval, traumatic experiences are associated with fear-based responses (Sherin & Nemeroff, 2011). In PTSD, the PFC, which aids thinking and decision-making, fails to help the amygdala make sense of the stimuli in situations where there is no actual threat, resulting in symptoms of PTSD such as hypervigilance (Sherin & Nemeroff, 2011). In the altered stress response, as the brain continues to perceive threats even when a threat no longer exists, cortisol remains elevated, leading to negative changes in the hippocampal neurons.

The hippocampus and prefrontal cortex inhibit the HPA while the amygdala stimulates the HPA axis. Children and adolescents with PTSD already show brain changes—a smaller prefrontal cortex, smaller gray matter and cerebellum, and a larger the amygdala (Keding & Herringa, 2015; Milani et al., 2017). The combination of these brain changes results in deficits in the prefrontal cortex's ability in modulating activation of the amygdala in response to traumatic reminders/triggers (Table 18.3).

TABLE 18.3 General differences between Stress and Trauma

	Stress	Trauma
Event and recollection	Nonaversive Usual or expected Part of normal life	Aversive Unusual, unexpected, or extreme Not an expected part of normal life
Stress response	Ordered Functional Generally, resolves following removal of stressor	Disordered Nonfunctional Persists even when the stressor has stopped
Feeling of control	Generally Preserved	Lost in variable degrees

CLINICAL MANIFESTATIONS

Stress is the body's reaction to a challenge or demand. It results in a feeling of emotional or physical tension. In short bursts, stress can be positive, such as by helping us avoid danger or meet deadlines. Stress can be positive or transient or negative or sustained (i.e., prolonged beyond the presence of the stressful event; see Figure 18.2). Traumatic stress is the body's response to trauma exposure or reminders. It can come from external sources (such as trauma reminders in the environment; for Miguel, an example of a trauma reminder was seeing older boys) or internal sources, sometimes called private events, including flashbacks in the form of thoughts, images, or deep-seated emotions related to past trauma stress response.

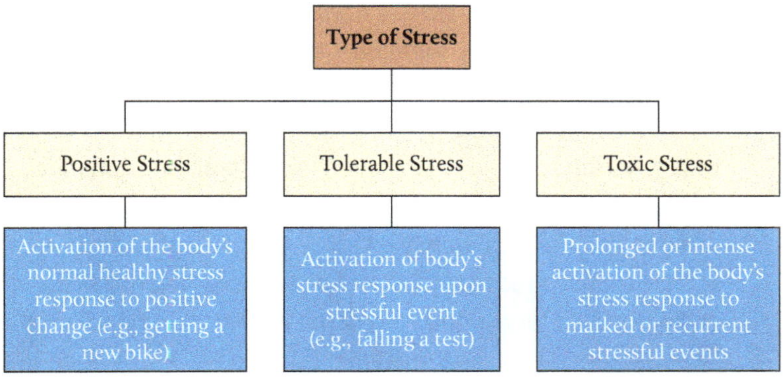

FIGURE 18.2 Different categories of stress.

How the event(s) is/are experienced is connected to the individual's developmental stage at the time of the trauma, their beliefs, their family, their culture, their exposure, and other social experiences. Some individuals do not recognize their experiences to be unusual or harmful until much later when they learn this from external sources. How the event(s) is/are coded in memory, particularly emotionally, and attached to meaning influences subsequent emotions and behavior. Negative emotions experienced at the time of the traumatic event, including shame, guilt, humiliation, betrayal, emotional numbness, fear, and terror, often shape the experience of the event. This influences the emotions that show up and the degree of psychological and physiological disruption that ensues, causing the specific trauma- and stressor-related symptoms, including anger, irritability, and aggression.

Trauma is hinged on an individual's personal experience and interpretation of the event. Different individuals may understand and experience the same event or critical components of the event differently with resultant varying effects. Autobiographical memory can be subject to reconstruction, which may affect the recall of encounters with trauma. Thus, individuals' representations or memories of their past experiences significantly contribute

> **KEY POINT**
>
> The three E's of trauma include event, experience, and effect. Individual trauma results from an event, series of events, or set of circumstances that is experienced by an individual as physically or emotionally harmful or life threatening and that has lasting adverse effects on the individual's functioning and mental, physical, social, emotional, or spiritual well-being.

to later psychopathology (Scott et al., 2010). This is in keeping with the three Es of trauma: event, experience, and effect. When these are followed by the shattering of the individual's trust and sense of safety, they indicate the presence of trauma (SAMHSA, 2014).

After exposure to a traumatic event, the onset of traumatic stress symptoms can occur immediately, soon after the event or may be delayed in onset. The long-lasting effects are a critical component of trauma and trauma treatment. They may occur immediately, may have a delayed onset, or may seemingly acquiesce until triggered by trauma reminders. In the face of perceived threat, danger, or trauma reminders, the brain triggers a cascade of events in other organs, resulting in a physiological stress response, including the release of stress hormones that cause these symptoms. Physical symptoms include increased muscle tension, trembling, palpitations, pupillary dilatation, feeling of choking, nausea, and gastrointestinal upset; emotional symptoms include fear or anxiety, sadness or depression, irritability or anger, and guilt; behavioral manifestations include avoidance of thoughts, reminders, or places associated with the trauma, isolating, or aggressive acts. When the threat is significant, it can result in the fear, fight, or freeze response. With toxic stress, responses can be dampened or heightened, and a freeze response (akin to playing possum) can occur. The resulting symptoms include negative emotions of anxiety, dysphoria, irritability, or dread; sleep disruption; and dissociative symptoms, including derealization and depersonalization.

Symptoms of traumatic stress are experienced and can be categorized into four main domains: intrusion, avoidance, hyperarousal, and alterations in mood and cognition (APA, 2013). Symptoms often vary by age. In very young children, flashbacks can occur via reenactment of their trauma experience, through play, through interaction with others or through actions during dissociative periods. For example, a child with a history of burns may be observed swatting away imaginary flames while in a daze. Children with abuse could repeat these abusive acts during play on dolls or other children. While children also have symptoms in these domains, they may present differently according to the child's developmental stage. For example, children may depict aspects of the traumatic event in drawings, develop problems in school, or regress to an earlier stage of functioning (such as reverting to thumb sucking, the loss of previously acquired language, or bedwetting; Gore et al., 2020).

The age of the individual at the time of experiencing a traumatic event is related to the risk of developing PTSD. Younger children are at a higher risk of developing PTSD, making children particularly vulnerable to the effects of certain types of trauma. Children exposed to traumatic or adverse experiences may develop disordered patterns of relating to people or impaired attachment. Problems in attachment may result in disorders, including RAD and DSED.

Traumatic experiences hinder development. Children who have experienced significant trauma experience have more progressive shortening of their telomere—a marker of premature aging (Shalev et al., 2013). In addition, children who have experienced trauma show cognitive and language delay, poor memory, behavioral regulation, and executive function (Bellis et al., 2009). Trauma also impacts development across multiple domains (e.g., cognitive, social, emotional), which can manifest as other comorbid disorders and an accumulative deficit of multiple coping skills. Van der Kolk coined the term *developmental trauma* to describe symptoms that develop in children who have traumatic experiences and problems in the emotional, attentional, and relational domains, yet they do not meet the criteria for PTSD (van der Kolk, 2007; van Der Kolk et al., 2019). It is important to note that in children, symptoms of PTSD may resemble ADHD. On the other hand, children with ADHD are also at increased risk of experiencing ACEs and other trauma, and as such, asking about trauma is clinically important. Adolescents with PTSD start to have symptoms similar to adults. They may disclose having problems with sleeping, nightmares, isolation from peers, frequent crying, and an inability to focus or concentrate at school with consequent failing grades (Gore et al., 2020). Adolescents may also present with depression and truancy and may begin to experiment with substances to avoid painful emotional symptoms.

QUICK POINT

Traumatic experiences hinder development. Children who have experienced significant trauma experience have more progressive shortening of their telomere—a marker of premature aging (Shalev et al., 2013).

Adults who have been exposed to abuse may exhibit deficits in executive dysfunction and working memory (Dodaj et al., 2017). Elderly individuals who are experiencing abuse may present with signs of neglect. These include untreated pressure sores, poor hygiene, lack of medical aids such as a walker or cane, unexplained injuries such as burns, fractures or lacerations, unexplained sexually transmitted diseases, delay in seeking medical treatment following an injury, laboratory findings that do not fit with the history provided, depression, and isolation (Bond & Butler, 2013).

Reactive Attachment Disorder and Disinhibited Social Engagement Disorder

Reactive attachment disorder (RAD) and disinhibited social engagement disorder (DSED) arise in the setting of severe neglect in the early years of life. Children who develop these disorders have been deprived of basic needs, such as leaving a baby hungry for hours, leaving a baby soiled for hours, consistent failure to comfort a crying baby, failure to cuddle a baby for a long time, and inconsistent and multiple caregivers. As a result, children fail to master Erikson's first stage of psychosocial development (trust versus mistrust). Children with RAD are withdrawn, do not express a wide range of affect/emotions, and are avoidant of behaviors that seek comfort or respond aggressively to behaviors meant to provide comfort, such as touch. Exposure to severe neglect can predispose to developmental delay (Spratt et al., 2012) and stereotypies, which may be comorbid in children with RAD and DSED. It is important, however, to identify developmental delay to provide appropriate treatment.

Due to the deficits in social relationships, autism spectrum disorder needs to be ruled out in children suspected to have RAD. Children with autism display repetitive, restricted behaviors and interests, which are not seen in RAD. Children with DSED do not show selective attachment behavior to primary caretakers. Instead, they exhibit overfamiliarity and inappropriate behaviors toward strangers. In children younger than 5, these behaviors may present as attention-seeking behaviors. Adolescents with DSED have significant problems in their relationships with peers arising from conflict and maintenance of poor boundaries. Impulsivity seen in DSED may raise concern for attention-deficit/ hyperactivity disorder. However, children with DSED without ADHD do not have problems with attention or hyperactivity.

KEY POINT

Adjustment disorders occur following an identifiable stressor. The emotional and behavioral response exceeds what is typically expected in a particular situation and is accompanied by significant functional impairment. Symptoms of adjustment disorder occur within 3 months of the event and usually resolve within 6 months after the stressful event has stopped or passed.

Adjustment Disorder

Adjustment disorders occur following an identifiable stressor and are distinct from normal negative reactions to bad events because the emotional and behavioral response is out of proportion to what is typically expected in a particular situation and is associated with significant functional impairment (APA, 2013). Symptoms occur within 3 months of the event and usually resolve within 6 months after the stressful event has stopped or passed. Symptoms arising from an adjustment disorder may interfere with functioning in school or at work, interfere with relationships, and interfere with treatment adherence.

KEY POINT

Acute stress disorder symptoms begin within three days after the traumatic event and resolve within 1 month.

Acute Stress Disorder

At least nine or more acute stress disorder symptoms persist for more than 3 days following the traumatic event and last up to a month (APA, 2013). Patients experience intrusive symptoms: repeated disturbing images about the event, nightmares; avoidance of any situation, place, or people that remind you of the event, experiencing physical symptoms such as sweating, palpitations, and gastrointestinal upset when reminded of the event; and developing negative patterns of thinking related to the event.

Posttraumatic Stress Disorder

Acute stress disorder and posttraumatic stress disorder (PTSD) share similar symptoms. Symptoms that persist beyond a month meet the criteria for PTSD. In addition to symptoms in the four domains (intrusion, avoidance, hyperarousal, and alterations in cognitions and mood), people with PTSD may experience paranoia or pseudo-hallucinatory phenomena characterized by the sensation of hearing whispers or one's thoughts (Brewin & Patel, 2010).

Risk factors for the development of PTSD include the severity of the traumatic event, the type of trauma (e.g., rape or exposure to war or combat), prior exposure to a traumatic event, history of child abuse, substance use, history of mental illness, lack of support systems, gender, exposure to adversity, and poor coping strategies. Emerging research suggests that there may be biological vulnerability that predisposes to disordered stress response and development of PTSD, such as finding low cortisol levels at the time of traumatic exposure in people who later developed PTSD (Sherin & Nemeroff, 2011).

CLINICAL TIP

PTSD symptoms in the four domains (intrusion, avoidance, hyperarousal, and alterations in cognitions and mood). People with PTSD may experience paranoia or pseudo-hallucinatory phenomena characterized by the sensation of hearing whispers or one's thoughts (Brewin & Patel, 2010).

DIAGNOSIS

Differential diagnoses following a traumatic or stressful experience include adjustment disorder, acute stress disorder, posttraumatic stress disorder, reactive attachment disorder, disinhibited social engagement disorder, another specified trauma- or stressor-related disorder, and unspecified trauma- or stressor-related disorder.

A diagnosis is made based on clinical assessment. According to the *DSM-5*, a diagnosis of ASD is made when a person develops nine or more symptoms, including intrusion, hyperarousal, and avoidance immediately following the event and lasting at least 3 days but not more than 1 month (APA, 2013). The criteria for PTSD require one or more symptoms of intrusion, one or more symptoms of avoidance, two or more symptoms of alterations in mood and cognition, and two or more symptoms of alterations in arousal (APA, 2013). In addition, symptoms need to have been present for at least 1 month following exposure, cause significant impairment in functioning, and are not attributable to the effects of a substance or a medical condition. In children 6 years or younger, the criteria for PTSD require one or more symptoms of intrusion, one or more symptoms of avoidance or alterations in mood and cognition, and two or more symptoms of alterations in arousal (APA, 2013). Like adults, symptoms need to be present for at least a month with accompanying impairment in social relationships and school functioning.

The diagnoses for RAD, DSED, and adjustment disorders are made when specific criteria are met according to the DSM (APA, 2013). Children younger than 9 months old do not have the developmental capacity to form selective attachments. As such, the diagnosis of RAD and DSED cannot be made before a child is 9 months old (APA, 2013).

> **MEMORY TIP**
>
> ***Post Traumatic Stress Disorder**, useful mnemonic*
>
> **TRRAAUMA**
>
> **T**—Traumatic event experienced, witnessed, or confronted by actual or threatened serious injury or threat to the physical integrity of self or others
> **R**—Response included intense horror, fear, or helplessness
> **R**—Reexperiencing by intrusive thoughts, nightmares, flashbacks, or recollection of traumatic memories and images.
> **A**—Avoidance of physical reminders (e.g., people, places, things associated with the traumatic experience) and emotions (e.g., emotional numbing, dissociation, detachment from others, and flattening of affect; loss of interest; and lack of motivation)
> **A**—Alterations in cognitions and mood negatively: lack of focus, loss of memory for event, depressed mood, negative cognitions of self, others, or the world
> **U**—Unable to function: distress or functional impairment in social, occupational, or interpersonal functioning
> **M**—Month: symptoms last longer than 1 month
> **A**—Arousal: hypervigilance, exaggerated startled reaction, poor sleep and concentration, or irritable mood
>
> *(Adapted from Khouzam, 2001)*

Assessing Trauma

A comprehensive assessment is necessary to determine accurate diagnosis and comorbid disorders and inform appropriate management. Firstly, this includes a thorough psychiatric interview. Comorbid disorders, such as substance use disorder or borderline personality disorder, need to be treated concurrently to ensure successful outcomes. In conjunction with a clinical assessment, psychometrically validated measures can be used to monitor improvement in treatment. These include CAPS-CA (clinician-administered PTSD Scale), UCLA PTSD reaction index for *DSM-4*, child PTSD symptom scale (CPSS), trauma symptom checklist for children (TSCC), trauma symptom inventory-2 (TSI-2), ASC-kids (for acute stress disorder). The goal of treatment is to reduce or eliminate posttraumatic symptoms of intrusion; hyperarousal, such as problems with sleep; and mood changes.

Treatment

The past, including the events and experience of traumatic events cannot be undone. However, the future, including living and thriving with trauma, can be intentionally done. The odds of recovery from trauma are strongly increased when adequate treatment is received. The goal of treatment is to reduce or eliminate posttraumatic symptoms of intrusion, hyperarousal, such as problems with sleep, and mood changes and improve functioning. A trauma-informed care approach should be employed in addressing symptoms. This starts from the initial contact of the patient and family; being observant to individual needs of the patient, which vary by type of abuse; current symptomatology; areas of functional impairment; and family dynamics. The mainstay of trauma treatment is psychosocial. However, medications play a pivotal role in treating trauma in many individuals.

PSYCHOPHARMACOLOGY

Medications are indicated when therapy alone is not sufficient, symptoms are severe and significantly impairing, and safety toward self or others is of concern. The different classes of medications used for PTSD include SSRIs, SNRIs, alpha-2 agonists, alpha antagonists, and neuroleptics. SSRIs have been shown to be effective in reducing symptoms of PTSD. Several SSRI medications are FDA approved for treating PTSD in adults, including sertraline and paroxetine. However, other SSRIs, including fluoxetine, citalopram, and escitalopram, have been used, with fluoxetine having the most evidence for use. Despite different medication trials, only about two thirds of patients respond to SSRI medications, and one third of patients show clinical remission of symptoms (Gu et al., 2016; Steckler & Risbrough, 2012). Among the SNRI medications, venlafaxine ER has shown efficacy in treating PTSD in randomized controlled trials. In children and adolescents, the evidence for SSRI medications is limited, and SSRIs are used to treat comorbid disorders such as anxiety and depression. Atypical antipsychotics are best used as adjunctive therapies and are generally not recommended for monotherapy or first-line treatments. Risperidone and Seroquel have been the most studied. Risperidone can be helpful in reducing intrusive symptoms (Adetunji et al., 2005), while Seroquel appears helpful in addressing sleep-related problems among patients with PTSD. Prazosin, an alpha-antagonist, has been useful for reducing intrusive symptoms, such as nightmares and hyperarousal symptoms (Simon & Rousseau, 2017). Alpha-2 agonists include guanfacine and clonidine, both of which have limited evidence for use in treating PTSD but may be useful in patients with residual hyperarousal and sleep-related symptoms (Belkin & Schwartz, 2015).

QUICK POINT

The past, including the events and experience of traumatic events cannot be undone. However, the future including living and thriving with trauma can be intentionally done. The odds of recovery from trauma are strongly increased when adequate treatment is received.

CLINICAL TIP

Medications are indicated when therapy alone is not sufficient, symptoms are severe and significantly impairing, and safety toward self or others is of concern.

PSYCHOTHERAPY

Psychotherapy is the primary modality of treatment used to target trauma-related disorders in children and is the recommended first-line treatment in adults. Evidence-based psychotherapy treatments for adults include CBT, cognitive processing therapy (CPT), and prolonged exposure (PE; Guideline Development Panel for the Treatment of PTSD in Adults & American Psychological Association, 2019; Watkins et al., 2018). Evidence-based treatment for children and adolescents include child and family traumatic stress intervention (CFTSI), trauma-focused cognitive behavioral therapy (TF-CBT), child–parent psychotherapy (CPP), and parent–child interaction therapy (PCIT). TF-CBT is considered the gold

KEY POINT

Psychotherapy is the primary modality of treatment used to target trauma-related disorders in children and is the recommended first-line treatment in adults. There are several evidence-based psychotherapies that are effective in treating trauma. Of these, trauma-focused cognitive behavior therapy, (TF-CBT) is considered the gold standard.

standard of treatment of trauma in children (The National Child Traumatic Stress Network, n.d.). TF-CBT is a family-focused treatment involving both the traumatized child or teen and their parents. All forms of therapy include psychoeducation that helps that patient and their family (with children) understand the relationship between the traumatic experience and its symptoms.

CBT targets PSTD by addressing negative, unhelpful thoughts that perpetuate fear and hyperarousal symptoms by helping patients challenge untrue beliefs known as distortions. Distortions include overgeneralizations, such as "the world is a bad place." Similarly, CPT helps patients evaluate unhelpful thinking patterns and teaches them how to change these thought patterns. Both CPT and CBT are based on the notion that thoughts, feelings, and behaviors are interrelated and that a change in one's thoughts can also serve to reduce unhelpful negative emotions. Prolonged exposure addresses the intense negative emotions (e.g., fear and shame) triggered when patients recall the traumatic event. By reviewing the trauma in a controlled and supportive environment in therapy, patients learn to reduce the association of these negative emotions with memories of the traumatic event.

Child and family traumatic stress intervention (CFTSI) is an evidence-based family intervention for children and adolescents (Berkowitz et al., 2011; Epstein et al., 2017). CFTSI is indicated within the first 30–45 days following a traumatic event's experience or disclosure. The treatment involves the child or adolescent and a caregiver. CFTSI targets peritraumatic symptoms by improving communication between child and caregiver, supporting the family, and teaching coping strategies to manage symptoms. CFTSI is a brief treatment that occurs over five to eight sessions and has been shown to effectively reduce peritraumatic symptoms. TF-CBT is a longer-term treatment for children and their caregivers (Kliethermes et al., 2017). CPP is also a long-term treatment, typically lasting 1 year and is indicated for children and adolescents aged 0–6 years (Reyes et al., 2017). CPP targets traumatic symptoms by addressing and strengthening the relationship between the child and parent as a medium to improve the child's functioning in multiple domains (Reyes et al., 2017).

Other Treatments

Other treatments that have been used in trauma treatment include eye movement desensitization and reprocessing therapy (EMDR; Chen et al., 2018), eclectic psychotherapy (BEP; Lindauer et al., 2005), and narrative exposure therapy (NET; Lely et al., 2019).

MEDICAL CONSIDERATIONS

Children, adolescents, and elders are at increased risk of physical abuse. In certain situations, it may be readily evident that abuse has occurred. However, in certain circumstances, it may be challenging to determine if abuse has occurred. Vagueness or inconsistencies about how the individual sustained the injury can point to a possible abuse case (Kellogg,

2007; Kodner & Wetherton, 2013). The physical examination may reveal bruises, bite marks, scalp hematomas, burn marks, rib, and other skeletal fractures (Kellogg, 2007; Kodner & Wetherton, 2013). Imaging may reveal multiple fractures, brain bleeds, or bowel rupture (Kellogg, 2007; Kodner & Wetherton, 2013). During medical encounters, some patients with a history of trauma may experience intense anxiety and emotional distress, which may trigger symptoms. These include unexpected physical contact, some physical examination maneuvers, vaginal examinations, Pap smear procedures, interactions with health care workers of the opposite sex, and so on.

TRAUMA-INFORMED CARE (TIC)

Trauma-informed care, or a trauma-informed approach, refers to the context of the delivery of health care services in a manner that facilitates effective engagement and care of individuals, including those with trauma histories. Health care workers and systems with a trauma-informed approach exhibit helpful behaviors that engage patients. SAMHSA (2015) has defined four main components that define trauma-informed care, which are known as the four Rs (see Table 18.3). A trauma-informed approach reflects adherence to six key principles rather than a prescribed set of practices or procedures.

TABLE 18.4 The Four Rs: Defining Components in a Trauma-Informed Approach

Realize	*Realizing* the impact of trauma while understanding potential paths of recovery and resilience
Recognize	*Recognizing* signs and symptoms of trauma in patients, families, staff, and others
Respond	*Responding* and fully integrating knowledge about trauma into policies, procedures, and practices
Resist retraumatization	Actively *resisting retraumatization*

Source: Substance Abuse and Mental Health Services Administration. (2014). (SAMHSA, 2014)

CLINICAL TIP

During medical encounters, some patients with a history of trauma may experience intense anxiety and emotional distress, which may trigger symptoms. These include unexpected physical contact, some physical examination maneuvers, vaginal examinations, Pap smear procedures, interactions with health care workers of the opposite sex, and so on.

QUICK POINT

With appropriate supports and intervention, people can overcome traumatic experiences.

KEY POINT

The four Rs of trauma-informed care or approach are:

- *Realizing* the impact of trauma while understanding potential paths of recovery and resilience
- *Recognizing* signs and symptoms of trauma in patients, families, staff, and others
- *Responding* and fully integrating knowledge about trauma into policies, procedures, and practices
- Actively *resisting retraumatization*

TABLE 18.5 Key Principles of a Trauma-Informed Approach

Principle	Application
Trauma awareness and acknowledgment	• Increase staff awareness of the prevalence and effects of trauma/ ACEs on substance use, mental health, and physical health • Educate staff on how trauma and ACEs affect life experiences • Recognize the effect of trauma and ACEs on a patient's development and coping strategies in daily life (e.g., with difficult or challenging patient encounters)
Safety and trustworthiness	• Support patients and help them feel they are in a safe place • Recognize the need for emotional and physical safety (during communication avoid disrespect, impatient or angry undertones, raised voice tones, fast-paced speech; respect the need for personal space) • Avoid interventions that might trigger or retraumatize a patient (e.g., inform of physical touch if needed as part of a procedure, etc.) • Design services that maximize access and participation by trauma survivors (allow reasonable flexibility in scheduling) to facilitate continuity of care • Promote cultural competence with respect to a person's context (e.g., financial instability, dependents' care, and work-related constraints) and life experiences
Peer support	• Ask, "What happened to this patient?" as opposed to, "What's wrong with this patient?" • Express empathy. This promotes a therapeutic milieu, which facilitates healing and recovery • Support a patient's self-efficacy and sense of empowerment • Provide the space to discuss patient strengths even within context of discussing their symptoms and pathology
Collaboration and mutuality	• Realize everyone has a role and a part to play, including the patient and their family members • Engage in two-way conversations • Develop a collaborative relationship (e.g., "We will work this through together")
Empowerment, voice, and choice	• Ask directly and listen for patient input in decisions affecting their treatment • Seek feedback and involve patients when designing and evaluating services
Cultural, historical, and gender issues	• Increase cultural sensitivity awareness in staff • Incorporate processes that are sensitive to a patient's culture, ethnicity, and social and personal identity • Incorporate processes that are sensitive to trauma associated with group marginalization

SUMMARY

Exposure to traumatic events is common and can result in significant mental health disorders if not prevented, identified, and treated. Traumatic events can occur at any age. Biological, psychological, and social factors increase the risk of developing PTSD. Providers need to be aware of the trauma-related symptomatology to provide early screening and trauma-informed care, as neglecting to address this hinders response and recovery from comorbid disorders. Psychotherapy is the treatment of choice for PTSD, particularly among children and adolescents.

RESOURCES

1 https://www.samhsa.gov/trauma-violence

2 https://www.ptsd.va.gov/understand/index.asp

3 https://www.nctsn.org

4 https://istss.org/home

5 www.nationalcenterdvtraumamh.org

REFERENCES

Adetunji, B., Mathews, M., Williams, A., Budur, K., Mathews, M., Mahmud, J., & Osinowo, T. (2005). Use of antipsychotics in the treatment of post-traumatic stress disorder. *Psychiatry (Edgmont), 2*(4), 43–47.

Afifi, T. O., Taillieu, T., Zamorski, M. A., Turner, S., Cheung, K., & Sareen, J. (2016). Association of child abuse exposure with suicidal ideation, suicide plans, and suicide attempts in military personnel and the general population in Canada. *JAMA Psychiatry, 73*(3), 229–238. https://doi.org/10.1001/jamapsychiatry.2015.2732

American Psychiatric Association. (2013). *Diagnostic and statistical manual of mental disorders* (5th ed.).

Belkin, M. R., & Schwartz, T. L. (2015). Alpha-2 receptor agonists for the treatment of post-traumatic stress disorder. *Drugs in Context, 4*, 212286. https://doi.org/10.7573/dic.212286

Benjet, C., Bromet, E., Karam, E. G., Kessler, R. C., McLaughlin, K. A., Ruscio, A. M., Shahly, V., Stein, D. J., Petukhova, M., Hill, E., Alonso, J., Atwoli, L., Bunting, B., Bruffaerts, R., Caldas-de-Almeida, J. M., de Girolamo, G., Florescu, S., Gureje, O., Huang, Y., ... & Koenen, K. C. (2016). The epidemiology of traumatic event exposure worldwide: Results from the World Mental Health Survey Consortium. *Psychological Medicine, 46*(2), 327–343. https://doi.org/10.1017/S0033291715001981

Berenz, E. C., Amstadter, A. B., Aggen, S. H., Knudsen, G. P., Reichborn-Kjennerud, T., Gardner, C. O., & Kendler, K. S. (2013). Childhood trauma and personality disorder criterion counts: A co-twin control analysis. *Journal of Abnormal Psychology, 122*(4), 1070–1076. https://doi.org/10.1037/a0034238

Berkowitz, S. J., Stover, C. S., & Marans, S. R. (2011). The child and family traumatic stress intervention: Secondary prevention for youth at risk of developing PTSD. *Journal of Child Psychology and Psychiatry, 52*(6), 676–685. https://doi.org/10.1111/j.1469-7610.2010.02321.x

Berkowsky, R. W. (2020). Elder mistreatment and psychological well-being among older Americans. *International Journal of Environmental Research and Public Health, 17*(20). https://doi.org/10.3390/ijerph17207525

Blais, R. K., Brignone, E., Maguen, S., Carter, M. E., Fargo, J. D., & Gundlapalli, A. V. (2017). Military sexual trauma is associated with post-deployment eating disorders among Afghanistan and Iraq veterans. *The International Journal of Eating Disorders, 50*(7), 808–816. https://doi.org/10.1002/eat.22705

Bond, M. C., & Butler, K. H. (2013). Elder abuse and neglect: Definitions, epidemiology, and approaches to emergency department screening. *Clinics in Geriatric Medicine, 29*(1), 257–273. https://doi.org/10.1016/j.cger.2012.09.004

Breiding, M. J., Smith, S. G., Basile, K. C., Walters, M. L., Chen, J., & Merrick, M. T. (2014). *Prevalence and characteristics of sexual violence, stalking, and intimate partner violence victimization—National Intimate Partner and Sexual Violence Survey, United States, 2011*. Centers for Disease Control and Prevention. https://www.cdc.gov/mmwr/preview/mmwrhtml/ss6308a1.htm

Brewin, C. R., & Patel, T. (2010). Auditory pseudohallucinations in United Kingdom war veterans and civilians with post-traumatic stress disorder. *The Journal of Clinical Psychiatry, 71*(4), 419–425. https://doi.org/10.4088/JCP.09m05469blu

Casey, P., Maracy, M., Kelly, B. D., Lehtinen, V., Ayuso-Mateos, J.-L., Dalgard, O. S., & Dowrick, C. (2006). Can adjustment disorder and depressive episode be distinguished? *Journal of Affective Disorders, 92*(2), 291–297. https://doi.org/10.1016/j.jad.2006.01.021

Centers for Disease Control and Prevention. (2020, February 11). *Sex trafficking*. https://www.cdc.gov/violenceprevention/sexualviolence/trafficking.html

Chen, R., Gillespie, A., Zhao, Y., Xu, Y., Ren, Y., & McLean, L. (2018). The efficacy of eye movement desensitization and reprocessing in children and adults who have experienced complex childhood trauma: A systematic review of randomized controlled trials. *Frontiers in Psychology, 9*. https://doi.org/10.3389/fpsyg.2018.00534

Chu, B., Marwaha, K., Sanvictores, T., & Ayers, D. (2020). *Physiology, stress reaction*. StatPearls. http://www.ncbi.nlm.nih.gov/books/NBK541120/

De Bellis, M. D., Hooper, S. R., Spratt, E. G., & Woolley, D. P. (2009). Neuropsychological findings in childhood neglect and their relationships to pediatric PTSD. *Journal of the International Neuropsychological Society: JINS, 15*(6), 868–878. https://doi.org/10.1017/S1355617709990464

Dodaj, A., Krajina, M., Sesar, K., & Šimić, N. (2017). The effects of maltreatment in childhood on working memory capacity in adulthood. *Europe's Journal of Psychology, 13*(4), 618–632. https://doi.org/10.5964/ejop.v13i4.1373

Dong, X. Q. (2015). Elder abuse: Systematic review and implications for practice. *Journal of the American Geriatrics Society, 63*(6), 1214–1238. https://doi.org/10.1111/jgs.13454

Dovydaitis, T. (2010). Human trafficking: The role of the health care provider. *Journal of Midwifery & Women's Health, 55*(5), 462–467. https://doi.org/10.1016/j.jmwh.2009.12.017

Dunn, E. C., Nishimi, K., Powers, A., & Bradley, B. (2017). Is the developmental timing of trauma exposure associated with depressive and post-traumatic stress disorder symptoms in adulthood? *Journal of Psychiatric Research, 84*, 119–127. https://doi.org/10.1016/j.jpsychires.2016.09.004

Epstein, C., Hahn, H., Berkowitz, S., & Marans, S. (2017). The Child and Family Traumatic Stress Intervention. In M. A. Landolt, M. Cloitre, & U. Schnyder (Eds.), *Evidence-based treatments for trauma-related disorders in children and adolescents* (pp. 145–166). Springer. https://doi.org/10.1007/978-3-319-46138-0_7

Finkelhor, D., Ormrod, R., Turner, H., & Hamby, S. L. (2005). The victimization of children and youth: A comprehensive, national survey. *Child Maltreatment, 10*(1), 5–25. https://doi.org/10.1177/1077559504271287

Garza, K., & Jovanovic, T. (2017). Impact of gender on child and adolescent PTSD. *Current Psychiatry Reports, 19*(11), 87. https://doi.org/10.1007/s11920-017-0830-6

Gleason, M. M., Fox, N. A., Drury, S., Smyke, A., Egger, H. L., Nelson, C. A., Gregas, M. C., & Zeanah, C. H. (2011). Validity of evidence-derived criteria for reactive attachment disorder: Indiscriminately social/disinhibited and emotionally withdrawn/inhibited types. *Journal of the American Academy of Child and Adolescent Psychiatry, 50*(3), 216–231.e3. https://doi.org/10.1016/j.jaac.2010.12.012

Gore, T. A., Lucas, J. Z., & Lubit, R. H. (2020). *Post-traumatic stress disorder: Practice essentials, background, etiology*. https://emedicine.medscape.com/article/288154-overview#a1

Gu, W., Wang, C., Li, Z., Wang, Z., & Zhang, X. (2016). Pharmacotherapies for posttraumatic stress disorder: A meta-analysis. *The Journal of Nervous and Mental Disease, 204*(5), 331–338. https://doi.org/10.1097/NMD.0000000000000478

Guideline Development Panel for the Treatment of PTSD in Adults & American Psychological Association. (2019). Summary of the clinical practice guideline for the treatment of post-traumatic stress disorder (PTSD) in adults. *The American Psychologist, 74*(5), 596–607. https://doi.org/10.1037/amp0000473

Hillis, S., Mercy, J., Amobi, A., & Kress, H. (2016). Global prevalence of past-year violence against children: A systematic review and minimum estimates. *Pediatrics, 137*(3). https://doi.org/10.1542/peds.2015-4079

Keding, T. J., & Herringa, R. J. (2015). Abnormal structure of fear circuitry in pediatric post-traumatic stress disorder. *Neuropsychopharmacology: Official Publication of the American College of Neuropsychopharmacology, 40*(3), 537–545. https://doi.org/10.1038/npp.2014.239

Kellogg, N. D. (2007). Evaluation of suspected child physical abuse. *Pediatrics, 119*(6), 1232–1241. https://doi.org/10.1542/peds.2007-0883

Kessler, R. C., Sonnega, A., Bromet, E., Hughes, M., & Nelson, C. B. (1995). Post-traumatic stress disorder in the National Comorbidity Survey. *Archives of General Psychiatry, 52*(12), 1048–1060. https://doi.org/10.1001/archpsyc.1995.03950240066012

Khouzam H. R. (2001). A simple mnemonic for the diagnostic criteria for post-traumatic stress disorder. *The Western Journal of Medicine, 174*(6), 424. https://doi.org/10.1136/ewjm.174.6.424

Kilpatrick, D. G., Resnick, H. S., Milanak, M. E., Miller, M. W., Keyes, K. M., & Friedman, M. J. (2013). National estimates of exposure to traumatic events and PTSD prevalence using DSM-IV and DSM-5 criteria. *Journal of Traumatic Stress, 26*(5), 537–547. https://doi.org/10.1002/jts.21848

Kliethermes, M. D., Drewry, K., & Wamser-Nanney, R. (2017). Trauma-focused cognitive behavioral therapy. In M. A. Landolt, M. Cloitre, & U. Schnyder (Eds.), *Evidence-based treatments for trauma-related disorders in children and adolescents* (pp. 167–186). Springer. https://doi.org/10.1007/978-3-319-46138-0_8

Kodner, C., & Wetherton, A. (2013). Diagnosis and management of physical abuse in Children. *American Family Physician, 88*(10), 669–675.

Lely, J. C. G., Smid, G. E., Jongedijk, R. A., W Knipscheer, J., & Kleber, R. J. (2019). The effectiveness of narrative exposure therapy: A review, meta-analysis and meta-regression analysis. *European Journal of Psychotraumatology, 10*(1), 1550344. https://doi.org/10.1080/20008198.2018.1550344

Lindauer, R. J. L., Gersons, B. P. R., van Meijel, E. P. M., Blom, K., Carlier, I. V. E., Vrijlandt, I., & Olff, M. (2005). Effects of brief eclectic psychotherapy in patients with post-traumatic stress disorder: Randomized clinical trial. *Journal of Traumatic Stress, 18*(3), 205–212. https://doi.org/10.1002/jts.20029

Lloyd, T. (2020). *The major effects of untreated childhood trauma: A systematic review* [Dissertation, Northcentral University]. https://search.proquest.com/docview/2455972085/abstract/49C86C89E7A7406DPQ/1

Maercker, A., Forstmeier, S., Pielmaier, L., Spangenberg, L., Brähler, E., & Glaesmer, H. (2012). Adjustment disorders: Prevalence in a representative nationwide survey in Germany. *Social Psychiatry and Psychiatric Epidemiology, 47*(11), 1745–1752. https://doi.org/10.1007/s00127-012-0493-x

Martin, A., Volkmar, F. R., & Bloch, M. H (Eds.). (2017). *Lewis's child and adolescent psychiatry: A comprehensive textbook* (5th edition). Wolters Kluwer Health.

McLaughlin, K. A., Koenen, K. C., Hill, E. D., Petukhova, M., Sampson, N. A., Zaslavsky, A. M., & Kessler, R. C. (2013). Trauma exposure and post-traumatic stress disorder in a national sample of adolescents. *Journal of the American Academy of Child and Adolescent Psychiatry, 52*(8), P815–830.e14. https://doi.org/10.1016/j.jaac.2013.05.011

Mcnutt, L.-A., Carlson, B. E., Persaud, M., & Postmus, J. (2002). Cumulative abuse experiences, physical health and health behaviors. *Annals of Epidemiology, 12*(2), 123–130. https://doi.org/10.1016/S1047-2797(01)00243-5

Milani, A. C. C., Hoffmann, E. V., Fossaluza, V., Jackowski, A. P., & Mello, M. F. (2017). Does pediatric post-traumatic stress disorder alter the brain? Systematic review and meta-analysis of structural and functional magnetic resonance imaging studies. *Psychiatry and Clinical Neurosciences, 71*(3), 154–169. https://doi.org/10.1111/pcn.12473

National Center for Injury Prevention and Control, & Division of Violence Prevention. (2014). *Understanding child maltreatment 2014 - cdc.gov*. https://www.cdc.gov/violenceprevention/pdf/CM-Factsheet-2013.pdf

National Child Traumatic Stress Network. (n.d.). *Home page*. https://www.nctsn.org/

O'Brien, B. S., & Sher, L. (2013). Military sexual trauma as a determinant in the development of mental and physical illness in male and female veterans. *International Journal of Adolescent Medicine and Health, 25*(3), 269–274. https://doi.org/10.1515/ijamh-2013-0061

Reyes, V., Stone, B. J., Dimmler, M. H., & Lieberman, A. F. (2017). Child–parent psychotherapy: An evidence-based treatment for infants and young children. In M. A. Landolt, M. Cloitre, & U. Schnyder (Eds.), *Evidence-based treatments for trauma-related disorders in children and adolescents* (pp. 321–340). Springer. https://doi.org/10.1007/978-3-319-46138-0_15

Ryan, A. T., Daruwala, S. E., Perera, K. U., Lee-Tauler, S. Y., Tucker, J., Grammer, G., Weaver, J., & Ghahramanlou-Holloway, M. (2020). The relationship between trauma exposure and psychiatric hospitalization for suicide ideation or suicide attempt among patients admitted to a military treatment setting. *International Journal of Environmental Research and Public Health, 17*(8), 2729. https://doi.org/10.3390/ijerph17082729

Saltzman, L. E., Fanslow, J. L., McMahon, P. M., & Shelley, G. A. (1999). *Intimate partner violence surveillance: Uniform definitions and recommended data elements*. https://stacks.cdc.gov/view/cdc/7537

Sanz-Barbero, B., Barón, N., & Vives-Cases, C. (2019). Prevalence, associated factors, and health impact of intimate partner violence against women in different life stages. *PLOS ONE, 14*(10), e0221049. https://doi.org/10.1371/journal.pone.0221049

Scott, K. M., Smith, D. R., & Ellis, P. M. (2010). Prospectively ascertained child maltreatment and its association with DSM-IV mental disorders in young adults. *Archives of General Psychiatry, 67*(7), 712–719. https://doi.org/10.1001/archgenpsychiatry.2010.71

Seim, A. R., Jozefiak, T., Wichstrøm, L., & Kayed, N. S. (2020). Validity of reactive attachment disorder and disinhibited social engagement disorder in adolescence. *European Child & Adolescent Psychiatry, 29*(10), 1465–1476. https://doi.org/10.1007/s00787-019-01456-9

Shalev, I., Moffitt, T. E., Sugden, K., Williams, B., Houts, R. M., Danese, A., Mill, J., Arseneault, L., & Caspi, A. (2013). Exposure to violence during childhood is associated with telomere erosion from 5 to 10 years of age: A longitudinal study. *Molecular Psychiatry, 18*(5), 576–581. https://doi.org/10.1038/mp.2012.32

Sherin, J. E., & Nemeroff, C. B. (2011). Post-traumatic stress disorder: The neurobiological impact of psychological trauma. *Dialogues in Clinical Neuroscience, 13*(3), 263–278.

Simon, P. Y. R., & Rousseau, P.-F. (2017). Treatment of post-traumatic stress disorders with the alpha-1 adrenergic antagonist Prazosin. *Canadian Journal of Psychiatry, 62*(3), 186–198. https://doi.org/10.1177/0706743716659275

Smith, S. G., Fowler, K. A., & Niolon, P. H. (2014). Intimate partner homicide and corollary victims in 16 states: National Violent Death Reporting System, 2003–2009. *American Journal of Public Health, 104*(3), 461–466. https://doi.org/10.2105/AJPH.2013.301582

Spratt, E. G., Friedenberg, S. L., Swenson, C. C., Larosa, A., De Bellis, M. D., Macias, M. M., Summer, A. P., Hulsey, T. C., Runyan, D. K., & Brady, K. T. (2012). The effects of early neglect on cognitive, language, and behavioral functioning in childhood. *Psychology, 3*(2), 175–182. https://doi.org/10.4236/psych.2012.32026

Steckler, T., & Risbrough, V. (2012). Pharmacological treatment of PTSD—established and new approaches. *Neuropharmacology, 62*(2), 617–627. https://doi.org/10.1016/j.neuropharm.2011.06.012

Substance Abuse and Mental Health Services Administration. (2014). SAMHSA's concept of trauma and guidance for a trauma-informed approach. HHS publication no. (SMA) 14-4884. Substance Abuse and Mental Health Services Administration.

Substance Abuse and Mental Health Services Administration. (2019). *Trauma and violence.* https://www.samhsa.gov/trauma-violence

Sundermann, J. M., Chu, A. T., & DePrince, A. P. (2013). Cumulative violence exposure, emotional nonacceptance, and mental health symptoms in a community sample of women. *Journal of Trauma & Dissociation: The Official Journal of the International Society for the Study of Dissociation (ISSD), 14*(1), 69–83. https://doi.org/10.1080/15299732.2012.710186

Sundquist, J., Ohlsson, H., Sundquist, K., & Kendler, K. S. (2017). Common adult psychiatric disorders in Swedish primary care where most mental health patients are treated. *BMC Psychiatry, 17*(1), 235. https://doi.org/10.1186/s12888-017-1381-4

Tedeschi, R. G., & Calhoun, L. G. (1996). The posttraumatic growth inventory: Measuring the positive legacy of trauma. *Journal of Traumatic Stress, 9*(3), 455–471. https://doi.org/10.1007/BF02103658

Tsigos, C., Kyrou, I., Kassi, E., & Chrousos, G. P. (2000). Stress: Endocrine physiology and pathophysiology. In K. R. Feingold, B. Anawalt, A. Boyce, G. Chrousos, W. W. de Herder, K. Dungan, A. Grossman, J. M. Hershman, H. J. Hofland, G. Kaltsas, C. Koch, P. Kopp, M. Korbonits, R. McLachlan, J. E. Morley, M. New, J. Purnell, F. Singer, C. A. Stratakis, ... & D. P. Wilson (Eds.). *Endotext.* http://www.ncbi.nlm.nih.gov/books/NBK278995/

van der Kolk, B. (2007). The developmental impact of childhood trauma. In L. J. Kirmayer, R. Lemelson, & M. Barad. *Understanding trauma: Integrating biological, clinical, and cultural perspectives.* https://doi.org/10.1017/CBO9780511500008.016

van der Kolk, B., Ford, J. D., & Spinazzola, J. (2019). Comorbidity of developmental trauma disorder (DTD) and post-traumatic stress disorder: Findings from the DTD field trial. *European Journal of Psychotraumatology, 10*(1). https://doi.org/10.1080/20008198.2018.1562841

Watkins, L. E., Sprang, K. R., & Rothbaum, B. O. (2018). Treating PTSD: A review of evidence-based psychotherapy interventions. *Frontiers in Behavioral Neuroscience, 12*, 258. https://doi.org/10.3389/fnbeh.2018.00258

Wilson, L. C. (2018). The prevalence of military sexual trauma: A meta-analysis. *Trauma, Violence & Abuse, 19*(5), 584–597. https://doi.org/10.1177/1524838016683459

Wolff, K. B., & Mills, P. D. (2016). Reporting military sexual trauma: A mixed-methods study of women veterans' experiences who served from World War II to the war in Afghanistan. *Military Medicine, 181*(8), 840–848. https://doi.org/10.7205/MILMED-D-15-00404

Yaseen, Y. A. (2017). Adjustment disorder: Prevalence, sociodemographic risk factors, and its subtypes in outpatient psychiatric clinic. *Asian Journal of Psychiatry, 28*, 82–85. https://doi.org/10.1016/j.ajp.2017.03.012

CHAPTER 19

Thought and Psychotic Disorders[1]

Olaoluwa Okusaga, M.D. and John Coverdale, M.D.

> *"And those who were seen dancing were thought to be insane by those who could not hear the music."*
>
> — Friedrich Nietzsche

OBJECTIVES

At the end of this chapter, students will be able to do the following:

- understand the symptoms of thought and psychotic disorders
- review and differentiate between types of primary psychotic disorders
- summarize secondary psychotic disorders

DEFINITIONS AND KEY CONCEPTS

The words *psychosis* or *psychotic* (an adjective) are often used to describe individuals presenting with some form of bizarre, abnormal, or unusual behavior. According to the U.S. National Institute of Mental Health (NIMH), "The word *psychosis* is used to describe conditions that affect the mind, where there has been some loss of contact with reality." (NIMH, 2020), Psychosis is not a specific diagnosis, but a term used to indicate the presence of certain symptoms. Based on the *Diagnostic and Statistical Manual of Mental Disorders* (5th ed.; *DSM-5*, American Psychiatric Association [APA], 2013), a person is said to be experiencing psychosis (i.e., having a psychotic episode) if the person has one or more of the following signs and symptoms:

- delusions
- hallucinations

1 Readers may also see "Psychopharmacology" (Chapter 31) for related material.

- disorganized speech (a reflection of disorganized thought process)
- grossly disorganized or catatonic behavior
- negative symptoms

It is also important to make a distinction between primary psychosis and secondary psychosis. Primary psychosis is psychosis that occurs without any clearly identified inducing agent/condition, while secondary psychosis is psychosis that can be attributed to an identified agent/condition (e.g., illicit drugs, prescribed medications, or medical conditions). Primary psychosis is generally synonymous with a primary psychotic disorder, such as schizophrenia. An important difference between primary psychosis and secondary psychosis is that secondary psychosis is expected to resolve after the inducing agent or condition is removed. For example, cocaine-induced psychosis is expected to resolve after a person stops using cocaine and the cocaine clears from the person's body. However, and especially in cases of illicit drug-induced psychosis, some individuals continue to experience psychosis after the inducing agent is removed, which suggests that they have developed a psychotic disorder that has become independent of the use of illicit substances.

KEY POINT

Thought disorders are a group of mental health disorders characterized by unusual, disorganized, or bizarre thoughts, speech, or behavior.

QUICK POINT

Psychosis often begins in late teens to mid-20s. About three out of 100 people will experience psychosis at some time in their lives. About 100,000 adolescents and young adults in the United States experience first-episode psychosis each year (U.S. Department of Health and Human Services, n.d.).

INTRODUCTION

The term *psychosis* was introduced by Canstatt in 1841 (Bürgy, 2008), and for most of the second half of the 19th century it was a nonspecific term synonymous with *mental illness* or *insanity*. Afterward, in 1899, Emil Kraepelin introduced the term *dementia praecox* (now replaced with *schizophrenia*) to describe certain individuals with early onset psychosis and deteriorating clinical course. The concept of psychosis has undergone several iterations over the past 100 years, and every health care professional who uses the term should understand its meaning and ramifications.

The Symptoms of Psychosis

The first step toward an understanding of the concept of thought disorder and psychosis is to fully grasp the distinction between *content* of thought and *form* (or process) of thought. The content of thought (i.e., thought content) refers to the thoughts and ideas contained in a person's mind. An example of an abnormal thought content is a delusion that is a fixed, false belief impervious to reason. On the other hand, form/process of thought (i.e., thought process) refers to the structure of a person's thought without reference to the content. Disorganized, illogical thinking are examples of abnormal thought processes. In psychiatric practice, the term *thought disorder* denotes abnormal thought content, thought process, or both (e.g., a patient who expresses delusional ideas but also disorganized in thinking; Oyebode, 2015). In practice, inferences on a person's thought are based on the person's speech.

CLINICAL TIP

Thought content and process involve but refer to different aspects of thought. *Thought content* refers to the thoughts or ideas contained in a person's mind. *Thought process* refers to how these thoughts are expressed.

CASE VIGNETTE A

A 28-year-old woman lives alone and (for no apparent reason) becomes convinced that her neighbors are FBI agents who are spying on her and monitoring her movements in and outside her home even though she does not have any evidence to support this belief. She clearly communicates her conviction of being monitored in a logical and coherent manner that is easy to comprehend. She is said to have a disorder of thought content rather than a disorder of thought process.

CASE VIGNETTE B

A 20-year-old man who was born and raised in Texas presents with disorganized speech that is difficult to comprehend because there is no clear connection between one expressed thought and another (i.e., nonlinear and illogical). He is described as having a disorder of thought process. Note that, when specifically referring to disorganized thinking (i.e., disorder of thought processes), the term *formal thought disorder* is also used.

Description of the Symptoms That Characterize Psychosis

Delusions

These are beliefs that are false but held with such tenacity that even in the light of significant conflicting evidence the false beliefs are not relinquished. Different types of delusions are listed in Table 19.1. Delusions are also categorized as bizarre if they are implausible and inconsistent with normal human experiences (e.g., delusion of being abducted by aliens from Mars) or nonbizarre if they are plausible (e.g., delusion of being spied on by the FBI).

KEY POINT

Delusions are fixed false beliefs that are impervious to reason. A delusion is a form of abnormal thought content.

TABLE 19.1 Different Types of Delusions

Types of delusions	
Paranoid delusions	A patient believes that they are being persecuted and may be suspicious and distrustful of others.
Grandiose delusions	A patient has an inflated and often unrealistic estimation of their abilities or uniqueness and feels superior to others.
Erotomanic delusions	The patient believes that another person is in love with them.
Delusions of reference (referential delusion)	The patient believes that statements made, behavior exhibited by people, or other cues in the environment have meanings or personal significance (when they actually do not; e.g., immediately after the doctor scratched his forehead the patient spontaneously became convinced independent of evidence to the contrary that the head scratching meant that the doctor concluded that they are stupid).
Nihilistic delusions	A patient believes that a catastrophic event has occurred (e.g., the patient believes that their internal organs are rotten or decomposed, they have ceased to exist, or the world has ended).
Somatic delusions	The patient becomes convinced, without evidence, that their organs, bodily functions, or appearance are grossly abnormal.
Thought insertions	The patient believes that some external agent is putting thoughts into their head.
Thought withdrawals	The patient believes that some outside agent is removing their thoughts.
Delusions of control	A patient believes that an outside agent or force is controlling their actions.

KEY POINT

Hallucinations are false sensory perceptions. In this case, there is no actual sensory stimulus, but the individual perceives that there is. On the other hand, illusions are misinterpretations of true sensory stimulus. There is a sensory stimulus, but it is misinterpreted as something it is not.

Hallucinations

These are defined as sensory perceptions in the absence of any external sensory stimulus—for example, hearing "voices" (an auditory perception) when there is nobody around talking. Hallucinations can involve all five sensory modalities (i.e., auditory, visual, olfactory, gustatory, and tactile). Auditory hallucinations, especially voices talking to the patient (second-person auditory hallucinations) or voices talking among themselves and referring to the patient as "he," "she," or "they" (third-person auditory hallucinations), are more often associated with primary mental illnesses, while visual, olfactory, gustatory, and tactile hallucinations should raise suspicion of a secondary psychosis (Waters & Fernyhough, 2017). Two types of hallucinatory experiences that are also worth describing are hypnagogic and hypnopompic hallucinations. Hypnagogic hallucinations are usually transient visual or auditory hallucinatory experiences (e.g., a person's name being called) that occur while a person is dozing off to sleep, while hypnopompic hallucinations are experienced while waking up. Both hypnagogic and hypnopompic hallucinations occur in healthy individuals and are not associated with any mental illness.

Disorganized Speech

This is speech that lacks coherence or is excessively vague and difficult to comprehend. As mentioned earlier, speech enables inferences to be made about a person's thinking, and as such, disorganized speech enables a description of the type of thought disorder a person is experiencing. *Tangential thinking* is characterized by a patient not giving direct answers to questions (even though they seem to understand the question) or who skirts around the topic and brings up other unrelated and irrelevant topics without returning to the original question. In *derailment* or *looseness of associations*, the patient initially starts talking about a specific topic but (either midsentence or between sentences) veers off topic onto either remotely related or totally unrelated topics. *Word salad* describes an extreme form of formal thought disorder in which speech is reduced to meaningless words and phrases that make speech incomprehensible given a severe loosening of associations. Tangentiality, derailment, and word salad are different types of loose associations. *Neologisms* are new words or phrases invented by the patient that have idiosyncratic, personal meaning to the patient. *Circumstantial thinking* is a relatively less severe form of thought disorder in which the patient gives excessively detailed and often unnecessary information that hinders the patient from getting to the point, but the patient eventually answers the original question.

Grossly Disorganized or Catatonic Behavior

Disorganized behavior characteristic of psychosis can present as bizarre, unpredictable, inappropriate responses that affect the person's ability to function in society. Catatonic behavior is characterized by abnormalities in the manner of relating to the environment and increased muscle tone. Catatonic behavior includes mutism (i.e., very little or absent verbal response not due to aphasia), stupor (i.e., absent psychomotor activity), echolalia (i.e., automatic repetition of interviewer's speech), echopraxia (i.e., automatic repetition of the interviewer's movements), and posturing (i.e., patient spontaneously assumes and maintains a posture against gravity for an abnormally prolonged duration). See Chapter 32, "Neuromodulation Treatments in Psychiatry."

MEMORY TIP

***Catatonia**, useful mnemonic*

WIRED 'N MIRED

W—Waxy flexibility/catalepsy
I—Immobility
R—Refusal to eat or drink
E—Excitement
D—Deadpan staring
N—Negativism
M—Mutism
I—Impulsivity
R—Rigidity
E—Echolalia/echopraxia
D—Direct observation of symptoms by clinic staff in the past day or week

(Carroll, 2008)

Negative Symptoms

Negative symptoms are so named because, unlike the first four symptoms described (which are also referred to as positive symptoms), they represent a deficit of features that are present in normal healthy individuals. Examples of negative symptoms include lack of variability in emotional expression (affective blunting), reduced speech and reduced content of speech (poverty of speech and poverty of content of speech), inability to initiate purposeful actions (loss of volition), and indifference to social interactions (loss of sociality).

PRIMARY PSYCHOTIC DISORDERS

Brief Psychotic Disorder

The *DSM-5* (APA, 2013) criteria for diagnosing brief psychotic disorder require the presence of one or more of delusions, hallucinations, disorganized speech, or grossly disorganized or catatonic behavior.

Psychotic symptoms that last 1 day to 1 month (Figure 19.1) with return to premorbid functional status are the two essential features of this condition. The effects of drugs of abuse, medications, and other medical or psychiatric conditions must be ruled out before making a diagnosis of brief psychotic disorder.

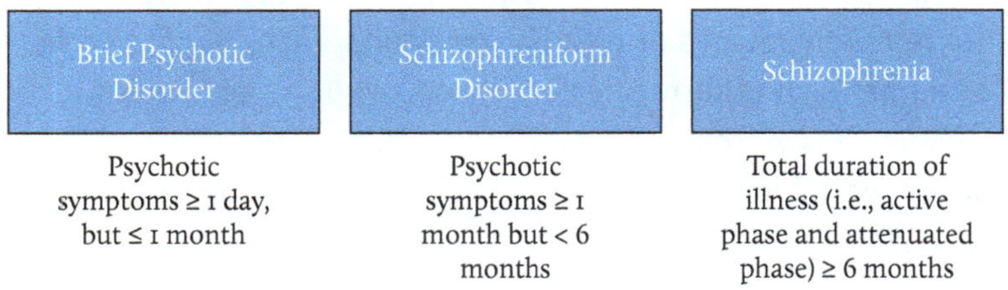
Brief Psychotic Disorder
Schizophreniform Disorder
Schizophrenia
Psychotic symptoms ≥ 1 day, but ≤ 1 month
Psychotic symptoms ≥ 1 month but < 6 months
Total duration of illness (i.e., active phase and attenuated phase) ≥ 6 months

FIGURE 19.1 Differentiating between the psychotic disorders based on the duration of psychotic symptoms. Figure 19.1 legend: The primary psychotic disorders are differentiated based on the duration of psychotic symptoms. Psychotic symptoms last a day to a month in a brief psychotic disorder, at least a month but less than 6 months in schizophreniform disorder, and 6 months or greater in schizophrenia.

Epidemiology

It is estimated that 9% of new cases of psychosis in the United States can be attributed to brief psychotic disorder (Susser et al., 1995). Brief psychotic disorder is twice as common in females than males. Brief psychotic disorder is seen across the life span, but the mean age of onset is mid-30s. Certain personality disorders (e.g., paranoid, schizotypal, or borderline personality disorder) can predispose a person to developing brief psychotic disorder.

Clinical Manifestations

In addition to the psychotic symptoms, individuals diagnosed with brief psychotic disorder may exhibit mood lability, confusion, and emotional turbulence. They may exhibit poor judgment and insight; therefore, steps to prevent harm to self and others in these cases should be taken. Sometimes the onset of symptoms coincides with significantly stressful events in the patient's life (in this case, a specifier—"with marked stressor[s]"—is added; i.e., a brief psychotic disorder with marked stressor). Onset of symptoms could also be during pregnancy or within 4 weeks postpartum (brief psychotic disorder with peripartum onset).

Treatment

Antipsychotic medications are prescribed for distressing psychotic symptoms. Benzodiazepines can also be prescribed (short term) for their calming properties. Supportive psychotherapy (i.e., empathic listening, encouraging the patient to elaborate on their concerns and reorienting to reality, and providing education and advice as to appropriate behaviors) should also be offered.

Schizophreniform Disorder

The *DSM-5* (APA, 2013) diagnostic criteria for schizophreniform disorder are the same as schizophrenia (please see the section on schizophrenia) with two exceptions: (a) the entire duration of illness for schizophreniform disorder is at least 1 month but less than 6 months (Figure 19.1) and (2) impaired social and occupational function could be present but is not required to make a diagnosis of schizophreniform disorder. In cases in which a patient's symptoms have not resolved and the duration of illness is more than 1 month (ruling out brief psychotic disorder) but less than 6 months, "schizophreniform disorder (provisional)" can be diagnosed, since it is not known if the patient's symptoms would resolve before the 6-month mark or progress beyond 6 months, when the diagnosis will change to schizophrenia. The estimated lifetime prevalence of schizophreniform disorder ranges between 0.05–0.07%. There is limited data regarding the pathophysiology and neurobiology of schizophreniform disorder. In terms of treatment, the same principles of treatment of psychosis in schizophrenia apply (please refer to the section on schizophrenia).

Schizophrenia

Schizophrenia, based on the *DSM-5* (APA, 2013) criteria, is defined by the presence of two or more symptoms of psychosis, including delusions, hallucinations, disorganized speech, grossly disorganized or catatonic behavior, and negative symptoms. Note that at least one of the symptoms must be delusions, hallucinations, or disorganized speech and that the psychotic symptoms must be present for a significant portion of a one-month period (referred to as "active-phase symptoms" and can last less than a month if the patient is treated). Continuous signs of the illness must persist for a minimum of 6 months (e.g., after the active phase, residual, attenuated psychotic symptoms, such as paranoia, odd beliefs, and behavior persist for at least five more months; see Figure 19.1). In addition, onset of psychotic symptoms is associated with a decline in several domains of functioning, including (but not limited to) self-care, social, academic, and occupational functioning. To make a diagnosis of schizophrenia, other mental disorders (including schizoaffective disorder, bipolar, or depressive disorder with psychotic features), the effects of a substance (medication or drug of abuse), and a medical condition, must have been ruled out.

> **MEMORY TIP**
>
> ***Schizophreniform Disorder***, *useful mnemonic*
>
> **Delusions Herald Schizophrenic's Bad News Delusions Herald Schizophrenic's Bad News**
>
> **D**—**D**elusions
> **H**—**H**allucinations
> **S**—**S**peech disorganization
> **B**—**B**ehavior disorganization
> **N**—**N**egative symptoms

Epidemiology and Genetics

The lifetime prevalence of schizophrenia is approximately 0.7% (Owen et al., 2016). The age of onset of symptoms of schizophrenia is earlier in men (18–25 years) than women (21–30 years). Schizophrenia increases the risk of suicide with a lifetime risk of 4–5%. Epidemiologic studies have found an association between the following environmental factors and schizophrenia, although in some cases these are tenuous: maternal infections and nutritional deficiencies during pregnancy, intrauterine growth retardation, obstetric complications, being born in late winter or early spring, childhood adversity, immigration (first and second generation), being born or raised in cities, advanced paternal age, and cannabis use. Cannabis use is an important risk factor well supported by evidence and is particularly important because it is a factor that can be modified. Genetics has also been found to play a role in the development of symptoms of schizophrenia. The risk of developing schizophrenia in individuals with various genetic loading for schizophrenia is as follows: 10% in individuals who have a sibling with schizophrenia; 5–6% in individuals who have one parent with schizophrenia; 46% in individuals who have both parents with schizophrenia.

> **KEY POINT**
>
> Dysregulation in the dopamine neurotransmission is the main neurobiological cause of psychotic disorders. In schizophrenia, increased dopaminergic neurotransmission in the mesolimbic pathway is linked to positive symptoms (e.g., hallucinations and delusions), while decreased dopaminergic neurotransmission in the mesocortical pathway is linked to negative symptoms (e.g., apathy, avolition, and anhedonia).

Neurobiology

Dysregulated dopamine neurotransmission has been implicated in the genesis of psychotic symptoms (McCutcheon et al., 2020). Specifically, increased dopaminergic neurotransmission in the mesolimbic pathway (the pathway involving dopamine-producing cells in the ventral tegmental area in the midbrain, which project to the striatum, hippocampus, and amygdala) is thought to be related to the development of positive symptoms (hallucinations and delusions). Decreased dopaminergic neurotransmission in the mesocortical pathway (dopamine-producing cells in the ventral tegmental area in the midbrain, which project to the prefrontal cortex) is postulated to underly negative and cognitive symptoms of schizophrenia. In addition, abnormalities in the N-methyl-D-aspartate (NMDA) glutamate transmission are also postulated to be related to the negative and cognitive symptoms of schizophrenia. Finally, chronic low-grade inflammatory processes and oxidative stress, which modulate the development and maintenance of synaptic connectivity, have also been implicated in the pathophysiology of schizophrenia.

The Stress-Vulnerability Model

Although the etiology of schizophrenia remains unknown, the stress–vulnerability hypothesis represents current thinking on the development of schizophrenia. The stress–vulnerability model posits that emotionally stressful events add to biological vulnerabilities in lowering the threshold for the development of schizophrenia and in lowering the likelihood of a reoccurrence of an illness episode. Two major sources of stress include ambient stressors, those that are associated with the home or living situation, and stressful life events. The ability to cope with these effectively reduces the risk of clinical morbidities (Falloon, 1986).

Clinical Manifestations

The signs and symptoms observed in patients with schizophrenia can be categorized into three main domains: positive, negative, and cognitive. Positive symptoms, the most dramatic symptom domain, include delusions, hallucinations, disorganized speech, and behaviors. Negative symptoms include blunting of emotional reactivity, social withdrawal, and alogia. Cognitive symptoms of schizophrenia include impaired selective attention, working memory, learning, and executive function. Agitation, anxiety, and demoralization are other symptoms with which patients may also present.

Treatment

Pharmacological Treatment

Antipsychotic medications are the mainstay schizophrenia treatment (APA, 2020). Apart from clozapine, which is approved for treatment-resistant schizophrenia (i.e., cases that fail to respond to at least two antipsychotic medications prescribed at optimal doses for an adequate duration), first-generation (also called typical or conventional) and second-generation (also called atypical) antipsychotics are generally equally effective for treating psychosis. However, first- and second-generation antipsychotics differ in their side effect profile with first-generation agents being more likely associated with extra-pyramidal side effects (EPS), such as acute dystonia, akathisia, parkinsonism, and tardive dyskinesia, while second-generation agents are more likely associated with metabolic syndrome (truncal obesity, glucose intolerance, dyslipidemia, and elevated blood pressure). Nowadays, more patients are started on and maintained on second-generation antipsychotics with fewer patients receiving the first-generation antipsychotics (this is probably because most practitioners want to avoid EPS, especially tardive dyskinesia). It is important to note that even though the risk of EPS is less in second-generation antipsychotics, this may still occur. Adjunctive medications used in treating schizophrenia include mood stabilizers (e.g., to target aggressiveness, impulsiveness and associated mood or affective symptoms), benzodiazepines (e.g., to target short term for anxiety, agitation, and insomnia), and antidepressants (e.g., to target associated depressive symptoms).

Psychological Treatments

Psychotherapies that have been reported to be beneficial for patients with schizophrenia include supportive psychotherapy and cognitive behavioral therapy (CBT) for psychosis (Eells, 2000). Of note, CBT for psychosis was recently found to have robust and stable efficacy for psychosis.

Social Interventions

Interventions that address the patient's social needs have also been found to be effective, especially for keeping patients well after the acute psychotic phase resolves. Social interventions include provision of housing, social skills training, vocational rehabilitation and supported employment. Other interventions that are beneficial include psychoeducation, cognitive remediation, family interventions, and intensive case management. One important and very well evidenced strategy comprehensively integrates the pharmacological approaches with psychosocial interventions. The psychosocial interventions involve patients and their primary care providers and include psychoeducation, early warning signs management, problem-solving skills training, communication skills training, social skills training, and specific cognitive behavioral strategies for addressing residual delusions (Coverdale, 2015; Falloon Coverdale et al., 1998; Falloon, Held et al., 1998). Moreover, psychiatric services should be closely integrated with other services relevant to treating biopsychosocial vulnerabilities. These include primary care and relevant medical services, nursing, pharmacies, occupational therapy, cognitive behavioral therapy, chemical dependency services, social work and rehabilitative services, and other allied professionals.

Schizoaffective Disorder

CLINICAL TIP

Schizoaffective disorders patient have the presence of psychotic symptoms (for at least 2 weeks) in the absence of a major mood episode.

Schizoaffective disorder is closely related to schizophrenia but is distinct based on the presence of mood episodes. The *DSM-5* (APA, 2013) diagnostic criteria for schizoaffective disorder include two or more of the five symptoms of psychosis (for 1 month or less if treated) required for schizophrenia, concurrent with a major mood episode (manic or depressive episode). In addition, the patient must have a history of psychosis (hallucinations or delusions) for 2 or more weeks in the absence of a major mood episode. The effects of substances (illicit drugs or medication) and general medical conditions must also be ruled out. There are two subtypes of schizoaffective disorder: bipolar type and depressive type. The bipolar subtype is diagnosed if the patient has had a manic episode (major depressive episodes may have also occurred), while the depressive subtype is diagnosed if the patient has only experienced depressive episodes. Figure 19.2 is a diagrammatic representation of differences between mood disorders with psychotic symptoms, schizophrenia, and schizoaffective disorder.

Epidemiology

The estimated lifetime prevalence of schizoaffective disorder is around 0.3% (Perälä et al., 2007), and it appears to occur more often in women than men. As in schizophrenia, the onset of the illness is later in women than men. The depressive subtype appears to be more common in the elderly and the bipolar type in younger individuals.

Neurobiology

The neurobiology of schizoaffective disorder has not been as well studied as for schizophrenia. Nevertheless, available studies indicate that cognitive impairment and brain grey matter volume loss, comparable to that seen in schizophrenia, are also present in schizoaffective disorder.

Clinical Manifestations

As in schizophrenia, patients with schizoaffective disorder experience positive, cognitive, and negative symptoms in addition to symptoms of a mood episode (e.g., depression or mania). Depressive episodes are associated with suicidal ideation and suicide attempt.

Treatment

Antipsychotic medications are prescribed to target psychotic symptoms, but they also target mood symptoms. However, antidepressants, mood stabilizers, and anxiolytic medications are also often prescribed. The psychological and social interventions that were discussed under the section on schizophrenia are similarly applicable to schizoaffective disorder.

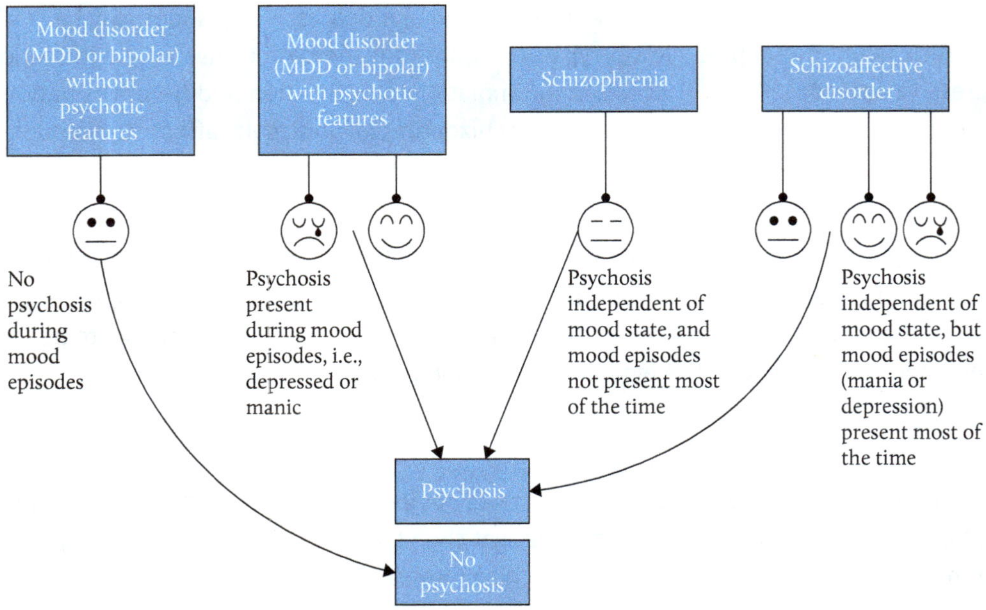

FIGURE 19.2 Distinguishing between a mood disorder with psychotic symptoms, schizophrenia, and a schizoaffective disorder. Although patients with mood disorder (i.e., MDD or bipolar disorder) can present with psychotic symptoms, it is important to note that patients with primary mood disorders experience psychotic symptoms only during mood episodes (severe depression or mania) and not when euthymic. However, patients with schizophrenia experience psychotic symptoms that are independent of their mood state. Although patients with schizophrenia can experience episodes of depression, in general, mood episodes are not present most of the time. On the contrary, patients with schizoaffective disorder experience recurrent mood episodes, including depression and mania, but unlike patients with mood disorders, they experience psychotic symptoms during mood episodes and when euthymic. MDD = major depressive disorder; Bipolar = bipolar disorder.

Delusional Disorder

According to *DSM-5* (APA, 2013), delusional disorder requires the presence of one or more delusions for 1 month or longer without ever meeting criteria for schizophrenia. If an individual diagnosed with delusional disorder experiences hallucinations, the hallucinations must not be prominent and must be consistent with the theme of the delusions (e.g., a patient with a delusion of having her baby kidnapped reports hearing a baby crying). Behavior must not be grossly bizarre.

Epidemiology

Estimated lifetime prevalence of delusional disorder is 0.2% (Perälä et al., 2007). Mean age of onset is approximately 40 years with persecutory and jealous delusions being more prevalent in males, while erotomanic delusions are more common in females. Patients will present with various types of delusional themes.

Neurobiology

In addition to dysregulated dopamine neurotransmission in the mesolimbic pathway (please refer to the section on schizophrenia), abnormal activity and impaired brain circuit connection in the dorsolateral prefrontal cortex, left orbitofrontal cortex, and hippocampus are also involved in the formation, development, and maintenance of delusions. Impaired glutamate neurotransmission is also implicated in the development of delusions (Arjmand et al., 2020).

Clinical Manifestations

Since global functioning of patients with delusional disorder is generally higher than patients with schizophrenia or schizoaffective disorder (Muñoz-Negro et al., 2018), persons with delusional disorder may seem normal until they start expressing or acting on their delusions. Delusions can result in interpersonal difficulties at home, work, and school. Anger, irritability, and aggressive and violent behavior secondary to delusions are sometimes seen. Patients may also engage in lawsuits due to their delusional conviction of being unjustly wronged.

Treatment

Delusional disorder is a difficult disorder to treat. Due to poor insight, patients may not show up for treatment, since they may not appreciate that they have a mental disorder. Establishing a good working alliance and rapport with the patient should be an important goal of treatment. Patients might be more willing to take antipsychotic medications if the emphasis is not on treating psychosis (delusions) but other associated symptom domains, such as mood, insomnia, and anxiety. Antipsychotic medications are the mainstay of treatment, although delusional thinking is difficult to diminish and to eliminate. Should a good rapport become established, the clinician can tactfully point out the disruptions in the patient's life, due to the delusions in assisting the patient toward living a fulfilled life even in the context of ongoing delusional thinking.

MEMORY TIP

Delusional Disorder, *useful mnemonic*

DeluSIONAL

Delu—**Delu**sion/s
S—**S**chizophrenia A criteria not met
I—**I**mpairment of functioning is absent
O—**O**dd or bizarre behavior absent
N—**N**ot due to substance or another medical condition
A—**A**bsence of mood episodes and if occurred are brief relative to the duration of delusional periods
L—**L**asts one month or more

(Kadiyala, 2019)

SECONDARY PSYCHOTIC DISORDERS

Substance- or Medication-Induced Psychotic Disorder

Substance- or medication-induced psychotic disorder is psychosis that results from exposure to a drug of abuse (e.g., marijuana, cocaine, or amphetamines) or prescribed medication (e.g., dexamethasone). The *DSM-5* (APA, 2013) criteria for substance- or medication-induced psychotic disorder include the presence of either hallucinations or delusions (or both), with evidence that onset of the psychotic symptoms followed exposure to a substance or medication that can produce the symptoms. Other psychotic disorders such as schizophrenia or schizoaffective disorder must be ruled out before making a diagnosis of substance- or medication-induced psychotic disorder. It is important to note that substance- or medication-induced psychotic disorder should not be diagnosed if the individual is aware that the hallucinations that they are experiencing are due to substance or medication; in this instance "substance intoxication or withdrawal with perceptual disturbances" should be diagnosed.

Epidemiology

The lifetime prevalence of substance- or medication-induced psychotic disorder is not known. However, longitudinal studies of the different substance-induced psychotic disorders indicate that cannabis-induced psychotic disorder is noteworthy because it is associated with the highest risk of conversion to schizophrenia. Indeed, almost half of patients (47%) with cannabis-induced psychotic disorder end up with a future diagnosis of schizophrenia (Starzer et al., 2018).

Neurobiology

Substance-/medication-induced psychotic disorder involves several neurotransmitters, including dopamine (e.g., amphetamines), NMDA (e.g., phencyclidine), cannabinoid (e.g., cannabis), and serotonin (e.g., lysergic acid diethylamide).

Clinical Manifestations

The hallmark of substance- or medication-induced psychotic disorder is the temporal relationship between use of the substance or medication and the onset of delusions or hallucinations. Evidence of exposure to substances or medication can be from the history (self-report or collateral information), physical examination (substance injection marks), or laboratory findings (urine toxicological analysis). Substance- or medication-induced psychotic disorder should be suspected in all cases of psychosis, especially when symptoms are rapid in onset, when there is not a relevant family history, or when an older person develops delusions and hallucinations for the first time, since primary psychotic disorders usually occur earlier in life (20s and 30s).

Treatment

In substance- or medication-induced psychotic disorder, psychosis is expected to resolve after the substance or medication that induced the psychotic episode is removed. However, antipsychotic agents are used to facilitate recovery, especially when the psychosis is severe or when there are safety issues. Antipsychotic medications and other adjunctive medications may be discontinued once psychosis resolves, although it is important to be alert for the reemergence of psychosis, especially should the patient continue to use illicit substances. Psychosocial interventions, such as AA (Alcoholics Anonymous) and NA (Narcotics Anonymous) meetings, are also required to address substance use disorder.

CLINICAL TIP

The hallmark of substance- or medication-induced psychotic disorder is the temporal relationship between use of the substance or medication and the onset of delusions or hallucinations.

Psychotic Disorder Due to Another Medical Condition

Sometimes, psychosis (hallucinations and/or delusions) is secondary to a known medical or neurological condition in which case psychotic disorder due to another medical condition is diagnosed. Note that this diagnosis is generally not made if the individual appreciates that the hallucinations are due to the medical or neurological condition (i.e., intact perception of reality). Since psychosis secondary to a medical condition can present with features similar to psychosis due to a primary mental illness, it is routine practice to take a standard and thorough history and to carry out appropriate physical examination and laboratory workup (e.g., blood, urine and imaging studies, as indicated) in all cases of psychosis. A list of some of the medical and neurological conditions that can present with psychosis is presented in Table 19.2.

Clinical Manifestations

Hallucinations associated with psychotic disorder due to another medical condition can involve any sensory modality, but visual and olfactory hallucinations should raise suspicion of a psychosis secondary to a general medical condition (e.g., olfactory hallucinations seen in temporal lobe epilepsy). An important consideration in the clinical manifestation of psychotic disorder due to another medical condition is the temporal relationship between the onset or exacerbation of the medical condition and the appearance of hallucinations and delusions (Marsh, 1997; Merritt et al., 2020). Psychosis could be transient or recurrent (waxing and waning with periods of exacerbations and remission of the medical condition) or assume a protracted course (e.g., chronic interictal psychosis observed in epilepsy). An older age of onset or atypical symptoms is also

TABLE 19.2 Medical Disorders That Can Present With Psychotic Symptoms

Neurologic disorders	Epilepsy Parkinson's disease CNS tumors Aura of migraine Normal pressure hydrocephalus Multiple sclerosis Traumatic brain injury (TBI) Auditory or visual nerve injury
Infectious diseases	Lyme disease Brucellosis Toxoplasmosis Rabies Cerebral malaria Cytomegalovirus Epstein–Barr virus Borna (human retrovirus) Herpes simplex encephalitis Syphilis HIV
Rheumatologic disorders	Systemic lupus erythematosus Antiphospholipid syndrome Sarcoidosis
Autoimmune disorders	Hashimoto encephalopathy Paraneoplastic limbic encephalitis Limbic encephalitis Anti N-methyl-D-aspartate receptor (anti-NMDAR) encephalitis
Endocrine disorders	Hypothyroidism (myxedema psychosis) Hyperthyroidism Cushing disease Pheochromocytoma
Metabolic disorders	Acute intermittent porphyria Tay–Sachs disease Niemann–Pick disease type C Wilson disease
Nutritional deficiencies	Vitamin B12 deficiency Thiamin deficiency Niacin deficiency

common in psychosis secondary to a medical condition (e.g., first-episode psychosis in a child/adolescent or an elderly individual). A lack of a family history, concomitant medical problems, and a sudden onset of symptoms might also alert the clinician to conducting an assiduous search for medical contributory causes.

Treatment

Treatment of the underlying medical condition is the main treatment approach for psychosis secondary to a medical condition. The novel antipsychotic pimavanserin is approved for psychosis in Parkinson's disease.

Psychosis in Delirium and Dementia

Psychotic symptoms are seen in some patients with delirium or dementia (major neurocognitive disorder). The onset of hallucinations and delusions in delirium is acute but likely to be insidious in dementia (Karameh et al., 2019). Furthermore, the psychosis of delirium is expected to resolve once delirium resolves, but in dementia psychosis tends to be chronic. Antipsychotics are not approved for psychosis in either delirium or dementia but are often prescribed off-label. Psychosis presenting for the first time in an elderly individual should prompt evaluation for delirium or dementia and for other underlying medical causes of psychosis.

SUMMARY

Thought and psychotic disorders are a group of psychiatric disorders that cause abnormal thinking and perceptions. The symptoms can be brief or long lasting, often resulting in a permanent change in the individual's life trajectory. Like other major psychiatric disorders, there is a genetic component that increases an individual's risk of developing the disorder. Some medical conditions, medications, and substances can cause or contribute to the occurrence of psychotic symptoms. Individuals with psychotic symptoms may or may not be aware that their symptoms do not reflect the reality around them. Treatments for psychotic disorders include medications and psychosocial interventions.

RESOURCES

1 https://medlineplus.gov/psychoticdisorders.html#:~:text=Psychotic%20disorders%20are%20severe%20mental,symptoms%20are%20delusions%20and%20hallucinations.

2 https://www.nimh.nih.gov/health/publications/understanding-psychosis/index.shtml

3 https://www.nimh.nih.gov/health/topics/schizophrenia/index.shtml

REFERENCES

American Psychiatric Association. (2013). *Diagnostic and statistical manual of mental disorders.* https://doi.org/10.1176/appi.books.9780890425596.x00diagnosticclassification

American Psychiatric Association. (2020). *The American Psychiatric Association practice guideline for the treatment of patients with schizophrenia.* https://doi.org/10.1176/appi.books.9780890424841

Arjmand, S., Kohlmeier, K. A., Behzadi, M., Ilaghi, M., Mazhari, S., & Shabani, M. (2020). Looking into a deluded brain through a neuroimaging lens. *Neuroscientist, 27(*1), 72–87. https://doi.org/10.1177/1073858420936172

Bürgy, M. (2008). The concept of psychosis: Historical and phenomenological aspects. *Schizophrenia Bulletin, 34*, 1200–1210. https://doi.org/10.1093/schbul/sbm136

Carroll, B. T., Kirkhart, R., Ahuja, N., Soovere, I., Lauterbach, E. C., Dhossche, D., & Talbert, R. (2008). Katatonia: A new conceptual understanding of catatonia and a new rating scale. *Psychiatry, 5*(12), 42–50.

Coverdale, J. H., Roberts, L. W., Balon, R., Beresin, E. V., Tait, G. R., & Louie, A. K. (2015). Integrated care in community settings and psychiatric training. *Academic Psychiatry, 39*, 419–421. https://doi.org/10.1007/s40596-015-0363-4

Ebert, A., & Bär, K. J. (2010). Emil Kraepelin: A pioneer of scientific understanding of psychiatry and psychopharmacology. *Indian Journal of Psychiatry, 52*, 191–192. https://doi.org/10.4103/0019-5545.64591

Eells T. D. (2000). Psychotherapy of schizophrenia. *The Journal of Psychotherapy Practice and Research, 9*(4), 250–254.

Falloon, I. R. H. (1986). Family stress and schizophrenia: Theory and practice. *Psychiatric Clinics of North America, 9*, 182. https://doi.org/10.1016/s0193-953x(18)30642-7

Falloon, I. R. H., Coverdale, J. H., Laidlaw, T. M., Merry, S., Kydd, R. R., & Morosini, P. (1998). Early intervention for schizophrenic disorders. *British Journal of Psychiatry, 172*(S33), 33–38. https://doi.org/10.1192/s0007125000297638

Falloon, I. R. H., Held, T., Roncone, R., Coverdale, J. H., & Laidlaw, T. M. (1998). Optimal treatment strategies to enhance recovery from schizophrenia. *Australian & New Zealand Journal of Psychiatry, 32*(1), 43–49. https://doi.org/10.3109/00048679809062704

Kadiyala,P. K. (2020). Mnemonics for diagnostic criteria of DSM V mental disorders: a scoping review. *General Psychiatry, 33*:e100109. https://www.doi.org/10.1136/ gpsych-2019-100109

Karameh, W. K., Murari, G., Schweizer, T. A., Munoz, D. G., & Fischer, C. E. (2019). Psychosis in neurodegenerative disorders: Recent developments. *Current Opinion in Psychiatry, 32*, 117–122. https://doi.org/10.1097/YCO.0000000000000476

Marsh, C. M. (1997). Psychiatric presentations of medical illness. *Psychiatric Clinics of North America, 20*(1), 181–204. https://doi.org/10.1016/S0193-953X(05)70400-7

McCutcheon, R. A., Reis Marques, T., & Howes, O. D. (2020, February 1). Schizophrenia: An overview. *JAMA Psychiatry, 77*, 201–210. https://doi.org/10.1001/jamapsychiatry.2019.3360

Merritt, J., Tanguturi, Y., Fuchs, C., & Cundiff, A. W. (2020). Medical etiologies of secondary psychosis in children and adolescents. *Child and Adolescent Psychiatric Clinics of North America, 29*, 29–42. https://doi.org/10.1016/j.chc.2019.08.005

Muñoz-Negro, J. E., Ibáñez-Casas, I., de Portugal, E., Lozano-Gutiérrez, V., Martínez-Leal, R., & Cervilla, J. A. (2018). A psychopathological comparison between delusional disorder and schizophrenia. *Canadian Journal of Psychiatry, 63*(1), 12–19. https://doi.org/10.1177/0706743717706347

Owen, M. J., Sawa, A., & Mortensen, P. B. (2016). Schizophrenia. *The Lancet, 388*(10039), 86–97. https://doi.org/10.1016/S0140-6736(15)01121-6

Oyebode, F. (2015). *Sims' symptoms in the mind: Textbook of descriptive psychopathology* (5th ed). Elsevier.

Perälä, J., Suvisaari, J., Saarni, S. I., Kuoppasalmi, K., Isometsä, E., Pirkola, S., Partonen, T., Tuulio-Henriksson, A., Hintikka, J., Kieseppä, T., Härkänen, T., Koskinen, S., Lönnqvist, J. (2007). Lifetime prevalence of psychotic and bipolar I disorders in a general population. *Archives of General Psychiatry, 64*(1), 19–28. https://doi.org/10.1001/archpsyc.64.1.19

Starzer, M. S. K., Nordentoft, M., & Hjorthøj, C. (2018). Rates and predictors of conversion to schizophrenia or bipolar disorder following substance-induced psychosis. *American Journal of Psychiatry, 175*(4), 343–350. https://doi.org/10.1176/appi.ajp.2017.17020223

Susser, E., Fennig, S., Jandorf, L., Amador, X., & Bromet, E. (1995). Epidemiology, diagnosis, and course of brief psychoses. *American Journal of Psychiatry, 152*(12), 1743–1748. https://doi.org/10.1176/ajp.152.12.1743

U.S. Department of Health and Human Services. (2020). *What is psychosis?* National Institute of Mental Health. NIH Publication No. 20-MH-8110 Retrieved January 16, 2022, from https://www.nimh.nih.gov/sites/default/files/documents/health/publications/understanding-psychosis/20-mh-8110-understandpsychosis.pdf

Waters, F., Blom, J. D., Dang-Vu, T. T., Cheyne, A. J., Alderson-Day, B., Woodruff, P., & Collerton, D. (2016). What is the link between hallucinations, dreams, and hypnagogic-hypnopompic experiences? *Schizophrenia Bulletin, 42*(5), 1098–1109. https://doi.org/10.1093/schbul/sbw076

Waters, F., & Fernyhough, C. (2017). Hallucinations: A systematic review of points of similarity and difference across diagnostic classes. *Schizophrenia Bulletin, 43*, 32–43. https://doi.org/10.1093/schbul/sbw132

CHAPTER 20

Depressive Disorders[1]

Nandhini Madhanagopal, M.D.; Kammarauche Asuzu, M.D., M.H.S.; Edore Onigu-Otite, M.D.; and Asim Shah, M.D.

"Mental pain is less dramatic than physical pain, but it is more common and also harder to bear. The frequent attempt to conceal mental pain increases the burden: It is easier to say, 'My tooth is aching' than to say 'My heart is broken."

— C.S. Lewis

OBJECTIVES

At the end of this chapter, students will be able to do the following:

- describe the epidemiology, etiology, clinical features, diagnosis, and treatment of depressive disorders
- review the roles of neurotransmitters, endocrine pathways, and the significance of the hippocampus in depression and mood disorders

CASE VIGNETTE

John is a 33-year-old adult male who presents to the ER today feeling suicidal. His past psychiatry history reveals that as a child he was a cheerful kid. This all changed in his teens. His parents complained he had lost his bubbly personality. He became irritable, complained about almost everything, had low self-esteem, found little to no pleasure in anything, and avoided going out. His sleep, appetite, and energy all seemed to vary from week to week. He was gloomy, felt his friends no longer liked him, and was sensitive to their comments, often feeling they were rejecting him. This went on for over a year. His pediatrician referred him to a psychiatrist who diagnosed him with persistent depressive

---

1 Readers may also see "Depression in the Medically Ill" (Chapter 21), "Adjustment- and Grief-Related Disorders" (Chapter 22), and "Suicide" (Chapter 34) for related material.

disorder. With regular attendance to therapy, his symptoms reduced but never quite went away. He continued to function well and graduated high school successfully. He made it through college and seemed to do well.

At age 19, soon after starting college, he became very depressed. He presented to the students' counseling office and began therapy. At his first session, he revealed that he no longer wanted to live. He did not have a plan to kill himself. However, the therapist promptly referred him to see a psychiatrist, who started him on Sertraline. Sertraline was titrated over 6 weeks to 150 mg with good response. He was maintained on this dose for over a year, after which he was successfully tapered off.

At age 24, he got a new job, which involved moving out of town away from his family. This was stressful for him. About 3 months after the move, he suffered a recurrence of depression. He presented to a psychiatrist and resumed Sertraline. Soon after this, he got married and had a good supportive marriage. He felt happy and went off his meds.

About 6 months ago, he and his wife began to have problems in their relationship. John gradually became sour and cynical about everything. Unbeknownst to him, he was experiencing his third major depressive episode. His wife felt he was no longer fun to be around. Last week, she informed him she would be filing for a divorce. John got even more depressed. For the past 3 days, John has heard voices telling him he is worthless and that he should kill himself, and he had the thought of purchasing a gun for this purpose.

Today, John is evaluated in the ER, diagnosed with major depressive disorder that is recurrent and severe with psychotic features. He has his first psychiatric inpatient hospitalization. He is treated with duloxetine and quetiapine as an adjunct. Because this is his third major depressive episode, he is advised to continue antidepressants as a maintenance treatment and regularly attends therapy. Five years later, John and his wife are happily married with children and doing well. They are stunned by the difference adequate treatment has made in their family life.

DEFINITIONS AND KEY CONCEPTS

Depressive disorders are a heterogeneous diagnostic group and among the most common mental condition you will encounter in medicine. The term *depression* is derived from the Latin word *deprimere*, which means "to press down." Depression is a disorder that causes a persistent feeling of sadness or lack of interest to the extent that it interferes with daily life. Major depressive disorder, also called unipolar depression, or clinical depression, is the most known of the depressive disorders. However, many other types of depressive disorders exist, each with specific diagnostic criteria.

INTRODUCTION

The use of the word *depression* has evolved, often including a "lowering of spirit." Depression was viewed as a spiritual, rather than physical, condition, which was managed by priests rather than physicians. In ancient Greece, depression was thought to be an imbalance in the four humors and excess of melas (dark) and kholé (bile). Hippocrates described a condition called melancholia, which was characterized by protracted "fears and despondencies" due to an excess of melas (dark) and kholé (bile) in the spleen. The treatment methods used included bloodletting, exercise, bath, and diet. Subsequent authors highlighted the social and psychological causes of depression. Several explanations of depression were given, including laziness, lack of caring, a disturbance of the soul due to moral conflict within the patient, involving low spirits and lethargy and usually linked to isolation (Reynolds & Wilson, 2013).

KEY POINT

The medical and biological explanations of depression include genetics, neurotransmitter systems, hormones, and brain circuits. Psychological and social factors play a prominent role in initiating and maintaining the state of depression. In addition to medications, psychotherapy and social interventions continue to play a main role in the treatment of depression.

The term *depression* as it is used today first appeared in the 19th century when Emil Kraepelin, a German psychiatrist, used it to distinguish depression originating from primary mood disorders from dementia praecox (a term used for schizophrenia at that time) in 1895. Since then, the term *depression* has gained increased currency in medical language.

The medical model of depression emerged in the late 1900s, and biological explanations of depression, including genetics, neurotransmitters, hormones, and brain circuits, came into play. This influenced the conceptualization and understanding of depressive illnesses as well as its treatment.

The *DSM-5* lists nine conditions under depressive disorders (Figure 20.1), which include major depressive disorder (MDD), persistent depressive disorder (also known as dysthymia), disruptive mood dysregulation disorder (DMDD), premenstrual dysphoric disorder, substance- or medication-induced depressive disorder, depressive disorder due to another medical condition, another specified depressive disorder, and an unspecified depressive disorder. In addition, there are other conditions with prominent depressive symptoms, including adjustment disorders, grief, and bereavement (see chapter 22). Depression may present in many ways, each with overlapping yet distinct qualifiers. This chapter focuses on addressing MDD, other depressive disorders, as designated by the *DSM-5*. The various ways depression may present within the context of medical illnesses is contained in Chapter 21.

KEY POINT

Psychological and social factors play a prominent role in initiating and maintaining the state of depression. Psychotherapy and social interventions continue to play a main role in the treatment of depression.

Psychological and social factors play a prominent role in initiating and maintaining the state of depression. Psychotherapy and social interventions continue to play a main role in the treatment of depression. Sigmund Freud, in 1917, and other psychologists proposed theories, in the early and late 1900s, to describe depression in terms of psychodynamic and cognitive–behavioral principles, respectively.

EPIDEMIOLOGY

Globally, depression is one of the most common mental health ailments worldwide. According to the World Health Organization (WHO), more than 264 million people suffer from depression. Depression is a leading cause of disability worldwide and contributes significantly to the overall global burden of disease. Nearly 800,000 people die of suicide every year, and suicide is the second leading cause of death in 15- to 29-year-olds (WHO, 2020). Notably, depression is a major, but not the only, cause of suicide (see Chapter 34). Despite the destructive impact on the individual, family, and society, depression remains underdiagnosed for many reasons, including mental health stigma. Nevertheless, roughly 10% of ambulatory visits have depression noted on their medical records (Katon, 1992).

QUICK POINT

Depression is a leading cause of disability worldwide and contributes significantly to the overall global burden of disease. Nearly 800,000 people die of suicide every year, and suicide is the second leading cause of death in 15- to 29-year-olds (WHO, 2020). Notably, depression is a major, but not the only, cause of suicide

TYPES OF DEPRESSIVE DISORDERS

Major Depressive Disorder

Major depressive disorder (MDD) is one of the most common disabling psychiatric disorders in the United States. The prevalence rate of major depressive episodes among U.S. adults, based on the 2017 National Survey on Drug Use and Health (NSDUH), was 17.3 million (NSDUH, 2019). The prevalence was higher in females, adults aged 18–25 years, and adults reporting two or more races. In 2017, 11 million U.S. adults had at least one major depressive episode with severe impairment, and approximately 35% of adults with major depressive episode did not receive any treatment (NIMH, 2019).

Epidemiology

Results from a national study of 36,309 individuals collected in 2012–2013 show the lifetime prevalence of MDD was 20.6%; on average, depressive episodes lasted 6 months; most episodes were moderate to severe depression; and more than 75% reported anxious distress (Hasin et al., 2018). More than 13% attempted suicide during their severe major depressive episode. MDD is the leading cause of death by suicide worldwide (Hasin et al., 2018). About two thirds of patients with MDD contemplate suicide, and 10–15% die of suicide (Hasin et al., 2018). Suicide associated with depression occurs more commonly in elderly individuals, and psychosis is a common manifestation in this age group (Hasin et al., 2018). The course of MDD is variable. Cohort studies show that at 2 years after the initial diagnosis, 58% recovered, and 21% still experienced significant depressive symptoms.

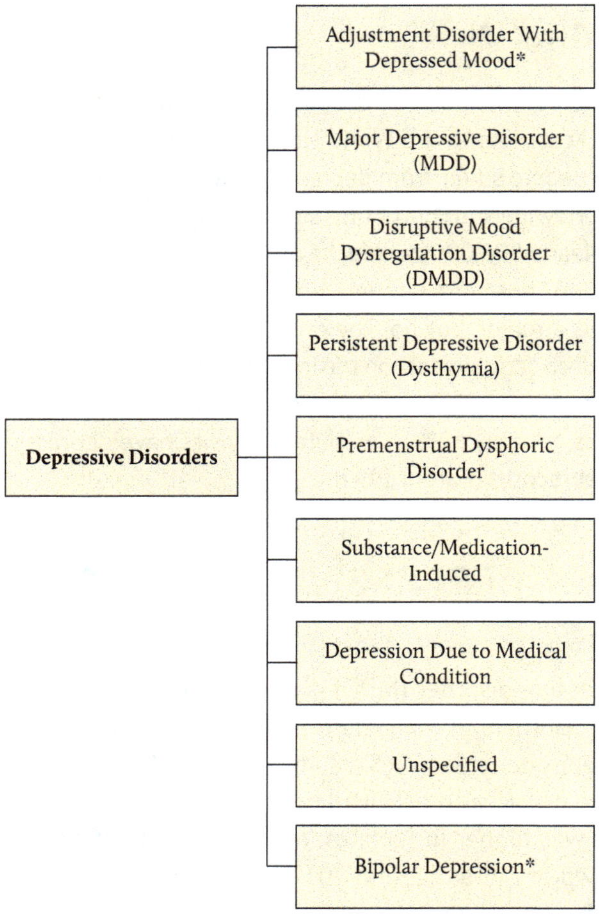

FIGURE 20.1 Types of depressive disorders. (See Chapters 22 and 23 for further information on adjustment- and grief-related disorders and bipolar spectrum disorders, respectively.)

> **QUICK POINT**
>
> The lifetime prevalence of MDD was 20.6%; on average, depressive episodes lasted 6 months; most episodes were moderate to severe depression; and more than 75% reported anxious distress (Hasin et al., 2018). More than 13% attempted suicide during their severe major depressive episode. MDD is the leading cause of death by suicide worldwide (Hasin et al., 2018).

At 6-year follow-ups, the recovery rate decreased to 17%, and patients who still experienced active major depressive disorder symptoms (i.e., did not achieve remission) increased to 55% (Hasin et al., 2018; Verduijn et al., 2017).

Age

The mean age of onset of a first major depressive episode is 32.5 years with 50% of all patients having an onset between 20 and 50 years. Between 2005 and 2017, in youth, the rate of depression in adolescents increased from 8.7% to 13.2% among adolescents aged 12 to 17 and from 8.1% to 13.2% among young adults aged 18–25 (Center for Behavioral Health Statistics and Quality, 2018). Serious psychological distress and suicide-related outcomes (i.e., suicidal ideations, plans, attempts, and deaths by suicide) had also increased among young adults. Cultural trends, including an increase in the use of electronic devices, digital media, and sleep disturbances, are proposed as the causes of elevated depression and suicide-related outcomes.

Gender

MDD is twice as common in females than in males. Factors that increase the risk of depression in women include hormonal changes and disproportionate psychosocial factors, including gender-based violence, socioeconomic disadvantage, and income inequality (Burt & Stein, 2002). Puberty marks the onset of increased risk of depression in females, followed by the postpartum and perimenopausal periods. Pregnancy does not increase the risk of depression (Burt & Stein, 2002). However, if patients discontinue antidepressants during pregnancy, they are prone to developing recurrent depressive episodes (Burt & Stein, 2002).

Marital Status

The prevalence of MDD is higher in separated, divorced, and widowed individuals. This increased prevalence is bidirectional; there is an increased risk of marital disruption in those with MDD, and those who are separated or divorced are at a higher risk for MDD (Bulloch et al., 2009). This relationship between depression and marital status is modified by gender and age. Compared to men, the odds of depression in women declines with age for those who are single, separated, or divorced (Bulloch et al., 2017).

Race

Studies indicate the lifetime prevalence of MDD among Caucasians was 17.9% and 10.4% in African Americans. Caucasians are likely to suffer from acute episodes of MDD, while minority populations are more likely to suffer from chronic, severe, and debilitating depression that causes significant impairment in daily functioning. Despite the advances in the treatment of depression, racial and ethnic disparities in medication use among Hispanics and African Americans primarily relate to lack of health insurance and access to mental health resources. African Americans and Hispanic patients also discontinue treatment prematurely due to multiple reasons, including mistrust of providers, cultural perception of mental illness and social stigma surrounding mental health (Bailey et al., 2019).

Comorbidity

MDD is often comorbid with other conditions, including anxiety disorders, such as generalized anxiety disorder and panic disorder; substance use disorders, such as alcohol use and nicotine use disorders; trauma- and stressor-related disorders, such as posttraumatic stress disorder (PTSD); and personality disorders, such as borderline, antisocial, and schizotypal personality disorders. Anxiety disorders are the most frequent comorbid psychiatric illness with some studies showing comorbid anxiety in up to 75% of individuals with MDD. Poor academic/work

CLINICAL TIP

MDD is often comorbid with other conditions. Anxiety disorders are the most frequent comorbid psychiatric illness with some studies showing comorbid anxiety in up to 75% of individuals with MDD. Other disorders include alcohol and substance use disorders; trauma- and stressor-related disorders, such as posttraumatic stress disorder (PTSD); and personality disorders, such as borderline and antisocial personality disorders.

performance, high suicide risk, and poor social outcomes complicate individuals with comorbid MDD and ADHD (McIntosh et al., 2009). The prevalence of MDD comorbid with ADHD ranges between 9% and 50% across different studies. Substance use disorder commonly co-occurs with MDD. Comorbid MDD and substance use disorder lead to increased hospitalization rates and relapse, elevated suicide risks, and delayed recovery (Quello et al., 2005).

Clinical Features and Diagnosis of MDD

MDD is a syndromic cluster of symptoms with the presence of depressed mood (or irritability in youth) or anhedonia (loss of interest or pleasure) being the core symptom. Additional symptoms include neurovegetative symptoms (e.g., disturbances in sleep, appetite, psychomotor activity, and energy) and feelings of worthlessness or excessive guilt, decreased concentration, and thoughts of death or dying. These symptoms of MDD include depressed mood or anhedonia, occurring most days and lasting 2 weeks or longer, or irritable mood in a child. The acronym *SIGECAPS* summarizes the rest of the symptoms (Figure 20.2).

The *DSM-5* provides the criteria for the diagnosis of major depressive episode (MDE). To meet criteria for MDD, symptoms should be present for 2 weeks or longer. A patient with MDD should have a total of five out of nine symptoms. Depressed mood is usually reported by patients as feeling sad, empty, and hopeless. Patients may describe themselves as lethargic, unable to get things done, either because they feel lethargic or lack the motivation to do things. They are often unable to experience pleasure and lose their drive. Fatigue is often more common in women. Insomnia is a frequent symptom of depression with over half of depressed patients reporting varying combinations of early, middle, or late insomnia. Neuropsychological deficits documented in older depressed patients include disturbances in attention, memory (correlates with reduced hippocampal volume), executive function, and psychomotor speed. Sexual dysfunction in depressed patients is common with more than two thirds of women and men with depression reporting decreased libido. The prevalence of sexual dysfunction increased with the severity and duration of the episode (Kennedy, 2008).

MEMORY TIP

Depression, *useful mnemonic*

DEPRESSION
D—Depressed mood
E—Energy loss or fatigue
P—Pleasure lost
R—Retardation or excitation
E—Eating changes (i.e., appetite/weight)
S—Sleep changes
S—Suicidal thoughts
I—"I'm a failure" (i.e., loss of confidence)
O—"Only me to blame" (i.e., guilt)
N—No concentration

(Blenkiron, 2006)

Mood

- Depressed or Anhedonic
- Irritable (in child/adolescent)

Sleep

- Increase
- Decrease
- Disruption

Interest (loss of) / Anhedonia

- Decreased
- Loss of pleasure
- Non-reactive mood (mood unable to respond to pleasurable events)

Guilt / Worthlessness

- Excessive
- Inappropriate

Energy

- Increased
- Decreased

Concentration

- Difficulty focusing

Appetite

- Increase
- Decrease

Psychomotor

- Increase (Agitation)
- Decrease (Retardation)

Suicidal Ideation

- Passive / Active
- Acute / Chronic

FIGURE 20.2 SIGECAPS for diagnostic symptoms of MDE (major depressive episode). To meet the criteria for MDD, a patient should have five symptoms, including depressed (irritable mood in a child/adolescent) or anhedonia (loss of pleasure) and four out of the eight SIGECAPS.

The severity of MDD is based on the number of symptoms and the degree of functional impairment. Some features invariably qualify for severe depression, including the presence of suicidal ideation and psychotic symptoms. The specifiers or depression are depicted in Figure 20.3. Each specifier has different criteria as spelled out in the *DSM-5*.

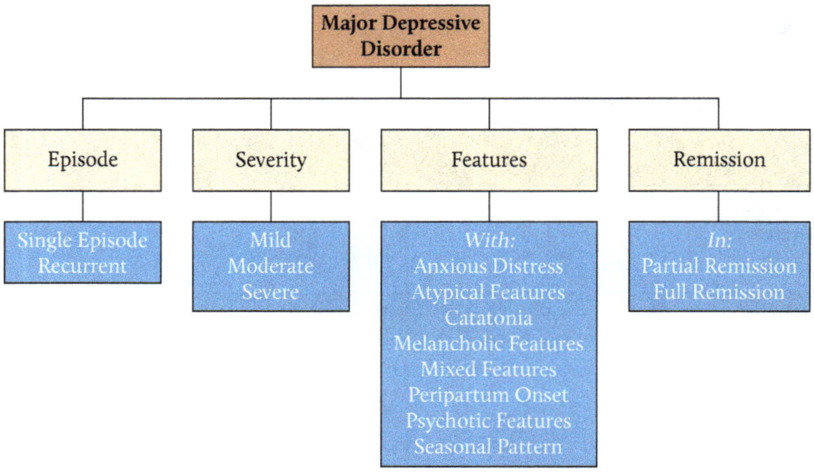

FIGURE 20.3 Major depressive disorder qualifiers.

With Anxious Distress

MDD with anxious distress specifier is diagnosed when a patient meets two out of the five symptoms (feeling keyed up, feeling restless, poor concentration due to worry, fear that something awful may happen, and feelings that one might lose control of themself) during most days of a major depressive episode or persistent depressive disorder.

With Mixed Features

MDD patients who have three out of the seven hypomanic or manic symptoms during most days of a MDD with symptoms manifesting as a change from the person's usual behavior. Diagnosis of the mixed features specifier is a significant risk factor for the diagnosis of bipolar 1 and bipolar 2 disorder.

With Melancholic Features

MDD patients are diagnosed with melancholic features when they meet one core criteria: anhedonia or lack of reactivity to usual pleasurable stimuli and have three or more of the six symptoms, including profound despondency, moroseness, early morning awakening with depression regularly worse in the mornings, marked psychomotor agitation or retardation, significant anorexia or weight loss, and excessive or inappropriate guilt. The near complete absence of capacity of pleasure and psychomotor changes are characteristic features. This specifier is more frequent among inpatients, less likely to occur in mild depressive episode, and more likely to occur in those with psychotic features.

With Atypical Features

MDD with atypical features is diagnosed when a patient presents with mood reactivity and two out of the four symptoms (significant weight gain or increase in appetite, hypersomnia, leaden paralysis, and a longstanding pattern of interpersonal rejection sensitivity resulting in impairment), and criteria for melancholic or catatonia specifiers are not met in the same episode.

With Psychotic Features

Patients with MDD who have delusions and/or hallucinations are diagnosed with the psychotic features specifier. Based on whether the delusions and hallucination are in line with the depressed mood it is further classified into mood-congruent and mood-incongruent psychotic features. Psychotic depression is associated with significant mortality and morbidity.

With Catatonia

The catatonia specifier is applied when patients with MDD present with catatonic features for the most part of the major depressive episode. Patients with catatonia exhibit more severe depressive symptoms and have greater cognitive impairment and a higher frequency of family history of mood disorders.

With Peripartum Onset

Development of mood symptoms in major depression during pregnancy or in the 4 weeks following delivery are diagnosed with MDD with peripartum onset; 3–6% of women develop MDD during pregnancy or in the 4 weeks following delivery. Severe anxiety, panic attacks, and psychotic features may be associated. Risk of recurrence of postpartum psychosis in subsequent delivery is 30%–50%.

With Seasonal Pattern

The characteristic feature of this specifier is the onset and remission of major depressive episodes at particular times of the year. In most cases, the episodes begin in fall or winter and remit in spring. To meet criteria, patients should have had two episodes of MDD in the last 2 years with temporal seasonal relationships.

Persistent Depressive Disorder (Dysthymia)

Dysthymia was conceptualized in *DSM-3* and *DSM-4* and was characterized by milder symptoms not meeting full criteria for MDD but lasting two years or longer. *DSM-5* combined dysthymia and chronic depression into persistent depressive disorder. Persistent depressive disorder in the *DSM-5* encompasses dysthymia, MDD superimposed on dysthymia, and chronic

MEMORY TIP

Persistent Depressive Disorder (Dysthymia), *useful mnemonic*

HE'S 2 SAD
H—Hopelessness
E—Energy loss or fatigue
'S—Self-esteem is low

2—2 years minimum of depressed mood most of the day for more days than not (one year in children/adolescents)

S—Sleep is increased or decreased
A—Appetite is increased or decreased
D—Decision-making or concentration is impaired

(Christman, 2008)

MDD. Genetic factors, a history of childhood maltreatment, and environmental stressors predispose to persistent depression. Individuals with persistent depressive disorder have an earlier onset of depressive symptoms and high comorbidity with anxiety and personality disorders. Psychologically, patients with dysthymia engage in ruminations and pessimistic thinking processes, and present with avoidant, submissive, and hostile interpersonal styles. They suffer from poor social network and support and greater functional impairment and have higher suicide rate (Schramm et al., 2020; Uher, 2014).

Disruptive Mood Dysregulation Disorder (DMDD)

Disruptive mood dysregulation (DMDD) is a new diagnosis that was introduced in the *DSM-5* under the depressive disorders category. The primary aim of adding DMDD to *DSM-5* was to decrease the misdiagnosis of bipolar disorder and thereby the use of psychotropics in children and adolescents with chronic irritability. DMDD is the only diagnosis in the *DSM-5* under depressive disorders that requires the onset of the illness in childhood. The core symptoms of DMDD include severe temper outbursts disproportionate to the trigger and nonepisodic irritability. The prevalence of DMDD in the community, according to the Great Smoky Mountains study sample, is about 4.4% (Baweja et al., 2016). The prevalence is higher in clinical samples and highly comorbid with disorders associated with disruptive behavior, such as ADHD and conduct disorder. Patients who meet criteria for both DMDD and ODD (oppositional defiant disorder) should receive a diagnosis of only DMDD.

Premenstrual Dysphoric Disorder

Premenstrual dysphoric disorder (PMDD) is characterized by psychiatric and/or somatic symptoms that occur typically during the luteal phase of the menstrual cycle and resolve after menstruation. While 20% to 25% of women experience moderate to severe premenstrual syndrome (PMS), only about with 5% of women meet the criteria for PMDD (Lanza di Scalea & Pearlstein, 2017). PMDD is distinguished from PMS by the severity of symptoms and functional impairment. PMDD is often comorbid with anxiety disorders and mood disorders. A recent longitudinal study determined that MDD is the most prevalent lifetime psychiatric disorder in women with PMDD (Kepple et al., 2016). Some studies suggest PMDD may be a risk factor for developing depression in the postpartum and perimenopausal period. The etiology of PMDD is multifactorial, including abnormal response to normal fluctuations of the hypothalamic–pituitary–gonadal axis, genetic factors (polymorphism of ESR1 gene), abnormal serotonin system, and dysfunction of the hypothalamic–pituitary–adrenal axis.

Substance- or Medication-Induced Depressive Disorder

Mood disorders and substance use disorders (SUD) frequently co-occur and are often dually diagnosed. Substance- or medication-induced depressive disorder is defined as a prominent and persistent depressed mood or anhedonia in the context of intoxication or withdrawal of a substance or exposure to a medication, and the involved substance or medication should be capable of causing these symptoms. The substances commonly implicated are alcohol, cocaine, opioids, and marijuana. The medications implicated with moderate to strong evidence include alpha interferon, corticosteroids, varenicline, and isotretinoin lead to depression (Blanco et al., 2012). Additional information on this is contained in Chapter 29.

Depressive Disorder Due to Another Medical Condition

Depression could be an early manifestation of a medical illness. Depressive symptoms are common; however, only limited patients meet criteria for MDD. Some of the hypotheses about how medical illness leads to depressive symptoms include structural changes in the brain, as in stroke, and alterations in neurotransmitters, as in Cushing's disease. In a systematic review, symptoms of MDD were observed prior to the onset of illness or in the early phase of the illness in Cushing's syndrome, multiple sclerosis, Parkinson's disease and meningiomas. Depressive symptoms were seen in hypothyroidism, primary hyperparathyroidism, lung cancer, pancreatic cancer, Wilson's disease, and AIDS (Cosci et al., 2015). (For further discussion, see Chapter 21.)

NEUROPATHOLOGY

Biologic Factors

Role of Bioamines

A major hypothesis about the development of depression focuses on the deficiency of biogenic amines, specifically serotonin, norepinephrine, and dopamine in the central nervous system.

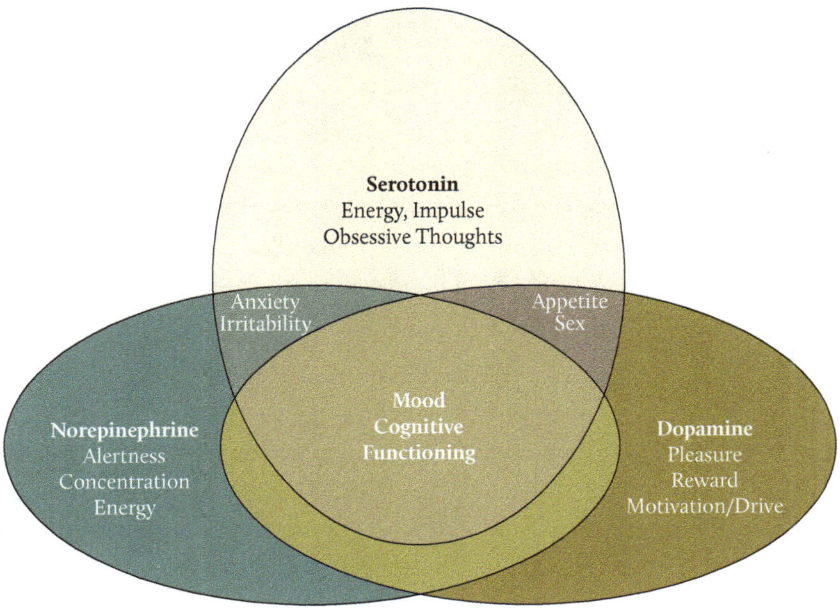

FIGURE 20.4. Functions of monoamine neurotransmitters involved in depression.

Serotonin is the most studied biogenic amine associated with depression with most evidence from the tryptophan depletion studies leading to decreased serotonin syntheses and development of depressive symptoms in those who are at high risk. Besides the use of SSRIs for the treatment of depression, decreased CSF serotonin metabolite levels in patients with suicidal impulses indicate that serotonin is involved in the pathophysiology of depression. Serotonin 1A receptor dysfunction has also been found in patients with depression.

Decreased NE (norepinephrine) receptor density in locus coeruleus in depressed patients and efficacy of treatment of depression by medications, such as venlafaxine, which targets the noradrenergic receptors, points to the importance of dysfunction of central noradrenergic mechanisms in depression. Along with serotonin and norepinephrine, dopamine is another neurotransmitter whose depletion is associated with depressive symptoms. Moreover, drugs that increase dopamine concentration, such as bupropion and amphetamines, help with depression (Hasler, 2010). More recent research has resulted in NMDA and glutamate receptor modulators, such as ketamine, being recently approved for treatment-resistant depression in adults.

Genetic Factors

Twin studies help us delineate genetic from environmental factors: nature versus nurture. Based on twin studies, the heritability of major depression is likely in the range of 31–42%, whereas it is twice high at 70% for schizophrenia and bipolar disorder. The role of environmental stress has been a huge focus and has indicated that it is the susceptibility to depression that is being inherited. Gene-mapping studies have identified strong links to unipolar depression and cAMP response element-binding protein (CREB1) on chromosome 2. Subjects who experienced adverse childhood events had a much higher risk of developing depression when they carried a variant of the serotonin transporter gene, whereas other genes acted as a protective factor (Brigitta, 2002).

QUICK POINT

Elevated hypothalamic–pituitary–adrenal axis (HPA) activity is characteristic of chronic stress and is noted in 40–60% of depressed inpatients and 20–40% of depressed outpatients.

Stress Hormones and Inflammation

Elevated hypothalamic–pituitary–adrenal axis (HPA) activity is characteristic of chronic stress and is noted in 40–60% of depressed inpatients and 20–40% of depressed outpatients. Under normal circumstances, exogenous corticosteroids, such as dexamethasone, suppress early morning cortisol. Dexamethasone is a potent glucocorticoid that normally suppresses HPA activity. In individuals with depression, due to elevated HPA activity, this suppression is lacking and is indicative of impaired feedback inhibition of the HPA axis. A positive dexamethasone test is the nonsuppression of cortisol at 8 a.m. the following morning after administration of dexamethasone. The dexamethasone suppression test is a sensitive measure of dysregulated HPA axis activity in depression; however, the specificity of the test to depression is low.

The link between the immune system and neurological changes has been established by studies. Depression occurs as a side effect of recombinant interferon administration in 30% of people. Clinical data indicates that cytokines play a role in the pathophysiology of a subgroup of depressed individuals who have comorbid physical illnesses.

Neuroanatomy and Depression

The hippocampus, amygdala, and prefrontal cortex have been widely studied in relation to depression. The hippocampus has long been implicated in the structural neuropathology of depression and response to stress. It is a part of the limbic system and has a central role in learning and memory. The hippocampus is important for neuroplasticity and is one of two brain locations where neurogenesis continues in the adult brain (the other being the olfactory bulb). It is posited that smaller hippocampal volume may be a trait characteristic of depression. Depression is associated with smaller hippocampal volumes. Stress plays a key role in depression. Stress suppresses brain-derived neurotrophic factor (BDNF), resulting in sluggish production of new neurons in the hippocampus in low mood states. Depression is associated with *hippocampal atrophy.* Atrophy correlates with the *duration of depression* (Bremner, et al., 2000; Shah, et al, 1998). Emerging data suggest a correlation between *remission of depression* and *restoration of normal hippocampal volume (*Sheline, et al., 1998). It is posited that depressed mood only improves as nerves grow and form new connections, a process that takes weeks and possibly coincides with the length of treatment needed to see symptom-response in depressed patients. Animal studies show antidepressants increase growth and branching of nerve cells in the hippocampus.

Neuroimaging findings in depression are heterogeneous due to the diversity of imaging methods used and studies with small sample sizes. Most available evidence points to the structural and functional abnormality of the subgenual cingulate cortex in MDD. Functional MRI has identified decreased activity at rest and relative lack of activation during negative emotions and increase in activity following treatment with SSRIs in lateral, temporal, and frontal cortices, the insula, and the cerebellum.

The primary function of the prefrontal cortex is to integrate complex sensorimotor information with motivation and affect. Large brain volume reductions in MDD were noted in the ventromedial prefrontal cortex, particularly in the left anterior cingulate and in the orbitofrontal cortex. Moderate volume reductions were observed in the lateral prefrontal cortex, striatum, and hippocampus.

QUICK POINT

Stress can precipitate major depressive episodes. The hippocampus plays a key role in depression. Stress decreases BDNF synthesis in the hippocampus. Treatment with antidepressant and electroconvulsive therapy (ECT) increases BDNF in the hippocampus.

Neurotrophins and Depression

Neuroplasticity is defined as the structural changes in neurons impacting synaptic transmission. Neuroplasticity is impaired in MDD, and SSRIs and brain stimulation have been shown to enhance neuroplasticity to mediate recovery in depressed individuals. Brain-derived neurotrophic factor is one of the neurotrophic factors involved in the maintenance and survival of neurons and in synaptic plasticity (figure 20.5). Multiple studies show that BDNF expression is decreased in depressed individuals, and it correlates with the severity of depression. Stress decreases BDNF synthesis in the hippocampus, and treatment with antidepressant and electroconvulsive therapy (ECT) increases it (Figure 20.5).

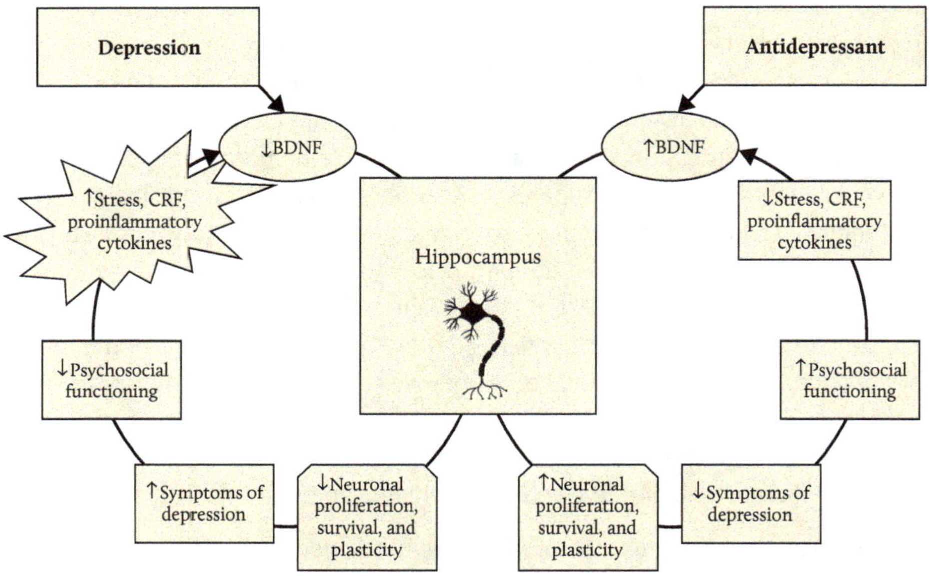

FIGURE 20.5 Suppression of brain-derived neurotrophic factor (BDNF) by depression and stress and the effect of antidepressants. BDNF plays a key role in the proper growth and maintenance of healthy neurons. Chronic stress is thought to decreases expression of BDNF genes, which reduces the availability of BDNF in the brain, particularly in the hippocampus. This can lead to neuronal degeneration by apoptosis. Antidepressants are thought to increase the expression of BDNF, resulting in regeneration of previously shriveled neurons.

Source: https://www.pxfuel.com/en/free-photo-jrxih.

Psychosocial Factors

Psychosocial factors play a big role in symptom onset, progression, ability to access and maintain treatment and the support needed to identify, treat, and support individuals with depression. Identifying and managing psychosocial factors impacts patient outcomes both directly and indirectly.

Psychosocial Stress

Stressful life events play a major role among the nongenetic causes of susceptibility to MDD. These events are usually adverse childhood experiences and ongoing interpersonal challenges, including childhood sexual abuse, other trauma, loss of a parent before age 11, and, in adults, marital problems. Men are more likely to develop depression after a divorce and work difficulties, whereas women are more vulnerable to stress in their social relationships, such as difficulty with getting along with an individual, serious illness, and death. It is notable that stressful life events frequently predate the first episode of depression. The resulting changes in the central nervous system predispose the individual to further depressive episodes, even in the absence of an external stressor. The efficacy of psychotherapies addressing interpersonal difficulties, such as interpersonal psychotherapy, cognitive behavioral therapy, and psychodynamic psychotherapy, in treating depression also supports the role of stressful life events in the development of depression.

Psychodynamic Theories of Depression

Depression is understood in the psychodynamic theories as follows: Freud conceptualized depression as stemming from the loss or rejection by a parent or parental figure with the repressed anger toward the lost person being turned inward toward the self. This leads to low self-esteem, predisposing the individual to depression. Melanie Klein described depressive illness as one that arises from an inability to adequately resolve internal conflicts. John Bowlby construed depression in children as stemming from insecure attachment to primary caregivers.

Cognitive Theories of Depression

Behavioral theorists understand the behavior of humans as a response to an environmental stimulus. Engaging in avoidant behaviors prevents individuals from experiencing rewards and positive reinforcement in their environment, leading to the development and maintenance of depression. Behavioral activation is a personalized treatment that addresses depression by increasing engagement in pleasurable activities and decreasing engagement in activities that maintain depression.

Cognitive theorists posit that various thought processes contribute to the initiation, maintenance, and recurrence of depression. Aaron Beck postulated that individuals predisposed to depression have memory organizations that lead them to view their environment negatively. When experiencing a stressful life event, these individuals are susceptible to developing automatic negative thoughts about the self, environment, and future, termed the cognitive triad and accompanying negative mood. Individuals with MDD develop cognitive bias (unhelpful thinking patterns), leading to discounting their accomplishments and positive aspects of a situation. The affective interference hypothesis proposes that patients with depression display cognitive deficits in attention and memory that allow engagement in negative thoughts.

CLINICAL MANIFESTATIONS IN SPECIAL AGE GROUPS

Depression in Children and Adolescents

> **CLINICAL TIP**
>
> Children with depression may manifest with irritable rather than depressed mood. They may report somatic symptoms, such as stomach or headaches that do not respond to typical medical treatment.

The clinical picture of depression in children and adolescents is similar to adults; however, some differences are observed based on the emotional, physical, social, and cognitive developmental stage. Children with depression may manifest with: irritable mood rather than depressed mood; somatic symptoms, including pain that does not respond to typical treatment; and low self-esteem or worthlessness, rather than guilt. They may be observed to be socially withdrawn and interact less with family and friends. Children with depression show low frustration tolerance and reduced ability to function well during regular activities at home, in school, or during extracurricular activities. Importantly, children with depression may initiate alcohol or drug use in their early teenage years, often to mitigate their depressive symptoms. Depressed adolescents present with higher rates of sleep and appetite disturbance and delusions and are more prone to suicidal ideations and acts (Birmaher & Brent, 2007).

Depression in the Elderly

Depression in the elderly is associated with disability, increased mortality, and poorer outcomes from physical illness. According to the WHO, people older than 65 years more commonly attempt suicide compared to any other age group and are more likely to die of suicide. The increase in suicide rate for White men is striking, as it peaks in older age to more than four times the nation's overall age-adjusted rate of suicide (Conwell et al., 2011). Elderly patients with depression present with somatic complaints, unwarranted fear that they are seriously ill, feelings of worthlessness rather than guilt, more psychomotor retardation, and manifested psychotic delusions. In the elderly, depression is associated with cognitive and functional impairment and an increased risk of dementia. It is important to diagnose and treat depression adequately in this population (Rodda et al., 2011).

SCREENING FOR DEPRESSION

The U.S. Preventive Services Task Force (USPSTF) and American Academy of Family Physicians recommend screening for depression in the adult population. Patient Health Questionnaire (PHQ) 2 and PHQ 9 scales have been well validated for screening depression. The sensitivity of PHQ 2 and PHQ 9 scales are comparable, but PHQ is more specific (91–94%) compared to PHQ 2 (78–92%). If screening for depression is positive, then a clinical interview is conducted to confirm the diagnosis of depression using the *DSM-5*. The USPSTF (2016) also recommends screening children and adolescents (12–18 years of age). The USPSTF, American Academy of Family Physicians, American Academy of Pediatrics, and American Academy of Obstetricians and Gynecologists recommend screening all postpartum women for depression. Women should be screened at least once during the perinatal period by using the PHQ 2, PHQ 9, or Edinburgh Postnatal Depression rating scale (EDPS). In older adults, the Geriatric Depression Scale (GDS) is used.

CLINICAL TIP

The Patient Health Questionnaire (PHQ) 9 and the modified PHQ-A for adolescents are commonly used screening tools for depression in primary care settings.

The Hamilton rating scale for depression (HAM-D) and the Montgomery–Asberg Depression Rating Scale (MADRS) are commonly used clinician-rated scales. Both are well-validated scales; they are commonly used to monitor response to electroconvulsive therapy (ECT). Examples of self-administered scales that have been validated include the Quick Inventory of Depressive Symptomatology (QID-SR) and the Beck Depression Inventory (BDI).

KEY POINT

Various treatment modalities are used to treat depressive symptoms and are often based on the severity of symptoms. This includes psychopharmacologic agents (medications); psychotherapy; and neurostimulation, such as ECT, transcranial magnetic stimulation (TMS), and ketamine for medication-resistant depression.

TREATMENT

Various treatment modalities are used to treat depressive symptoms and are often based on the severity of symptoms (Figure 20.6). This includes psychopharmacologic agents; psychotherapy; and neurostimulation, such as ECT, transcranial magnetic stimulation (TMS), and ketamine.

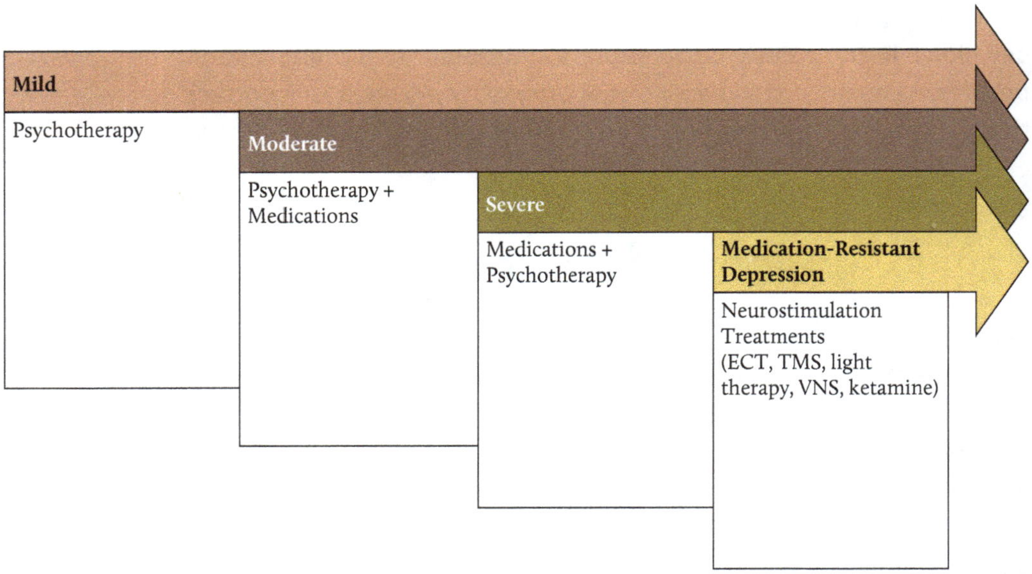

FIGURE 20.6 Treatment of MDD, based on severity of symptoms.

> **CLINICAL TIP**
>
> Treatment of depression with medications or brain stimulation occurs along three phases:
>
> 1. Acute phase of treatment
> 2. Continuation phase of treatment
> 3. Maintenance phase of treatment

Establishing a therapeutic alliance is a salient and primary component of treatment for any psychiatric illness. It is important to collaborate with the patient regarding treatment preferences and concerns and tailor the treatment to the individual, taking their psychosocial and medical history into account. Completing a full diagnostic assessment, which includes a risk and safety assessment, is essential. Completing a suicide risk assessment for all patients with depressive disorder includes eliciting a detailed history of suicidal thoughts, intents, plans, and attempts. It includes assessing risk and protective factors, the history of suicide attempts, and family history of suicide. For adult patients, assessing the patient's ability to care for self and dependents within the context of their depressive symptoms is essential. A determination on the appropriate level of treatment setting is based on the diagnostic and safety assessment findings, the severity of symptoms, available support, and the patient's functional impairment. Keeping this in mind, the least restrictive setting that assures safety and leads to improvement in depression should be considered. Collaborating care with other physicians and mental health care workers involved in the patient's care provides additional support for the patient's treatment and resources for psychosocial treatment and intervention. Providing psychoeducation about depression and its treatment for the patient and their family members and monitoring the patient closely for treatment response, side effects to medications, and symptom resolution or worsening, including suicidal ideation, is an essential component of treatment. Treatment of MDD occurs along three phases (see Figure 20.7):

1. *The acute phase*—The acute phase of treatment aims to attain remission of depressive symptoms and return to the baseline level of functioning. Depending on the severity of symptoms, comorbid psychiatric and medical illness, functional impairment, patient preference, and past treatment trials, this may take up to 3 months to achieve. In the acute phase, treatment modalities used include medications, psychotherapy, a combination of medication and psychotherapy, or additional neurostimulation therapies if indicated. Such neurostimulation treatments are usually employed for treatment-resistant depression and include electroconvulsive therapy (ECT), transcranial magnetic stimulation (TMS), ketamine treatment, and light therapy.
2. *Continuation phase*—During this phase, the patient is monitored for relapse of depression. It is recommended that first episode uncomplicated MDD patients who respond satisfactorily to antidepressant treatment should continue the same medications for 6–9 months after achieving remission. Several studies have documented cognitive behavioral therapy (CBT) may effectively prevent relapses following treatment with an antidepressant.

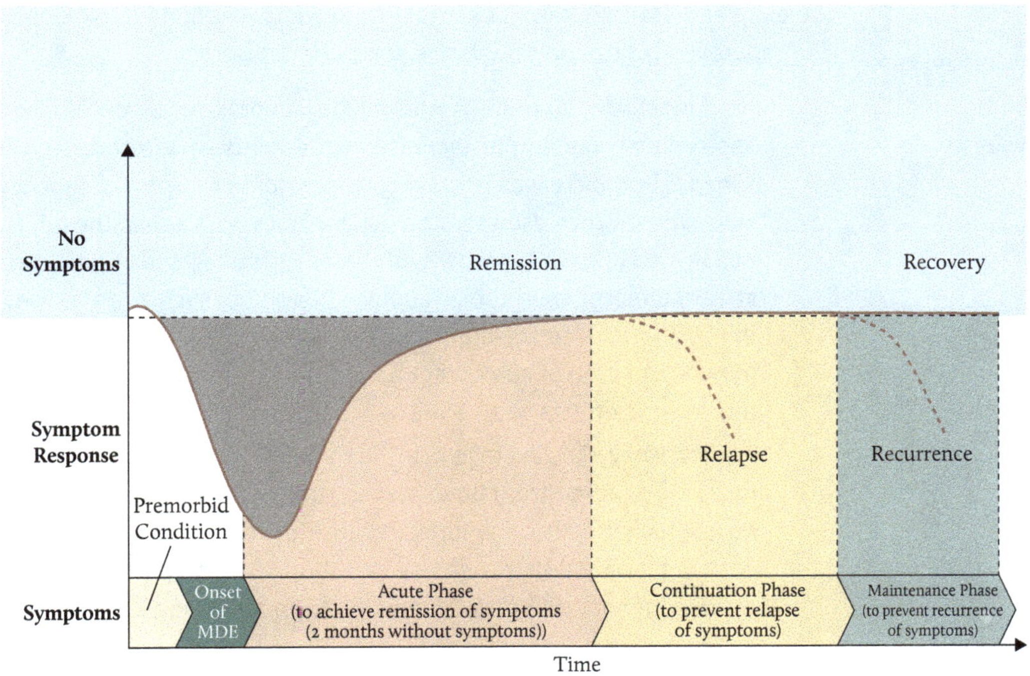

FIGURE 20.7 Treatment phases for major depressive disorder.

3. *Maintenance phase*—Patients with three or more major depressive episodes or have chronic MDD should go on to the maintenance phase to reduce the risk of recurrence of depression. Additionally, patients at a high risk of recurrence, such as early age of onset, ongoing psychosocial stressors, family history of mood disorder, and residual symptoms, should be considered for maintenance treatment. It is recommended that the same treatment modalities (e.g., antidepressant, psychotherapy, or ECT) that induced and maintained remission in the continuation phase should be used in the maintenance phase.

Psychopharmacology

Various psychopharmacologic agents are used in the treatment of depression (see Figure 20.8). The list of antidepressant medications continues to expand.

CLINICAL TIP

Depression differs from person to person. Similar to antibiotics, different antidepressants are indicated with different clinical data. Individual responses to antidepressants vary sometimes based on differential metabolism due to genetic polymorphism.

Selective Serotonin Reuptake Inhibitors (SSRIs)

SSRIs are the most commonly prescribed antidepressants. They are favorable medications to use due to their low side effect profile and wide therapeutic range when compared to other major classes of antidepressants. They include fluoxetine (Prozac), sertraline (Zoloft), paroxetine (Paxil), citalopram (Celexa), and escitalopram (Lexapro). Notably, fluvoxamine (Luvox) is an SSRI approved for treating obsessive compulsive disorder.

- *Mechanism of action*—SSRIs prevent the reuptake of serotonin from the synapse, leading to increased availability of serotonin in the synapse and increased postsynaptic serotonin receptor occupancy. However, the increased serotonin alone does not explain the effects of SSRIs, as it takes 2–4 weeks for therapeutic effects to occur. Downstream effects of serotonin reuptake inhibition, such as an increase in BDNF-mediated signaling and modulation of serotonin receptors (downregulation of autoreceptor, 5HT1A) explain the time taken for therapeutic effects of an SSRI.
- *Pharmacology*—The average half-life for SSRIs is 20–30 hours. Hence, most SSRIs, aside from fluvoxamine, are prescribed as a once daily dose. Fluoxetine has the longest half-life among SSRIs at 1–3 days with single administration. Its metabolite, norfluoxetine, has an even longer half-life of 4–16 days. Fluvoxamine has a short half-life at 15 hours.
- *Use in pregnancy*—SSRIs are the most studied antidepressant class for use in pregnancy. SSRIs carry a potential risk of persistent pulmonary hypertension of the newborn (PPHN). Some SSRIs, such as

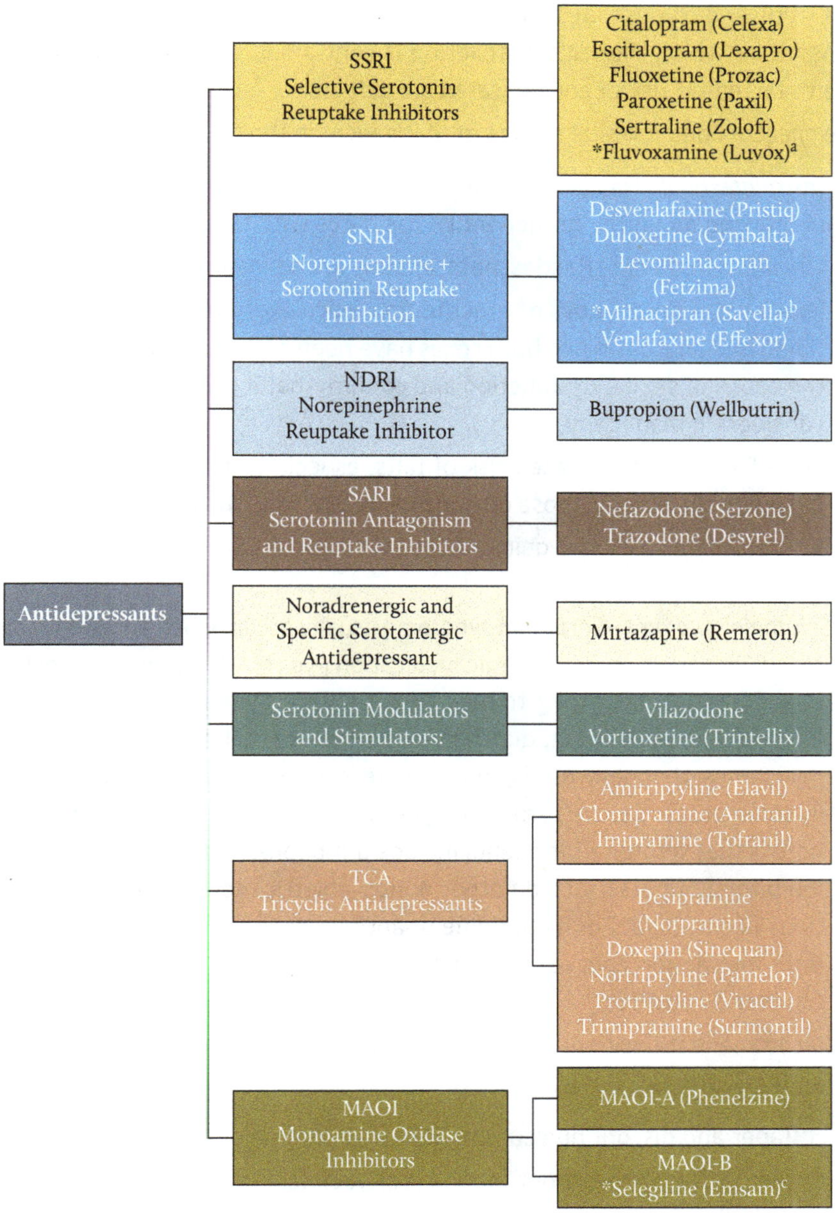

FIGURE 20.8 Antidepressants used in depressive disorders (FDA approved). Although classified as antidepressants, this medication is not currently FDA approved for treating depression. This medication is FDA approved for treating additional conditions: (a) obsessive compulsive disorder, (b) fibromyalgia, (c) Parkinsonism.

sertraline and citalopram, can be used with caution in pregnancy and lactation if the benefits outweigh the risks. Paroxetine is contraindicated for use during pregnancy due to increased risk of congenital heart defects.

- *Side effects*—Common side effects of SSRIs include the following:
    - *Gastrointestinal*—Nausea, vomiting, and diarrhea are common in the first few weeks of starting an SSRI. This generally dissipates with time.
    - *Activation/insomnia*—Restlessness, akathisia, and insomnia can occur.
    - *Sexual side effects*—Loss of erectile and ejaculatory function in men and loss of libido and anorgasmia in both sexes have been reported. It is important to explore the cause of sexual dysfunction and confirm that it is medication induced prior to considering management.
    - *Falls*—There is an increased risk of falls, especially in those who are at high risk, including the elderly; those on benzodiazepine; and those on multiple medications.
    - *Weight changes*—Weight gain is noted with some SSRIs. Fluoxetine may cause an initial weight loss.
    - *Serotonin syndrome*—Serotonin syndrome usually occurs when an SSRI is administered along with another serotonergic medication (e.g., MAOI [monoamine oxidase inhibitors], linezolid [antibiotic], tramadol [pain killer]). Symptoms of serotonin syndrome include abdominal pain, diarrhea, sweating, mental status changes, tremor and myoclonus, rhabdomyolysis, renal failure, cardiovascular complications, and death in some cases. Severe serotonin syndrome can be lethal. Clinically important to note is that serotonergic agents include antidepressants (e.g., monoamine oxidase inhibitors) but also include other nonpsychiatric medications (e.g., pain medications like tramadol or meperidine or antibiotics like Linezolid). Using an updated drug-interaction checker can prevent the occurrence of serotonin syndrome (see Chapter 31 and 38).
    - Recommendations to prevent serotonin syndrome while switching from an SSRI to an MAOI are as follows:
        - Taper and discontinue current SSRI over 2–4 weeks.
        - Start a 2-week "washout" period (between last dose of SSRI and first dose of an MAOI). It is important to note that the washout period is 5 weeks if the patient was on fluoxetine due to its long half-life.
        - Start new MAOI.
    - *Discontinuation syndrome*—SSRIs should not be abruptly discontinued, especially after four or more weeks of treatment. The discontinuation syndrome symptoms include flu-like symptoms, such as nausea, chills, headache, body ache, paresthesia, "electric shock-like" phenomena, and insomnia. Discontinuation symptoms occur more frequently with antidepressants, such as paroxetine, venlafaxine, desvenlafaxine, and duloxetine, which all have shorter half-lives and less with bupropion, mirtazapine, and fluoxetine, which have relatively long half-lives.

Serotonin Norepinephrine Reuptake Inhibitors (SNRIs)

SNRIs include venlafaxine, desvenlafaxine, duloxetine, milnacipran, and levomilnacipran. They act by inhibiting reuptake of both serotonin and norepinephrine at the synapse. The side effect profile is similar to those with SSRIs, and additionally, the side effects that reflect noradrenergic activity, such as elevated blood pressure and pulse rate, dilated pupils, excessive sweating, and dry mouth. As with SSRIs, sudden discontinuation of SNRIs should be avoided to prevent discontinuation syndrome.

- *Bupropion*—Bupropion acts by dopamine and norepinephrine reuptake inhibition. Due to its lack of effect on the serotonergic system, bupropion lacks the side effects of SSRIs. Side effects of bupropion include headaches, tremors, seizures, insomnia, gastrointestinal upset, and agitation. The risk of seizures can be decreased by not using high doses (not more than 450 mg/day); avoid use in patients with high risk of seizures. Avoid use in anorexia and bulimia nervosa due to increased risk of seizures.
- *Mirtazapine*—Mirtazapine exerts antidepressant effects by antagonizing central presynaptic alpha-2 adrenergic receptors, which leads to increased release of serotonin and norepinephrine. It also acts as an antagonist at H1 histamine receptors, producing sedation and calming effects, and at 5-HT2A, 5-HT2C, and 5-HT3 serotonin receptors. The most common side effects include dry mouth, sedation, and weight gain. Mirtazapine is commonly used in patients with depression with insomnia and weight loss. Mirtazapine significantly improved both nausea and vomiting in gastroparetics after 2 and 4 weeks of treatment and is the drug of choice in cancer patients, due to its M3 muscarinic receptor activity.
- *Trazodone*—Trazodone works as an antidepressant by its inhibitory action on both serotonin transporter and antagonist action at the 5-HT2 receptor. The most common side effect is sedation. Trazodone is used in patients with depression with insomnia. Trazodone also causes cardiovascular side effects, including orthostasis, especially in elderly individuals. Priapism (persistent painful penile erection) is a rare (occurs in 0.01–0.1% of those on trazodone) but serious side effect.
- *Nefazodone*—Nefazodone acts by inhibiting the neuronal reuptake of serotonin and acts as an antagonist at the 5-HT2 receptor. Nefazodone was discontinued due to drug-induced hepatic injury associated with risk of need for hepatic transplant or even death.
- *Vilazodone*—Vilazodone exhibits antidepressant action by selective inhibition of serotonin reuptake. It also acts as a partial agonist at 5-HT1A receptors. Vilazodone is FDA approved for treatment of MDD in adults. It may be especially useful in patients who develop sexual dysfunction, weight gain, or increased blood pressure on an SSRI or SNRI.
- *Vortioxetine*—Vortioxetine is a mechanism of action and inhibits neuronal reuptake of serotonin and acts as an agonist at the 5-HT1A receptor and an antagonist at the 5-HT3 receptor. The FDA approved vortioxetine for the treatment of MDD in adults. Regarding side effects, it has less propensity to cause weight gain and sexual dysfunction.
- *Tricyclic and tetracyclic antidepressants (TCA)*—Imipramine is the first tricyclic antidepressant that was approved by the FDA in 1959 for the treatment of MDD. Eventually,

the FDA approved doxepin, amoxapine, desipramine, nortriptyline, and protriptyline for the treatment of MDD and clomipramine for the treatment of OCD in patients aged 10 and above. Off-label use of TCA include migraine headaches, neuropathic pain, enuresis, insomnia, and fibromyalgia. TCAs exert their effect via inhibition of serotonin and norepinephrine reuptake from the synaptic cleft. The various side effects of TCAs are due to their multiple antagonistic action at various receptors; sedation, increased appetite, and weight gain are due to a blockade of the H1 histaminergic receptor; dry mouth, blurred vision, confusion, urinary retention, and constipation are due to the M1 cholinergic receptor blockade; and orthostatic hypotension and dizziness are due to the alpha-1 adrenergic receptor blockade. TCAs can cause cardiovascular complications, including cardiac arrhythmias and sudden cardiac death, especially in patients with preexisting cardiac issues, due to their membrane-stabilizing effect on the myocardium by blocking the fast sodium channels on the cardiac myocyte. TCAs also lower seizure threshold. These side effects make TCA less tolerable compared to other antidepressants and dangerous in an overdose. Some studies document that TCAs are superior to SSRIs in treatment of depressed patients who are hospitalized and in the treatment of severe depression and patients with melancholic depression (Anderson, 1998; Perry, 1996).

Monoamine Oxidase Inhibitors (MAOIs)

Monoamine oxidase (MAO) is the enzyme that metabolizes monoamine neurotransmitters and inactivates them. Monoamine oxidase inhibitors (MAOI) were first introduced in the 1950s. There are two MOA enzyme isomers: MAO-A and MAO-B. Inhibition of MAO-A is responsible for antidepressant action, and inhibition of both MAO-A and MAO-B theoretically leads to greater increase of monoamine neurotransmitters in the synapse.

The MAO inhibitors currently available in the United States are both MAO-A and -B inhibitors: oral MAO inhibitors include tranylcypromine, phenelzine, and isocarboxazid. Selegiline (Emsam), an MAOI-B, is the only transdermal MAOI and is mostly prescribed for treating Parkinsonism, for which it is FDA approved.

Side effects of MAOI include cholinergic side effects (e.g., dry mouth, nausea, and urinary hesitancy), orthostatic hypotension, dizziness, weight gain, and myoclonic jerks. Hypertensive crises and serotonin syndrome are serious adverse effects, which can result in medical emergencies. Hypertensive crisis occurs due to inhibition of tyramine metabolism in the gut by the MAO-A inhibitor, leading to increased tyramine entering circulation and increasing levels of norepinephrine. This causes rapid increase in blood pressure and can lead to stroke or death from cerebral hemorrhage. Therefore, patients taking MAOI are instructed to avoid foods rich in tyramine, such as aged cheeses; aged meats; spoiled meat, fish, and poultry; broad bean pods; concentrated yeast extract; sauerkraut; tofu; soy beans; and tap beer (Culpepper, 2013; Thase, 2012).

Due to the food and drug interactions with MAOI inhibitors, their use is restricted to treat patients who do not respond to other antidepressants (e.g., SSRIs, SNRIs, bupropion, mirtazapine, etc.), and studies have shown that MAOI are particularly effective for atypical depression (Liebowitz et al., 1988).

Adjunctive Medications

In patients with MDD experiencing partial response, several medications may augment treatment response. These include atypical antipsychotics such as aripriprazole (Abilify), lurasidone (Latuda), extended-release quetiapine (Seroquel), olanzapine/fluoxetine combination (Symbyax), and brexiprazole (Rexulti). Other adjunctive agents sometimes used include omega-3 fatty acids and lithium.

Psychotherapy

Psychotherapy is an important part of treatment for depression. Depressive disorder symptoms can occur with or without a clear preceding stressful life experience and are often worsened or perpetuated by psychosocial factors. On the other hand, patients with depression may have difficulty managing stress, resulting in perpetuation or increase in stress and depressive symptoms. Various forms of psychotherapy are used to treat patients with depressive symptoms to address psychological factors related to their illness, support them through their experience of depression, and to manage their stresses more optimally.

CLINICAL TIP

Psychotherapy is an effective mode of treatment for depressive disorders. It is often used alone for mild depression or in conjunction with medications. Importantly, psychotherapy helps address stress and functioning. Stress is a major factor, which can precipitate or perpetuate depressive symptoms if left unaddressed.

Cognitive and Behavioral Therapy (CBT)

In the treatment of depressed patients, both cognitive (focusing on negative automatic thoughts) and behavioral (behavioral activation) therapy are used in combination. In a meta-analysis, CBT was reported to have similar efficacy to treat depression as other empirically supported therapies (interpersonal therapy [IPT] and behavioral therapy). Studies comparing pharmacotherapy and psychotherapy found the results inconsistent. It is unclear if CBT is less effective for patients with severe depression.

i. *Behavioral therapy*—Behavioral activation is one of the interventions of behavioral therapy. Techniques include activity scheduling, social skills training, problem-solving, scheduling enjoyable activities, and minimizing unpleasant activities. In a randomized controlled trial, behavioral activation was comparable to antidepressant medications in severely depressed patients (Dimidjian, 2006).

Interpersonal Therapy (IPT)

The focus of IPT is on the current life changes such as losses (grief, bereavement), role dispute (maintenance of depressive symptoms is due to nonreciprocal role expectations between patient and an important person in their life), role transitions (maintenance of depressive symptoms is due to difficulty coping with transition in social roles), social isolation, and other interpersonal factors that may contribute to a patient's depression.

IPT has been found effective for treating depression in primary care patients as well as patients with severe depression. IPT can be used as a monthly maintenance therapy to prevent relapse. IPT studies also show the treatment is beneficial for specific patient populations, including HIV-positive patients, patients with obsessive personality traits, and patients and who are single and not living with others.

Psychodynamic Psychotherapy

Psychodynamic psychotherapy encompasses both short-term (brief) and long-term interventions. Evidence supports use of psychodynamic psychotherapy in the treatment of depression; however, its effects compared to placebo and nonactive control treatments are modest. The goal of psychodynamic psychotherapy is to understand the complex interplay between aspects of an individual's relationship (based on their personality style, childhood experiences, psychological vulnerability, etc.) with their environment—either internal or external. The goal of psychodynamic psychotherapy is to modify the patient's underlying psychological conflicts, which increase their vulnerability to depressive affect and development of MDD (Fonagy, 2015).

Other Treatments

Other treatments include ECT, TMS, vagus nerve stimulation (VNS), phototherapy, and ketamine, deep brain stimulation (DBS) and are covered in the chapter on neurostimulation.

SUMMARY

Depression is a complex disorder, stemming from many factors, including faulty mood regulation by the brain, genetic vulnerability, stressful life events, medications, and medical problems. Depression can be a debilitating chronic illness that affects the individual, their family, and the community, due to its impact on functioning. Recently, some studies have focused on identifying biological and behavioral markers for diagnosing subtypes of depression and treatment response. New directions to advance therapeutic options for depression include studies exploring opioid system modulators and adjunctive treatment with intranasal ketamine for treatment-resistant depression.

RESOURCES

1 https://www.nimh.nih.gov/health/topics/depression/index.shtml

2 https://www.psychiatry.org/patients-families/depression

3 https://www.aacap.org/aacap/Resources_for_Primary_Care/CAP_Resources_for_Medical_Student_Educators.aspx

4 https://www.aacap.org/aacap/Families_and_Youth/Resource_Centers/Depression_Resource_Center/Home.aspx

REFERENCES

Anderson, I. M. (1998). SSRIS versus tricyclic antidepressants in depressed inpatients: A meta-analysis of efficacy and tolerability. *Depression and Anxiety, 7*(1), 11–17.

Bailey, R. K., Mokonogho, J., & Kumar, A. (2019). *Racial and ethnic differences in depression: Current perspectives.* Dove Press.

Baweja, R., Mayes, S. D., Hameed, U., & Waxmonsky, J. G. (2016). Disruptive mood dysregulation disorder: Current insights. *Neuropsychiatric Disease and Treatment, 2016*(12), 2115–2124. https://doi.org/10.2147/NDT.S100312

Birmaher, B., & Brent, D. (2007). Practice parameter for the assessment and treatment of children and adolescents with depressive disorders. *Journal of the American Academy of Child & Adolescent Psychiatry, 46*(11), 1503–1526. https://doi.org/10.1097/chi.0b013e318145ae1c

Blanco, C., Alegría, A. A., Liu, S.-M., Secades-Villa, R., Sugaya, L., Davies, C., & Nunes, E. V. (2012). Differences among major depressive disorder with and without co-occurring substance use disorders and substance-induced depressive disorder: Results fom the National Epidemiologic Survey on Alcohol and Related Conditions. *The Journal of Clinical Psychiatry, 73*(6), 865–873. https://doi.org/10.4088/JCP.10m06673

Blenkiron P. (2006). A mnemonic for depression. *BMJ, 332*(7540), 551.

Brigitta, B. (2002). Pathophysiology of depression and mechanisms of treatment. *Dialogues in Clinical Neuroscience, 4*(1), 7–20.

Bulloch, A. G., Williams, J. V., Lavorato, D. H., & Patten, S. B. (2009). The relationship between major depression and marital disruption is bidirectional. *Depression and Anxiety, 26*(12), 1172–1177. https://doi.org/10.1002/da.20618

Bulloch, A. G. M., Williams, J. V. A., Lavorato, D. H., & Patten, S. B. (2017). The depression and marital status relationship is modified by both age and gender. *Journal of Affective Disorders, 223*, 65–68. https://doi.org/10.1016/j.jad.2017.06.007

Burt, V. K., & Stein, K. (2002). Epidemiology of depression throughout the female life cycle. *The Journal of Clinical Psychiatry, 63*(7), 9–15.

Center for Behavioral Health Statistics and Quality. (2018). *2017 national survey on drug use and health final analytic file codebook, substance abuse and mental health services administration.*

Christman D. S. (2008). *"HE'S 2 SAD" detects dysthymic disorder.* https://cdn.mdedge.com/files/s3fs-public/Document/September-2017/0703CP_Pearls.pdf.

Conwell, Y., Van Orden, K., & Caine, E. D. (2011). Suicide in older adults. *Psychiatric Clinics of North America, 34*(2), 451–468. https://doi.org/10.1016/j.psc.2011.02.002

Cosci, F., Fava, G. A., & Sonino, N. (2015). Mood and anxiety disorders as early manifestations of medical illness: A systematic review. *Psychotherapy and Psychosomatics, 84*(1), 22–29. https://doi.org/10.1159/000367913

Culpepper, L. (2013). Reducing the burden of difficult-to-treat major depressive disorder: Revisiting monoamine oxidase inhibitor therapy. *The Primary Care Companion for CNS Disorders, 15*(5). https://doi.org/10.4088/PCC.13r01515

Dimidjian, S. (2006). Randomized trial of behavioral activation, cognitive therapy, and antidepressant medication in the acute treatment of adults with major depression. *Journal of Consulting and Clinical Psychology, 74*(4), 658–670. https://doi.org/10.1037%2F0022-006X.74.4.658

Fonagy, P. (2015). The effectiveness of psychodynamic psychotherapies: An update. *World Psychiatry, 14*(2), 137–150. https://doi.org/10.1002/wps.20235

Hasin, D. S., Sarvet, A. L., Meyers, J. L., Saha, T. D., Ruan, W. J., Stohl, M., & Grant, B. F. (2018). Epidemiology of adult DSM-5 major depressive disorder and its specifiers in the United States. *JAMA Psychiatry, 75*(4), 336. https://doi.org/10.1001/jamapsychiatry.2017.4602

Hasler, G. (2010). Pathophysiology of depression: Do we have any solid evidence of interest to clinicians? *World Psychiatry, 9*(3), 155–161.

Katon, W., & Schulberg, H. (1992). Epidemiology of depression in primary care. *General hospital psychiatry, 14*(4), 237–247. https://doi.org/10.1016/0163-8343(92)90094-q

Kennedy, S. H. (2008). Core symptoms of major depressive disorder: Relevance to diagnosis and treatment. *Dialogues in Clinical Neuroscience, 10*(3), 271–277.

Kepple, A. L., Lee, E. E., Haq, N., Rubinow, D. R., & Schmidt, P. J. (2016). History of postpartum depression in a clinic-based sample of women with premenstrual dysphoric disorder. *The Journal of Clinical Psychiatry, 77*(4), 415–420. https://doi.org/10.4088/JCP.15m09779

Lanza di Scalea, T., & Pearlstein, T. (2017). Premenstrual dysphoric disorder. *Psychiatric Clinics of North America, 40*(2), 201–216. https://doi.org/10.1016/j.psc.2017.01.002

Liebowitz, M. R., Quitkin, F. M., Stewart, J. W., McGrath, P. J., Harrison, W. M., Markowitz, J. S., Rabkin, J. G., Tricamo, E., Goetz, D. M., & Klein, D. F. (1988). Antidepressant specificity in atypical depression. *Archives of General Psychiatry, 45*(2), 129–137. https://doi.org/10.1001/archpsyc.1988.01800260037004

Lloyd-Williams, M., & Friedman, T. (2001). Depression in palliative care patients—a prospective study. *European journal of cancer care, 10*(4), 270–274. https://doi.org/10.1046/j.1365-2354.2001.00290.x

McIntosh, D., Kutcher, S., Binder, C., Levitt, A., Fallu, A., & Rosenbluth, M. (2009). Adult ADHD and comorbid depression: A consensus-derived diagnostic algorithm for ADHD. *Neuropsychiatric Disease and Treatment, 5*, 137–150. https://doi.org/10.2147/NDT.S4720

National Institute of Mental Health. (2019). *Major depression.* https://www.nimh.nih.gov/health/statistics/major-depression.shtml

Perry, P. J. (1996). Pharmacotherapy for major depression with melancholic features: Relative efficacy of tricyclic versus selective serotonin reuptake inhibitor antidepressants. *Journal of Affective Disorders, 39*(1), 1–6. https://doi.org/10.1016/0165-0327(96)00014-6

Quello, S. B., Brady, K. T., & Sonne, S. C. (2005). Mood disorders and substance use disorder: A complex comorbidity. *Science & Practice Perspectives, 3*(1), 13–21.

Reynolds, E. H., & Wilson, J. V. K. (2013). Depression and anxiety. *Babylon: Journal of the Royal Society of Medicine, 106*(12), 478–481. https://doi.org/10.1177/0141076813486262

Rodda, J., Walker, Z., & Carter, J. (2011). Depression in older adults. *BMJ, 343.* https://doi.org/10.1136/bmj.d5219

Schramm, E., Klein, D. N., Elsaesser, M., Furukawa, T. A., & Domschke, K. (2020). Review of dysthymia and persistent depressive disorder: History, correlates, and clinical implications. *Lancet Psychiatry, 7*(9), 801–812. https://doi.org/10.1016/S2215-0366(20)30099-7

Thase, M. E. (2012). The role of monoamine oxidase inhibitors in depression treatment guidelines. *The Journal of Clinical Psychiatry, 73*(1), 10–16. https://doi.org/10.4088/JCP.11096su1c.02

Uher, R. (2014, July 31). Persistent depressive disorder, dysthymia, and chronic depression: Update on diagnosis, treatment. *Psychiatric Times.* https://www.psychiatrictimes.com/view/persistent-depressive-disorder-dysthymia-and-chronic-depression-update-diagnosis-treatment

U.S. Preventative Services Task Force. (2016, January 26). Final recommendation statement: Depression in adults: Screening. https://www.uspreventiveservicestaskforce.org/uspstf/document/RecommendationStatementFinal/depression-in-adults-screening

Verduijn, J., Verhoeven, J. E., Milaneschi, Y., Schoevers, R. A., van Hemert, A. M., Beekman, A. T. F., & Penninx, B. W. J. H. (2017). Reconsidering the prognosis of major depressive disorder across diagnostic boundaries: Full recovery is the exception rather than the rule. *BMC Medicine, 15*(1), 215. https://doi.org/10.1186/s12916-017-0972-8

World Health Organization. (2020). *Depression.* https://www.who.int/news-room/fact-sheets/detail/depression

CHAPTER 21

Depression in the Medically Ill[1]

Nandhini Madhanagopal, M.D.; Kammarauche Asuzu, M.D., M.H.S.; Edore Onigu-Otite, M.D.; and Asim Shah, M.D.

> *"Depression is, in part, grief for your own life not turning out how it should; grief for your own needs not being met."*
>
> — Johann Hari

OBJECTIVES

At the end of this chapter, students will be able to do the following:

- describe the epidemiology, clinical features, diagnosis, and treatment of depressive disorders in medically ill patients
- review the impact of depression on the medical illness and vice versa

CASE VIGNETTE

Mr. K was a 57-year-old male brought by his wife to his primary care physician (PCP), complaining that he was depressed. He was usually the life of the party, but recently, although outwardly he put on a show, privately, once the crowds left, his mood was sour, he lacked interest or motivation in his usual hobbies, had unexplained crying spells, lost appetite, and interacted little if at all with his family and pets. Mr. K had a history of alcohol and drug use. At different points in his life, he had become depressed, often while drinking. With intervention, by way of completing several drug rehab programs, he became abstinent, and his depressive symptoms always went away. Mr. K had been sober now for about 15 years. His PCP diagnosed him with primary depression and started him on an antidepressant. His depressive symptoms improved, and he became his usual cheerful self.

(continued)

1 Readers may also see "Depressive Disorders" (Chapter 20) and "Adjustment- and Grief-Related Disorders" (Chapter 22) for related material.

Three years later, he was back in his PCP's office, this time because his movement had become slow, and he began to have memory problems. After a full neurological assessment, he was diagnosed with Parkinson's disease and started on methyldopa. Mr. K had a difficult time adjusting to this new diagnosis. From his viewpoint, the life he enjoyed was changing for the worse, never to return. The roles were now reversed. Instead of him cheering others up, those who knew his diagnosis felt his loss and tried to cheer him up. To please them for their effort, Mr. K often forced himself to act like he was laughing when he was silently weeping within. He found this new life difficult to bear, stopped working as a volunteer at his local YMCA, and became more recluse. With support and encouragement from close family and friends and regular attendance to psychotherapy, he improved moderately over the next 5 months.

Within the next year, his mental health deteriorated rather rapidly. Mr. K became severely depressed again and began to see "floating fairies" in his house. Within his home, he relocated his bedroom to a room he felt he saw the floating fairies in less. He gradually became more homebound and stayed in his room. His memory now failed him, and he hardly recognized some family members, including his grandchildren. Mr. K grew increasingly paranoid and scared whenever people came to visit him. One fateful morning, his wife walked into his bedroom, devastated to find Mr. K had committed suicide. An autopsy showed he had Lewy bodies in his brain. A new diagnosis, Lewy body dementia, was added to his diagnosis postmortem.

COMMENTARY

Over the course of his life and medical illnesses, Mr. K. manifested different types of depressive disorders. At the first visit to his PCP, Mr. K met criteria for *major depressive disorder, single episode, moderate severity*. With the history of alcohol and drug use directly linked to prior depressive symptoms, he had a history of *substance- or medication-induced depressive disorder*. Although methyldopa has depression listed as a side effect, for Mr. K, there was no evidence that this was the case. Nevertheless, after receiving the diagnosis of Parkinson's disease, Mr. K grieved the loss of his old life. He had trouble adjusting to the stressor of receiving a serious diagnosis and the subsequent treatment and functional decline this would bring to his life. This could have been an *expected response to receiving a serious medical diagnosis* or an adjustment disorder. In this case, Mr. K stopped working and stopped taking visitors, and this lasted about 5 months, which implies more functional impairment. As such, it is more likely to have been an *adjustment disorder with depressed mood*. His depressive symptoms worsened to include psychotic symptoms and suicidal thinking. At this point, Mr. K meets criteria for *major depressive disorder, recurrent episode, severe, with psychotic features*. Parkinson's disease is associated with depression, as is Lewy body dementia, which is also associated with psychotic features. Given this, Mr. K also met the criteria for *depression due to medical condition*.

DEFINITIONS AND KEY CONCEPTS

Depression is a collection of symptoms that encompass depressed mood or anhedonia and neurovegetative symptoms, which may include emotional, somatic, and cognitive symptoms. Medical illnesses may present with somatic and cognitive symptoms, making it challenging to diagnose depression in medically ill patients.

KEY POINT

Depression is a collection of symptoms that encompass depressed mood or anhedonia and neurovegetative symptoms, which may include emotional, somatic, and cognitive symptoms. Medical illnesses may present with somatic and cognitive symptoms, making it challenging to diagnose depression in medically ill patients.

INTRODUCTION

Depression is often under recognized and therefore undertreated in medical settings (Rosenblat, 2020). Historically, the role of physical symptoms in the diagnosis of depression has been documented. Wernicke named the physical symptoms associated with mood disorders as "vital depression," and Bleuler noted that physical symptoms are very common in depression and may mask the underlying psychological condition (Thom et al., 2019). Depression can manifest as a systemic illness whose pathophysiology overlaps with other systemic medical illnesses (Thom, 2019). In modern times, depression has been found to be a proinflammatory condition, which results in a chronic, low-grade inflammatory response with reflex activation of the compensatory anti-inflammatory system (Beurel, 2020). Major depressive disorder is associated with a systemic immune activation, including abnormality in inflammatory markers, immune cell numbers, and antibody titers (Gibney and Drexhage, 2013). Having a major depressive disorder increases the vulnerability to major medical disorders, such as cardiovascular disease, stroke, diabetes, autoimmune disease, and various cancers (Benros et al., 2013; Windle and Windle, 2013; Bortolato et al., 2017). Depression also predisposes patients to poor health behaviors such as sedentary lifestyle, obesity, smoking, and poor adherence to medical treatment. Given the above, major depressive disorder is associated with significant reduction in life span not only from suicide but also significantly from medical disease.

QUICK POINT

Depression has been associated with chronic low-grade inflammatory response with reflex activation of the compensatory anti-inflammatory system (Beurel, 2020).

EPIDEMIOLOGY

The point prevalence of depression increases from 2% to 4% in the community to 5% to 10% in primary care outpatients and 10% to 14% in medically hospitalized patients (Katon & Schulberg, 1992). Major depression is frequently comorbid with multiple sclerosis (MS). The lifetime prevalence of major depression in MS is about 19% to 54% (Skokou et al., 2012). Diabetes is identified as an independent risk factor for the development of major

QUICK POINT

The point prevalence of depression increases from 2% to 4% in the community to 5% to 10% in primary care outpatients and 10% to 14% in medically hospitalized patients (Katon & Schulberg, 1992).

depression; the prevalence of depression among diabetics is 12% to 18% (Ali et al., 2006). Similarly, depression is found in 15% to 23% of patients with coronary heart disease (Spijkerman et al., 2005). Major depression is commonly comorbid with other medical conditions, such as cancer, chronic kidney disease, and chronic pain.

CLINICAL MANIFESTATIONS

Patients with medical diagnoses often experience depressive symptoms. Depression in medical illness manifests in different ways. While a transient mild to moderate low mood state can be considered a normal reaction to receiving a medical diagnosis, more severe depressive symptoms can also be experienced. Within the context of medical illness, depression can be primary, secondary to the medical condition, secondary to substance use or medications used to treat the condition, or an adjustment disorder based on receiving the diagnosis of a medical condition (Figure 21.1). To meet criteria for depression secondary to medical conditions, a direct pathophysiological relationship should be established. A diagnosis of MDD or adjustment disorder is given if the mood disturbance is not the direct pathophysiological consequence of a medical condition based on the patient's history, physical examination, and laboratory findings.

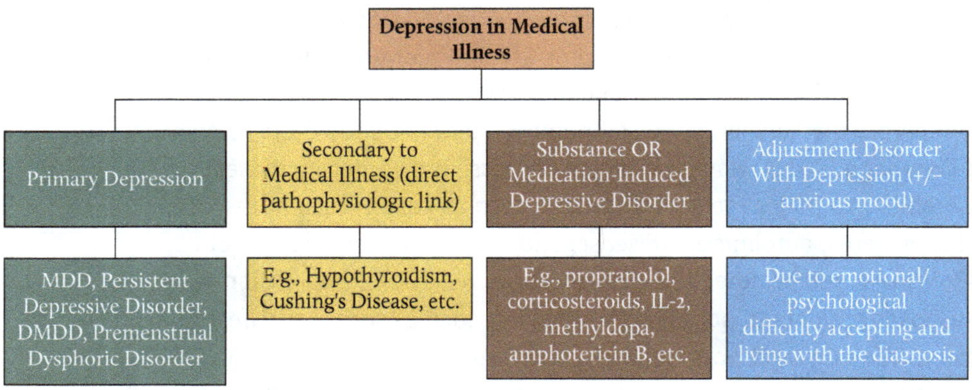

FIGURE 21.1 Types of depression experienced in medical illness.

The impact of depression is comparable to other chronic medical diseases, such as diabetes, arthritis, or hypertension. Chronic medical conditions affect patients' lives, sometimes causing chronic pain, disability, and disruption in the individual or family's life. Depression is an independent source of suffering, disruption in daily life, and disability. Co-occurring depression can worsen the effects of medical illness. Depression increases the risk of treatment nonadherence. Depressed patients are three times more likely to be noncompliant with medical treatment recommendations when compared to patients without depression (DiMatteo et al., 2000). Depressive symptoms are associated with treatment noncompliance in patients with chronic medical conditions, including HIV-AIDS, diabetes, and hypertension (Crockett et al., 2020). Individuals with a lifetime history of depression have higher health care usage (Lee et al., 2020). Patients with chronic medical diseases often have depression, which places them at increased risk of negative health behaviors and negative treatment outcomes.

Primary Depression in Patients With Medical Illness

It is essential to distinguish between the normal response to a serious medical illness from primary depression. It has been studied that health care providers may assume depression to be a "normal" response in patients with serious medical illnesses, leading to delay in diagnosis and treatment (Endicott, 1984). It is well documented that depressive disorders negatively impact health outcomes and lead to increased mortality (Tufo et al., 1970). Personal and family history of depression and the timing of depressive symptom onset and symptom severity can help diagnose depression in this population. The validity of a single question item (i.e., asking the patient, "Are you depressed?") was superior to brief screening questionnaires for depression in terminally ill patients (Chochinov et al., 1997).

Depression Secondary to Medical Illness

Medical illnesses must be assessed for whenever a patient presents with psychiatric symptoms, especially when the review of general medical illness is positive. A study that examined depression and thyroid issues recommended that assessing for signs and symptoms and risk factors for hypo- and hyperthyroidism, but routine testing was not indicated (Briggs et al., 1993). It is important to note that depressive symptoms due to medical illness tend not to respond to antidepressants but improve with treatment of the underlying medical illness. It is worth noting that the list of medical conditions causing depression is never complete. (See the "Management of Depression in Medically Ill Patients" section for further information.) Medical conditions linked to depression are shown in Table 21.1.

TABLE 21.1 Medical Conditions With Pathophysiologic Links to Depression

Endocrine disorders	Neurological disorders	Rheumatic disorders	Malignant diseases	Metabolic disorders	Viral infections
Hypothyroidism	Parkinson's disease	Systemic lupus erythematosus	Pancreatic cancer	Vitamin B12 deficiency	Hepatitis
Cushing's disease	Huntington's disease	Rheumatoid arthritis	Lung cancer	Vitamin D deficiency	Infectious mononucleosis
Addison's disease	Dementia, Alzheimer's, Lewy body, and HIV	Arthritis	Gastric cancer	Wilson's disease	Herpes simplex
Diabetes mellitus	Traumatic brain injury	Back pain	Meningioma	Hartnup disease	COVID-19

> **CLINICAL TIP**
>
> Depression can worsen medical conditions in many ways. Depression is associated with increased medical and psychiatric symptom burden, higher medical costs, lower motivation to get well, nonadherence to treatment, and, ultimately, increased morbidity and mortality.

Substance- or Medication-Induced Depression

Distinguishing a primary depressive disorder from a substance-induced mood disorder can be challenging. Transient substance-induced depressive symptoms can be differentiated by monitoring the patient during a period of abstinence (determined based on the half-life of the substance used) or obtaining history. Individuals with primary depressive disorders more likely present with a family history of depression, the onset of depressive symptoms before the onset of substance use, and persistent depressive symptoms during prolonged periods of abstinence. Often, patients receive a dual diagnosis (i.e., both a primary depressive disorder and a substance-induced depressive disorder) with optimal treatment of both conditions providing the best treatment outcomes (Myrick et al., 2004). Medications linked to depression are shown in Table 21.2 (Rogers & Pies, 2008).

TABLE 21.2 Medications Linked to Depression

Medications acting on the nervous system	Medications acting on GIT	Chemotherapeutic agents	Medications acting on CVS	Others
Antiparkinsonian drugs: methyldopa	Omeprazole	Procarbazine	Propranolol	Corticosteroids
Anticonvulsants: barbiturates and benzodiazepines	Esomeprazole	L-Asparaginase	Metoprolol	Endogenous and exogenous cytokines (i.e., interferon-alfa and aldesleukin [interleukin-2])
Cyclobenzaprine	Ranitidine	Tamoxifen	Atenolol	Anticholinergic drugs
Baclofen	Famotidine	Asparaginase	Enalapril	Antifungal: amphotericin B
Triptans	Cimetidine	Temozolomide	Telmisartan	Statins and cholesterol-lowering drugs

Adjustment Disorder With Depressed Mood

Adjustment disorder is almost three times as common as major depressive disorder (13.7% versus 5.1%) in acutely medically ill patients (Silverstone, 1996). Dynamic points in the illness—diagnosis, treatment response, a relapse or recurrence of the disease, a change in prognosis, and a move to chronically ill or terminally ill state—could be acute stressors (Rackley & Bostwick, 2012) when patients are vulnerable for adjustment disorder (see Chapter 22).

Differential Diagnosis

Hypoactive delirium is a common differential diagnosis for depression in medically ill patients. Up to 40% of medically hospitalized patients referred to consult–liaison psychiatry for concerns of depressive symptoms were diagnosed with delirium (Farrell & Ganzini, 1995). Patients with hypoactive delirium may present with emotional withdrawal, motivation, sleep disturbances, and affective flattening. Fluctuation in consciousness, acute onset of symptoms, disorientation, and inattention on cognitive examination points toward a diagnosis of delirium.

Dementia may also present with withdrawn behavior, motivation, lack of interest in self-care, and affective blunting, making it hard to differentiate from depression. Obtaining collateral from family and friends regarding the patient's recent baseline and a thorough history and mental status examination with cognitive assessment may help establish a diagnosis of dementia.

DEPRESSION AND DIABETES

The incidence of depression is 24% higher in people with diabetes (Nouwen et al., 2010). Depression is associated with noncompliance (e.g., poorer diet, less medication compliance, higher functional impairment, and higher health care costs on diabetic patients; Ciechanowski et al., 2000). The association between depression and diabetes is bidirectional in that each disease predisposes the patient to the other. A randomized controlled study showed that CBT with diabetes education outperformed (85% remittance versus 27% in the control group) diabetes education alone. Patients in the intervention group also had significantly lower glycosylated hemoglobin A1C during the 6-month follow-up (Thom et al., 2019).

QUICK POINT

The prevalence of depression among diabetics is 12% to 18%, and the incidence of depression is higher (by 24%) than in nondiabetics. The association between depression and diabetes is bidirectional in that each disease predisposes the patient to the other (Nouwen et al., 2010).

DEPRESSION AND PAIN

Pain is said to be the fifth vital sign. Depression can cause or worsen pain. Conversely, chronic pain is associated with depression. Over 25% of patients with pain as a complaint have depressive symptoms. About 65% of patients with depression complain of pain (Bair et al., 2003). The impact of chronic pain on a person's life also contributes to depression. Patients with chronic pain conditions often experience a loss of independence, lack of physical movement/exercise, sleep disruption due to pain, sexual problems due to pain, and lower productivity/income, all of which increase vulnerability to depression.

DEPRESSION AND CANCER

> **QUICK POINT**
>
> A diagnosis of depression and higher levels of depressive symptoms is linked to increased mortality risk in cancer patients (Pinquart, 2010). Depression in patients with cancer is believed to equally affect men and women. The pooled mean prevalence of depression in patients with cancer ranges from 8%–24%, going from about 3% in patients with lung cancer to 31% in patients with cancer of the digestive tract (Krebber, 2014).

A substantial body of literature suggests that a diagnosis of depression and higher levels of depressive symptoms is linked to elevated mortality in cancer patients. This includes studies on patients with depression before cancer diagnosis and studies that assessed depression following cancer diagnosis (Pinquart, 2010). Depression affects about over 10% of patients with cancer and is believed to equally affect men and women. The pooled mean prevalence of depression in patients with cancer ranges from 8%–24%, going from about 3% in patients with lung cancer to 31% in patients with cancer of the digestive tract (Krebber, 2014). Depression is highest during treatment and is estimated to be around 14%. Post-cancer depression diagnosis remains of concern. A diagnosis of depression and higher levels of depressive symptoms predicted elevated mortality in patients with cancer. Mortality rates have been found to be up to 25% higher in patients with depressive symptoms (Satin, 2009). Notably, the depression–mortality association was weaker in younger samples. Factors affecting depression-related cancer mortality include treatment delay, treatment nonadherence, somatic symptoms (pain, fatigue, and dyspnea associated with psychological distress and level of depression), health risk behaviors, and the effect of depression on immune functioning, which may lead to initiation and progression of neoplastic processes. (Lloyd-Williams, 2001).

MANAGEMENT OF DEPRESSION IN MEDICALLY ILL PATIENTS

Depression in medically ill patients is associated with worse medical symptoms, poor adherence to treatment, greater health care utilization, and ultimately worse patient outcomes. Identifying, then managing depression improves patient outcomes in medical patients. Medications are used to treat depression in the medically ill where antidepressant side effects can be beneficial for some medical symptoms. In addition, psychological and social factors impact depression in many ways. For the medically ill patient with depression, including counseling or other specific forms of psychotherapy in addition to being a treatment for depression, helps them cope with their medical illness and improves stress management and potentially functioning through their illness.

Medications

The choice of antidepressant in treating major depression in the medically ill is similar to that in the nonmedically ill population. SSRIs, SNRIs, bupropion, and mirtazapine are initial choices due to their similar efficacy. However, the following special considerations should be kept in mind (Rackley & Bostwick, 2012; Thom et al., 2019):

- Side effects or added benefits of antidepressants should be considered while choosing antidepressants. For example, mirtazapine is used for treating insomnia alongside depression, and tricyclic antidepressants (TCAs) and duloxetine can be considered if patients with depression have comorbid neuropathic pain.
- Serotonin syndrome is another concern when starting a serotonergic antidepressant in medically ill patients, especially for those who are on medications such as linezolid and tramadol. Using short-acting SSRIs, such as sertraline or bupropion, a nonserotonergic antidepressant, should be considered to treat major depression.
- Cytochrome p450 (CYP 450) enzyme effects: It is important to keep in mind that the psychotropics impact CYP 450 enzymes, which play an important role in metabolizing antibiotics, antiepileptics, and antiretrovirals. The use of potent 2D6 enzyme inhibitors (fluoxetine and paroxetine) in patients taking tamoxifen led to increased risk of breast cancer recurrence, as tamoxifen required 2D6 to be converted to its active metabolite (Sideras et al., 2010).
- In patients with a history of GI bleeds, caution is advised with the use of SSRIs and SNRIs, as they may slightly increase the risk of bleeding, due to decreasing platelet function.
- Lithium, gabapentin, and topiramate are renally excreted and may need adjustments in renal failure patients.
- All antidepressants carry dose adjustment recommendations when used in patients with severe hepatic impairment.

Psychotherapy

Interpersonal psychotherapy and cognitive behavioral therapy (CBT) are the two most studied types of therapy in this patient population. Interpersonal therapy helps address the role transitions and role disputes that accompany chronic illnesses. In CBT, the cognitive part of therapy identifies and challenges the negative automatic thoughts regarding illness that perpetuate the depressed mood. The behavioral aspect of CBT helps patients engage in positively reinforcing behaviors, such as problem-solving and creating a list of priorities. One study found that modified brief CBT for patients with uncontrolled diabetes and comorbid depression significantly improved their medication adherence and depression scores (Safren et al., 2014). Modified CBT has been studied in the management of specific illnesses such as multiple sclerosis, Parkinson's disease, coronary artery disorders, and renal disease patients on dialysis.

CLINICAL TIP

Depression in patients with medical conditions:

- is not a normal state,
- is indicative of the need for treatment of depression,
- treatment for depression in medically ill patients is beneficial,
- promotes a less psychologically stressful course of treatment,
- enhances quality of life, and
- may lead to a more robust treatment outcome of the medical condition.

SUMMARY

Depression within the context of medical illness can take on many forms. In medical settings, screening for depression should be routinely done and referrals to mental health specialists considered. Treating depression in medical illness improves treatment outcomes, including the patient's quality of life.

RESOURCES

1 https://www.cdc.gov/tobacco/campaign/tips/diseases/depression-anxiety.html

2 https://adaa.org/understanding-anxiety/depression

REFERENCES

Ali, S., Stone, M. A., Peters, J. L., Davies, M. J., & Khunti, K. (2006). The prevalence of comorbid depression in adults with Type 2 diabetes: A systematic review and meta-analysis. *Diabetic Medicine: A Journal of the British Diabetic Association, 23*(11), 1165–1173. https://doi.org/10.1111/j.1464-5491.2006.01943.x

Bair, M. J., Robinson, R. L., Katon, W., & Kroenke, K. (2003). Depression and pain comorbidity: A literature review. *Archives of Internal Medicine, 163*(20), 2433–2445. https://doi.org/10.1001/archinte.163.20.2433

Beurel, E., Nemeroff, C. B., & Toups, M. (2020). *The bidirectional relationship of depression and inflammation: Double trouble*. Redirecting. https://doi.org/10.1016/j.neuron.2020.06.002.

Briggs, J., McBride, L., Hagino, O., Brown, W. A., & Bauer, M. S. (1993). Screening depressives for causative medical illness; the example of thyroid function testing: II. Hypothesis testing in ambulatory depressives. *Depression, 1*(4), 220–224. https://doi.org/10.1002/depr.3050010405

Chochinov, H. M., Wilson, K. G., Enns, M., & Lander, S. (1997). "Are you depressed?" Screening for depression in the terminally ill. *The American Journal of Psychiatry, 154*(5), 674–676. https://doi.org/10.1176/ajp.154.5.674

Ciechanowski, P. S., Katon, W. J., & Russo, J. E. (2000). Depression and diabetes: Impact of depressive symptoms on adherence, function, and costs. *Archives of Internal Medicine, 160*(21), 3278–3285. https://doi.org/10.1001/archinte.160.21.3278

Crockett, K. B., Entler, K. J., Brodie, E., Kempf, M.-C., Konkle-Parker, D., Wilson, T. E., Tien, P. C., Wingood, G., Neilands, T. B., Johnson, M. O., Weiser, S. D., Turan, J. M., & Turan, B. (2020). Brief report: Linking depressive symptoms to viral nonsuppression among women with HIV through adherence self-efficacy and ART adherence. *Journal of Acquired Immune Deficiency Syndromes (1999), 83*(4), 340–344. https://doi.org/10.1097/QAI.0000000000002268

DiMatteo, M. R., Lepper, H. S., & Croghan, T. W. (2000). Depression is a risk factor for non-compliance with medical treatment: Meta-analysis of the effects of anxiety and depression on patient adherence. *Archives of Internal Medicine, 160*(14), 2101–2107. https://doi.org/10.1001/archinte.160.14.2101

Endicott, J. (1984). Measurement of depression in patients with cancer. *Cancer, 53*(10), 2243–2249. https://doi.org/10.1002/cncr.1984.53.s10.2243

Farrell, K. R., & Ganzini, L. (1995). Misdiagnosing delirium as depression in medically ill elderly patients. *Archives of Internal Medicine, 155*(22), 2459–2464.

Gibney, S. M., & Drexhage, H. A. (n.d.). Evidence for a dysregulated immune system in the etiology of psychiatric disorders. *Journal of Neuroimmune Pharmacology: The Official Journal of the Society on NeuroImmune Pharmacology.* https://pubmed.ncbi.nlm.nih.gov/23645137/.

Katon, W., & Schulberg, H. (1992). Epidemiology of depression in primary care. *General Hospital Psychiatry, 14*(4), 237–247. https://doi.org/10.1016/0163-8343(92)90094-q

Lee, G. B., Kim, H. C., & Jung, S. J. (2020). Association between depression and disease-specific treatment. *Journal of Affective Disorders, 260*, 124–130. https://doi.org/10.1016/j.jad.2019.08.073

Lloyd-Williams, M., & Friedman, T. (2001). Depression in palliative care patients--a prospective study. *European Journal of Cancer Care, 10*(4), 270–274. https://doi.org/10.1046/j.1365-2354.2001.00290.x

Myrick, H., Cluver, J., Swavely, S., & Peters, H. (2004). Diagnosis and treatment of co-occurring affective disorders and substance use disorders. *Psychiatric Clinics of North America, 27*(4), 649–659. https://doi.org/10.1016/j.psc.2004.06.003

Nouwen, A., Winkley, K., Twisk, J., Lloyd, C. E., Peyrot, M., Ismail, K., Power, F., & European Depression in Diabetes (EDID) Research Consortium. (2010). Type 2 diabetes mellitus as a risk factor for the onset of depression: A systematic review and meta-analysis. *Diabetologia, 53*(12), 2480–2486. https://doi.org/10.1007/s00125-010-1874-x

Rackley, S., & Bostwick, J. M. (2012). Depression in medically ill patients. *The Psychiatric Clinics of North America, 35*(1), 231–247. https://doi.org/10.1016/j.psc.2011.11.001

Rogers, D., & Pies, R. (2008). General medical drugs associated with depression. *Psychiatry (Edgmont), 5*(12), 28–41.

Rosenblat, J. D., Kurdyak, P., Cosci, F., Berk, M., Maes, M., Brunoni, A. R., Li, M., Rodin, G., McIntyre, R. S., & Carvalho, A. F. (2020). Depression in the medically ill. *The Australian and New Zealand Journal of psychiatry, 54*(4), 346–366. https://doi.org/10.1177/0004867419888576

Safren, S. A., Gonzalez, J. S., Wexler, D. J., Psaros, C., Delahanty, L. M., Blashill, A. J., Margolina, A. I., & Cagliero, E. (2014). A randomized controlled trial of cognitive-behavioral therapy for adherence and depression (CBT-AD) in patients with uncontrolled type 2 diabetes. *Diabetes Care, 37*(3), 625–633. https://doi.org/10.2337/dc13-0816

Sideras, K., Ingle, J. N., Ames, M. M., Loprinzi, C. L., Mrazek, D. P., Black, J. L., Weinshilboum, R. M., Hawse, J. R., Spelsberg, T. C., & Goetz, M. P. (2010). Coprescription of tamoxifen and medications that inhibit CYP2D6. *Journal of Clinical Oncology: Official Journal of the American Society of Clinical Oncology, 28*(16), 2768–2776. https://doi.org/10.1200/JCO.2009.23.8931

Silverstone, P. H. (1996). Prevalence of psychiatric disorders in medical inpatients. *The Journal of Nervous and Mental Disease, 184*(1), 43–51. https://doi.org/10.1097/00005053-199601000-00008

Skokou, M., Soubasi, E., & Gourzis, P. (2012). Depression in multiple sclerosis: A review of assessment and treatment approaches in adult and pediatric populations. *ISRN Neurology.* https://doi.org/10.5402/2012/427102

Spijkerman, T., Jonge, P. de, Brink, R. H. S. van den, Jansen, J. H. C., May, J. F., Crijns, H. G. J. M., & Ormel, J. (2005). Depression following myocardial infarction: First-ever versus ongoing and recurrent episodes. *General Hospital Psychiatry: Psychiatry, Medicine and Primary Care, 27*(6), 411–417.

Thom, R., Silbersweig, D. A., & Boland, R. J. (2019). Major depressive disorder in medical illness: A review of assessment, prevalence, and treatment options. *Psychosomatic Medicine, 81*(3), 246–255. https://doi.org/10.1097/PSY.0000000000000678

Tufo, H. M., Ostfeld, A. M., & Shekelle, R. (1970). Central nervous system dysfunction following open-heart surgery. *JAMA, 212*(8), 1333–1340. https://doi.org/10.1001/jama.1970.03170210039006

CHAPTER 22

Adjustment- and Grief-Related Disorders[1]

Nandhini Madhanagopal, M.D.; Kirti Saxena, M.D.; and Edore Onigu-Otite, M.D.

> *"What is done is done. What is gone is gone. One of life's lessons is learning how to move on. It is okay to look back and think of fond memories but never stop moving forward."*
>
> — Gautam Buddha

OBJECTIVES

At the end of this chapter, students will be able to do the following:

- review types of adjustment disorders
- review types of grief
- distinguish between grief, bereavement, and depression

CASE VIGNETTE

Mrs. Z is a 41-year-old female with no past psychiatric history. She is married and has four children—three boys aged 5, 8, and 10 and a 3-year-old daughter. Her daughter was diagnosed with a neoplastic illness. All members of the family were investigated, and Mrs. Z was found to have a breast lump. Her daughter unfortunately passed away a few months after. Mrs. Z, while making funeral arrangements for her daughter, surprisingly inquired about an adult coffin as well. Her husband was upset! After the funeral, Mrs. Z did not follow up with her mammogram appointments. Two years later, she was diagnosed with

1 Readers may also see "Depressive Disorders" (Chapter 20), "Depression in the Medically Ill" (Chapter 21), and "Trauma- and Stressor-Related Disorders" (Chapter 18) for related material.

metastatic breast cancer. Despite receiving the best medical treatment, Mrs. Z died, leaving behind a husband and three young children. Her complicated grief, which interfered with her treatment compliance, had gone unnoticed.

DEFINITIONS AND KEY CONCEPTS

Adjustment disorder is a maladaptive emotional and/or behavioral response to an identifiable stressor that is out of proportion to the severity and intensity of the stressor. The symptoms of adjustment disorder occur within 3 months of the stressor and resolve in 6 months after the stressor has terminated, and the symptoms interfere with the individual's functioning. Adjustment disorder is postulated as a continuum of a normal adaptive response to a stressor but is delineated by the intensity of the distress and its resultant impairment (Maercker et al., 2013).

INTRODUCTION

Adjustment disorder is a frequently utilized diagnostic category and plays an important role in current health care utilization. In a global survey among psychiatrists by the World Health Organization (WHO) regarding the category of psychiatric illness they used at least once a week in their practice, adjustment disorder ranked seven out of 44 categories (Maercker & Lorenz, 2018). Adjustment disorder differs from the other diagnoses (such as depression) for which life stressors are a common factor because of the requirement of a stressor as an essential criterion. Other than posttraumatic stress disorder (PTSD) and substance use disorder, adjustment disorder is the only other disorder based on etiology in the current classifications (Casey & Jabbar, 2013).

ADJUSTMENT DISORDERS

Epidemiology

In the general population, the prevalence of adjustment disorder with clinically significant impairment was 0.9% (Maercker et al., 2012). Adjustment disorder is a common diagnosis in the emergency department and in the consult liaison psychiatry service. One study recorded adjustment disorder in 6.7% of the patients assessed in the emergency department over 1 year (Kropp et al., 2007). In acutely ill medical patients, adjustment disorder was almost three times more common (13.7%) than major depressive disorder (5.1%; Silverstone, 1996). Adjustment disorder was diagnosed in 12% of patients in the consult liaison psychiatry service, and the depressed mood was the most common subtype recorded (11.6%; Strain et al., 1998). Adjustment disorder is the most common diagnosis in the military and is very frequently diagnosed in children (Strain, 2019).

QUICK POINT

The neurobiology of adjustment disorder is closely linked to dysregulation in the hypothalamic pituitary adrenal (HPA) axis caused by experiencing a stressful event or condition.

Neurobiology

The neurobiology of adjustment disorder can be best understood by examining the effects of stress on the brain and the key role played by the HPA (hypothalamic pituitary adrenal) axis. The distress and disorder present when the need for adaptation exceeds the individual's capacity to maintain physiologic and psychologic equilibrium. A study documented significantly higher maximal binding capacity of platelet serotonin H2A receptor in patients with adjustment disorder. This finding was noted in other psychiatric patients with suicidality, and the study concluded that loss of control over suicidal impulses may be associated with decrease in availability of serotonin and upregulation of serotonin-2A receptors (Rao et al., 1998).

Higher levels of biological markers of oxidative stress (protein carbonyl and nitrosylated protein) were observed in individuals with adjustment disorder postexposure to psychological abuse at workplace (Di Rosa et al., 2009).

CLINICAL TIP

Symptoms of adjustment disorder include low mood, sadness, worry, anxiety, insomnia, poor concentration, irritability, and others. Examples of the stressors include changes in home, school, work environments, relationship changes, traumatic events, community disasters, new medical diagnoses, or disabilities.

Clinical Manifestations

Adjustment disorder cannot be diagnosed in the absence of a stressor. The stressful life event occurs in close proximity to the onset of symptoms, and, per the *DSM-5* criteria, symptom onset occurs within 3 months of the onset of the stressor. The nature and severity of the stressor has not been defined. The severity of the stressor can range from mild to severe; individual vulnerability determines development of an adjustment disorder (Casey & Bailey, 2011).

Psychosocial factors that predisposed individuals to adjustment disorder include insecure-fearful avoidant attachment style, low self-esteem, and poor social support (Ponizovsky et al., 2011). Symptoms of adjustment disorder include low mood, sadness, worry, anxiety, insomnia and poor concentration, irritability, and others. It is important to remember that some of the symptoms resemble major depressive disorder. The sad mood in adjustment disorder is predominant when individuals cognitively engage with the event; removal from the stressful situation is associated with improvement of symptoms (Casey & Bailey, 2011).

The natures of the stressors include the following:

- Change or move at home, school, or work
- Significant loss, including job, relationship, financial related
- Experiencing traumatic events—directly or indirectly
- Witnessing a natural disaster—directly or indirectly
- Receiving bad news (e.g., news of a significant medical diagnosis in self or close family or friends)
- Disability

Based on the predominant symptoms the subtypes of adjustment disorder are categorized based on disturbances in emotions or conduct (Figure 22.1).

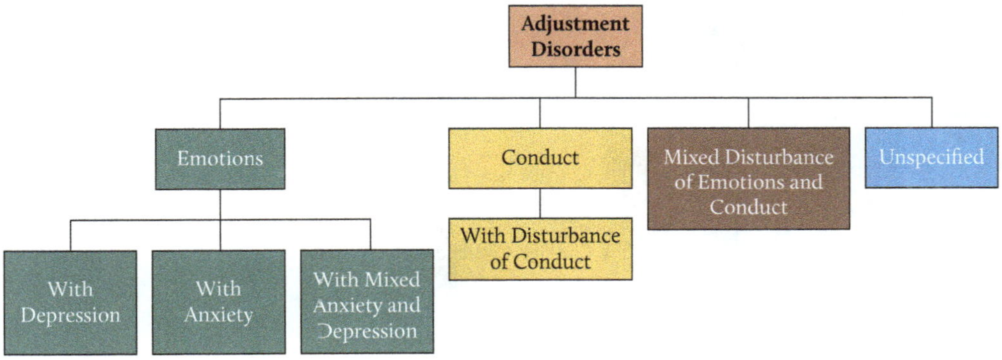

FIGURE 22.1 Types of adjustment disorders.

The depressive subtype is common in adults; disturbance of conduct and disturbance of conduct and emotion are more commonly diagnosed in children and adolescents.

Twenty-five percent of adolescents with adjustment disorder engage in suicidal behavior (Pelkonen et al., 2005), and this increases to 60% in adults (Kryzhanovskaya & Canterbury, 2001). Common risk factors for suicidality in adolescents include past psychiatric treatment, poor psychosocial functioning at admission to the hospital, suicide as a stressor, dysphoric mood, and psychomotor restlessness (Pelkonen et al., 2005). Adjustment disorder patients who attempted suicide had lower social status, were less educated, and were unmarried when compared to patients with major depressive disorder; about half of the patients had reported an unstable parental family and emotionally deprived childhood (Polyakova et al., 1998).

QUICK POINT

Adjustment disorder is a significant risk factor for suicidal behavior. Twenty-five percent of adolescents with adjustment disorder engage in suicidal behavior (Pelkonen et al., 2005), and this increases to 60% in adults (Kryzhanovskaya & Canterbury, 2001).

Differential Diagnosis

The common differential diagnoses of adjustment disorder include normal reaction to stress, major depressive disorder, generalized anxiety disorder, PTSD, acute stress reaction, substance use disorder, and dysthymia. Figure 22.2 is a useful algorithm to help work through differential diagnoses related to adjustment disorders. Notably, adjustment disorders can occur alongside other major psychiatric disorders. Additionally, acute and posttraumatic stress disorders can occur within context of loss associated with trauma (e.g., death of friends or family [loss] in a motor vehicle accident that involved or was witnessed by the patient [traumatic experience]). A traumatic response to grief that is sudden and expected, such as through violence or an accident, is sometimes called traumatic grief.

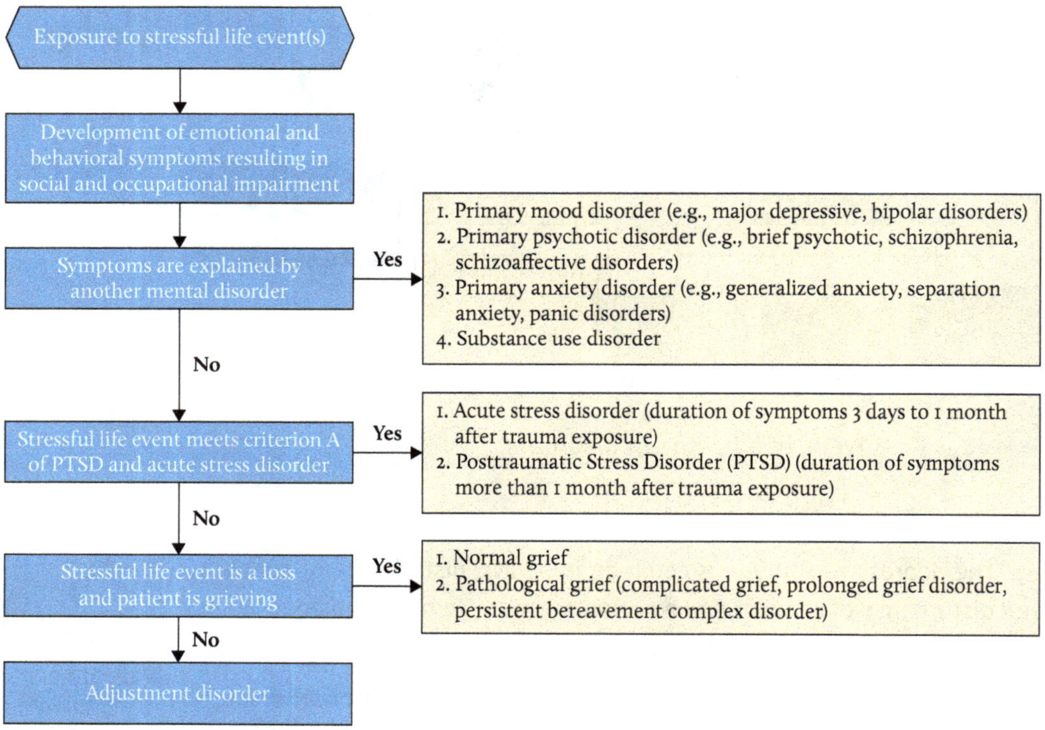

FIGURE 22.2 Differentiating adjustment and related disorders.

Comorbidity

Personality disorder and organic mental disorder were the most frequently identified comorbidities with adjustment disorder (Strain et al., 1998). In the same study, it was noted that patients with adjustment disorder had less past psychiatric illnesses and functioned better in line with the description of the disorder as a maladaptation to a stressor. Adults were found to have comorbid substance use disorder (Greenberg et al., 1995).

Course and Prognosis

Due to the temporal nature of the symptoms to the stressor in adjustment disorder, the symptoms resolve more quickly, and readmission rates are lower (Jones et al., 2002). However, as mentioned, patients with adjustment disorder engage in suicidal behavior. Up to 25% of male adolescents who die of by suicide carry a diagnosis of adjustment disorder (Lönnqvist et al., 1995). Studies posit that adults with adjustment disorder have a good long-term prognosis; however, adolescents are at an increased risk of being diagnosed with major psychiatric illness later in their life.

Diagnosis

Adjustment disorder is diagnosed using the *DSM-5* criteria. It requires the development of emotional or behavioral symptoms within context of experiencing a stressful event or condition. It requires the presence of an identifiable stressor with the onset of symptoms within 3 months of the stressor and a resolution of symptoms within 6 months of the cessation of the stressor.

KEY POINT

An adjustment disorder requires the presence of an identifiable stressor with the onset of symptoms within 3 months of the stressor and a resolution of symptoms within 6 months of the cessation of the stressor.

Treatment

Given that the symptoms resolve spontaneously unless the stressors continue and maintain the symptoms when prolonged therapy may be required, brief psychotherapy is regarded as the appropriate first line of treatment for adjustment disorder. Therapy types, including supportive, psychoeducational, cognitive, and psychodynamic therapy, have been tried with some success (Casey, 2009). Dialectical behavioral therapy is beneficial in those with suicidal and self-harm behaviors. Mirror therapy, a therapy that incorporates psychocorporeal, cognitive, and neurolinguistic components has shown to be effective in patients with adjustment disorder secondary to myocardial infarction (González-Jaimes & Turnbull-Plaza, 2003).

Pharmacological treatments have a limited role, apart from treatment of insomnia, anxiety, and panic attacks, in adjustment disorder with benzodiazepines. Though there is not much evidence, antidepressants have been prescribed for about 45% of patients diagnosed with adjustment disorder (Fernández et al., 2012). A study compared antidepressant, supportive psychotherapy, benzodiazepine, and placebo for the treatment of adjustment disorder and concluded that none of the treatment modalities had superior effect over others (De Leo, 1989). A stepped care approach to address adjustment disorder has been described (Domhardt & Baumeister, 2018).

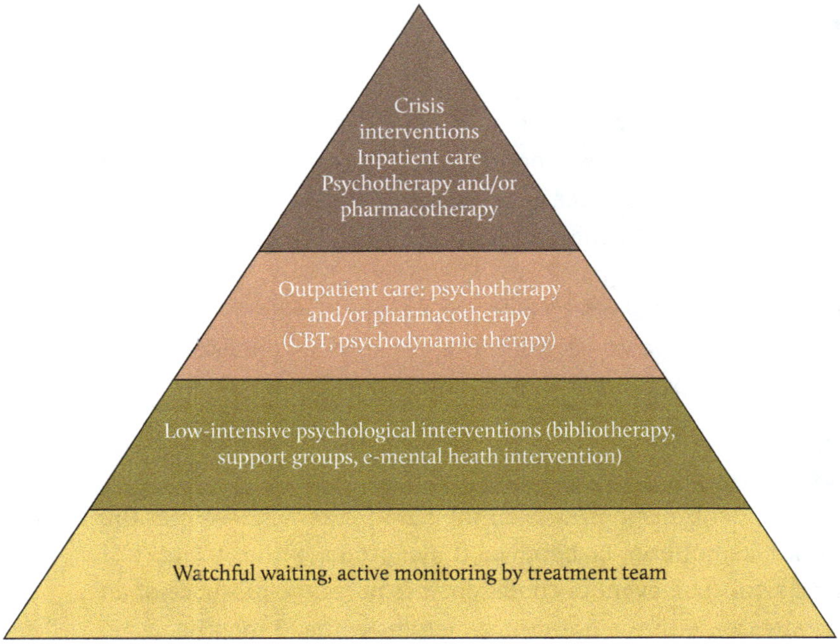

FIGURE 22.3 Treatment approach to adjustment disorders.

Adapted from Matthias Domhardt and Harald Baumeister, "Psychotherapy of Adjustment Disorders: Current State and Future Directions," The World Journal of Biological Psychiatry, vol. 19, no. s1, p. 527. Copyright © 2018 by Taylor & Francis Group. Adapted by Nandhini Madhanagopal, Kirti Saxena, and Edore Onigu-Otite.

Medical Considerations

Medical illness is one of the predominant stressors predisposing to the development of adjustment disorder. The prevalence of adjustment disorder in consultation-liaison psychiatric samples is high, ranging from 12.5% (Strain et al., 1998) to 18.5% (Foster & Oxman, 1994). In a study of psychiatric consultation for gynecological–obstetric inpatients, adjustment disorder was almost twice as common as mood disorders (Rigatelli et al., 2002). The prevalence of adjustment disorder was approximately 15.4% in palliative care settings and about 19.4% in oncology–hematology settings (Mitchell et al., 2011).

The psychological response of the patients to the medical illness, including worry, fear, dependency, helplessness, and pain, and the impairment in both physical and mental health directly from the medical illness leads to the high prevalence of adjustment disorder in this population. It is important to accurately diagnose adjustment disorder in the medical–surgical setting, as (a) the stressors may be prolonged due to consequences of the illness and (b) it gets patients who are distressed and dysfunctional, yet not meeting criteria for other psychiatric disorders, mental health care.

Despite the wide prevalence of adjustment disorder, there is a lack of specific assessment tools that can be used universally. Further studies to explore the culturally informed stepped care approach for treatment of this disorder are vital, especially given the mild mental health symptoms that may go unnoticed.

GRIEF-RELATED DISORDERS

Grief is an expected response to loss or bereavement. Grief-related disorders occur when the normal grief process becomes complicated, prolonged, or has an additional distinct element of trauma involved.

KEY POINT

Grief is an expected response to loss or bereavement. Grief-related disorders occur when the normal grief process becomes complicated, prolonged, or has an additional distinct element of trauma involved.

Definitions

- *Bereavement*—The experience of having lost someone close
- *Grief*—The reaction to bereavement, composed of thoughts, feelings, behaviors, and physiological changes that vary in pattern and intensity over time
- *Traumatic grief*—A traumatic response to grief that is sudden and expected, such as through violence or an accident
- *Mourning*—The public display of grief (Shear, 2012)

Normal Grief

This is the most common reaction to the loss of a significant other. It progresses from acute to integrated grief. Acute grief is characterized by intense psychological suffering, repeated thoughts of the deceased, sadness, loneliness, sleep and appetite changes, and a tendency to neglect daily life. Integrated grief encompasses the acceptance of loss, decreased intensity of suffering when remembering the deceased, and recommitment to life (Moayedoddin & Markowitz, 2015).

KEY POINT

The stages of grief, as originally conceptualized by Elisabeth Kübler-Ross, described patient responses when facing terminal illness. These five stages—denial, anger, bargaining, depression, and acceptance—are now often used as a model of bereavement adjustment.

The stages of grief, as originally conceptualized by Elisabeth Kübler-Ross, described patient responses when facing terminal illness. These five stages—denial, anger, bargaining, depression, and acceptance—are now often used as a model of bereavement adjustment (Table 22.1).

It is important to know that individuals do not all go through the stages and not always in the same sequence. A prospective research studied the five stages of grief and reported that during the 6 months after a loss, the disbelief of the loss of a significant other decreases and acceptance of the loss increases. Consequently, the intensity of the stages continues to diminish, and persistence of these stages after the 6-month period indicates a need for evaluation for abnormal grief (Maciejewski et al., 2007).

Normal grief can resemble a depressive episode or disorder. Distinguishing both conditions can be challenging. Table 22.1 contains a list of features that help differentiate between both conditions. Of note, both grief and a major depressive disorder can co-occur and require identification and treatment. The experience of loss can include a traumatic

TABLE 22.1 Stages of Grief and Loss

		Description	Sample patient comments
1.	Denial	Denial, usually temporary, is often manifested as disbelief. This may include shock, confusion, and avoidance	"No." "This isn't be happening." "I'm fine." "Everything's okay."
2.	Anger	Anger may be directed outward or inward. It may include frustration, irritability, and blame-seeking behaviors	"How could this happen?!" "It's not fair!" "Why did this happen?" "Who is to blame?"
3.	Bargaining	Bargaining comes from a mindset or hope, albeit misplaced, that the loss can somehow be deferred or delayed. It may be reflected in positive behaviors (e.g., "If I do good acts, I will live longer.") and struggling to find meaning for the loss coming at this time.	"I'll do anything to keep this from happening." "Just let me have more time." "Just let me live to see (an important event; e.g., my children graduate)."
4.	Depression	Depression is manifested by a sad mood and lack of motivation. The individual may feel sad, hopeless, and overwhelmed.	"I cannot bear this." "I'm too sad to do anything." "Why bother with anything?" "I'm going to die. What's the point in doing anything?"
5.	Acceptance	Acceptance brings a reckoning that the loss is/will/has happened. It may be manifested by peace (the calm after the storm), which is manifested in a decrease in anxiety. The individual begins to adapt to the loss, exploring and planning according to the new circumstances the loss brings.	"I acknowledge this has happened." "I cannot change it." "This is set to happen." "I must move on now." "I can't fight it; I may as well prepare for it."

component, particularly when the grief is sudden or involves violence or an accident. Identification and both components of grief and trauma are important in attaining optimal treatment outcomes.

Pathological Grief

Patterns of grief that do not run the normal course, that are prolonged (symptoms lasting more than 6 months), intense, and lead to impairment in functioning, have been described by different entities as "complicated grief," "prolonged grief disorder" by the ICD 11 guidelines, and "persistent complex bereavement disorder" by the *DSM-5*.

Complicated Grief

Only a small proportion of the people who grieve develop complicated grief with the prevalence ranging from 2.4% in Japan to 6.7% in Germany (Nakajima, 2018). Studies have shown that prevalence of complicated grief increase following traumatic events, such as homicide and terrorist attacks. Major depressive disorder and posttraumatic disorder frequently exist comorbidly with complicated grief (Nakajima, 2018).

Symptoms

Persistent intense acute grief is grief that has been present for more than 6 months is expected by others in the person's social or cultural environment. Some of the symptoms include the following:

- Persistent intense yearning or longing for the person who died
- Recurrent thoughts that it is unfair or meaningless to have to live when a loved one has died or a recurrent urge to die to join the deceased
- Frequent preoccupying thoughts about the person who died
- Persistent feeling of being shocked, dazed, or emotionally numb since the death
- Persistent difficulty trusting or caring about other people or feeling intensely envious of others who haven't experienced a similar loss
- Experiencing intense emotional or physiologic reactivity to memories of the person who died (Shear et al., 2011)

Many of these symptoms are similar to the acute phase of grief; however, the symptoms of complicated grief continue for a prolonged period of time (Nakajima, 2018). A study found that 43% of bereaved adults of the September 11 attack in New York met criteria for complicated grief 2.5 to 3.5 years after the event (Neria et al., 2007). Additionally, individuals with complicated grief suffer with poor physical health symptoms, such as high blood pressure, cancer, heart disease, headache, flu, various psychiatric problems, and reduced vitality (Prigerson et al., 1997; Silverman et al., 2000).

Prolonged Grief Disorder

ICD-11 defines prolonged grief disorder as a persistent and pervasive longing for the deceased and/or persistent and pervasive cognitive preoccupation with the deceased, combined with any of the 10 grief reactions representative of intensive emotional pain for at least 6 months after bereavement. Risk factors include history of trauma or loss, history of mood and anxiety disorders, being a caregiver for the deceased, insecure attachment, a violent cause of death, and lack of social support (Jordan & Litz, 2014).

Persistent Complex Bereavement Disorder

The *DSM-5* has included persistent complex bereavement disorder (PCBD) under "other specified trauma- and stressor-related disorder" in the section dedicated to conditions requiring further study. There is overlap between the PCBD and prolonged grief disorder diagnostic criteria; however, PCBD is diagnosed when the symptoms are present for at least 12 months after the death of a close other.

PCBD includes symptoms of separation distress (persistent longing for the deceased, preoccupation with the deceased), reactive distress to death (anger related to the loss, excessive avoidance of reminders of the loss), and social/identity disruption (desire to die to be with the deceased, feeling alone or detached from others since the death, or confusion about one's role in life).

TABLE 22.2 Differentiating Between Grief and Major Depressive Disorder

	More likely in complicated grief	More likely in major depression
Prevailing feeling	• Feelings of vacancy and loss directly due to the absence of the deceased	• Persistent sadness
Negative emotions	• Decrease with time • Decrease in intensity • Intermittent or come in waves (pangs of grief) • Associated with reminders	• May increase with time • May increase in intensity • Stable with fewer fluctuations • More pervasive; not limited to reminders
Positive emotions	• Able to experience positive emotions and humor	• Diminished or lack of ability to experience positive emotions or humor
Guilt or worthlessness	• Revolves around the deceased or circumstances around the loss	• More pervasive and global (not limited to the loss) • May feel a sense of worthlessness or experience the feeling of being a burden
Self-loathing	• Feeling of failing the deceased	• Feeling of failing in general (including others unrelated to the loss)

Treatment of Pathological Grief

Psychotherapy is the first line of treatment for pathological grief. Complicated grief treatment includes loss-focused cognitive behavioral techniques (repeated retelling of the story of the death, imagined conversation with the deceased, and work on memories) and restoration-focused interpersonal therapy strategies (enhance rapport building, restoring effective interpersonal functioning, and guided treatment termination; Shear et al., 2005).

Regarding pharmacotherapy, literature does not reveal a consensus that medications are helpful in the treatment of pathological grief. One study reported that complicated grief treatment is the treatment of choice for complicated grief and the addition of citalopram to complicated grief treatment optimized the treatment of co-occurring depressive symptoms (Shear et al., 2016).

CLINICAL TIP

Symptoms of grief and major depressive disorder overlap. A careful clinical interview and close follow up are essential to support the patient. Both conditions can also coexist in the same individual. It is important to treat major depressive disorder if a patient meets the criteria, including to prevent self-harm.

SUMMARY

The proportion of grieving individuals struggling from pathological grief is significant, and evidence points to the needs for mental health interventions to reduce morbidity. We need larger randomized controlled trials to ascertain the role of medications and other psychotherapeutic techniques for pathological grief. Given the need for effective interventions, it is also important to arrive at a consensus regarding the diagnosis and explore assessment tools to identify pathological grief.

RESOURCES

1 How to Cope With Death as a Future Doctor | Medical School Admissions Doctor | US News

2 Bereavement: MedlinePlus

3 Grief and Children (aacap.org)

4 Adjustment Disorder: What Is Adjustment Disorder? (10faq.com)

REFERENCES

Casey, P. (2009). Adjustment disorder: Epidemiology, diagnosis and treatment. *CNS Drugs, 23*(11), 927–938. https://doi.org/10.2165/11311000-000000000-00000

Casey, P., & Bailey, S. (2011). Adjustment disorders: The state of the art. *World Psychiatry, 10*(1), 11–18.

Casey, P., & Jabbar, F. (2013). Adjustment disorder considered. *Advances in Psychiatric Treatment, 19*(2), 99–107. https://doi.org/10.1192/apt.bp.111.010058

De Leo, D. (1989). Treatment of adjustment disorders: A comparative evaluation. *Psychological Reports, 64*(1), 51–54. https://doi.org/10.2466/pr0.1989.64.1.51

Di Rosa, A. E., Gangemi, S., Cristani, M., Fenga, C., Saitta, S., Abenavoli, E., Imbesi, S., Speciale, A., Minciullo, P. L., Spatari, G., Abbate, S., Saija, A., & Cimino, F. (2009). Serum levels of carbonylated and nitrosylated proteins in mobbing victims with workplace adjustment disorders. *Biological Psychology, 82*(3), 308–311. https://doi.org/10.1016/j.biopsycho.2009.09.005

Domhardt, M., & Baumeister, H. (2018). Psychotherapy of adjustment disorders: Current state and future directions. *The World Journal of Biological Psychiatry, 19*(1), S21–S35. https://doi.org/10.1080/15622975.2018.1467041

Fernández, A., Mendive, J. M., Salvador-Carulla, L., Rubio-Valera, M., Luciano, J. V., Pinto-Meza, A., Haro, J. M., Palao, D. J., Bellón, J. A., Serrano-Blanco, A., & DASMAP investigators. (2012). Adjustment disorders in primary care: Prevalence, recognition and use of services. *The British Journal of Psychiatry: The Journal of Mental Science, 201*, 137–142. https://doi.org/10.1192/bjp.bp.111.096305

Foster, P., & Oxman, T. (1994). A descriptive study of adjustment disorder diagnoses in general hospital patients. *Irish Journal of Psychological Medicine, 11*(4), 153–157. https://doi.org/10.1017/S0790966700001683

González-Jaimes, E. I., & Turnbull-Plaza, B. (2003). Selection of psychotherapeutic treatment for adjustment disorder with depressive mood due to acute myocardial infarction. *Archives of Medical Research, 34*(4), 298–304. https://doi.org/10.1016/S0188-4409(03)00051-1

Greenberg, W. M., Rosenfeld, D. N., & Ortega, E. A. (1995). Adjustment disorder as an admission diagnosis. *The American Journal of Psychiatry, 152*(3), 459–461. https://doi.org/10.1176/ajp.152.3.459

Jones, R., Yates, W. R., & Zhou, M. H. (2002). Readmission rates for adjustment disorders: Comparison with other mood disorders. *Journal of Affective Disorders, 71*(1–3), 199–203. https://doi.org/10.1016/s0165-0327(01)00390-1

Jordan, A. H., & Litz, B. T. (2014). Prolonged grief disorder: Diagnostic, assessment, and treatment considerations. *Professional Psychology: Research and Practice, 45*(3), 180–187. https://doi.org/10.1037/a0036836

Kropp, S., Andreis, C., te Wildt, B., Sieberer, M., Ziegenbein, M., & Huber, T. J. (2007). Characteristics of psychiatric patients in the accident and emergency department (ED). *Psychiatrische Praxis, 34*(2), 72–75. https://doi.org/10.1055/s-2005-915330

Kryzhanovskaya, L., & Canterbury, R. (2001). Suicidal behavior in patients with adjustment disorders. *Crisis, 22*(3), 125–131. https://doi.org/10.1027//0227-5910.22.3.125

Lönnqvist, J. K., Henriksson, M. M., Isometsä, E. T., Marttunen, M. J., Heikkinen, M. E., Aro, H. M., & Kuoppasalmi, K. I. (1995). Mental disorders and suicide prevention. *Psychiatry and Clinical Neurosciences, 49*(1), S111–116. https://doi.org/10.1111/j.1440-1819.1995.tb01912.x

Maciejewski, P. K., Maercker, A., Boelen, P. A., & Prigerson, H. G. (2016). "Prolonged grief disorder" and "persistent complex bereavement disorder," but not "complicated grief" are one and the same diagnostic entity: An analysis of data from the Yale Bereavement Study. *World Psychiatry: Official Journal of the World Psychiatric Association (WPA), 15*(3), 266–275. https://doi.org/10.1002/wps.20348

Maciejewski, P. K., Zhang, B., Block, S. D., & Prigerson, H. G. (2007). An empirical examination of the stage theory of grief. *JAMA, 297*(7), 716. https://doi.org/10.1001/jama.297.7.716

Maercker, A., Brewin, C. R., Bryant, R. A., Cloitre, M., van Ommeren, M., Jones, L. M., Humayan, A., Kagee, A., Llosa, A. E., Rousseau, C., Somasundaram, D. J., Souza, R., Suzuki, Y., Weissbecker, I., Wessely, S. C., First, M. B., & Reed, G. M. (2013). Diagnosis and classification of disorders specifically associated with stress: Proposals for ICD-11. *World Psychiatry, 12*(3), 198–206. https://doi.org/10.1002/wps.20057

Maercker, A., Forstmeier, S., Pielmaier, L., Spangenberg, L., Brähler, E., & Glaesmer, H. (2012). Adjustment disorders: Prevalence in a representative nationwide survey in Germany. *Social Psychiatry and Psychiatric Epidemiology, 47*(11), 1745–1752. https://doi.org/10.1007/s00127-012-0493-x

Maercker, A., & Lorenz, L. (2018). Adjustment disorder diagnosis: Improving clinical utility. *The World Journal of Biological Psychiatry: The Official Journal of the World Federation of Societies of Biological Psychiatry, 19*(1), S3–S13. https://doi.org/10.1080/15622975.2018.1449967

Mitchell, A. J., Chan, M., Bhatti, H., Halton, M., Grassi, L., Johansen, C., & Meader, N. (2011). Prevalence of depression, anxiety, and adjustment disorder in oncological, haematological, and palliative-care settings: A meta-analysis of 94 interview-based studies. *Lancet: Oncology, 12*(2), 160–174. https://doi.org/10.1016/S1470-2045(11)70002-X

Moayedoddin, B., & Markowitz, J. C. (2015). Abnormal grief: Should we consider a more patient-centered approach? *American Journal of Psychotherapy, 69*(4), 361–378. https://doi.org/10.1176/appi.psychotherapy.2015.69.4.361

Nakajima, S. (2018). Complicated grief: Recent developments in diagnostic criteria and treatment. *Philosophical Transactions of the Royal Society of London. Series B, Biological Sciences, 373*(1754). https://doi.org/10.1098/rstb.2017.0273

Neria, Y., Gross, R., Litz, B., Maguen, S., Insel, B., Seirmarco, G., Rosenfeld, H., Suh, E. J., Kishon, R., Cook, J., & Marshall, R. D. (2007). Prevalence and psychological correlates of complicated grief among bereaved adults 2.5–3.5 years after September 11th attacks. *Journal of Traumatic Stress, 20*(3), 251–262. https://doi.org/10.1002/jts.20223

Pelkonen, M., Marttunen, M., Henriksson, M., & Lönnqvist, J. (2005). Suicidality in adjustment disorder—Clinical characteristics of adolescent outpatients. *European Child & Adolescent Psychiatry, 14*(3), 174–180. https://doi.org/10.1007/s00787-005-0457-8

Polyakova, I., Knobler, H. Y., Ambrumova, A., & Lerner, V. (1998). Characteristics of suicidal attempts in major depression versus adjustment reactions. *Journal of Affective Disorders, 47*(1), 159–167. https://doi.org/10.1016/S0165-0327(97)00137-7

Ponizovsky, A. M., Levov, K., Schultz, Y., & Radomislensky, I. (2011). Attachment insecurity and psychological resources associated with adjustment disorders. *The American Journal of Orthopsychiatry, 81*(2), 265–276. https://doi.org/10.1111/j.1939-0025.2011.01095.x

Prigerson, H. G., Bierhals, A. J., Kasl, S. V., Reynolds, C. F., Shear, M. K., Day, N., Beery, L. C., Newsom, J. T., & Jacobs, S. (1997). Traumatic grief as a risk factor for mental and physical morbidity. *The American Journal of Psychiatry, 154*(5), 616–623. https://doi.org/10.1176/ajp.154.5.616

Rao, M. L., Hawellek, B., Papassotiropoulos, A., Deister, A., & Frahnert, C. (1998). Upregulation of the platelet Serotonin2A receptor and low blood serotonin in suicidal psychiatric patients. *Neuropsychobiology, 38*(2), 84–89. https://doi.org/10.1159/000026522

Rigatelli, M., Galeazzi, G. M., & Palmieri, G. (2002). Consultation-liaison psychiatry in obstetrics and gynecology. *Journal of Psychosomatic Obstetrics & Gynecology, 23*(3), 165–172. https://doi.org/10.3109/01674820209074669

Shear, K., Frank, E., Houck, P. R., & Reynolds, C. F. (2005). Treatment of complicated grief: A randomized controlled trial. *JAMA, 293*(21), 2601–2608. https://doi.org/10.1001/jama.293.21.2601

Shear, M. K. (2012). Getting straight about grief. *Depression and Anxiety, 29*(6), 461–464. https://doi.org/10.1002/da.21963

Shear, M. K., Reynolds, C. F., Simon, N. M., Zisook, S., Wang, Y., Mauro, C., Duan, N., Lebowitz, B., & Skritskaya, N. (2016). Optimizing treatment of complicated grief: A randomized clinical trial. *JAMA Psychiatry, 73*(7), 685–694. https://doi.org/10.1001/jamapsychiatry.2016.0892

Shear, M. K., Simon, N., Wall, M., Zisook, S., Neimeyer, R., Duan, N., Reynolds, C., Lebowitz, B., Sung, S., Ghesquiere, A., Gorscak, B., Clayton, P., Ito, M., Nakajima, S., Konishi, T., Melhem, N., Meert, K., Schiff, M., O'Connor, M.-F., . . . & Keshaviah, A. (2011). Complicated gried and related bereavement issues for DSM-5. *Depression and Anxiety, 28*(2), 103–117. https://doi.org/10.1002/da.20780

Silverman, G. K., Jacobs, S. C., Kasl, S. V., Shear, M. K., Maciejewski, P. K., Noaghiul, F. S., & Prigerson, H. G. (2000). Quality of life impairments associated with diagnostic criteria for traumatic grief. *Psychological Medicine, 30*(4), 857–862. https://doi.org/10.1017/s0033291799002524

Silverstone, P. H. (1996). Prevalence of psychiatric disorders in medical inpatients. *The Journal of Nervous and Mental Disease, 184*(1), 43–51. https://doi.org/10.1097/00005053-199601000-00008

Strain, J. J. (2019). The adjustment disorder diagnosis, its importance to liaison psychiatry, and its psychobiology. *International Journal of Environmental Research and Public Health, 16*(23). https://doi.org/10.3390/ijerph16234645

Strain, J. J., Smith, G. C., Hammer, J. S., McKenzie, D. P., Blumenfield, M., Muskin, P., Newstadt, G., Wallack, J., Wilner, A., & Schleifer, S. S. (1998). Adjustment disorder: A multisite study of its utilization and interventions in the consultation-liaison psychiatry setting. *General Hospital Psychiatry, 20*(3), 139–149. https://doi.org/10.1016/s0163-8343(98)00020-6

CHAPTER 23

Bipolar Spectrum Disorders[1]

Kirti Saxena, M.D.; Sherin Kurian, M.D.;

and Johanna Saxena, B.S., B.A.

> *"Which of my feelings are real? Which of the me's is me? The wild, impulsive, chaotic, energetic, and crazy one? Or the shy, withdrawn, desperate, suicidal, doomed, and tired one? Probably a bit of both, hopefully much that is neither."*
>
> — Kay Redfield Jamison.

OBJECTIVES

After reading this chapter, students will be able to do the following:

- review bipolar spectrum disorders
- discuss clinical features of bipolar I and II disorders
- review available treatments for bipolar disorders

CASE VIGNETTE

Jerry is a 29-year-old male who lives with his wife. At age 16, he first became depressed. He was diagnosed with major depressive disorder with psychotic features and hospitalized because he was suicidal. He was treated with an antidepressant and psychotherapy and recovered. In college, he had two further depressive episodes, which were promptly treated with antidepressants, and he did not need to be hospitalized. He graduated from college, got married, and moved into an apartment with his wife. He was successful at his job, where he has now been working for 2 years.

Jerry's wife notices some changes. Although he sleeps only 3 hours at night, he wakes up with abundant energy. He stays up all night writing a new novel, which he believes will

(continued)

1 Readers may also see "Depressive Disorders" (Chapter 20) for related material.

be the next bestseller. He suddenly had the brilliant idea of repainting their apartment's sitting room bright orange. He painted half of the room before he gets sidetracked to begin an art project. He completes several art projects within just 4 days. While painting, he believes God is directing his strokes. He is very confident that his paintings will sell for millions of dollars, his family will be set for life, and he will never need to work again.

Speaking of work, he has not been to work in the past week because he says he does not need the "coins" his salaried job pays him and would rather bet on the bundles coming from his art and writing. He has typed his resignation letter but has not discussed this yet with his wife. A car salesman dropped off the keys to an expensive car her husband just bought. As newly-weds, they certainly cannot afford this. She finds out that he used 2 years' worth of savings the couple had planned to use as a down payment for their first home to pay for this. When she confronts Jerry about it, he seems pleased and confidently assures her that they will be just fine. He is in a very good mood and speaking loud and fast. It is not easy to follow his train of thought and challenging to get a word in. Midsentence, he often bursts out crying and then begins screaming obscenities. His wife is alarmed. This change had gone on for 10 days now. She quits trying to make him see reason and calls their family doctor, who instructs them to proceed for an emergency psychiatry evaluation.

Jerry was hospitalized and diagnosed with bipolar I disorder (with psychotic features). He was started on lithium. He has been successfully maintained on lithium at a therapeutic level of 0.9mEq/L. He attends psychotherapy appointments regularly and has a reasonably stable and happy life with his wife and young kids.

DEFINITIONS AND KEY CONCEPTS

Bipolar spectrum disorders are a group of mood disorders characterized by episodes of mood extremes, including low (depressed), elevated (manic), or angry (irritable) mood states. These mood states are accompanied by cognitive and neurovegetative changes, such as in sleep, appetite, energy, and concentration.

INTRODUCTION

Bipolar disorder (BD) as a distinct entity was first diagnosed by Falret in the 1850s (Angst & Sellaro, 2000). Currently, the *Diagnostic and Statistical Manual of Mental Disorders*, 5th edition (*DSM-5*; APA, 2013) includes the category "bipolar and related disorders," which encompasses bipolar I, bipolar II, and cyclothymic disorders. Atypical bipolar-like phenomena that do not fit the noted subtypes are included in the "other specified and bipolar related disorder" category.

Since 1980, *DSM* criteria have specified that adult criteria can be used to diagnose mania in children, while taking age and developmental stage into consideration (Weller, 1995). Accordingly, structured and semi-structured interviews were developed, and researchers began to depend more on standardized criteria for diagnoses, using symptoms such as those

KEY POINT

Bipolar disorder is primarily a mood disorder that typically includes depressive, manic, or hypomanic episodes in the longitudinal manifestation of this disorder. Bipolar and related disorders encompass bipolar I, bipolar II, and cyclothymic disorders. Atypical bipolar-like phenomena that do not fit the noted subtypes are included in the "other specified and bipolar related disorder" category.

CLINICAL TIP

The onset of BD typically occurs at around the age of 20 years. An earlier onset is often associated with a poorer prognosis, longer treatment delays, more severe depressive episodes, and a higher prevalence of concurrent anxiety and substance use disorders (Joslyn et al., 2016). The first episode of BD is usually a depressive episode.

in the *Research Diagnostic Criteria* (Spitzer, 1979) and the *Diagnostic and Statistical Manual of Mental Disorders* (APA, 1980, 1987, 1994, 2000, 2013).

The *DSM-5* outlines the depressive, manic, and hypomanic episode criteria similar to the previous *DSM* version. However, symptoms of mixed episodes are replaced with a mixed-features specifier that can be used with any of the mood episodes (APA, 2013). This specifier is used when individuals concurrently experience full criteria for a manic episode and three symptoms of a depressive episode or when individuals experience full criteria for a depressive episode and three symptoms of a manic episode (Reed et al., 2019).

The onset of BD typically occurs at around the age of 20 years. An earlier onset is often associated with a poorer prognosis, longer treatment delays, more severe depressive episodes, and a higher prevalence of concurrent anxiety and substance use disorders (Joslyn et al., 2016). The first episode of BD is usually a depressive episode. Of note, in many persons with either bipolar I or bipolar II disorder, the depressive episodes may last considerably longer than manic or hypomanic episodes throughout the course of illness. For this reason, BD is often misclassified as major depressive disorder (Zimmerman et al., 2008). It is important to be aware that misdiagnosis and overdiagnosis of BD can occur; therefore, a careful evaluation is always warranted (Zimmerman et al., 2008).

EPIDEMIOLOGY

Bipolar disorders rank as the 17th leading source of disability among all diseases worldwide (Vigo et al., 2016). The World Mental Health Survey Initiative reported lifetime and 12-month prevalence estimates for bipolar disorders of 2.4% and 1.5%, respectively (Merikangas et al., 2011). Twelve-month prevalence of bipolar disorder, type I, across 11 countries ranged from 0.0% to 0.6%. The lifetime male-to-female prevalence ratio is approximately 1.1:1 (APA, 2013). In a recent meta-analysis (Van Meter et al., 2019), the average prevalence rate of bipolar spectrum disorders in the pediatric population was noted to be 3.9%.

This illness significantly impacts developmental, educational, and occupational milestones and affects cognitive and psychosocial dysfunction during acute episodes and in periods of remission (Miskowiak et al., 2018). Approximately 6% to 7% of individuals with BD commit suicide. Indeed, suicide rates among individuals with BD are 20 to 30 times higher than in the general population (Plans et al., 2019).

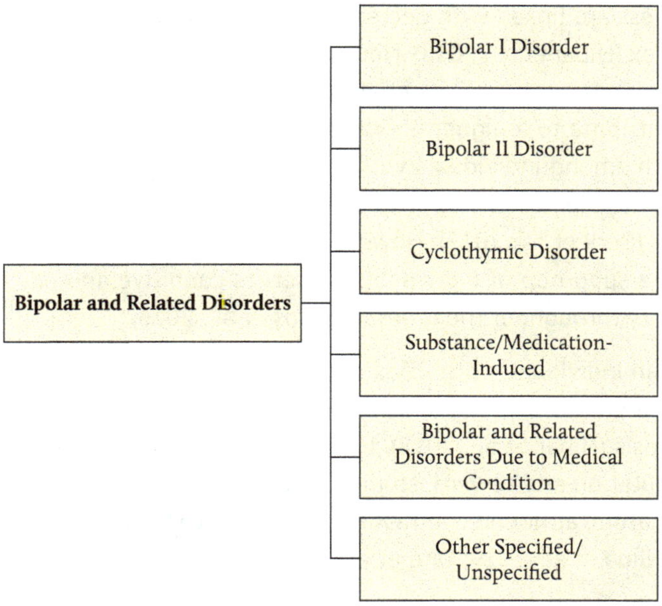

FIGURE 23.1 Bipolar and related disorders.

NEUROPATHOLOGY

Studies report BD having a strong genetic component. Indeed, twin studies show heritability rates (i.e., the extent to which the disorder can be explained by genetic factors) as high as 70–80% (Edvardsen et al., 2008; McGuffin et al., 2003). There is an increased risk of BD noted in first-degree relatives of individuals, including offspring (Gottesman et al., 2010). Notably, the risk of BD is significantly higher in children of parents diagnosed with BD versus offspring of parents with no psychiatric diagnoses (Duffy, 2019a; Rasic et al., 2014).

Epigenetic mechanisms encompass several pathways that can mediate gene-by-environment interactions and modulate gene expression and activity without altering the DNA sequence. These include DNA methylation, histone modifications, chromatin remodeling, and the actions of noncoding RNAs. Several of these have been suggested to play significant roles in the pathophysiology of BD, especially DNA methylation (Fries et al., 2016; Gaine et al., 2019; Ludwig & Dwivedi, 2016). In addition, several epigenetic alterations that may underlie risk/resilience mechanisms have been described in offspring of BD parents (Duffy, 2019b; Fries et al., 2017).

In individuals with BD, progressive changes in brain structure and cellular function, referred to as neuroprogression, have been observed (Berk et al.,

QUICK POINT

Bipolar disorders are ranked the 17th leading source of disability among all diseases worldwide (Vigo et al., 2016). The lifetime prevalence of bipolar disorder is about 2.5%. The lifetime male-to-female prevalence ratio is approximately 1.1:1 (APA, 2013). The average prevalence rate of bipolar spectrum disorders in the pediatric population was noted to be less than 4% (Van Meter et al., 2019).

KEY POINT

Individuals with bipolar disorder have a high rate of suicide. About 6% to 7% commit suicide. Suicide rates among individuals with bipolar disorder 20 to 30 times higher than in the general population (Plans et al., 2019)

KEY POINT

Bipolar disorder has a strong genetic component. The heritability rate (the extent to which genes impact the presence of a disorder) is as high as 70–80%. First degree relatives of individuals with bipolar disorder are at increased risk of the disorder (Edvardsen et al., 2008; McGuffin et al., 2003).

2011). Long periods of illness are linked with decreased cortical thickness in brain regions, such as the prefrontal cortex (Hibar et al., 2018). Neuroprogression may account for worsening cognitive and functional impairments (Berk et al., 2017). The mechanisms underpinning neuroprogression may contribute to a higher prevalence of coexisting medical conditions as well as premature death among individuals with BD (Morris et al., 2019). Furthermore, evidence indicates that as the bipolar illness progresses, the response to mood-stabilizing medications may decrease (Berk et al., 2017). However, with the course and trajectories of BD being heterogeneous, a subgroup of individuals preserves cognitive and psychosocial functioning and productivity throughout the illness (Passos et al., 2016).

A history of psychosis in individuals with BD is associated with reduced surface area in the right caudal anterior cingulate cortex and left inferior temporal gyrus compared with individuals without psychosis (Hibar et al., 2018). In regard to the volume of brain regions associated with mood regulation and reward, studies reported smaller amygdala and hippocampus and a larger striatum, although contrasting findings have been found (Caseras et al., 2013; Ho et al., 2019; Niida et al., 2019; Ong et al., 2012).

Neuroimaging studies have fostered some understanding of the pathophysiology of BD in adults (although there are mixed results from adult studies); however, less is known about the pathophysiology of BD in children. It has been reported that children with BD exhibit differences in the volumes of the hippocampus, caudate, or thalamus relative to healthy controls (Chang et al., 2005), and other studies suggest that smaller volume in the amygdala can be accompanied by smaller volume in the hippocampus in children with bipolar disorder (Blumberg et al., 2003). Other studies also reported that children and adolescents who experienced at least one manic or hypomanic episode have reduced grey matter volume in the left dorsolateral prefrontal cortex, the left accumbens, and the left amygdala (Dickstein et al., 2005) and that adolescents with bipolar disorder have decreased volume in the left superior temporal gyrus (Chen et al., 2004). Additional research is needed to clarify the neurobiology of BD in children and adolescents (Renk et al., 2014). Also, Chang et al. (2005) noted that there is a relationship between use of lithium and valproate and greater grey matter volume in the amygdala.

Furthermore, in children and adolescents with familial BD, smaller amygdalar volumes relative to healthy volunteers have been reported (Blumberg et al., 2003; Chang et al., 2005; Delbello et al., 2004). Also, children and adolescents with familial BD may have underlying abnormalities in the regulation of prefrontal–subcortical circuits. For example, Chang et al. (2004) found that children and adolescents with familial BD have greater activation in their bilateral anterior cingulate cortex, left putamen, left thalamus, left dorsolateral prefrontal cortex, and right inferior frontal gyrus during a visuospatial working memory task, whereas healthy volunteers have greater activation in their cerebellar vermis.

There are significant advances in technology and interesting neuroimaging findings associated with a psychiatric diagnosis (Favre et al., 2019) as well as the response to treatment and risk identification (Acuff et al., 2019; Webb et al., 2018). However, there is currently no direct clinical application of brain imaging in psychiatry (Scaini et al., 2020).

KEY POINT

Bipolar I disorder is characterized by manic and depressive episodes. Bipolar II disorder is characterized by episodes of hypomania and depression. The occurrence of at least one manic episode in a lifetime is considered consistent with the diagnosis of bipolar I disorder. The occurrence of at least one hypomanic episode in a lifetime is considered consistent with the diagnosis of bipolar II disorder.

CLINICAL MANIFESTATIONS AND DIAGNOSIS

Bipolar disorder type I is characterized by manic and depressive episodes. Bipolar II disorder is characterized by episodes of hypomania and depression. The occurrence of at least one hypomanic episode in a lifetime is considered consistent with the diagnosis of bipolar II disorder (Carvalho et al., 2020). Bipolar disorder type II can be challenging to diagnose, since hypomania can be easily missed, and the person gets a diagnosis of unipolar depression. Cyclothymic disorder is considered a subtype of bipolar disorder, characterized by a chronic presentation of low-grade alternating depressive and hypomanic symptoms (lasting for at least two years in adults and one full year in children) that do not meet the criteria for hypomania or major depressive episodes.

TABLE 23.1 Bipolar Disorder Episodes Criteria

	Bipolar disorder				
Episode	**Manic**	**Hypomanic**	**Mixed**	**Depressive**	**Other specified/ unspecified***
Criteria requirement	Full criteria for manic episode	Full criteria for hypomanic episode	Full criteria of manic plus three features of depressive episode or full criteria for depressive episode plus three features of manic episode	Full criteria for major depressive episode	Elevated mood symptoms are clinically significant but do not meet full criteria for mania, hypomania, depression, mixed, or cyclothymia. Criteria for bipolar disorder are met, but a suspicion of symptoms caused by recreational drugs, alcohol, or a neurological disorder is present. Experienced a manic or mixed episode after having been previously diagnosed with either schizophrenia or a psychotic episode.

TABLE 23.1 *(Continued)*

	Bipolar disorder				
Episode	**Manic**	**Hypomanic**	**Mixed**	**Depressive**	**Other specified/ unspecified***
Mood state	Elevated or irritable mood and increased activity or energy present most of the day	Elevated or irritable mood and increased activity or energy present most of the day	Full criteria of manic plus three features of depressive episode or full criteria for depressive episode plus three features of manic episode	Depressed mood most of the day nearly every day (children and adolescents' moods can be irritable) or anhedonia (loss of interest or pleasure)	Manic, hypomanic, depressive, or mixed features
Duration	At least one week and present most of the day	At least four consecutive days and present most of the day	At least one week (manic episode) At least 2 weeks (depressive episode)	At least 2 weeks	Variable
Symptoms	Three (or more) of the following symptoms (four if the mood is only irritable) are present: • Grandiosity • Decreased need for sleep • Increased talkativeness or pressured speech • Flight of ideas or racing thoughts • Distractibility	Three (or more) of the following symptoms (four if the mood is only irritable) are present: • Grandiosity • Decreased need for sleep • Increased talkativeness or pressured speech • Flight of ideas or racing thoughts • Distractibility	As above	Four (or more) of the following symptoms: • Significant decrease in interest in all, or almost all, activities most of the day • Significant weight loss when not dieting, weight gain, or decrease or increase in appetite nearly every day (in children, failure to make expected weight gain) • Insomnia or hypersomnia nearly every day • Psychomotor agitation or retardation nearly every day • Fatigue or loss of energy nearly every day • Feelings of worthlessness or excessive or inappropriate guilt nearly every day	Variable

(continued)

TABLE 23.1 *(Continued)*

Episode	Bipolar disorder: Manic	Hypomanic	Mixed	Depressive	Other specified/ unspecified*
	• Increased goal-directed activity or psychomotor agitation • Impulsive, reckless behaviors	• Increased goal-directed activity or psychomotor agitation • Impulsive, reckless behaviors		• Diminished ability to concentrate nearly every day • Recurrent thoughts of death, recurrent suicidal ideation without a specific plan or a suicide attempt or a specific plan for committing suicide	
Functional impairment	The mood disturbance and associated behaviors cause significant impairment in social or occupational functioning and may require necessitate hospitalization. There may be psychotic features.	The episode is associated with a change in functioning that is not characteristic of the individual when not symptomatic.	The symptoms cause clinically significant distress or impairment in social, occupational, or other important areas of functioning.		The symptoms cause clinically significant distress or impairment in social, occupational, or other important areas of functioning.
		The disturbance in mood and the change in functioning are observable by others.			
		The episode is not severe enough to cause significant impairment in social or occupational functioning or to require hospitalization.			

TABLE 23.1 *(Continued)*

	Bipolar disorder				
Episode	**Manic**	**Hypomanic**	**Mixed**	**Depressive**	**Other specified/ unspecified***
Exclusion criteria	Episode is not due to the effects of drug abuse, a medication, or to a medical condition.	The episode is not due to the effects of a drug of abuse or a medication.	The depression is not due to the effects of a substance or another medical condition.		
		The episode is not severe enough to cause significant impairment in social or occupational functioning or to require hospitalization.	Symptoms clearly attributable to another medical condition are *not* to be considered.		
		If there are psychotic features, then it is a manic episode.			
Distinguishing factors	Criteria met for one manic episode.	Criteria *not* met for one manic episode.		Criteria met for one manic episode (distinguishes BD depressed episode from MDD).	
		Criteria may be met for MDE.			
		No psychotic features			
		No hospitalization			

Note: Refer to DSM-5 for full criteria.

In the *DSM-5*, the diagnostic criteria for bipolar I, bipolar II, and major depression have a "mixed features" specifier. During an episode of major depression, the mixed-state specifier requires the presence of at least three manic/hypomanic (Table 23.1) symptoms together with the depressive episode. At least three of these symptoms must be present nearly every day during the most recent 2 weeks of the major depressive episode. During an episode of mania or hypomania, using the specifier requires the presence of at least three symptoms of depression together with the manic/hypomanic episode. At least three depressive symptoms must be present nearly every day during the most recent week of a manic episode or during the most recent 4 days of a hypomanic episode.

Diagnostic criteria require that individuals with bipolar depression (Table 23.1) have a history of at least one manic episode and present with either a depressed mood most of the day, nearly every day, or a loss of interest and pleasure in all activities (anhedonia); additional symptoms may include weight loss, insomnia, psychomotor agitation or retardation, feelings of worthlessness or guilt, decreased ability to concentrate, and recurrent thoughts of death or suicidal ideation. Depressive symptoms must be severe enough to cause clinically significant distress and impairment in social or occupational functioning. The criteria for a bipolar depressive episode are the same as those for a unipolar depressive episode, which can complicate the diagnosis; thus, establishment of an accurate history of mania or hypomania is crucial (McIntyre & Calabrese, 2019).

The key feature distinguishing bipolar disorders from unipolar depressive disorders is the occurrence of manic or hypomanic symptoms. Having a manic or hypomanic episode will give one a diagnosis of bipolar disorder. Bipolar disorder is an episodic mood disorder, so one needs to recognize noticeable mood changes with associated symptoms. The mood changes can be an irritable mood or elevated, expansive, and euphoric mood. Together with change in mood and increased energy, symptoms associated with mania and hypomania include inflated self-esteem or grandiosity, decreased need for sleep, increased talkativeness, pressured speech, racing thoughts, distractibility, increase in goal-directed activity, and impulsive behaviors. The *DSM-5* duration criterion for a manic episode is one week and for a hypomanic episode is at least 4 days. Clinically, a hypomanic episode is less severe than a manic episode.

After establishing a noticeable change in mood, associated symptoms of mania or hypomania need to be ascertained. In regard to decreased need for sleep, pertinent questions to ask include, "Do you feel tired?" and "Do you feel like you need to sleep?". Staying up late at night and sleeping the next day does not construe a decreased need for sleep. So this symptom needs to be carefully ascertained. Indeed, decreased need for sleep is distinct from insomnia in which the individual is unable to sleep even though they want to. In manic episodes, individuals may go for days without sleep and not feel tired. Examples of an increase in goal-directed activity include organizing

MEMORY TIP

Mania, *useful mnemonic*

DIG FAST

D—Distractibility
I—Indiscretion
G—Grandiosity
F—Flight of ideas
A—Activity increase
S—Sleep deficit
T—Talkativeness

MEMORY TIP

Hypomania, *useful mnemonic*

TAD HIGH

T—Talkative
A—Attention deficit
D—Decreased need for sleep
H—High self-esteem or grandiosity
I—Ideas that race
G—Goal-directed activity increased
H—High-risk activity

(Caplan, 2008)

MEMORY TIP

Depressive Episode, useful mnemonic

SIG: E CAPS

S—Suicidal thoughts
I—Interests decreased
G—Guilt
E—Energy decreased
C—Concentration decreased
A—Appetite disturbance (increased or decreased)
P—Psychomotor changes (agitation or retardation)
S—Sleep disturbance (increased or decreased)

the furniture, writing a novel, and spending hours doing these activities. Impulsive behaviors can include running across the street without looking, spending a lot of money, sexual indiscretions, and engaging in alcohol and substance use, which leads to problems. Grandiosity is a symptom that can be hard to assess. In a younger child, it may present as the child stating they can teach the class better than their teacher and the child believing this. An adolescent may believe they are an exceptional singer or musician but in reality do not sing or play an instrument well.

A manic episode usually warrants hospitalization, since it significantly impacts daily functioning. Further, when mania is present with psychotic symptoms, such as delusions and hallucinations, functioning can be severely impaired to the point that hospitalization is needed. A careful evaluation of suicidal thought and behaviors is required both in the manic and depressive phases of the bipolar illness.

Family members living with the adult or child with bipolar disorder will notice these changes. The person affected with the illness may not feel there is a difference in mood and associated symptoms. Therefore, history from the persons living with or who know the person well is needed.

In children and adolescents, an accurate diagnosis of bipolar disorder can be challenging. However, assessing for episodic mood changes and associated manic or hypomanic symptoms, together with a history from caregivers, will help ascertain the diagnosis.

KEY POINT

The criteria for a bipolar depressive episode are the same as those for a unipolar depressive episode. Thus, it is critical to get an accurate history of mania or hypomania in the patient's lifetime.

KEY POINT

Patients with mood or affective disorders often suffer periods of depression. The presence of at least one episode of manic episode makes the diagnosis bipolar I disorder. The absence of a manic episode but the presence of at least one episode of hypomanic episode makes the diagnosis bipolar II disorder. The absence of a manic episode and the absence of a hypomanic episode in a patient with major depression makes the diagnosis unipolar depression (i.e., major depressive disorder)

CLINICAL TIP

Individuals with BD may lack insight, including during mood episodes. Obtaining and factoring in collateral information from family members can be invaluable in reaching a true assessment of the severity of their symptoms and functioning.

Medical- or Substance-Induced Considerations

Bipolar disorders require differentiation from substance- or medication-induced bipolar and related disorder; substance intoxication or substance-induced delirium; and medication adverse effects. During antidepressant treatment (e.g., medication or electroconvulsive therapy), a manic episode that emerges but persists at a fully syndromal level beyond the physiological effect of that treatment is sufficient to diagnose bipolar I. For a bipolar II diagnosis, a hypomanic episode that emerges during antidepressant treatment (e.g., medication or electroconvulsive therapy) but persists at a fully syndromal level beyond the physiological effect of that treatment is sufficient evidence only if preceded by a major depressive episode.

The essential feature of bipolar and related disorder due to another medical condition is the presence of manic or hypomanic symptoms predominating in the clinical picture that is attributable to another medical condition. In most cases the manic or hypomanic picture may appear during the initial presentation of the medical condition (i.e., within 1 month);

however, there are exceptions, especially in chronic medical conditions that might worsen or relapse and herald the appearance of the manic or hypomanic picture. Bipolar and related disorder due to another medical condition is not diagnosed when the manic or hypomanic episodes definitely precede the medical condition, since the proper diagnosis then would be BD (except if the preceding manic or hypomanic episode was associated with ingestion of a substance or medication). The diagnosis of bipolar disorder should not be made during the course of a delirium, since delirium can occur in individuals with medical conditions or after ingestion of substances or medications. After the delirium clears, a careful evaluation for mania or hypomania can be performed. Also, medical conditions may be treated with medications (e.g., steroids or alpha-interferon) that can induce depressive or manic symptoms (APA, 2013). A careful and systematic history to know whether there is a medical cause for the mania or hypomania is required in all instances.

CLINICAL TIP

In children and adolescents, an accurate diagnosis of bipolar disorder can be challenging. This is more difficult if their baseline mood is irritable. Determining a change from baseline mood state is the key, while excluding other psychosocial stressors that could account for this is crucial. Thus, carefully assessing for episodic mood changes that are different from their baseline, associated manic or hypomanic symptoms, and a history from caregivers helps clarify the diagnosis.

COMORBIDITY

Bipolar disorder is a highly comorbid disorder. The most frequent co-occurring mental health disorders are anxiety (estimated to be present in 71% of persons with BD), substance use (56%), personality disorders (36%), and attention-deficit/hyperactivity disorder (10 to 20%; Carvalho et al., 2020). Chronic medical conditions are more prevalent among individuals with BD than in the general population. These include metabolic syndrome (affecting 37% of patients with BD; Vancampfort et al., 2013), migraine (35%; Fornaro & Stubbs, 2015), obesity (21%; Krishnan, 2005), type 2 diabetes mellitus (14%; Vancampfort et al., 2016), and cardiovascular disease (Weiner et al., 2011). Individuals with BD have approximately twice the risk of death (Walker et al., 2015), which is attributable to both suicide and higher rates of physical diseases in this population (Hayes et al., 2015; Kessing et al., 2015). Alcohol use disorder is present in more than half of individuals whose symptoms meet criteria for BD. Indeed, monitoring and interventions for physical health conditions among individuals with BD is important (Firth et al., 2019).

QUICK POINT

Bipolar disorder has a high comorbidity with other mental health disorders including anxiety, substance use, personality disorders, and attention deficit disorders.

In individuals with BD type II, approximately 60% have three or more comorbid mental health disorders. Anxiety and substance use disorders occur in individuals with bipolar II disorder at a higher rate than in the general population. About 14% have at least one lifetime history of eating disorders with binge eating disorder being more common (APA, 2013). Notably, there is a higher rate of co-occurring anxiety disorders in children and adolescents with bipolar II disorder compared with those with bipolar

I disorder with the anxiety disorder most often predating the onset of the manic or hypomanic episode.

TREATMENT

QUICK POINT

Chronic medical conditions, such as metabolic syndrome, migraine, type II diabetes mellitus, and cardiovascular disease, are more prevalent among individuals with BD than in the general population.

The treatment approach for BD includes not only reducing the symptoms of mania and depression but being aware of the psychosocial factors that contribute to maintaining and exacerbating the overall illness. These include academic, social, peer and family relationships. Therefore, a comprehensive approach is needed when developing a treatment plan for individuals with BD.

Factors affecting the choice of treatment include patient and family preference, coexisting medical and psychiatric conditions, and prior response to treatments, including adverse effects. The safety of patients during acute affective episodes should be assured, in particular by assessing if they are at risk of suicide or harming themselves or others and, if so, by implementing measures to reduce the risk.

CLINICAL TIP

The treatment approach for BD includes not only reducing the symptoms of mania and depression but proactively mitigating stressors that can precipitate mood episodes and exacerbate the overall illness.

It is important to discuss evidence-based pharmacological and nonpharmacological treatments with patients and parents/legal guardians (in case of children and adolescents) and explain the importance of a comprehensive treatment plan. This includes medication management, psychotherapy, and consultation/communication with the school. The importance of compliance with treatment (both medication and therapy) needs to be addressed (Fountoulakis et al., 2020; Hidalgo-Mazzei et al., 2019).

Acute Mania

Pharmacologic treatment with antipsychotic agents or mood stabilizers is the mainstay of treatment for manic and hypomanic episodes. There are mood stabilizers and antipsychotic agents approved by the Food and Drug Administration (FDA) for the management of bipolar disorder (see Table 23.2).

Medications need to be initiated systematically. Monotherapy is the goal of treatment. However, for the treatment of BD, more than one mood stabilizer may be required for adequate stabilization of mood symptoms. Indeed, a combination of an antipsychotic agent and a mood stabilizer appears to be more efficacious than either medication alone, especially for severe mania (Grand & Vieta, 2015).

Other antipsychotic drugs that are not FDA approved but have been effective in the management of acute mania, such as haloperidol and paliperidone, have been used. For patients with refractory mania and aggressive behavior or psychotic symptoms, bifrontal electroconvulsive therapy (ECT), either as monotherapy or as an adjunctive treatment, has been reported to be effective (Fountoulakis et al., 2020).

Acute Depression

Presently there are four psychotropics currently approved by the FDA (see Table 23.2) for the management of depressive episodes in adults with bipolar disorder and two in children with bipolar depression. For individuals with treatment resistant bipolar depression, electroconvulsive therapy (ECT) has been effective (Hidalgo-Mazzei et al., 2019).

Maintenance Treatment

Maintenance treatment is important due to the chronic and recurring nature of BD. Such treatment should be started shortly after the onset of illness, aimed at preventing the emergence of affective episodes and burdensome affective symptoms and often requiring a combination of pharmacologic, psychological, and lifestyle interventions (Carvalho et al., 2020).

Lithium is one of the most effective medications for the prevention of both depressive and manic recurrences in BD. Evidence has suggested that lithium may have a protective effect against suicidal behavior in adults with BD (Cipriani et al., 2013; Tondo et al., 2016). The combination of quetiapine–lithium or quetiapine–divalproex and quetiapine alone have also been shown in trial to be effective maintenance treatments for BD (Miura et al., 2014). In pediatric bipolar disorder, a meta-analysis showed that lithium, anticonvulsant agents, and antipsychotic agents may reduce long-term morbidity (Yee et al., 2019). Maintenance ECT may be considered for individuals with BD who do not have a response to pharmacotherapy.

QUICK POINT

Lithium is one of the most effective medications for the prevention of both depressive and manic recurrences in BD. Evidence has suggested that lithium may have a protective effect against suicidal behavior in adults with BD (Cipriani et al., 2013; Tondo et al., 2016).

Psychotherapy

The combination of medication management and therapy constitutes a comprehensive treatment plan for the treatment of BD. Psychoeducation, cognitive behavioral therapy (CBT), family-focused therapy, dialectical behavioral therapy, mindfulness-based CBT, and interpersonal and social rhythm therapy (the incorporation of regular daily activities to restore circadian processes and improve mood) are all helpful psychotherapeutic approaches (Chatterton et al., 2017).

There is support for the efficacy of adjunctive family-focused psycho-education and skills-based interventions for youth with bipolar spectrum disorders (BPSD). This includes psychoeducational psychotherapy (PEP), family-focused tre ment, and child- and family-focused cognitive behavioral therapy (Fristad & MacPhers 2014; West et al., 2014). Notably, PEP has the strongest evidence for treating youth youn than 12 years of age with BPSD (Fristad, 2006; Fristad & MacPherson, 2014; Fristad et 2002, 2003, 2009; Mendenhall et al., 2009). Furthermore, these evidence-based psycho cial treatments are efficacious and may prevent relapses and recurrences of major affect episodes (Salcedo et al., 2016).

Adverse Effects

There are potential adverse effects associated with the medications used to treat the syr toms of BD. It is important to educate the patient and families about the adverse effects to monitor patients throughout treatment. Despite the long-term efficacy of lithium, s effects can occur, including renal impairment, hypothyroidism, polydipsia, polyuria, trem and an increase in peripheral calcium and parathyroid hormone levels (McKnight et al., 20 Liver enzyme levels are monitored regularly in patients treated with either divalproex carbamazepine because of the risk of liver toxicity. Weight and metabolic measures are m itored in patients receiving atypical antipsychotic drugs (Carvalho et al., 2020). For wom of childbearing age with BD, particularly during the first trimester of pregnancy, divalpro and carbamazepine are teratogens and are, therefore, not recommended. Also, there is a of congenital cardiac defects associated with the use of lithium during pregnancy. There high risk of relapse during pregnancy and in the postpartum period if mood-stabilizing m ications are abruptly discontinued. Therefore, in advance of a planned pregnancy, decisi need to be made regarding medication continuation (Anmella et al., 2019).

TABLE 23.2 FDA-Approved Medications for Bipolar Disorder

Drug	Phase of illness	Age	Adverse effects
Mood stabilizers			
Lithium	• Mania or mixed features • Maintenance therapy	• Adults • Children: 7–17	• Headache • Vomiting • Gastrointestinal discomfort • Hypothyroidism • Increased calcium levels • Reduced renal function
Antipsychotic medications			
Aripiprazole	• Mania or mixed features • Maintenance therapy	• Adults • Children: 10–17	• Akathisia • Weight gain • Extrapyramidal symptoms (EPS)

(continu

TABLE 23.2 (*Continued*)

Drug	Phase of illness	Age	Adverse effects
Risperidone	• Mania or mixed features • Maintenance therapy	• Adults • Children: 10–17	• Weight gain • Elevated metabolic parameters • Increased prolactin • Extrapyramidal symptoms (EPS)
Quetiapine	• Mania or mixed features • Bipolar depression (adults) • Maintenance therapy (adults)	• Adults • Children: 10–17	• Drowsiness • Weight gain • Metabolic abnormalities
Asenapine	• Mania or mixed features	• Adults • Children: 10–17	• Akathisia • Drowsiness • Risk of metabolic syndrome
Ziprasidone	• Mania or mixed features	• Adults	• Prolonged QTc interval on ECG • Akathisia • Hypotension
Olanzapine	• Mania or mixed features • Maintenance therapy	• Adults • Children: 13–17	• Weight gain • Drowsiness • Increased metabolic parameters
Cariprazine	• Mania or mixed features • Bipolar depression	• Adults	• Akathisia
Chlorpromazine	• Mania or mixed features	• Adults	• Risk of switch to depression • Sedation • Extrapyramidal symptoms
Olanzapine–fluoxetine	• Bipolar depression	• Adults • Children: 10–17	• Weight gain • Increased appetite • Drowsiness • Hyperlipidemia
Lurasidone	• Bipolar depression	• Adults • Children: 10–17	• Nausea • Sedation • EPS • Tardive dyskinesia
Anticonvulsants/ mood stabilizers			
Carbamazepine	• Mania or mixed features	• Adults	• CYP450 induction • Liver toxicity • Agranulocytosis, rash • Teratogenic effects

Drug	Phase of illness	Age	Adverse effects
Divalproex sodium	• Mania or mixed features	• Adults	• CYP450 inhibition • Teratogenic effects • Liver toxicity • Tremors • Thrombocytopenia • Polycystic ovarian syndrome • Menstrual abnormalities • Hirsutism in adolescent girls
Lamotrigine	• Maintenance therapy	• Adults	• Rash • Stevens–Johnson syndrome

SUMMARY

Bipolar disorder is a serious illness that significantly impacts the quality of life of an individual. Accurate diagnoses are crucial to implement the correct treatment plan. A comprehensive treatment approach is warranted during periods of acute episodes and during maintenance phases. Although the underlying pathophysiology of bipolar disorder is currently not known, evidence-based assessments and treatments are available for clinicians as they partner with individuals who have bipolar disorder.

RESOURCES

1 Bipolar Disorder Resource Center (aacap.org)

2 NIMH » Bipolar Disorder (nih.gov)

3 Bipolar disorder | NAMI: National Alliance on Mental Illness

REFERENCES

Acuff, H. E., Versace, A., Bertocci, M. A., Ladouceur, C. D., Hanford, L. C., Manelis, A., Monk, K., Bonar, L., McCaffrey, A., Goldstein, B. I., Goldstein, T. R., Sakolsky, D., Axelson, D., Birmaher, B., & Phillips, M. L. (2019). Baseline and follow-up activity and functional connectivity in reward neural circuitries in offspring at risk for bipolar disorder. *Neuropsychopharmacology: Official Publication of the American College of Neuropsychopharmacology, 44*(9), 1570–1578. https://doi.org/10.1038/s41386-019-0339-2

American Psychiatric Association. (1980). *Diagnostic and statistical manual of mental disorders* (3rd ed.).

American Psychiatric Association. (1987). *Diagnostic and statistical manual of mental disorders* (3rd ed. rev.).

American Psychiatric Association. (1994). *Diagnostic and statistical manual of mental disorders* (4th ed.).

American Psychiatric Association. (2000). *Diagnostic and statistical manual of mental disorders* (4th ed. rev.)

American Psychiatric Association. (2013). *Diagnostic and statistical manual of mental disorders* (5th ed.).

Angst, J., & Sellaro, R. (2000). Historical perspectives and natural history of bipolar disorder. *Biological psychiatry, 48*, 445–457.

Anmella G., Pacchiarotti I., Cubała W. J., Dudek D., Maina G., Thomas P., & Vieta E. (2019). Expert advice on the management of valproate in women with bipolar disorder at childbearing age. *European neuropsychopharmacology : the journal of the European College of Neuropsychopharmacology, 29*, 1199–2120.

Berk M., Kapczinski F., Andreazza A. C., Dean O. M., Giorlando F., Maes M., Yücel M., Gama C. S., Dodd S., Dean B., Magalhães P. V., Amminger P., McGorry P., & Malhi G. S. (2011). Pathways underlying neuroprogression in bipolar disorder: Focus on inflammation, oxidative stress and neurotrophic factors. *Neuroscience and Biobehavioral Reviews, 35*, 804–817.

Berk M., Post R., Ratheesh A., Gliddon E., Singh A., Vieta E., Carvalho A.F., Ashton M. M., Berk L., Cotton S. M., McGorry P. D., Fernandes B. S., Yatham L. N., & Dodd S. (2017). Staging in bipolar disorder: From theoretical framework to clinical utility. *World Psychiatry, 16*, 236–244.

Blumberg H. P., Kaufman J., Martin A., Whiteman R., Zhang J. H., Gore J. C., Charney D. S., Krystal J. H., & Peterson B. S. (2003). Amygdala and hippocampal volumes in adolescents and adults with bipolar disorder. *Archives of General Psychiatry, 60*(12), 1201–1208.

Caplan, J. P., & Stern, T. A. (2008). *Mnemonics in a mnutshell: 32 aids to psychiatric diagnosis*. Retrieved April 9, 2022, from https://cdn.mdedge.com/files/s3fs-public/Document/September-2017/0710CP_Article2.pdf

Carvalho, A. F., Firth, J., & Vieta, E. (2020). Bipolar disorder. *The New England Journal of Medicine, 383*(1), 58–66. https://doi.org/10.1056/NEJMra1906193

Caseras, X., Lawrence, N. S., Murphy, K., Wise, R. G., & Phillips, M. L. (2013). Ventral striatum activity in response to reward: Differences between bipolar I and II disorders. *The American Journal of Psychiatry, , 170*, 533–541.

Chang, K., Adleman, N. E., Dienes, K., Simeonova, D. I., Menon, V., & Reiss, A. (2004). Anomalous prefrontal-subcortical activation in familial pediatric bipolar disorder: A functional magnetic resonance imaging investigation. *Archives of General Psychiatry, 61*(8), 781–792.

Chang, K., Karchemskiy, A., Barnea-Goraly, N., Garrett, A., Simeonova, D. I., & Reiss, A. (2005). Reduced amygdalar gray matter volume in familial pediatric bipolar disorder. *Journal of the American Academy of Child and Adolescent Psychiatry, 44*(6), 565–573.

Chatterton, M. L., Stockings, E., Berk, M., Barendregt, J. J., Carter, R., & Mihalopoulos, C. (2017). Psychosocial therapies for the adjunctive treatment of bipolar disorder in adults: Network meta-analysis. *The British Journal of Psychiatry: The Journal of Mental Science, , 210*, 333–341.

Chen, H. H., Nicoletti, M. A., Hatch, J. P., Sassi R. B., Axelson D., Brambilla P., Monkul E. S., Keshavan M. S., Ryan N. D., Birmaher B., & Soares J. C. (2004). Abnormal left superior temporal gyrus volumes in children and adolescents with bipolar disorder: A magnetic resonance imaging study. *Neuroscience Letters, 36*(1), 365–368.

Cipriani, A., Hawton, K., Stockton, S., & Geddes, J. R. (2013). Lithium in the prevention of suicide in mood disorders: Updated systematic review and meta-analysis. *BMJ, 346*, f3646–3658.

DelBello, M. P., Zimmerman, M. E., Mills, N. P., Getz, G. E., & Strakowski, S. M. (2004). Magnetic resonance imaging analysis of amygdala and other subcortical brain regions in adolescents with bipolar disorder. *Bipolar Disorders, 6*(1), 43–52.

Dickstein, D. P., Milham, M. P., Nugent, A. C., Drevets W. C., Charney D. S., Pine D. S., Leibenluft E. (2005). Frontotemporal alterations in pediatric bipolar disorder: Results of a voxel-based morphometry study. *Archives of General Psychiatry, 62*(7), 734–741.

Duffy, A., Goodday, S., Keown-Stoneman, C., & Grof, P. (2019a). The emergent course of bipolar disorder: Observations over two decades from the Canadian high-risk offspring cohort. *American Journal of Psychiatry, , 176*, 720–729.

Duffy, A., Goodday, S. M., Keown-Stoneman, C., Scotti, M., Maitra, M., Nagy, C., Horrocks J., Turecki G. (2019b). Epigenetic markers in inflammation-related genes associated with mood disorder: A cross-sectional and longitudinal study in high-risk offspring of bipolar parents. *International Journal of Bipolar Disorders, 7*, 17.

Edvardsen, J., Torgersen, S., Roysamb, E., Lygren, S., Skre, I., Onstad, S., Oien P.A. (2008). Heritability of bipolar spectrum disorders. Unity or heterogeneity? *Journal of Affective Disorders, 106*, 229–240.

Favre, P., Pauling, M., Stout, J., Hozer, F., Sarrazin, S., Abé, C., Alda, M., Alloza, C., Alonso-Lana, S., Andreassen, O. A., Baune, B. T., Benedetti, F., Busatto, G. F., Canales-Rodríguez, E. J., Caseras, X., Chaim-Avancini, T. M., Ching, C. R. K., Dannlowski, U., Deppe, M., & Eyler, L. T. (2019). Widespread white matter microstructural abnormalities in bipolar disorder: evidence from mega- and meta-analyses across 3033 individuals. *Neuropsychopharmacology, 44*(13), 2285–2293. https://doi.org/10.1038/s41386-019-0485-6

Firth, J., Siddiqi, N., Koyanagi, A., Siskind, D., Rosenbaum, S., Galletly, C., Allan, S., Caneo, C., Carney, R., Carvalho, A. F., Chatterton, M. L., Correll, C. U., Curtis, J., Gaughran, F., Heald, A., Hoare, E., Jackson, S. E., Kisely, S., Lovell, K., ... Stubbs, B. (2019). The Lancet psychiatry commission: A blueprint for protecting physical health in people with mental illness. *Lancet: Psychiatry, 6*, 675–712.

Fornaro, M., & Stubbs, B. (2015). A meta-analysis investigating the prevalence and moderators of migraines among people with bipolar disorder. *Journal of Affective Disorders, 178*, 88–97.

Fountoulakis, K. N., Yatham, L. N., Grunze, H., Vieta, E., Young, A. H., Blier, P., Tohen, M., Kasper, S., Moeller, H. J. (2020). The CINP guidelines on the definition and evidence-based interventions for treatment-resistant bipolar disorder. *The International Journal of Neuropsychopharmacology, , 23*, 230–256.

Fries, G. R., Li, Q., McAlpin, B., Rein, T., Walss-Bass, C., Soares, J. C., Quevedo, J. (2016). The role of DNA methylation in the pathophysiology and treatment of bipolar disorder. *Neuroscience and Biobehavioral Reviews, 68*, 474–488.

Fries, G. R., Quevedo, J., Zeni, C. P., Kazimi, I. F., Zunta-Soares, G., Spiker, D. E., Bowden, C.L., Walss-Bass C., Soares, J. C. (2017). Integrated transcriptome and methylome analysis in youth at high risk for bipolar disorder: A preliminary analysis. *Translational Psychiatry, 7*, e1059.

Fristad, M. A. (2006). Psychoeducational treatment for school-aged children with bipolar disorder. *Development and Psychopathology, 18*, 1289–1306.

Fristad, M. A., Goldberg-Arnold, J. S., & Gavazzi, S. M. (2002). Multifamily psychoeducation groups (MFPG) for families of children with bipolar disorder. *Bipolar Disorders, 4*(4), 254–262. https://doi.org/10.1034/j.1399-5618.2002.09073.x

Fristad, M. A., Goldberg-Arnold, J. S., & Gavazzi, S. M. (2003). Multi-family psychoeducation groups in the treatment of children with mood disorders. *Journal of Marital and Family Therapy, 29*(4), 491–504. https://doi.org/10.1111/j.1752-0606.2003.tb01691.x

Fristad, M. A., & MacPherson, H. A. (2014). Evidence-based psychosocial treatments for child and adolescent bipolar spectrum disorders. *Journal of Clinical Child and Adolescent Psychology: The Official Journal for the Society of Clinical Child and Adolescent Psychology, American Psychological Association, Division 53, , 43*(3), 339–355. https://doi.org/10.1080/15374416.2013.822309

Fristad, M. A., Verducci, J. S., Walters, K., & Young, M. E. (2009). Impact of multifamily psychoeducational psychotherapy in treating children aged 8 to 12 years with mood disorders. *Archives of General Psychiatry, 66*(9), 1013–1021. https://doi.org/10.1001/archgenpsychiatry.2009.112

Gaine, M. E., Seifuddin, F., Sabunciyan, S., Lee, R. S., Benke, K. S., Monson, E. T., Zandi, P. P., Potash, J. B., & Willour, V. L. (2019). Differentially methylated regions in bipolar disorder and suicide. *American Journal of Medical Genetics. Part B, Neuropsychiatric Genetics : The Official Publication of the International Society of Psychiatric Genetics, 180*, 496–507.

Gottesman, I. I., Laursen, T. M., Bertelsen, A., & Mortensen, P. B. (2010). Severe mental disorders in offspring with 2 psychiatrically ill parents. *Archives of General Psychiatry, 67*, 252–257.

Grande, I., & Vieta, E. (2015). Pharmacotherapy of acute mania: Monotherapy or combination therapy with mood stabilizers and antipsychotics? *CNS Drugs, 29*, 221–227.

Hayes, J. F., Miles, J., Walters, K., King, M., & Osborn, D. P. J. (2015). A systematic review and meta-analysis of premature mortality in bipolar affective disorder. *Acta Psychiatrica Scandinavica, , 131*, 417–425.

Hibar, D. P., Westlye, L. T., Doan, N. T., Jahanshad, N., Cheung, J. W., Ching, C. R. K., Versace, A., Bilderbeck, A. C., Uhlmann, A., Mwangi, B., Krämer, B., Overs, B., Hartberg, C. B., Abé, C., Dima, D., Grotegerd, D., Sprooten, E., Bøen, E., Jimenez, E., & Howells, F. M. (2017). Cortical abnormalities in bipolar disorder: an MRI analysis of 6503 individuals from the ENIGMA Bipolar Disorder Working Group. *Molecular Psychiatry, 23*(4), 932–942.

Hidalgo-Mazzei, D., Berk, M., Cipriani, A., Cleare, A. J., Florio, A. D., Dietch, D., Geddes, J. R., Goodwin, G. M., Grunze, H., Hayes, J. F., Jones, I., Kasper, S., Macritchie, K., McAllister-Williams, R. H., Morriss, R., Nayrouz, S., Pappa, S., Soares, J. C., Smith, D. J., Suppes, T., Talbot P., Vieta, E., Watson, S., Watson, S. Yatham, L.N., Young, A. H., Stokes, P. R. A. (2019). Treatment-resistant and multi-therapy-resistant criteria for bipolar depression: Consensus definition. *The British Journal of Psychiatry: The Journal of Mental Science, 214*, 27–35.

Ho, N. F., Chong, P. L., Lee, D. R., Chew, Q. H., Chen, G., & Sim, K. (2019). The amygdala in schizophrenia and bipolar disorder: A synthesis of structural MRI, diffusion tensor imaging, and resting-state functional connectivity findings. *Harvard Review of Psychiatry, ,* 27, 150–164.

Joslyn, C., Hawes, D. J., Hunt, C., & Mitchell, P. B. (2016). Is age of onset associated with severity, prognosis, and clinical features in bipolar disorder? A meta-analytic review. *Bipolar Disorders, 18*, 389–403.

Kessing, L. V., Vradi, E., McIntyre, R. S., & Andersen, P. K. (2015). Causes of decreased life expectancy over the life span in bipolar disorder. *Journal of Affective Disorders, 180*, 142–147.

Krishnan, K. R. R. (2005). Psychiatric and medical comorbidities of bipolar disorder. *Psychosomatic Medicine, , 67*, 1–8.

Ludwig, B., & Dwivedi, Y. (2016). Dissecting bipolar disorder complexity through epigenomic approach. *Molecular Psychiatry, 21*, 1490–1498.

McGuffin, P., Rijsdijk, F., Andrew, M., Sham, P., Katz, R., & Cardno, A. (2003). The heritability of bipolar affective disorder and the genetic relationship to unipolar depression. *Archives of General Psychiatry, 60*, 497–502.

McIntyre, R. S., & Calabrese, J. R. (2019). Bipolar depression: The clinical characteristics and unmet needs of a complex disorder. *Current Medical Research and Opinion, 35*(11), 1993–2005. https://doi.org/10.1080/03007995.2019.1636017

McKnight, R. F., Adida, M., Budge, K., Stockton, S., Goodwin, G. M., & Geddes, J. R. (2012). Lithium toxicity profile: A systematic review and meta-analysis. *Lancet, 379*, 721–728.

Mendenhall, A. N., & Fristad, M. A., & Early, T. J. (2009). Factors influencing service utilization and mood symptom severity in children with mood disorders: Effects of multifamily psychoeducation groups (MFPGs). *Journal of Consulting and Clinical Psychology, 77*, 463–473.

Merikangas, K. R., Jin, R., He, J-P., Kessler, R. C., Lee, S., Sampson, N. A., Viana, M. C., Andrade, L. H., Hu, C., Karam, E. G., Ladea, M., Medina-Mora, M. E., Ono, Y., Posada-Villa, J., Sagar, R., Wells, J. E., Zarkov, Z. (2011). Prevalence and correlates of bipolar spectrum disorder in the World Mental Health Survey Initiative. *Archives of General Psychiatry, 68*(3), 241–251. https://doi.org/10.1001/archgenpsychiatry.2011.12

Miskowiak, K., Burdick, K., Martinez-Aran, A., Bonnin, C., Bowie, C., Carvalho, A., Gallagher, P., Lafer, B., López-Jaramillo, C., Sumiyoshi, T., McIntyre, R., Schaffer, A., Porter, R., Purdon, S., Torres, I., Yatham, L., Young, A., Kessing, L., & Vieta, E. (2018). Assessing and addressing cognitive impairment in bipolar disorder: The International Society for Bipolar Disorders Targeting Cognition Task Force recommendations for clinicians. *Bipolar Disorders, 20*, 184–194.

Miura, T., Noma, H., Furukawa, T. A., Mitsuyasu, H., Tanaka, S., Stockton, S., Salanti, G., Motomura, K., Shimano-Katsuki, S., Leucht, S., Cipriani, A., Geddes, J. R., & Kanba, S. (2014). Comparative efficacy and tolerability of pharmacological treatments in the maintenance treatment of bipolar disorder: A systematic review and network meta-analysis. *Lancet: Psychiatry, 1*, 351–359.

Morris, G., Puri, B. K., Walker, A. J., Maes, M., Carvalho, A. F., Bortolasci, C. C., Walder, K., & Berk, M. (2019). Shared pathways for neuroprogression and somatoprogression in neuropsychiatric disorders. *Neuroscience & Biobehavioral Reviews, 107*(107), 862–882. https://doi.org/10.1016/j.neubiorev.2019.09.025

Niida, R., Yamagata, B., Matsuda, H., Niida, A., Uechi, A., Kito, S., & Mimura, M. (2018). Regional brain volume reductions in major depressive disorder and bipolar disorder: An analysis by voxel-based morphometry. *International Journal of Geriatric Psychiatry, 34*(1), 186–192.

Ong, D., Walterfang, M., Malhi, G. S., Styner, M., Velakoulis, D., & Pantelis, C. (2012). Size and shape of the caudate nucleus in individuals with bipolar affective disorder. *The Australian and New Zealand Journal of Psychiatry, 46*, 340–351.

Passos, I. C., Mwangi, B., Vieta, E., Berk, M., & Kapczinski, F. (2016). Areas of controversy in neuroprogression in bipolar disorder. *Acta Psychiatrica Scandinavica, , 134*, 91–103.

Plans, L., Barrot, C., Nieto, E., Rios, J., Schulze, T. G., Papiol, S., Mitjans, M., Vieta, E., & Benabarre, A. (2019). Association between completed suicide and bipolar disorder: A systematic review of the literature. *Journal of Affective Disorders, 242*(242), 111–122.

Rasic, D., Hajek, T., Alda, M., & Uher, R. (2014). Risk of mental illness in offspring of parents with schizophrenia, bipolar disorder, and major depressive disorder: A meta-analysis of family high-risk studies. *Schizophrenia Bulletin, , 40*, 28–38.

Reed, G. M., First, M. B., Kogan, C. S., Hyman, S. E., Gureje, O., Gaebel, W., Maj, M., Stein, D. J., Maercker, A., Tyrer, P., Claudino, A., Garralda, E., Salvador-Carulla, L., Ray, R., Saunders, J. B., Dua, T., Poznyak, V., Medina-Mora, M. E., Pike, K. M., & Ayuso-Mateos, J. L. (2019). Innovations and changes in the ICD-11 classification of mental, behavioural and neurodevelopmental disorders. *World Psychiatry, 18*(1), 3–19.

Renk, K., White, R., Lauer, B. A., McSwiggan, M., Puff, J., & Lowell, A. (2014). Bipolar disorder in children. *Psychiatry Journal, 2014*(928685). https://doi.org/10.1155/2014/928685

Salcedo, S., Gold, A. K., Sheikh, S., Marcus, P. H., Nierenberg, A. A., Deckersbach, T., & Sylvia, L. G. (2016). Empirically supported psychosocial interventions for bipolar disorder: Current state of the research. *Journal of Affective Disorders, 201*(201), 203–214.

Scaini, G., Valvassori, S. S., Diaz, A. P., Lima, C. N., Benevenuto, D., Fries, G. R., & Quevedo, J. (2020). Neurobiology of bipolar disorders: A review of genetic components, signaling pathways, biochemical changes, and neuroimaging findings. *Revista brasileira de psiquiatria (Brazilian Journal of Psychiatry), 42*(5), 536–551. https://doi.org/10.1590/1516-4446-2019-0732

Spitzer, R. L., Endicott, J., & Williams, J. B. (1979). Research diagnostic criteria. *Archives of General Psychiatry, 36*(12), 1381–1383.

Spitzer, R. L., Endicott, J., & Williams, J. B. (1979). Research diagnostic criteria. *Archives of General Psychiatry, 36*(12), 1381–1383.

Tondo, L., Alda, M., Bauer, M., Bergink, V., Grof, P., Hajek, T., Lewitka, U., Licht, R. W., Manchia, M., Müller-Oerlinghausen, B., Nielsen, R. E., Selo, M., Simhandl, C., & Baldessarini, R. J. (2019). Clinical use of lithium salts: Guide for users and prescribers. *International Journal of Bipolar Disorders, 7*(1).

Vancampfort, D., Correll, C. U., Galling, B., Probst, M., De Hert, M., Ward, P. B., Rosenbaum, S., Gaughran, F., Lally, J., & Stubbs, B. (2016). Diabetes mellitus in people with schizophrenia, bipolar disorder and major depressive disorder: A systematic review and large scale meta-analysis. *World Psychiatry, 15*(2), 166–174.

Vancampfort, D., Vansteelandt, K., Correll, C. U., Mitchell, A. J., De Herdt, A., Sienaert, P., Probst, M., & De Hert, M. (2013). Metabolic syndrome and metabolic abnormalities in bipolar disorder: A meta-analysis of prevalence rates and moderators. *American Journal of Psychiatry, 170*(3), 265–274.

Van Meter, A., Moreira, A. L. R., & Youngstrom, E. (2019). Updated meta-analysis of epidemiologic studies of pediatric bipolar disorder. *The Journal of Clinical Psychiatry, 80*(3), 18r12180. https://doi.org/10.4088/JCP.18r12180

Vigo, D., Thornicroft, G., & Atun, R. (2016). Estimating the true global burden of mental illness. *Lancet: Psychiatry, 3*, 171–178.

Walker, E. R., McGee, R. E., & Druss, B. G. (2015). Mortality in mental disorders and global disease burden implications: A systematic review and meta-analysis. *JAMA Psychiatry, 72*, 334–341.

Webb, C. A., Olson, E. A., Killgore, W. D., Pizzagalli, D. A., Rauch, S. L., & Rosso, I. M. (2018). Rostral anterior cingulate cortex morphology predicts treatment response to internet-based cognitive behavioral therapy for depression. *Biological psychiatry. Cognitive Neuroscience and Neuroimaging, 3*, 255–262.

Weiner, M., Warren, L., & Fiedorowicz, J. G. (2011). Cardiovascular morbidity and mortality in bipolar disorder. *Annals of Clinical Psychiatry: The Official Journal of the American Academy of Clinical Psychiatrists, , 23*, 40–47.

Weller, E. B., Weller, R. A., & Fristad, M. A. (1995). Bipolar disorder in children: Misdiagnosis, underdiagnosis, and future directions. *Journal of the American Academy of Child and Adolescent Psychiatry, 34*(6), 709–714.

West, A. E., Weinstein, S. M., Peters, A. T., Katz, A. C., Henry, D. B., Cruz, R. A., & Pavuluri, M. N. (2014). Child- and Family-Focused Cognitive-Behavioral Therapy for Pediatric Bipolar Disorder: A Randomized Clinical Trial. *Journal of the American Academy of Child & Adolescent Psychiatry, 53*(11), 1168-1178.e1.

Yee, C. S., Hawken, E. R., Baldessarini, R. J., & Vázquez, G. H. (2019). Maintenance pharmacological treatment of juvenile bipolar disorder: Review and meta-analyses. *International Journal of Neuropsychopharmacology, 22*, 531–540.

Zimmerman, M., Ruggero, C. J., Chelminski, I., & Young, D. (2008). Is bipolar disorder overdiagnosed? *The Journal of Clinical Psychiatry, 69*, 935–940.

CHAPTER 24

Eating Disorders

Rachel Wolfe, Ph.D. and Sindhu Idicula, M.D.

> *"We turn skeletons into goddesses and look to them as if they might teach us how not to need."*
>
> — Marya Hornbacher

OBJECTIVES

At the end of this chapter, students will be able to do the following:

- describe the epidemiology, neuropathology, comorbidity of anorexia nervosa, bulimia nervosa, binge eating disorder, and avoidant restrictive feeding disorder
- identify anorexia nervosa (AN), bulimia nervosa (BN), binge eating disorder (BED), and avoidant-restrictive food intake disorder (ARFID), using clinical information and *DSM-5* diagnostic criteria
- recognize reasons for immediate hospitalization and appropriate treatment and management of AN, BN, BED, and ARFID

DEFINITIONS AND KEY CONCEPTS

Anorexia nervosa is an eating disorder characterized by weight loss or lack of appropriate weight gain in growing children and distorted body image. *Bulimia nervosa* is an eating disorder characterized by a cycle of bingeing and compensatory purging. *Binge eating disorder* is an eating disorder characterized by bingeing with no compensatory purging. A *binge* is an episode of eating large quantities of food (more than most people would eat) in a discrete period of time, often quickly and to the point of discomfort, with a feeling of loss of control. A *purge* is an episode of inappropriate compensatory behavior to prevent weight gain, such as self-induced vomiting, misuse of medicines (laxatives, diuretics, or others), fasting, or excessive exercise.

INTRODUCTION

Eating disorders (EDs) are complex psychiatric conditions that place their victims at risk for medical comorbidities. Individuals with EDs struggle with problematic behaviors and beliefs around food and the shape and size of the body (in some cases). Medical consequences can result that arise from starvation, purging, and other behaviors, making them one of the most lethal psychiatric conditions (Arcelus et al., 2011; Campbell, 2014).

Primary care clinicians are often the front lines of identifying EDs, leaving them with the task of providing appropriate guidance to the patient and family about the next steps. Timely diagnosis and intervention are crucial in treating EDs.

The aim of this chapter is to provide an overview of four major EDs: anorexia nervosa (AN), bulimia nervosa (BN), avoidant-restrictive food intake disorder (ARFID), and binge eating disorder (BED). It is hoped that by the end of this chapter the reader has gained the knowledge to identify and tentatively diagnose EDs and provide guidance to patients regarding treatment approaches that will best address their needs.

CLINICAL TIP

Patients with ED often present first to their primary care providers (PCP). PCPs often have the task of identifying the symptoms and providing appropriate guidance to the patient and family about the next steps.

EPIDEMIOLOGY

TABLE 24.1 Epidemiology of Eating Disorders

	Average age of onset	Lifetime prevalence
Anorexia nervosa	Adolescence or young adulthood	0.9–2% females 0.1–0.3% males
Bulimia nervosa	Adolescence or young adulthood	1.1–4.6% females 0.1–0.5% males
Binge eating disorder	Young adulthood	0.2–3.5% females 0.9–2% males

Adapted from American Psychiatric Association, 2013; Stice and Bohon, 2012.

QUICK POINT

Population studies found the lifetime prevalence of eating disorders was 2.7%. Eating disorders are over twice as prevalent among females (3.8%) than males (1.5%). Females with bulimia nervosa and binge eating disorder sought treatment more than males. However, males with anorexia nervosa sought treatment more often than females (Hudson, 2007).

CLINICAL MANIFESTATIONS

Often, EDs are first identified through their primary care physician (PCP). This can occur in a variety of ways. In some instances, the patient and/or parent does not directly report concerns for an ED. In fact, in restrictive EDs, adolescents attending a medical visit may do the following:

- demonstrate a significant change in weight or shift in their typical growth curve
- report irregularities in their menstrual cycle (or amenorrhea)
- complain of unexplained symptoms, such as hair loss, cold intolerance, or fatigue
- report gastrointestinal symptoms, such as early satiety, constipation, or lack of appetite

Given the secretive nature of EDs, the patient may conceal that they are purposefully trying to control aspects of their shape and size through food restriction and/or engaging in bouts of overeating. They can be masterful at presenting the illusion of eating meals throughout the day when they are not. Thus, parents do not always suspect an ED either. As the physician, it is important to ask key questions about EDs, both with the parent present and alone with the adolescent patient.

Adult patients with EDs may be more forthcoming in medical visits regarding their relationship with their bodies and food. Presenting medical concerns may be like those listed in adolescents. Additional concerns about fertility could arise as well.

QUICK POINT

Over half of patients with eating disorders have a comorbid psychiatric disorder. The highest comorbidity is with anxiety disorders followed by mood disorders, impulse control disorders, and substance use disorders (Hudson, 2007).

KEY POINT

Anorexia nervosa (AN) is characterized by an inaccurate perception of body shape and size that leads to significantly low weight status relative to age or growth curve or fear of weight gain or becoming fat (or behavior geared toward weight loss or preventing weight gain). There is not a BMI minimum requirement for someone to be diagnosed with AN.

Anorexia Nervosa

Diagnostic Criteria

The hallmarks of AN are significantly low weight status relative to age or growth curve, fear of weight gain or becoming fat (or behavior geared toward weight loss or preventing weight gain), and inaccurate perception of body shape and size. There is not a BMI minimum requirement for someone to be diagnosed with AN. It is important to consider growth curve and medical complications resulting from weight loss when making the diagnosis. This is particularly important for individuals who may have been previously overweight. AN can be classified as restricting type or binge–purge type (APA, 2013).

Treatment

Psychopharmacology

The mainstay of treatment for AN is nutritional support and psychotherapy. AN has no FDA-approved psychopharmacological agent used for treatment. Studies have shown that SSRIs, despite much anticipation, show little improvement. Typically they are used for significant comorbid depression or anxiety, unless these symptoms are a result of starvation itself (Frank & Shott, 2016).

Psychotherapy

The gold standard treatment for AN in teens is family-based therapy (FBT; Lock et al., 2013). FBT is a treatment modality that aims to provide the tools necessary for parents to manage refeeding, weight restoration, and ED behaviors at home. It is a stepped approach in which autonomy is systematically returned to the teen as they make progress in their ability to meet nutritional needs and reduce problem behaviors. Cognitive behavioral therapy (CBT) is another effective treatment method that can be conducted individually with a teen or adult patient (Fairburn, 2008). CBT focuses on the ED mindset and related behavioral patterns that can maintain EDs through replacing ED thoughts with more logical ones and changing ED-maintaining behaviors.

MEMORY TIP

Anorexia, *useful mnemonic*

ANOREXIA

A—Amenorrhea
N—No organic factors account for weight loss
O—Obviously thin but feels fat
R—Refusal to maintain normal body weight
E—Epigastric
X—X-symptoms (peculiar symptoms)
I—Intense fears of gaining weight
A—Always thinking of food

(Nursing.com, n.d.a.)

CASE VIGNETTE

Flor is a 15-year-old female who is diagnosed with AN, restricting type. She developed her ED the summer before sophomore year, wanting to be ready for bikini season. Flor successfully reached a weight loss goal she had set about 2 weeks before a scheduled vacation. Fearing regaining the weight, she continued her diet and exercise routine. She became obsessed with her weight and began weighing twice daily. Any mild increase in weight led to distress. She became even more restrictive in her eating, cutting all carbohydrates except fruit. When vacation occurred, Flor ate only fruit, grilled chicken, and steamed vegetables at the resort, and she had low energy and was irritable. Flor's parents started realizing something was wrong. They were stunned at her thinness when they saw Flor in her bikini. They confronted Flor, who vehemently denied that there was anything wrong. From then on, her parents noticed what she was eating, and Flo became more secretive, filling her plate with food and then getting rid of it without their notice, either trashing it or feeding it to the dog. When forced to eat more or eat "fattening" food, she'd sneak in extra exercise to burn it off. She began measuring her legs and wrists with her hands to monitor weight.

Bulimia Nervosa

Diagnostic Criteria

Bulimia nervosa is characterized by an overemphasis on weight and shape concerns that lead to a pattern of binging, purging, and most often both. Binges are experienced as consuming an objectively large amount of food while feeling completely out of control. Purges are compensatory in nature and can include vomiting, abuse of laxatives, exercise, or extreme caloric restriction. Individuals with bulimia nervosa are usually within a normal or above-normal weight limit, which differentiates them with the diagnosis of anorexia nervosa, binge-purge type (APA, 2013).

KEY POINT

Bulimia nervosa (BN) is characterized by an overemphasis on weight and shape concerns that lead to a pattern of binging, purging, and most often both. Individuals with bulimia nervosa are usually within a normal or above-normal weight limit, which differentiates them those with the diagnosis of anorexia nervosa, binge-purge type.

Treatment

Psychopharmacology

Individuals with bulimia nervosa may be treated using fluoxetine or Prozac. Fluoxetine has been shown to work independently of its antidepressant properties and works to reduce binge eating and vomiting episodes. A typical dose is 60 mg (Couturier, 2007).

MEMORY TIP

***Bulimia**, useful mnemonic*

BULIMIA

B—Binge eating
U—Under strict dieting
L—Lacks control/overeating
I—Induced vomiting
M—Minimum of 1 binge eating episodes per week for 3 months
I—Increased/persistent concern of body size
A—Abuse of diuretics and laxatives

(Adapted from Nursing.com, n.d.b.)

Psychotherapy

Cognitive behavioral therapy is the most effective treatment for bulimia nervosa, as it targets cognitive weight and shape concerns while also teaching strategies for management of binge and purge urges. A primary focus of CBT for bulimia nervosa is to establish a regular eating routine to reduce urges to binge (and thus reduce the subsequent urge to purge; Fairburn, 2008).

CASE VIGNETTE

Marisol is a 19-year-old female with bulimia nervosa. Marisol remembers being obsessed with her appearance as early as she can remember. By 12 years old, she developed a pattern of significantly restricting, impulsively binging, and throwing up. Her weight fluctuated frequently, which only intensified her obsession with her body. When Marisol's weight would fluctuate upward, Marisol's mother would make comments about her needing to exercise more and watch what she eats. Sometimes Marisol's pediatrician would also note increases in weight and encourage her to eat healthier. These experiences created a sense of shame around eating food, and Marisol became quite secretive with her binging. When she was old enough to drive, she would go to her favorite fast-food restaurant and binge in the parking lot. She felt incredible guilt and shame after binges, and the only thing that would relieve her guilt was to vomit. Now that Marisol is 19 and in college, her binging behavior has begun to include alcohol.

Binge Eating Disorder

Diagnostic Criteria

Binge eating disorder (BED) is characterized by recurrent episodes of overeating in which the individual feels out of control. The binge is not followed by a compensatory behavior. BED is not driven by weight or shape concerns (APA, 2013).

> **KEY POINT**
>
> Binge eating disorder (BED) is not driven by weight or shape concerns. BED is characterized by recurrent episodes of overeating in which the individual feels out of control.

Treatment

Psychopharmacology

Various medications have been tried for the treatment of BED, including medications used for depression, epilepsy, obesity, and attention-deficit/hyperactivity disorder (ADHD). They all had their limitations related to efficacy and side effects and were used off-label. The FDA approved lisdexamfetamine, or Vyvanse, as a medication for treating moderate to severe BED in adults in 2015. It is a prodrug stimulant medication that is also used for ADHD. Lisdexamfetamine works on the dopamine and norepinephrine systems in the brain, which are important systems in regulating eating behavior and reward (Guerdjikova, 2016).

Psychotherapy

The treatment for BED is cognitive behavioral therapy (Fairburn, 2013). CBT is an effective treatment for BED because it addresses both cognitive errors that can exacerbate binge eating behavior, such as all-or-nothing thinking, and helps create a behavioral plan to decrease environmental triggers and other behaviors that can drive binge eating. Interpersonal psychotherapy (IPT), with a focus on improving interpersonal relationships, has also been shown to be a helpful treatment for BED (Fairburn, 2013).

CASE VIGNETTE

Tanner is a 36-year-old male with a history of obesity and depressed mood. Tanner began to develop a complicated relationship with food during adolescence. He had struggled with being overweight since childhood. He was self-conscious and sometimes felt shame when eating "unhealthy" foods around other people because he believed that because he was obese, he should never eat them. He often set lofty goals to eat "clean" and tried several different fad diets. He would go a few days on these restrictive diets, often feeling hungry and deprived. He would then lose control and eat upward of 3,000 calories of his favorite foods. He would then feel severe guilt and promise himself it was the last time. This pattern continued for several years, only worsening his relationship with food.

Other Eating Disorders

KEY POINT

Avoidant restrictive food intake disorder (ARFID) is a restrictive ED that, unlike anorexia and bulimia, is not driven by weight or shape concerns. ARFID goes beyond general pickiness and can result in medical complications and the need for hospitalization.

Avoidant restrictive food intake disorder (ARFID) is a restrictive ED that, unlike anorexia and bulimia, is not driven by weight or shape concerns. Individuals (usually children and adolescents) with this disorder develop an aversion to eating or avoid food groups that results in weight loss, malnutrition, nutritional deficits, or a drop from the child's normal growth curve. ARFID goes beyond general pickiness and can result in medical complications and the need for hospitalization (APA, 2013).

Sometimes problematic eating behavior does not fit cleanly into one of the other *DSM-5* diagnostic categories for EDs. An individual who is at a normal weight but is engaging in restrictive eating and has disturbance in weight or shape perception, for example, could be diagnosed with atypical AN if impairment and distress are evident (APA, 2013).

THE MULTIDISCIPLINARY TREATMENT APPROACH

CLINICAL TIP

A multidisciplinary approach to treatment, including medical oversight, psychological treatment, psychiatric medication management, and nutritional guidance, is the most optimal approach to management of patients with ED.

It is widely accepted that the appropriate treatment of EDs take a multidisciplinary approach, including medical oversight, psychological treatment, and nutritional guidance, among others. Even for an individual who is stable and receiving less insensitive treatment, the multidisciplinary team continues to be of high importance and provides robust support in which all aspects of the ED are managed in unison. This is beneficial, as it allows for closer monitoring and early detection of relapse.

MEDICAL CONSIDERATIONS

EDs and malnutrition have significant impacts on every organ system. Studied with a group of healthy volunteers in the Minnesota Starvation Study, we now have a better understanding of how starvation can have a profound impact on the body. Additionally, bingeing and purging also have independent effects.

TABLE 24.2 Common Medical Complications of Eating Disorders (Rosen, 2010)

Neurological	• Cortical atrophy • Syncope • Cognitive impairment
Psychiatric	• Anxiety • Obsessive–compulsive symptoms • Depression
Fluid and electrolytes	• Dehydration • Electrolyte abnormalities • Decreased calcium, sodium, potassium, magnesium, and phosphate
Cardiovascular	• Bradycardia • Hypotension • Prolonged QTc
Endocrine	• Sick euthyroid syndrome • Growth retardation • Delayed puberty
Genitourinary	• Amenorrhea
Gastrointestinal	• Early satiety • Constipation • Gastroesophageal reflux
Dermatological	• Lanugo • Russell's sign—abrasions on knuckles from using fingers to induce vomiting
HEENT	• Enamel erosion • Parotid hypertrophy

One of the most critical clinical guidelines for physicians seeing patients with EDs is to promptly recognize when a patient requires immediate hospitalization. These reasons include both medical and psychiatric changes that may be life threatening. It is vital for a physician to monitor for these symptoms and swiftly intensify intervention when one of these issues arise. In the outpatient setting, patients who remain at an outpatient level of care may fall through the cracks and have worsening medical issues untreated.

TABLE 24.3 Medical and Psychiatric Changes Requiring Hospitalization

Reasons for Hospitalization
• Severe malnutrition—< 75% ideal body weight • Physiologic instability • Severe bradycardi—HR < 50 • Hypotension • Hypothermia • Severe orthostatic changes • Dehydration or electrolyte imbalance • Cardiac arrhythmias • Hematemesis • Suicidal or acute mental status changes

Adapted from Rosen, 2010.

SUMMARY

Eating disorders are psychological conditions often accompanied by medical comorbidities. Individuals with EDs often first present to their PCP. The PCP can play a critical role in identifying the ED and helping the patient move forward with appropriate treatment. All EDs, including BED, should be treated within a multidisciplinary framework with a team that includes a physician, behavioral health practitioner, registered dietitian, and sometimes others (such as psychiatry). Early identification, multidisciplinary treatment, and ongoing monitoring offer the individual with an ED the best chance at recovery.

RESOURCES

1 The Society for Adolescent Health and Medicine (2015). Position paper of the Society of Adolescent Health and Medicine: Medical management of restrictive eating disorders in adolescents and young adults. *Journal of Adolescent Health*, 56, 121-125. https://www.jahonline.org/article/S1054-139X%2814%2900686-7/fulltext

2 The American Academy of Eating Disorders (2016). Eating Disorders: A Medical Guide to Care, Third Edition. Academy for Eating Disorders. Reston, VA. https://www.aedweb.org/resources/online-library/publications/medical-care-standards

3 National Eating Disorder Association (xxxx). Parent tool kit. National Eating Disorder Association. New York, NY. https://www.nationaleatingdisorders.org/sites/default/files/Toolkits/ParentToolkit.pdf

4 Nationaleatingdisorders.org

5 https://www.nimh.nih.gov/health/statistics/eating-disorders

REFERENCES

American Psychiatric Association. (2013). *Diagnostic and statistical manual of mental disorders* (5th ed.).

Arcelus, J., Mitchell, A. J., Wales, J., & Nielsen, S. (2011). Mortality rates in patients with anorexia nervosa and other eating disorders: A meta-analysis of 36 studies. *Archives of General Psychiatry, 68*(7), 724–731.

Campbell, K., & Peebles, R. (2014). Eating disorders in children and adolescents: State of the art review. *Pediatrics, 134*(3), 582–592. https://doi.org/10.1542/peds.2014-0194

Couturier, J., & Lock, J. (2007). A review of medication use for children and adolescents with eating disorders. *Journal of the Canadian Academy of Child and Adolescent Psychiatry, 16*(4), 173–176.

Fairburn, C. (2008). *Cognitive behavior therapy and eating disorders*. Guilford.

Fairburn, C. (2013). *Overcoming binge eating*. Guilford.

Frank, G. K., & Shott, M. E. (2016). The role of psychotropic medications in the management of anorexia nervosa: Rationale, evidence and future prospects. *CNS Drugs, 30*(5), 419–442. https://doi.org/10.1007/s40263-016-0335-6

Guerdjikova, A. I., Mori, N., Casuto, L. S., & McElroy, S. L. (2016). Novel pharmacologic treatment in acute binge eating disorder - role of lisdexamfetamine. *Neuropsychiatric Disease and Treatment, 12*, 833–841. https://doi.org/10.2147/NDT.S80881

Hudson, J. I., Hiripi E., Pope H. G. Jr, & Kessler R. C. (2007). The prevalence and correlates of eating disorders in the National Comorbidity Survey Replication. *Biological Psychiatry, 61*(3), 348–58.

Lock, J., LeGrange, D., & Russell, G. (2013). *Treatment manual for anorexia nervosa: A family-based approach* (2nd ed.). Guilford.

NURSING.com. (n.d.a). Anorexia—signs and symptoms nursing mnemonic. Retrieved January 16, 2022, from https://nursing.com/lesson/nursing-mnemonics-anorexia/

NURSING.com. (n.d.b). Bulimia—signs and symptoms 1 nursing mnemonic. Retrieved January 16, 2022, from https://nursing.com/lesson/nursing-mnemonics-bulimia/

Rosen, D. (2010). Identification and management of eating disorders in children and adolescents. *Pediatrics, 126*(6), 1240–1253. https://doi.org/10.1542/peds.2010-2821

CHAPTER 25

Somatic Symptom and Related Disorders

Jin Han, M.D. and Sindhu Idicula, M.D.

> *"All emotions, even those that are suppressed and unexpressed, have physical effects. Unexpected emotions tend to stay in the body like small ticking bombs—they are illnesses in incubation"*
>
> — Marilyn Van M. Derbur

OBJECTIVES

At the end of this chapter, students will be able to do the following:

- describe the main diagnostic criteria for the somatic symptom and related disorders, including somatic symptom disorder (SSD), illness anxiety disorder (IAD), conversion disorder (IAD), and factitious disorder (FD)
- discuss the clinical implications of SSD, IAD, CD, and FD in terms of recognition and treatment strategies

CASE VIGNETTE

Alan is a 14-year-old boy, an only child of divorcing parents, who presented to his pediatrician with his mother with complaints of severe abdominal pain. He noted that the pain would come and go, was not associated with eating food, and noticed no associated symptoms. His mother had tried to change his diet, cutting out dairy and gluten, to no avail. Over the course of a few months, the pediatrician conducted an appropriate workup and sought consultation from a GI specialist, and workup results were unremarkable. He had undergone hospitalization for some of the workup and to help with acute pain and had sought additional opinions from other highly regarded institutions in the nation.

Alan was highly intelligent, did quite well when engaged in school, and was able to form strong alliances with the medical staff who cared for him in the hospital. He saw his father every few weeks but noted that his mother and father fought constantly. The pediatrician noted during an inpatient visit that the parents seemed rather engaged in his care while he was in the hospital with less hostility and animosity seen during those periods.

DEFINITIONS AND KEY CONCEPTS

Somatization occurs when psychological concerns are converted into physical symptoms. *Somatic symptom disorder* is a disorder with distressing somatic symptoms that disrupt function where there are excessive thoughts, feelings, or behaviors related to the symptoms. *Illness anxiety disorder* is a disorder where an individual has a preoccupation with having or acquiring a serious illness in the absence of symptoms. *Conversion disorder* is a disorder of altered voluntary motor or sensory function with significant functional impairment where there is an incompatibility between symptoms and recognized neurological or medical symptoms. *Factitious disorder* is a disorder where an individual falsifies physical or psychological signs or symptoms, typically in the absence of obvious external rewards.

INTRODUCTION

Somatic symptom and related disorders (SSRD) include forms of mental illness where emotional troubles express themselves within the body, creating symptoms, such as pain, that are associated with distress. Patients with these disorders often present to their primary care providers and other medical professional but less commonly to psychiatrists. The categories are shown in Table 25.1.

KEY POINT

Somatic symptom and related disorders (SSRD) include forms of mental illness where emotional troubles express themselves within the body, creating symptoms, such as pain, that are associated with distress. Patients with these disorders often present to their primary care providers and other medical professional but less commonly to psychiatrists.

The revisions in the *DSM-5* were meant to make this category less confusing, particularly to primary care practitioners, who are primarily the clinicians seeing this group of patients. In it, a key change was the elimination of the centrality of medically unexplained symptoms, as it is inappropriate to ascribe a mental health disorder solely because a physical disorder cannot be found. In addition, some individuals with a medical disorder have a comorbid mental health disorder, which may include a diagnosis in this category. With conversion disorder, medically unexplained symptoms remain a key feature. If symptoms are medically explainable, it is not possible to meet criteria because the symptoms would then be consistent with medical pathology (APA, 2013).

TABLE 25.1 Somatoform Disorders in *DSM-5*

Somatic symptom disorder (SSD; previously somatization disorder)
Illness anxiety disorder (previously hypochondriasis)
Conversion disorder
Psychological factors affecting other medical conditions
Factitious disorder (previously Munchausen's syndrome)
Other specified somatic symptom and related disorder
Unspecified somatic symptom and related disorder

Many factors contribute to SSRDs. These include both genetic and biological vulnerabilities (e.g., increased sensitivity to pain), early traumatic experiences (e.g., abuse, deprivation, or violence), and learning (e.g., attention received from being ill, lack of reinforcement of nonsomatic expressions of distress). In addition, in some cultures, there is a relative devaluing and stigmatization of psychological suffering compared to physical. (APA, 2013).

QUICK POINT

In the general population, the prevalence of SSDs is estimated to be about 5–7%, presenting across the life span and more represented in females (Harris et al., 2009; Kurlansik & Maffei, 2016). The prevalence in a primary care population is about 17% and may be higher in patient populations with functional disorders, such as fibromyalgia, irritable bowel syndrome, and chronic fatigue syndrome (Häuser et al., 2015).

In the general population, the prevalence of SSDs is estimated to be about 5–7%, presenting across the life span and more represented in females (Harris et al., 2009; Kurlansik & Maffei, 2016). The prevalence in a primary care population is about 17% and may be higher in patient populations with functional disorders, such as fibromyalgia, irritable bowel syndrome, and chronic fatigue syndrome (Häuser et al., 2015). A study of illness anxiety disorder (based on estimates of hypochondriasis) shows an estimate of 1–10% of the general population. There is difficulty in measuring the precise prevalence of conversion disorder, as it typically requires secondary care assessment, where it is found in about 5% of referrals to neurology and is estimated to occur in about 2 to 5 per 100,000 per year. The prevalence of factitious disorder is unknown due to the role of deception but is estimated to occur in about 1% of hospitalized patients (APA, 2013).

CLINICAL MANIFESTATIONS AND DIAGNOSIS

The assessment starts with taking a detailed biopsychosocial history from the patient, including a review of previous medical records, if available; a review of systems; and performing thorough physical and mental status examinations. Further collateral information from family and other clinicians that suggest significant impairment in daily functioning could be helpful such as summarizing patient's beliefs and feeling and coping behaviors, including their continuous efforts to get clarification about their symptomatology. It is also relevant to review previous diagnostic studies like laboratory tests and imaging to make sure appropriate the workup was done as part of the diagnostic process (Silverman et al., 2015). Further screening may also identify comorbid psychiatric conditions like major depressive disorder, generalized anxiety disorder, substance use disorder, and poor coping skills linked to underlying personality disorders (Bass & Halligan, 2014; Bekhuis et al., 2015; Han et al., 2016). Although not absolutely necessary, some clinicians may prefer to utilize self-reported questionnaire tools like the Patient Health Questionnaire-15 (PHfmunQ-15) or the Somatic Symptom Scale-8 (SSS-8) combined with the 12-item Somatic Symptom Disorder-B Criteria Scale to identify those patients at risk for somatic symptoms and related disorders (Toussaint et al., 2020).

Somatic Symptom Disorder

Somatic symptom disorder (SSD) is characterized by *at least one physical symptom* that disrupts the quality of daily life accompanied by *excessive thoughts, feelings or behaviors* lasting *for at least 6 months* (APA, 2013). The level of distress is significant, but lack of medical cause is not a requirement, and the symptoms can be associated with an underlying medical condition. Many patients with this condition are extremely concerned that they might have an underlying serious medical problem. It is estimated that the majority of those diagnosed with hypochondriasis in previous *DSM* versions would instead be included under this new diagnosis (Dimsdale, 2013). SSD can be categorized based on severity into mild, moderate, and severe. The specifier "with predominant pain" can be added as well.

Illness Anxiety Disorder

Illness anxiety disorder (IAD) is diagnosed when there is the *excessive preoccupation of having a serious illness*, but physical symptoms are minimal or not present at all, *lasting for at least 6 months* (APA, 2013). Some patients display care-seeking behaviors and others care-avoidant behaviors. The highlight of this condition is not the presence of the physical symptom, per se, but rather the presence of significant concern about having a serious illness. It is estimated that approximately a quarter of those patients diagnosed with hypochondriasis per *DSM-5-TR* meet criteria for this category (Dimsdale, 2013).

Conversion Disorder or Functional Neurological Symptom Disorder

Conversion disorder (CD) is diagnosed when a patient has *at least one symptom of altered voluntary motor or sensory function* causing significant

MEMORY TIP

Somatic Symptom Disorder, *useful mnemonic*

TEA

T—Thoughts: disproportionate and persistent about the seriousness of somatic symptoms
E—Emotions: persistently high anxiety about health or symptoms
A—Actions: excess time and energy devoted to these symptoms

(Kadiyala, 2020)

MEMORY TIP

Illness Anxiety Disorder, *useful mnemonic*

Persistent Search For Any Big Disease

P—Preoccupation of having or acquiring an illness
S—Somatic symptoms absent or of mild intensity/Significant preoccupation about the risk of a disease or developing a disease
F—For at least 6 months
A—Anxiety about health
B—Behavior; excessive health-related behaviors (care-seeking type) or maladaptive avoidance (care-avoidant type)
D—Disturbance not better explained by another mental disorder

(Kadiyala, 2020)

impairment in daily functioning, *but clinical workup is not compatible* with the possible neurological etiology. The identification of psychological stressors is not imperative to make this diagnosis (APA, 2013). This condition can be categorized based on the type of symptom, including but not limited to the following:

- weakness or paralysis
- abnormal movement
- swallowing symptoms
- speech symptoms
- attacks or seizures
- anesthesia or sensory loss
- special sensory symptoms
- mixed symptoms

Psychological Factors Affecting Other Medical Conditions

This condition captures a condition when some psychological or behavioral factors are influencing the course or outcome of an underlying medical illness.

Factitious Disorder

To make a factitious disorder (FD) diagnosis, the *falsification* of physical or psychological signs or symptoms or induction of injury or disease associated with identified deception is required. There are no clear external rewards, but there seem to be some emotional benefits of taking such roles. FD was previously called Munchausen's syndrome and is classified as "imposed to self" when the behavior is directed toward oneself or "imposed on another (by proxy)" when the actions are directed to another (APA, 2013).

Other Specified Somatic Symptom and Related Disorders

This diagnostic terminology can be used when full criteria is not met for any of the SSRDs because the minimum 6 months duration is not met or another criterion is not met (APA, 2013). "Pseudocyesis" is included in this category, and it is a syndrome seen in a female patient who is not pregnant or psychotic, per se, but she strongly believes in her ongoing gestation, and she could even display signs and symptoms related to it.

MEMORY TIP

Conversion Disorder, *useful mnemonic*

CONVERSION
C—Conscious control lacking
O—Organic etiology unproven
N—Neurological symptoms prevalent
V—Verisimilitude to physical illness
E—Etiologically
R—Related to
S—Stressor
I—Indifference may occur
O—Organic sequelae possible
N—Not culturally sanctioned

(Wiseman, 1993)

CLINICAL TIP

With conversion disorder, medically unexplained symptoms remain a key feature. If symptoms are medically explainable, it is not possible to meet criteria because the symptoms would then be consistent with medical pathology (APA, 2013).

KEY POINT

Factitious disorder is often called Munchausen's syndrome. A factitious disorder involves the ***falsification*** of physical or psychological signs or symptoms or induction of injury or disease associated with identified deception. While there are no clear external rewards, there seem to be some emotional benefits of taking such roles.

Unspecified Somatic Symptom and Related Disorders

This diagnosis is used when there is insufficient information to make more specified SSRDs (APA, 2013).

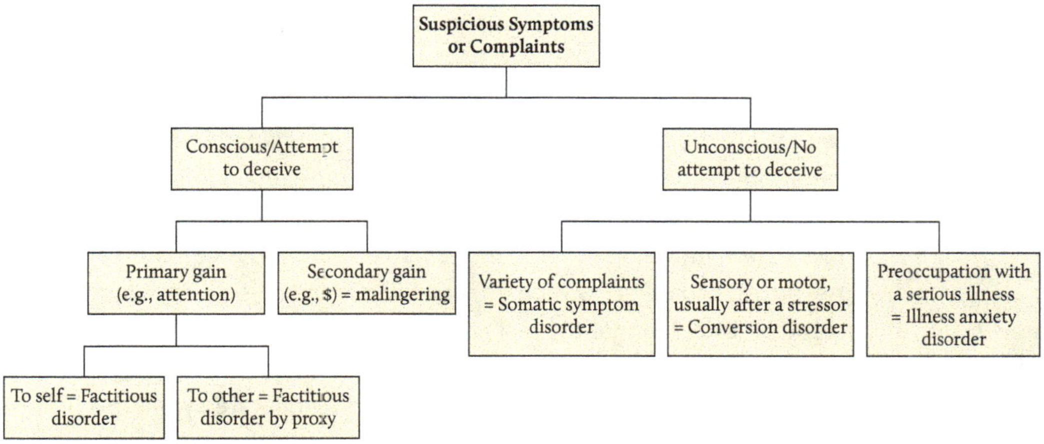

FIGURE 25.1 Algorithm for diagnosis of somatic symptoms and related disorders.

Note: Malingering is not within the *DSM-5* category for SSRDs but rather listed within "Other Conditions That May Be a Focus of Clinical Attention" (APA, 2013). It is characterized by intentional symptom(s) falsification or exaggeration to obtain obvious external benefits, such as money, certain addictive drugs, legal and financial compensation, placements, and others. This is not a mental disorder, and its likelihood increases in the context of medico-legal context, discrepancy of other evaluations and self-reported history, as well as antisocial traits.

TREATMENT

Psychopharmacology

There are no FDA-approved medications for any of the SSRDs, but clinicians should consider prescribing SSRIs and SNRIs (selective serotonin reuptake inhibitors or serotonin-norepinephrine reuptake inhibitors) or TCA (tricyclics antidepressants), based on evidence that it may provide some benefits for unexplained physical symptoms like pain (Kendrick et al., 2009; Teh et al., 2010). The use of antidepressants is particularly more relevant when comorbid depression and anxiety are identified during the assessment.

Psychotherapy

Some psychotherapeutic modalities, such as supportive psychotherapy, psychodynamic psychotherapy, family therapy, and others have been suggested, but cognitive behavioral therapy (CBT) is considered the most effective evidence-based approach (van Dessel et al., 2014).

CLINICAL CONSIDERATIONS

QUICK POINT

Most patients with somatoform disorders will be seen in primary care offices and emergency rooms. The primary care physician (PCP) plays an important role in guiding the therapeutic approach, and mental health providers are mainly collaborators and consultants.

CLINICAL TIP

Establishing rapport and trust with the patient are critical. Incorporating a language of support and validation of the patient's symptomatology and distress is important. Respectful and nonjudgmental communication and building a systematic approach with regular visits are the foundations of the treatment strategy.

The majority of patients with somatoform disorders will be seen in primary care offices and emergency rooms. The primary care physician (PCP) plays an important role in guiding the therapeutic approach and mental health providers are mainly collaborators and consultants. The PCP's efforts to establish good rapport and trust with the patient are critical, and it is important to incorporate a language of support and validation of the patient's symptomatology and distress. Respectful and nonjudgmental communication and building a systematic approach with regular visits are the key foundation of the treatment strategy. A judicious physical exam and diagnostic tests could be considered, and PCP should objectively communicate results reassuring that the test results rule out serious medical conditions, but the clinician will continue to work with the patient to help the patient to improve overall level of functioning and ameliorate symptoms (Croicu et al., 2014; Han et al., 2016). The PCP should be aware of and discuss the potential harm of performing unnecessary repetitive medical tests or procedures with the patient. Many patients with SSRD are not open to the idea of talking to a mental health provider, but the psychiatrist consult can be helpful for refractory cases for which further recommendations may facilitate rapport and strategies to help the patient (Morriss, 2012).

For patients with CD, the main intervention relies on psychoeducation, which embraces a similar approach to other SSRDs, validating patients' symptomatology, explaining the diagnostic process, and providing an ongoing collaboration to improve their functioning. Physical therapy is a reasonable alternative or add-on strategy if there are motor symptoms. CBT has been used as an adjunct intervention as well. Other interventions, like use of antidepressants, hypnosis, psychodynamic psychotherapy, and transcranial magnetic stimulation, have been used in refractory cases (O'Neal & Baslet, 2018; Stone & Edwards, 2012).

The management of FD imposed on self includes establishing a treatment team and incorporating regular visits. The PCP should continue to provide appropriate medical care but eventually should discuss this diagnosis in a respectful manner, emphasizing that the collaboration to address the condition will continue, but it is not uncommon for patients to react defensively and ultimately decide to look for another provider. The mental health provider remains a consultant, and psychotherapy can be offered (i.e., supportive or CBT). The FD imposed on others could be associated with a safety concern of a child or elderly person, so it is mandatory to report to appropriate protective agencies (Bass & Halligan, 2014).

SUMMARY

SSRDs include a variety of disorders where there may be psychological contribution to physical symptoms. They can be highly impairing and are often seen in primary care clinics. It is helpful as a primary care provider to use an appropriate physical exam and additional testing. Additionally, the use of empathy and objectivity (lack of judgment) is helpful in being able to form a strong therapeutic alliance necessary to help patients work toward recovery.

CLINICAL TIP

Building a systematic approach and regular scheduled visits are the foundations of the treatment strategy. A judicious physical exam and diagnostic tests could be considered, and the PCP should objectively communicate the results reassuring that the test results rule out serious medical conditions. The clinician can reassure the patient that they will continue to work with patient to help the patient to improve overall level of functioning and ameliorate symptoms.

RESOURCES

1. American Psychiatric Association. Diagnostic and Statistical Manual of Mental Disorders, Fifth Edition (DSM-5), American Psychiatric Association, Arlington, VA 2013.
2. Kurlansik, S. L., & Maffei, M. S. (2016). Somatic Symptom Disorder. American family physician, 93(1), 49–54.
3. Sharma, M. P., & Manjula, M. (2013). Behavioural and psychological management of somatic symptom disorders: an overview. International review of psychiatry (Abingdon, England), 25(1), 116–124. https://doi.org/10.3109/09540261.2012.746649

REFERENCES

American Psychiatric Association. (2013). *Diagnostic and statistical manual of mental disorders* (5th ed.).

Bass, C., & Halligan, P. (2014). Factitious disorders and malingering: Challenges for clinical assessment and management. *Lancet*, *383*(9926), 1422–1432. https://doi.org/10.1016/S0140-6736(13)62186-8

Bekhuis, E., Boschloo, L., Rosmalen, J. G., & Schoevers, R. A. (2015). Differential associations of specific depressive and anxiety disorders with somatic symptoms. *Journal of Psychosomatic Research*, , *78*(2), 116–122. https://doi.org/10.1016/j.jpsychores.2014.11.007

Croicu, C., Chwastiak, L., & Katon, W. (2014). Approach to the patient with multiple somatic symptoms. *The Medical Clinics of North America*, *98*(5), 1079–1095. https://doi.org/10.1016/j.mcna.2014.06.007

Dimsdale, J. E., Creed, F., Escobar, J., Sharpe, M., Wulsin, L., Barsky, A., Lee, S., Irwin, M. R., & Levenson, J. (2013). Somatic symptom disorder: An important change in DSM. *Journal of Psychosomatic Research*, *75*(3), 223–238. https://doi.org/10.1016/j.jpsychores.2013.06.033

Han, J. Y., French-Rosas, L., & Shah, A. A. (2016). Somatic symptom and related disorders overview, updates, and changes in the DSM-5. *Directions in Psychiatry*, *36*(1), 37–45.

Harris, A. M., Orav, E. J., Bates, D. W., & Barsky, A. J. (2009). Somatization increases disability independent of comorbidity. *Journal of General Internal Medicine, 24*(2), 155–161. https://doi.org/10.1007/s11606-008-0845-0

Häuser, W., Bialas, P., Welsch, K., & Wolfe, F. (2015). Construct validity and clinical utility of current research criteria of DSM-5 somatic symptom disorder diagnosis in patients with fibromyalgia syndrome. *Journal of Psychosomatic Research, 78*(6), 546–552. https://doi.org/10.1016/j.jpsychores.2015.03.151

Kadiyala P.K. (2020). Mnemonics for diagnostic criteria of DSM V mental disorders: A scoping review. *General Psychiatry, .14;33*(3):e100109.

Kendrick, T., Chatwin, J., Dowrick, C., Tylee, A., Morriss, R., Peveler, R., Leese, M., McCrone, P., Harris, T., Moore, M., Byng, R., Brown, G., Barthel, S., Mander, H., Ring, A., Kelly, V., Wallace, V., Gabbay, M., Craig, T., & Mann, A. (2009). Randomized controlled trial to determine the clinical effectiveness and cost-effectiveness of selective serotonin reuptake inhibitors plus supportive care, versus supportive care alone, for mild to moderate depression with somatic symptoms in primary care: The THREAD (THREshold for Antidepressant response) study. *Health Technology Assessment (Winchester, England), 13*(22). https://doi.org/10.3310/hta13220

Kurlansik, S. L., & Maffei, M. S. (2016). Somatic symptom disorder. *American Family Physician, 93*(1), 49–54.

Morriss, R. (2012). Role of mental health professionals in the management of functional somatic symptoms in primary care. *The British Journal of Psychiatry: The Journal of Mental Science, 200*(6), 444–445. https://doi.org/10.1192/bjp.bp.111.104083

O'Neal, M. A., & Baslet, G. (2018). Treatment for patients with a functional neurological disorder (conversion disorder): An integrated approach. *The American Journal of Psychiatry, 175*(4), 307–314. https://doi.org/10.1176/appi.ajp.2017.17040450

Silverman, J. J., Galanter, M., Jackson-Triche, M., Jacobs, D. G., Lomax, J. W., II, Riba, M. B., Tong, L. D., Watkins, K. E., Fochtmann, L. J., Rhoads, R. S., & Yager, J. (2015). The American Psychiatric Association practice guidelines for the psychiatric evaluation of adults. *American Journal of Psychiatry, 172*(8), 798–802. https://doi.org/10.1176/appi.ajp.2015.1720501

Stone, J., & Edwards, M. (2012). Trick or treat? Showing patients with functional (psychogenic) motor symptoms their physical signs. *Neurology, 79*(3), 282–284. https://doi.org/10.1212/WNL.0b013e31825fdf63

Teh, C. F., Zaslavsky, A. M., Reynolds, C. F., III, & Cleary, P. D. (2010). Effect of depression treatment on chronic pain outcomes. *Psychosomatic Medicine, 72*(1), 61–67. https://doi.org/10.1097/PSY.0b013e3181c2a7a8

Toussaint, A., Hüsing, P., Kohlmann, S., & Löwe, B. (2020). Detecting DSM-5 somatic symptom disorder: Criterion validity of the Patient Health Questionnaire-15 (PHQ-15) and the Somatic Symptom Scale-8 (SSS-8) in combination with the Somatic Symptom Disorder - B Criteria Scale (SSD-12). *Psychological Medicine, 50*(2), 324–333. https://doi.org/10.1017/S003329171900014X

van Dessel, N., den Boeft, M., van der Wouden, J. C., Kleinstäuber, M., Leone, S. S., Terluin, B., Numans, M. E., van der Horst, H. E., & van Marwijk, H. (2014). Non-pharmacological interventions for somatoform disorders and medically unexplained physical symptoms (MUPS) in adults. *The Cochrane Database of Systematic Reviews*, https://doi.org/10.1002/14651858.CD011142.pub2

Wiseman E. J. (1993). Conversion mnemonic. *The British Journal of Psychiatry: The Journal of Mental Science, 162*:272. https://www.doi.org/10.1192/bjp.162.2.272b. PMID: 8489608.

CHAPTER 26

Sleep Disorders

Zakaryia Irfanullah, M.D.; Hamza Khawaja, B.A.; and Imran Khawaja, M.D.

"Sleep is the best meditation."

— Dalai Lama

OBJECTIVES

After reading this chapter, students will be able to do the following:

- describe the stages of sleep
- understand the benefits of sleep for mental and physical health
- discuss common sleep disorders

CASE VIGNETTE

A 70-year-old woman, accompanied by her husband, presents to your clinic with excessive daytime somnolence complaints. She has a BMI of 34 kg/m^2. She has no psychiatric conditions. Her husband reports that she often snores loudly at night, and the patient admits that she doesn't feel well-rested upon awakening. You advise the patient to use a continuous positive airway pressure (CPAP) machine while sleeping. On follow-up, the patient and her spouse report significant improvement in symptoms. What condition is the patient most likely suffering from?

A. Insomnia
B. Obstructive sleep apnea
C. Willis-Ekbom disease
D. Narcolepsy

DEFINITIONS AND KEY CONCEPTS

Sleep is a regular, reoccurring, reversible state of loss of awareness with attenuated perceptual engagement from the environment, an elevated arousal threshold, and rapid reversibility.

INTRODUCTION

The prolific sleep researcher Allen Rechtschaffen (1971) remarked that "if sleep does not serve an absolutely vital function, then it is the biggest mistake the evolutionary process ever made." This is an astute observation, as sleep is a ubiquitous phenomenon exhibited by all higher species, yet it seemingly appears to be maladaptive. Sleeping humans cannot, for instance, protect themselves from danger, procreate, or engage in activities directly linked to prosperity. This apparent conundrum has given rise to a great deal of discussion and research over the ages. Our documented appreciation of this mysterious physiologic phenomenon dates back to as early as 350 BC when Aristotle asserted that "it is inevitable that every creature which wakes must also be capable of sleeping since it is impossible that it should continue actualizing its powers perpetually" (Beare, 2014).

Sleep science has continued to be an area of extensive research since the times of Aristotle's Lyceum. In the early 20th century, Nathaniel Kleitman, widely regarded as the father of American sleep research, pioneered several studies on sleep cycle regulation and the repercussions of sleep deprivation, which form the edifice of our modern conception of sleep physiology (Beare, 2014). Many of his students made strides in dream science and the study of rapid eye movement sleep (REM) and nonrapid eye movement sleep (NREM) sleep states. Today, we know that sleep serves a plethora of useful functions, we know that it is broken down into different stages, and we have also discovered a number of disorders associated with sleep. The rest of this chapter aims to distill these high-levels ideas.

SLEEP STAGES AND CYCLE

Contrary to popular belief, sleep is not a uniform state but rather two independent states: NREM and REM.

NREM Sleep

NREM sleep is further subdivided into three stages of increasing depth of responsiveness, known as stage N1, N2, and N3:

- *Stage N1* represents the transition from wake to sleep, which can be described as light sleep. The electroencephalogram (EEG) during N1 sleep demonstrates theta waves. Only 5–10% of total sleep time is spent in this stage in healthy adults, and it is commonly believed to be a transitory or segue stage from wakefulness to further stages of sleep.

- *Stage N2* represents deeper sleep and constitutes the majority of sleep time in healthy adults (45–55%). Teeth grinding can occur during this stage. Although theta waves predominate during the N2 stage, unique waveforms, such as sleep spindles and K complexes, appear. Although poorly understood, it is postulated that N2 sleep is most significant for the performance of procedural memory tasks, which include simple motor skills.
- *Stage N3*, or slow-wave sleep, represents the deepest stage of sleep. The term *slow wave* refers to delta waves (characterized by low frequency and high amplitude) on the EEG. Individuals are typically difficult to arouse during stage N3 sleep. Sleepwalking, night terrors, and bedwetting occur during this stage. Healthy adults spend 10–20% of total sleep time in N3 sleep, and this stage is the most critical for restoration and energy conservation.

REM Sleep

REM sleep is a state characterized by rapid eye movements. This stage most closely approximates the brain's EEG patterns associated with wakefulness. Patients have low muscle tone on EMG and low voltage, mixed pattern activity on EEG. This sleep state is associated with vivid emotional dreaming (though dream mentation can occur in NREM sleep). Healthy adults spend about 20–25% of total sleep time in REM sleep. It is worth noting that some medications can suppress REM sleep, and many psychiatric disorders impact REM sleep (Morrison, 2013). In adults, there are four to six sequential cycles in a full night's sleep. A cycle goes through N1, N2, N3, and REM with each cycle lasting approximately 90 minutes.

FUNCTIONS OF SLEEP

Physical Restoration

Despite ongoing research, there remains a paucity of evidence confirming the mechanisms by which sleep aids in growth and repair. A better paradigm would be to look at the evidence indicating deleterious effects on the body after short-term and long-term sleep deprivation. Studies have shown that chronically restricting sleep below optimum levels results in metabolic, endocrine, and immune dysregulation. Poor sleep is associated with increased appetite, weight gain, elevated blood pressure, and increased susceptibility to infections via an attenuated early immune response and poorer defense against oxidative stress (Weitzman et al., 1974)

Memory and Learning

Suboptimal sleep hampers memory formation. This can be extrapolated to say that sleep aids in memory formation, although, once again, the precise mechanism remains unclear (Belenky et al., 2003). What is particularly fascinating is that Goldstein and Walker (2014) concluded that sufficient sleep also removes the emotional aspect (particularly negatively-valenced

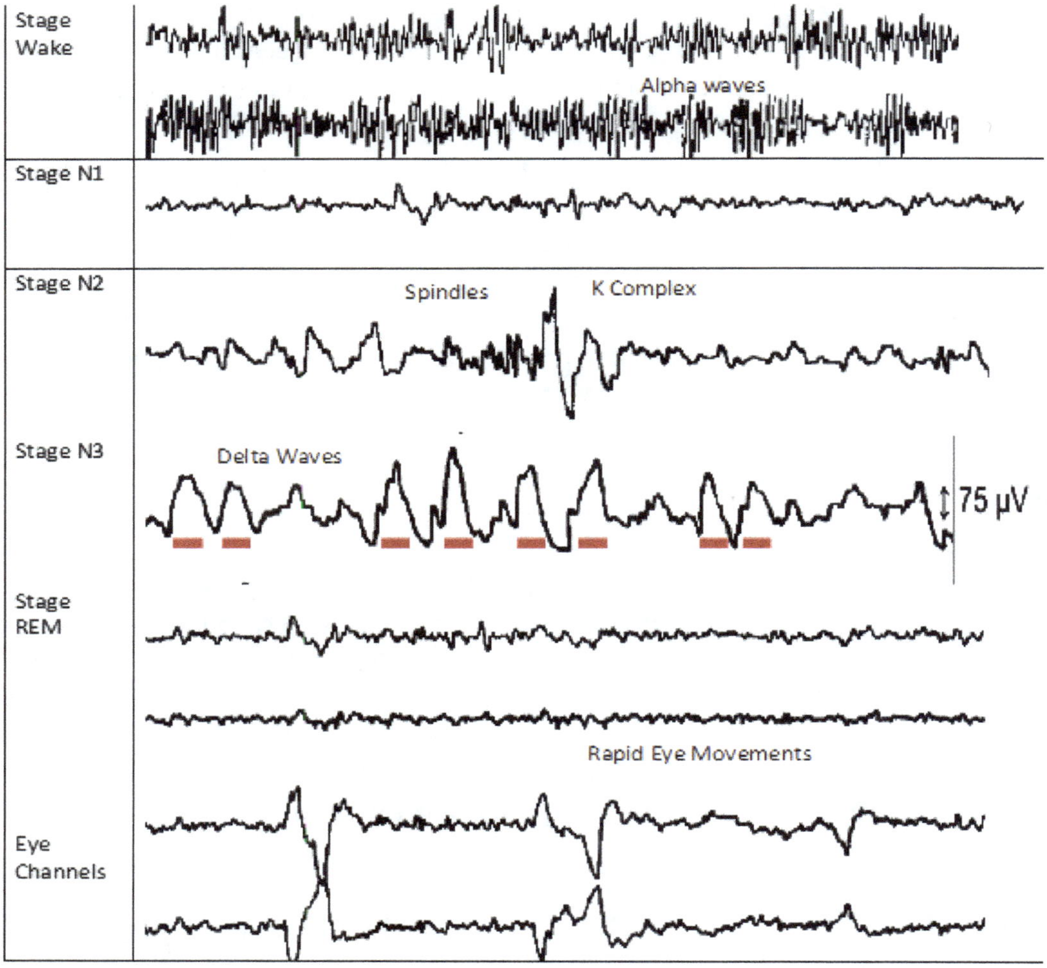

FIGURE 26.1 EEG waveforms in various sleep stages.

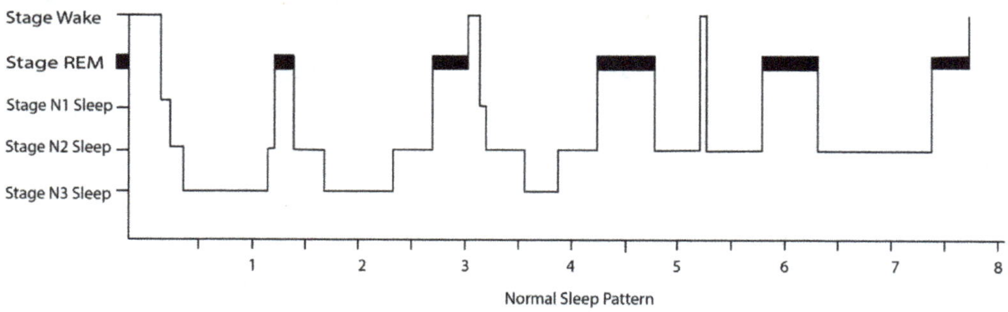

FIGURE 26.2 Hypnogram showing the passage through various sleep stages over the course of a night. Portions marked in black indicate REM sleep.

emotions) from memory. This depotentiates recall of traumatic memory over time in those with good sleep hygiene. It follows logically that individuals with chronic insomnia are less likely to forget the distressful emotions associated with certain memories. This is most evident in PTSD.

The theory that sleep serves as a time of neurogenesis—or restoration of local brain cells that have been active during periods of wakefulness—is gaining traction. Research over the last few decades has shown that new neurons are generated in selected areas of the adult mammalian brain. The function of these adult-born neurons is debatable. It is suggested that integration of new cells into the existing neuronal circuitry may be involved in memory processes and the regulation of emotions (Meerlo et al., 2009).

Neurocognitive Performance

Neurocognitive performance is impaired when sleep is restricted to suboptimal levels. Additionally, sleep deprivation demonstrates a dose response to performance impairment. That is to say, the more sleep we lose, the worse our objective performance is (Banks & Dinges, 2007). Sleep debt is cumulative. Interestingly, when Belenky et al. (2003) tested this, they found that the test subject's subjective perception of their sleep deprivation did not correlate with objective performance. More simply put, the test subjects were not able to successfully gauge how much sleep deprivation was affecting their ability to perform. This is an interesting manifestation of the Dunning–Kruger effect—our propensity to systematically overestimate our competence (in the context of sleep deprivation).

SLEEP REQUIREMENTS AND SLEEP DEBT

A discussion on the functions of sleep and the deleterious effects of sleep deprivation would be remiss without defining the parameters of optimal and suboptimal sleep and what constitutes sleep debt. The National Sleep Foundation recommends that, for healthy individuals without a sleep disorder, the appropriate sleep duration is 9–11 hours for school-aged children, 8–10 hours for teenagers, 7–9 hours for young adults, and 7–8 hours for older adults (Hirshkowitz et al., 2015). Sleep debt or deficit is the cumulative effect of not getting enough sleep. There are two types of sleep debt:

- *Total sleep debt*—results from being awake for 24 hours or more
- *Partial sleep debt*—not getting enough sleep (required for one's particular age group) over a specified period

KEY POINT

Chronically restricting sleep below optimum levels results in metabolic, endocrine, and immune dysregulation. Poor sleep is associated with increased appetite, weight gain, elevated blood pressure, and increased susceptibility to infections via an attenuated early immune response and poorer defense against oxidative stress.

QUICK POINT

Suboptimal sleep hampers memory formation. This can be extrapolated to say that sleep aids in memory formation, although the precise mechanism remains unclear (Belenky et al., 2003). The theory that sleep serves as a time of neurogenesis—or restoration of local brain cells that have been active during periods of wakefulness—is gaining traction.

KEY POINT

Neurocognitive performance is impaired when sleep is restricted to suboptimal levels. Additionally, sleep deprivation demonstrates a dose response to performance impairment. Simply put, the more sleep we lose, the worse our objective performance is.

TABLE 26.1 Recommended Sleep Times by Age

Age	Recommended amount of sleep (hours a day)
Newborns (0–3 months)	14–17
Infants (4–11 years)	12–15
Toddlers (1–2 years)	11–14
Preschoolers (3–5 years)	10–13
School-aged children (6–13 years)	10–11
Teenagers (14–17 years)	8–10
Young adults (18–25)	7–9
Adults (26–64)	7–9
Elderly adults (65+)	7–8

Adapted from Singh, 2021.

COMMON SLEEP DISORDERS

Sleep disorders are ubiquitous and carry a significant burden on society. As we illustrated earlier in this chapter, sleep is crucial for optimum performance, and, consequently, the repercussions of insufficient quality and quantity of sleep on our functionality are severe. Letting these disorders go undiagnosed and untreated can have a significant impact on the well-being of our patients. Most sleep disorders are treatable, and it is imperative that they be screened for in primary and mental health care settings.

Sleep-Related Breathing Disorders

The *DSM-5* recognizes three sleep-related breathing disorders: obstructive sleep apnea (OSA), central sleep apnea, and sleep-related hypoventilation (APA, 2013; Table 26.2).

OSA is estimated to be prevalent in 4% of adult men and 2% of adult women in the United States. Many overlapping symptoms with depression are increasingly recognized as an independent risk factor for hypertension and cardiovascular disease. Clinicians must remain vigilant in identifying patients with a constellation of symptoms consistent with OSA. OSA is a condition in which a person (generally, an obese person who snores loudly) frequently stops breathing for 10 seconds or more (apnea) or has shallow breathing (reduced airflow by ⩾ 30% for 10 seconds or more, which is accompanied by oxygen desaturation of ⩾ 4% [hypopnea]; Khawaja, S., 2015). This occurs due to obstruction of the upper (oropharyngeal) airway during sleep when there is a reduced motor tone of the pharyngeal muscles. OSA's *DSM-5* criteria require polysomnographic evidence of at least five obstructive apnea or hypopneas per hour of sleep accompanied by daytime sleepiness, fatigue, or unrefreshing sleep despite adequate

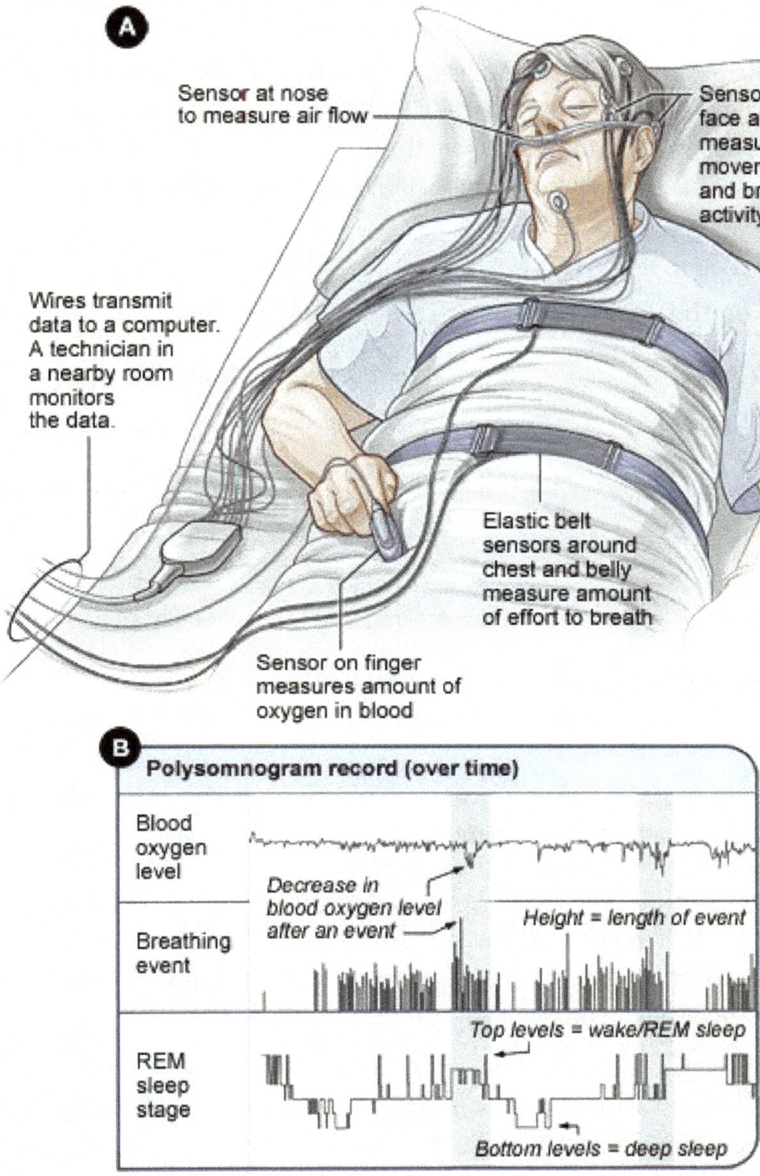

FIGURES 26.3A AND B The illustration shows a patient with the standard setup for a polysomnogram (sleep study). In figure a, the patient lies in a bed with sensors attached to the body. In figure b, the polysomnogram recording shows blood oxygen levels, breathing events, and REM sleep stage over time.

Source: https://commons.wikimedia.org/wiki/File:Sleep_studies.jpg.
Source: https://commons.wikimedia.org/wiki/File:Sleep_studies.jpg.

opportunities to sleep that are not better explained by a mental disorder or any other sleep disorder. Most treatments for OSA are designed to keep the upper airway open during sleep.

QUICK POINT

OSA is estimated to be prevalent in 4% of adult men and 2% of adult women in the United States. Many overlapping symptoms with depression are increasingly recognized as an independent risk factor for hypertension and cardiovascular disease.

Weight loss is typically helpful because it reduces the severity of the disease. Continuous positive airway pressure (CPAP) treatments are the mainstay of therapy for moderate to severe OSA as well as mild cases accompanied by daytime somnolence (Khawaja, 2015). Upper airway surgery has also shown good results in those in whom the primary cause of airway obstruction is a definitive craniofacial abnormality or upper airway obstruction.

TABLE 26.2 Obstructive Sleep Apnea: An Update for Mental Health Providers

Apnea	Cessation of airflow for ⩾ 10 seconds
Hypopnea	Reduction of airflow with resultant oxygen desaturation of ⩾ 4%
Apnea hypopnea index	Average frequency of apnea and hypopnea events per hour of sleep
Obstructive sleep apnea	AHI of ⩾ 15 or ⩾ 5 associated symptoms, such as excessive daytime sleepiness, impaired cognition, mood disorders, insomnia, hypertension, heart disease, or history of stroke
Central sleep apnea	AHI of ⩾ 5 with ⩾ 50% of the respiratory events occurring without any inspiratory effort—associated with symptoms of either excessive daytime sleepiness or disrupted sleep

Adapted from Khawaja and Hasmi, 2015.

Central sleep apnea is defined as the repetitive cessation of airflow during sleep due to reduced or lost ventilatory effort. Diagnosis requires cessation of respirations and ventilatory effort lasting at least 10 seconds on polysomnography.

QUICK POINT

Central apneas are present during NREM sleep and tend to resolve during REM sleep. Central sleep apneas are present in 25–40% of individuals with heart failure and 10% of stroke patients.

Central apneas are present during NREM sleep and tend to resolve during REM sleep. Central sleep apneas are present in 25–40% of individuals with heart failure and 10% of stroke patients. Primary central sleep apneas of unknown origin are rare. It is intuitive, then, that this condition's therapy is individualized, and the first step in management is treating the underlying condition.

Hypoventilation syndromes are marked by oxygen desaturation and elevated PaCO2 during sleep. The mechanisms responsible for the sleep-related increase in PaCO2 are myriad and include reduced minute ventilation, reduced tidal volume, suboptimal ventilation-perfusion relationships, and diminished respiratory load responsiveness. Once again, specific, individualized treatment, hand in hand with ventilatory assistance, is the mainstay of care.

Narcolepsy

The prevalence of narcolepsy (with or without cataplexy) is approximately 0.04%. The pentad of symptoms associated with narcolepsy include the following:

a. *Excessive daytime sleepiness*—Sleepiness during the day is considered excessive when it is subjectively severe and impacts daytime functioning. It can present as the inability to stay awake during the day and often unintentionally falling asleep. The latter is known as an irresistible sleep attack.

b. *Disturbed nighttime sleep*—Patients with narcolepsy have fragmented sleep architecture, particularly during REM sleep.

c. *Sleep paralysis*—This is defined as the complete inability to move for one or two minutes immediately after awakening.

d. *Hypnagogic/hypnopompic hallucinations*—Hallucinations are a sensory experience perceived in the absence of stimuli (e.g., hearing voices or seeing images that no one else can see). Experiencing hallucinations just before falling asleep (termed *hypnagogic*) or just before waking up (termed *hypnopompic*) is present in some patients with narcolepsy.

e. *Cataplexy*—This is the loss of muscle tone in response to a strong emotional stimulus (e.g., laughter, joy, or anger).

Beyond this pentad, several other conditions are associated with narcolepsy, including REM sleep behavior disorder, periodic limb movements, and sleep-disordered breathing. Age of symptom onset can occur from early childhood to late adulthood with a bimodal distribution occurring between 15 and 35 years. Most patients with narcolepsy have shown a decrease in the hypocretin (orexin) signaling in the lateral hypothalamus and CSF.

Treatment options for narcolepsy usually include education and behavioral modification. Stimulant medications, such as modafinil, armodafinil (the active R-enantiomer of modafinil), and more potent stimulants, such as methylphenidate amphetamines, have also shown strong results. A useful behavioral modification is regularizing sleep and scheduling naps one to three times a day. Moreover, it is essential to discuss avoiding jobs or activities in which sleep and alertness are priorities, such as jobs where shift work or significant driving are required.

The stimulant medications primarily act by increasing dopamine availability at the synaptic level to promote wakefulness. Modafinil and

MEMORY TIP

Hallucinations can occur in the interface between sleep and wake.

- Hypna**G**ogic hallucinations occur when a person is **G**oing to sleep.
- Hypno**P**ompic hallucinations occur when a person is waking up or **P**opping up from sleep.

armodafinil may also increase the availability of other monoamines and histamine, which may contribute to wakefulness-promoting properties. For cataplexy and other REM intrusion phenomena, treatments usually involve REM-suppressing medications that block the reuptake of serotonin and norepinephrine preferentially, such as serotonin–norepinephrine reuptake inhibitors or other tricyclic antidepressants with comparable activity. Selective serotonin reuptake inhibitors (SSRIs) with adrenergic activity, such as fluoxetine, have also been shown to be beneficial.

Restless Legs Syndrome (RLS)

Restless leg syndrome (RLS), also known as Willis–Ekbom disease (WED), is characterized by discomfort in the extremities and an urge to move. URGE (urge to move, rest-induced, gets better with activity, and evening and night worsening) is a helpful mnemonic (Figure 26.4).

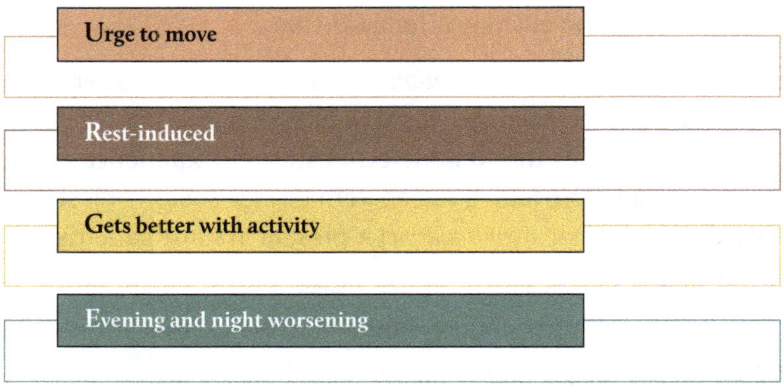

FIGURE 26.4 URGE: mnemonic for restless leg syndrome.

TABLE 26.3 Medications Used in Treating RLS

Medication class	Examples	Additional information
Anticonvulsants	Gabapentin, pregabalin, and gabapentin enacarbil	Gabapentin enacarbil is FDA approved for RLS
Benzodiazepines and benzodiazepine receptor agonists	Eszopilone, temazepam, zalephon, and zolpiderm	Not FDA approved
Ergot-derived dopaminergic agents	Pergolide and cabergoline	Pergolide (withdrawn from U.S. market due to risk of causing cardiac valvulopathy)
Iron supplements	Ferrous sulphate	May be useful in patients with low iron levels
Nonergot-derived dopaminergic agents	Levodopa, pramiprexole, ropinirole, and rotigotine	FDA approved
Opioids and opioid receptor agonists	Codeine, tramadol, and methadone	Potential for abuse present

It is present in 3–15% of the population with an increased likelihood in older patients, pregnant women, and individuals with anemia or uremia. The diagnosis is based on clinical history. RLS/WED is commonly comorbid with other psychiatric diagnoses, and psychotropic medications can affect RLS/WED symptomatology. Medications used in treatment of RLS are in Table 26.3.

Insomnia

Insomnia is the most prevalent of all sleep disorders with 30–50% of the population suffering from occasional insomnia and 10–30% suffering from chronic insomnia.

> **QUICK POINT**
>
> Insomnia is the most prevalent of all sleep disorders with 30–50% of the population suffering from occasional insomnia and 10–30% suffering from chronic insomnia.

It is characterized by either difficulty initiating sleep with a latency of 30 minutes or longer (sleep-onset insomnia), maintaining sleep (sleep-maintenance insomnia), early awakenings (terminal insomnia), or total sleep time less than 6 hours. All of these occur in the setting of adequate opportunity, condition, and time to sleep. It is associated with impairment of daytime function and increases the likelihood of accidents and the risk of developing comorbid psychiatric illnesses and leads to overall functional decline and diminished quality of life.

There are three main approaches to insomnia: institutionalizing strong sleep hygiene, cognitive behavioral therapy for insomnia (CBT-I), and hypnotic medications. The selection of a treatment approach should be made in collaboration with the patient. Some patients prefer to avoid medications, while others cannot make the time commitment or tolerate the temporarily increased fatigue required for CBT-I.

> **CLINICAL TIP**
>
> There are three main approaches to insomnia: institutionalizing strong sleep hygiene, cognitive behavioral therapy for insomnia (CBT-I), and hypnotic medications.

Medications approved by the FDA for insomnia treatment include several classes, including benzodiazepines and benzodiazepines receptor agonists (nonbenzodiazepines) in addition to other classes of drugs. These medications should be used cautiously as they increase the risk of falls, memory problems, and sleepwalking. CBT-I is considered the first line of treatment when available. Clinicians should use a shared decision-making approach, including discussing the benefits and harms of short-term use of medications for patients when CBT-I alone is not sufficient.

SUMMARY

The quest, initiated by the Greeks, to understand the central function of sleep continues to this day. Many theories elucidating the importance of sleep—many of which focus on the structural and neurobiological impacts of its deprivation—exist. Yet, the more we understand this complex evolutionary mechanism, the more we realize how much we have yet to discover. The definitive function of sleep and the determinants that affect the architecture and duration of sleep–wake cycles have yet to be uncovered. However, amid all this ambiguity, two things remain clear: deepening our understanding of sleep order and disorder is of paramount importance, and reducing the burden of common sleep disorders will go a long way in making us a more prosperous and productive society.

RESOURCES

1 Sleep Foundation

2 NHLBI Publications and Resources | NHLBI, NIH

3 American Sleep Association: Insomnia Sleep Apnea Narcolepsy & Snoring

REFERENCES

American Psychiatric Association. (2013). *Diagnostic and statistical manual of mental disorders* (5th ed.).

Banks, S., & Dinges, D. F. (2007). Behavioral and physiological consequences of sleep restriction. *Journal of Clinical Sleep Medicine, 3*(5), 519–528.

Beare, A. , 2014. *On sleep and sleeplessness*. http://classics.mit.edu/Aristotle/sleep.html

Belenky, G., Wesensten, N. J., Thorne, D. R., Thomas, M. L., Sing, H. C., Redmond, D. P., Russo, M. B., & Balkin, T. J. (2003). Patterns of performance degradation and restoration during sleep restriction and subsequent recovery: A sleep dose-response study. *Journal of Sleep Research, 12*(1), 1–12. https://doi.org/10.1046/j.1365-2869.2003.00337.x

Goldstein, A. N., & Walker, M. P. (2014). The role of sleep in emotional brain function. *Annual Review of Clinical Psychology,10*, 679–708. https://doi.org/10.1146/annurev-clinpsy-032813-153716

Hirshkowitz, M., Whiton, K., Albert, S. M., Alessi, C., Bruni, O., DonCarlos, L., Hazen, N., Herman, J., Katz, E. S., Kheirandish-Gozal, L., Neubauer, D. N., O'Donnell, A. E., Ohayon, M., Peever, J., Rawding, R., Sachdeva, R. C., Setters, B., Vitiello, M. V., Ware, J. C., & Adams Hillard, P. J. (2015). National Sleep Foundation's sleep time duration recommendations: methodology and results summary. *Sleep Health, 1*(1), 40–43. https://doi.org/10.1016/j.sleh.2014.12.010

Khawaja, I. S., Hashmi, A. E., Ebrahim, A., Ullevig, C., Shah, A., Hurwitz, T.D. (2015). *Psychiatric Annals, 1*(45).

Meerlo, P., Mistlberger, R. E., Jacobs, B. L., Heller, H. C., & McGinty, D. (2009). New neurons in the adult brain: The role of sleep and consequences of sleep loss. *Sleep Medicine Reviews, 13*(3), 187–194. https://doi.org/10.1016/j.smrv.2008.07.004

Morrison, A. R. (2013). Coming to grips with a "new" state of consciousness: The study of rapid-eye-movement sleep in the 1960s. *Journal of the History of the Neurosciences, 22*(4), 392–407. https://doi.org/10.1080/0964704x.2013.777230

Rechtschaffen A., Hunt, W. A. (Ed.). (1971). *The control of sleep*. Shenkman.

Weitzman, E. D., Nogeire, C., Perlow, M., Fukushima, D., Sassin, J., McGregor, P., & Hellman, L. (1974). Effects of a prolonged 3-hour sleep-wake cycle on sleep stages, plasma cortisol, growth hormone and body temperature in man. *J Clin Endocrinol Metab, 38*(6), 1018–1030. https://doi.org/10.1210/jcem-38-6-1018

CHAPTER 27

Delirium and Dementia[1]

Jose Ribas Roca, M.D.; Carla Benjjani, M.D.;

Lubna Khawaja, B.S., M.D.; and Asim Shah, M.D.

> *"The existence of forgetting has never been proven. We only know that some things do not come to our mind when we want them to."*
>
> — Friedrich Nietzsche

OBJECTIVES

At the end of this chapter, students will be able to do the following:

- review presentation and management of delirium
- review types and management of dementia
- distinguish between delirium and dementia

CASE VIGNETTE

Ms. K is an 85-year-old female who has a history of diabetes and hypertension and was diagnosed with dementia 2 years ago. She moved to an assisted living facility after a small fire at home caused by her leaving the stove on. She enjoys talking to other residents there and playing cards each afternoon. She is able to recognize family when they visit her about once per month but struggles with the names of her grandkids. The staff at her assisted living facility (ALF) sent her to the emergency room due to bizarre behavior. She started having conversations with her husband, who is long deceased, and complaining about spiders and snakes in her room at night. Her initial workup revealed a normal CBC, sodium of 131, glucose of 289, and urinalysis of 15 WBC per HPF and + leukocyte esterase. A diagnosis of delirium secondary to urinary tract infection (UTI) was made. She was

(continued)

1 Readers may also see "Geriatric Mental Health" (Chapter 40) for related material.

admitted for treatment with antibiotics, correction of her hyponatremia, and management of her elevated blood sugars. On her first night at the hospital, she became combative, accusing staff of trying to poison her with pills and trying to climb out of bed to leave the hospital. Her agitation was controlled with one dose of haloperidol (1 mg) with good results. The following day she could not remember any agitation the previous night, and she continued to comply with treatment for her UTI. She was discharged back to her ALF 2 days later with oral antibiotics.

DEFINITIONS AND KEY CONCEPTS

QUICK POINT

The *DSM-5* replaced the term *dementia* with "major neurocognitive disorder" (APA, 2013). This allowed the distinction from mild neurocognitive disorder (MCI), where individuals retain the ability to live independently.

Delirium is a clinical syndrome characterized by an acute onset of disturbance in attention, awareness, and cognition that fluctuates in severity throughout the day. The official definition in the *Diagnostic and Statistical Manual of Mental Disorders*, 5th edition (*DSM-5*; APA, 2013) also requires evidence of an underlying organic cause or causes.

Dementia is a syndrome in which there is a progressive deterioration in memory, thinking, behavior, and the ability to perform everyday activities. The decline in cognitive domains, including memory, language, and executive function must be severe enough to interfere with independent living. The *DSM-5* replaced the term *dementia* with "major neurocognitive disorder" (APA, 2013). This allowed the distinction from mild neurocognitive disorder (MCI), where individuals retain the ability to live independently. Notably, 5–10% of patients with MCI progress toward dementia each year.

INTRODUCTION

KEY POINT

Delirium is a significant driver of morbidity and mortality in the elderly, while dementia is a major cause of disability and dependency among the older population. The impact on caregivers, family, and society at large can be physical, psychological, social, and economic.

Delirium and dementia are an evolving public health challenge. Delirium is a significant driver of morbidity and mortality in the elderly, while dementia is a major cause of disability and dependency among the older population. The impact on caregivers, family, and society at large can be physical, psychological, social, and economic. Dementia is often mistakenly seen as an inevitable part of aging, rather than a disease process, resulting in barriers to diagnosis and care.

EPIDEMIOLOGY

Delirium can affect people of all ages but occurs more commonly in older persons. The prevalence of delirium varies widely by setting; its prevalence is 10%–15% among older adults in the emergency department and up to

50%–70% in intensive care units. The annual cost of delirium is estimated to be more than $164 billion annually in the United States alone (Oh et al., 2017).

Every three seconds, someone in the world develops dementia. In 2020, there were over 50 million people worldwide living with dementia, and it is expected that 152 million people will have dementia in 2050.

The main risk factor associated with dementia is age with prevalence doubling every five years after age 65. The annual global cost of dementia is now greater than 1 trillion USD. This includes unpaid care provided by family members, the costs of social care in the community and residential care settings, and the cost of medical care (Alzheimer's Disease International, n.d.).

Distinguishing between delirium and dementia is essential to providing effective treatment. When compared to patients who have no dementia, older adults who have dementia visit the ER more often, their visits are longer, and they are more frequently admitted to the hospital. Patients with dementia have higher numbers of comorbidities, receive more testing and interventions, have higher bills, and are more like to return to the ER (Inouye et al., 2014; Marcantonio, 2017). Patients with dementia are at high risk for developing delirium and all its attendant complications. Distinguishing features between dementia and delirium of both conditions are listed in Table 27.1.

KEY POINT

Dementia and delirium dementia are the most prevalent psychiatric illnesses in the elderly.

QUICK POINT

Every three seconds, someone in the world develops dementia. The main risk factor associated with dementia is age with prevalence doubling every five years after age 65. In 2020, there were over 50 million people worldwide living with dementia, and it is expected that 152 million people will have dementia in 2050.

TABLE 27.1 Differences Between Delirium and Dementia

	Delirium	Dementia
Age	Any	Late adulthood to elderly population
Onset	Sudden	Gradual
Vital signs	Fluctuate in some etiologies	Steady
Course	Rapid fluctuation of symptoms	Steady decline
Diurnal variation	Fluctuates through the day	Steady
Alertness and consciousness	Disturbed	Generally intact
Attention	Impaired	Generally intact until later stages
Memory	Poor working, immediate, and short-term memory	Poor short- to long-term memory
Delusions	Acute and fluctuating	More fixed and gradual
Sleep disturbance	Fragmented sleep–wake pattern; circadian rhythm is disrupted	Sleep–wake diurnal pattern changes
Outcome of treatment	Typically, completely resolves once underlying cause(s) are addressed	Treatments may slow progression or target behavioral symptoms

DELIRIUM

Neuropathology

> **CLINICAL TIP**
>
> Delirium is rarely caused by a single factor. Its occurrence depends on the relationship between patient vulnerability (predisposing factors) and exposure to noxious insults (precipitating factor).

Delirium is rarely caused by a single factor. Its occurrence depends on the relationship between patient vulnerability (predisposing factors; see Table 27.1) and exposure to noxious insults (precipitating factors; see Table 27.2). Thus, in a patient with underlying dementia and multiple chronic medical conditions, a relatively benign experience —such as a single dose of an over-the-counter (OTC) anticholinergic medication—may be enough to precipitate delirium. Conversely, in a young healthy patient, delirium will develop only after exposure to a series of noxious insults, such as severe illness, ICU stay, and multiple sedative medications. The fact that diverse etiologies share a similar clinical presentation raises the possibility of a final common pathway for delirium. This theorized pathway includes an acetylcholine deficiency and relative dopamine excess. These abnormalities account for deficits in attention and the emergence of hallucinations, respectively (Francis & Young, n.d.; Inouye et al., 2014; Marcantonio, 2017).

> **MEMORY TIP**
>
> ***Delirium***, *useful mnemonic*
>
> **DELIRIUM**
> **D**— Drugs
> **E**— Electrolyte disturbances
> **L**— Lack of drugs
> **I**— Infections
> **R**— Reduced sensory input
> **I**— Intracranial disorders
> **U**— Urinary and fecal disorders
> **M**—Myocardial and pulmonary disorders

TABLE 27.2 Delirium: Predisposing Factors

Older age (> 65 yrs)
Dementia or preexisting cognitive impairment
Functional impairment
Sensory impairment (e.g., visual and auditory)
History of delirium
History of transient ischemic attack or stroke
Severe illnesses' multiple comorbidities
Alcohol use

Clinical Manifestations

> **CLINICAL TIP**
>
> Key features of delirium include a disturbance of attention and consciousness. This typically develops within a short time and tends to fluctuate throughout the day. There is a change in the level of awareness and the ability to focus, sustain, or shift attention.

Delirium is generally transient. Key features of delirium include a disturbance of attention and consciousness. This typically develops within a short time and tends to fluctuate throughout the day. There is a change in the level of awareness and the ability to focus, sustain, or shift attention (APA, 2013). Patients are easily distractable, and their speech may become tangential and disorganized. Sometimes, this change in mental clarity may be subtle and may precede the more apparent signs of delirium by up to a day or more. Thus, when family members or caregivers say that the patient "isn't

TABLE 27.3 Delirium: Precipitating Factors

Medications
• Polypharmacy
• Sedative-hypnotics (e.g., narcotics and benzodiazepines)
• Psychoactive medications (e.g., antiemetics, antiepileptics, muscle relaxants, antihistamines, and tricyclic antidepressants)
• Steroids
• Anticholinergic medications
• Fluoroquinolones
Infections
• Urinary tract infections, pneumonia, sepsis
Metabolic/physiologic
• Electrolyte abnormalities (e.g., hypo-/hypernatremia, hypercalcemia, hypoglycemia, or metabolic acidosis)
• Endocrine abnormalities (e.g., hypo-/hyperthyroidism or hypercortisolism)
• Hepatic encephalopathy (e.g., hyperammonemia)
• Uremic encephalopathy (e.g., elevated BUN or creatinine)
• Dehydration or hyperthermia (e.g., neuroleptic malignant syndrome or serotonin syndrome)
• Hypertensive emergency, hypotension, or shock
• Hypoxemia or hypercapnea
Toxins/Drugs
• Intoxication (e.g., recreational or prescription drugs—use or overdose)
• Substance withdrawal (e.g., alcohol, benzodiazepines, or opioids)
Intracranial pathology
• Intracranial bleed
• TIA or stroke
• Meningitis or encephalitis
• Increased intracranial pressure
• Seizures (post ictal) or nonconvulsant status epilepticus
• Traumatic brain injury
Environmental
• Hospitalization, ICU admission, major surgery, or anesthesia
• Disturbance of sleep—wake cycle
• Immobility/physical restraints
Elimination
• Urinary or fecal incontinence
• Vomiting or diarrhea

quite acting right," the vigilant clinician should take these seriously, even if delirium is not evident on their exam.

Patients can appear withdrawn, less active, tired, drowsy, or lethargic. This hypoactive form of delirium is more common in the elderly, and subtle forms are easy to miss or mistake for depression. The hyperactive form presents with hypervigilance, insomnia, and agitation. This form is often accompanied by hallucinations and is more easily recognized by family and clinicians. It is commonly seen in cases of alcohol or sedative withdrawal.

Cognitive changes that often accompany delirium include memory loss, disorientation, difficulty with language and speech, and perceptual disturbances. Patients may misidentify persons and objects in their surroundings. They may have visual and auditory hallucinations, usually with a lack of insight. Hallucinations may be simple (e.g, shadows, vague shapes, or simple noises) or more complex (e.g., people, faces, or conversations). Delusions, including those persecutory or grandiose in nature, can be present. Other features include psychomotor agitation or retardation, sleep–wake reversals, irritability, anxiety, and emotional lability.

Delirium develops over hours to days. The acuteness of the presentation is the most helpful feature in differentiating delirium from dementia. Additionally, the features of delirium fluctuate over time: A hospitalized patient may appear relatively lucid during morning rounds and be more altered in the evening and at night. Another fact worth noting is that older patients with delirium often do not look sick apart from their behavioral change. Delirium may be the only finding suggesting acute illness in these older demented patients. Caregivers should be educated that sudden changes in mental functioning are not expected with most progressive dementias and require prompt medical attention (Francis & Young, n.d.; Inouye et al., 2014; Marcantonio, 2017).

Diagnosis

The two essential aspects to the diagnostic evaluation of delirium are as follows:

1. recognizing the symptoms of the disorder
2. assessing for underlying causes

Clinicians may readily observe behavioral problems or cognitive impairment but may wrongly attribute it to aging, dementia, or other mental disorders. It is sometimes misdiagnosed as psychosis when hallucinations and delusions are present or as depression when the presentation is hypoactive.

Due to the symptoms' fluctuating nature, clinicians need to examine the hospitalized patient at different times throughout the day and be attentive to input from caregivers and staff who can better observe these fluctuations. Clinicians should also establish the patient's baseline mental status, eliciting the timeline of any changes in cognition and consciousness when talking to caregivers, as patients may be too confused to provide this information. Clinicians should avoid assuming that illness, sleep loss, fatigue, or anxiety are causing the changes (Francis & Young, n.d.; Inouye et al., 2014; Marcantonio, 2017).

Bedside observation and exam should focus on physical findings suggesting underlying etiology, such as signs of infection, dehydration, focal neurologic deficits, and alcohol withdrawal. The Confusion Assessment Method (CAM) is the most widely used bedside delirium screening tool with a sensitivity above 94% and a specificity of 90–95% in diagnosing delirium. This test addresses the key features of delirium: disturbances in awareness, cognition, and attention. CAM has also been validated for the intensive care unit (ICU) setting and mechanically ventilated patients (Inouye et al., 1990).

TABLE 27.4 The Confusion and Assessment Method (CAM)

The presence of delirium requires features 1 *and* 2 with either feature 3 or 4
1. Acute change in mental status with a fluctuating course
2. Inattention
3. Disorganized thinking
4. Altered level of consciousness

Once the delirium diagnosis is established, the clinician should search for the underlying cause, remembering that delirium's multiple etiologies can be present in the same patient. The most common causes of delirium include fluid and electrolyte disturbances, infections, drug or alcohol toxicity, withdrawal from alcohol, benzodiazepines, selective serotonin reuptake inhibitors, liver and kidney failure, thyrotoxicosis, low perfusion states, and postoperative state, especially in older adults. Particular attention should be given to the patient's medication list and any recent changes in medications. Drug toxicity accounts for approximately 30% of all cases of delirium. Several commonly used medications have significant anticholinergic effects, which contribute to acetylcholine deficiency underlying in delirium.

CLINICAL TIP

The focus of treatment of delirium is to:

1. identify and address all modifiable risk factors,
2. provide supportive care, and
3. manage symptoms and behavioral disturbances.

Nonpharmacologic interventions are the cornerstone of preventing and managing behavioral problems in delirium (Figure 27.3).

Laboratory tests and imaging should be selected based on history and exam findings. Tests routinely required include a complete blood count, electrolytes, blood urea nitrogen, and creatinine. Liver function tests, urinalysis, urine cultures, chest radiography, and an electrocardiography are also often helpful. Additional tests in select situations include a toxicology screen, arterial blood gas and blood cultures, and, if seizures are suspected, an electroencephalography (EEG). In delirium, EEG typically shows a diffuse generalized slowing of the background rhythm. Cerebral imaging is indicated only when there is concern for head trauma or new focal neurologic deficits. Lumbar puncture with cerebrospinal fluid testing should be undertaken in patients with findings suggestive of meningitis or encephalitis.

Treatment

The focus of treatment of delirium is to:

1. identify and address all modifiable risk factors,
2. provide supportive care, and
3. manage symptoms and behavioral disturbances.

Common treatable conditions are infections, electrolyte and metabolic abnormalities, and offending medications. Supportive care should attend to the patient's hydration and nutrition to prevent constipation and urinary retention and get the patient out of bed and preferably walking. Behavioral problems, such as agitation, anxiety, restlessness, and combative behavior, pose a significant risk to a patient's safety, interfere with care, and are a source of significant distress for patients and their families. It is best to prevent the onset or escalation of behavior problems, as depicted in Figure 27.3. Supportive therapy and psychoeducation may be offered to family members, as they may be particularly distressed from witnessing delirium symptoms in their loved ones.

Nonpharmacologic interventions are the cornerstone of preventing and managing behavioral problems in delirium (Figure 27.3). Interventions include reorientation, maintaining hydration and nutrition, facilitating early mobilization (while preventing falls), and minimizing the use of restraints. Sitters are often required to ensure patient safety, know de-escalation techniques for agitated patients, and avoid restraints. Interventions to improve orientation include clocks/calendars, and sensory deprivation can be reduced by encouraging patients to wear eyeglasses and hearing aids. To address the circadian rhythm dysfunction, the patient's room should remain well-lit during the day and dark at night, and staff should avoid unnecessary vitals checks to allow uninterrupted sleep at night. Polypharmacy should be minimized with special attention toward anticholinergic drugs. Benzodiazepine agents should be avoided as they increase confusion, except in benzodiazepine or alcohol withdrawal, where they are indicated for treatment (Kishi, et al., 2016; Nikooie et al., 2019).

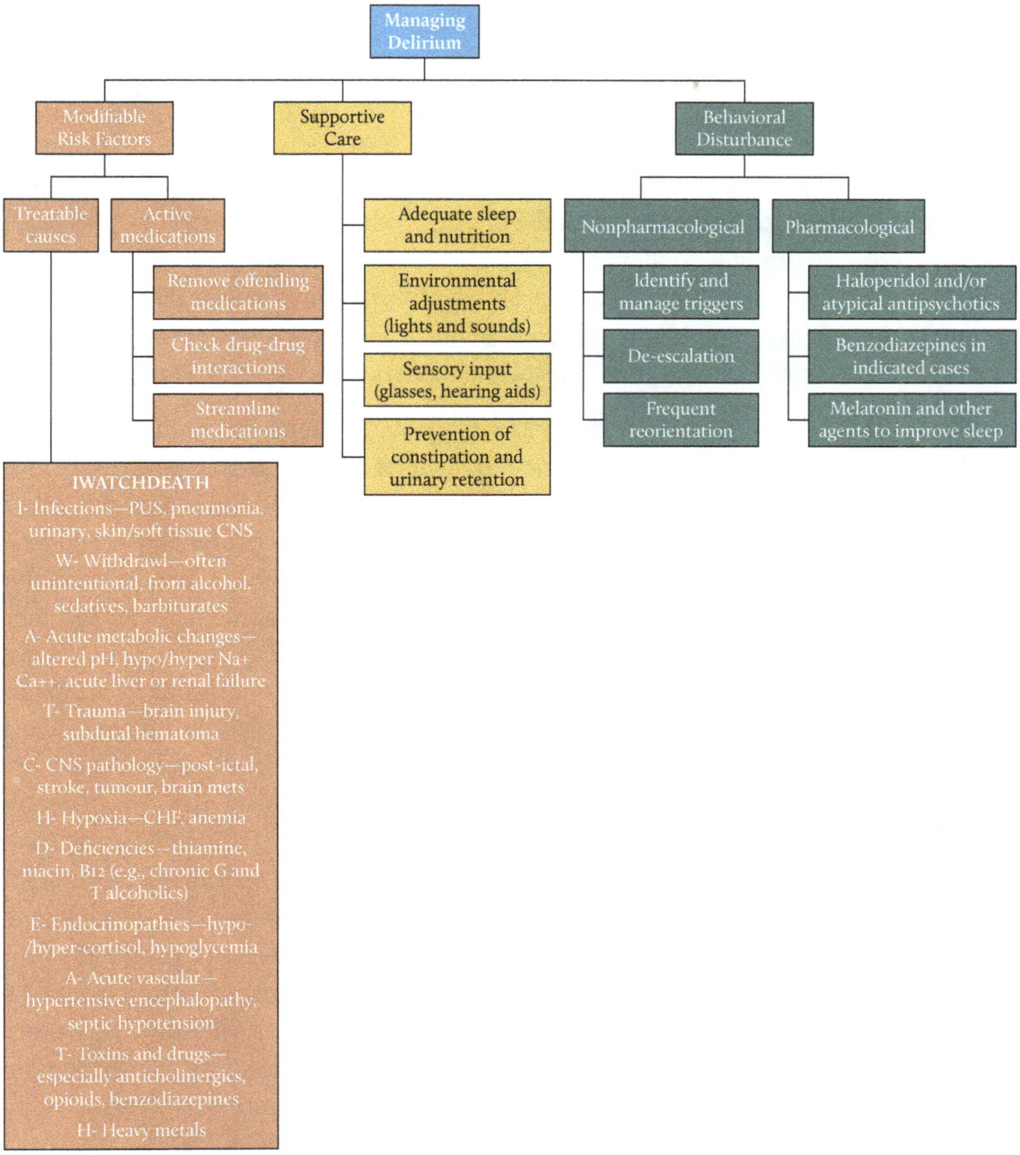

FIGURE 27.1 Overview of management of delirium.

DEMENTIA

The annual rates of progression from MCI to AD were estimated to range from 5% to 10% with higher estimates in clinical than community samples. The prevalence of dementia is higher in women, African American, and Latino populations when compared to White, non-Hispanic populations in the United States. In the United States, the most common subtype of neurocognitive disorder (NCD) is Alzheimer's (43.5%), followed by vascular (14.5%), Lewy

QUICK POINT

The annual rates of progression from MCI to AD were estimated to range from 5% to 10% with higher estimates in clinical than community samples.

body (5.4%), frontotemporal (1.0%), and alcohol-induced (0.7%; Goodman et al., 2017; Figure 27.2).

Neuropathology

Dementia is characterized by the loss of neurons within the gray matter, often due to the accumulation of protein, which damages the neuron. This results in cerebral atrophy, which becomes evident in imaging as narrowing of the gyri, widening of the sulci, and dilation of the ventricles (Figure 27.3). The *DSM-5* describes several types of major NCDs, each with different underlying neuropathology and clinical manifestations (APA, 2013; Figure 27.1).

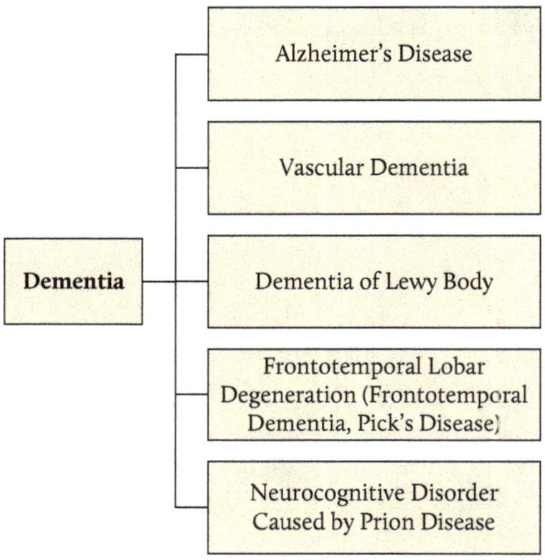

FIGURE 27.2 Types of major neurocognitive disorders.

- *Alzheimer's disease* (AD)—The neuropathologic hallmarks of AD are extracellular accumulation of amyloid plaques (i.e., neuritic plaques) and intracellular accumulation of neurofibrillary tangles (NFTs). The plaques are composed of Aβ peptide and the NFTs of hyperphosphorylated protein-tau (p-tau). These deposits first occur in the hippocampus and then spread to neocortical areas. They lead to loss of synapses and neurons and result in prominent cholinergic deficits. Polymorphisms in the apolipoprotein (APOE) gene affect the amount of Aβ protein deposited in the brain and, as a result, the risk of Alzheimer's disease. The E2 allele is thought to be protective, while the E4 allele accounts for as much as 50% of the attributable genetic risk of suffering this disease. Early-onset familial AD presentations are associated with presenilin 1 and presenilin 2 mutations located in chromosomes 14 and 1, respectively. Patients with Trisomy 21 develop Alzheimer's disease by age 40 because of the additional copy of the amyloid precursor protein (APP) gene located on chromosome 21 (Nowrangi et al., 2011).
- *Vascular dementia*—This is the second most common cause of dementia. It can result from both large and small vessel disease due to hypertension, atherosclerosis, or vasculitis. These pathologies can result in cerebral infarcts, hemorrhages, and chronic progressive white matter disease (Hugo & Ganguli, 2014).
- *Dementia of Lewy body*—These dementias are characterized by intracellular deposits of misfolded alpha-synuclein, referred to as Lewy bodies. Lewy body dementia (LBD or DLB), Parkinson's disease (PD), and Parkinson's disease dementia (PDD) may be linked to the same underlying abnormalities in the brain processing of

KEY POINT

Dementia is characterized by the loss of neurons within the gray matter, often due to the accumulation of protein, which damages the neuron. This results in cerebral atrophy, which becomes evident in imaging as narrowing of the gyri, widening of the sulci, and dilation of the ventricles.

alpha-synuclein. PD is characterized by a degenerative loss of dopaminergic neurons in the substantia nigra of the basal ganglia. PDD is characterized by Lewy bodies in the substantia nigra and develops late in Parkinson's disease (Hugo & Ganguli, 2014).

- *Frontotemporal lobar dementia* (FTD)—FTD is characterized by prominent atrophy and degeneration of cortical and subcortical structures within frontal and temporal regions of the brain. Most FTD cases are caused by intracellular aggregates of hyperphosphorylated tau or ubiquitin protein (Elahi & Miller, 2017; Hugo & Ganguli, 2014).
- *Neurocognitive disorder* (NCD) caused by prion disease—This is caused by the propagation of misfolded prion proteins that are normally expressed in the nervous system. Most cases are sporadic, and the misfolding of this protein occurs spontaneously. Damage to neurons and glial cells is characterized by intracellular vacuoles (spongy degeneration). The most common form is Creutzfeldt-Jakob disease (CJD), which also has a familial form (fCJD) with an autosomal dominant pattern of inheritance. The acquired form of prion disease, variant CJD (vCJD), results from consumption of cattle affected by bovine spongiform encephalopathy (mad cow disease; Elahi & Miller, 2017; Hugo & Ganguli, 2014).

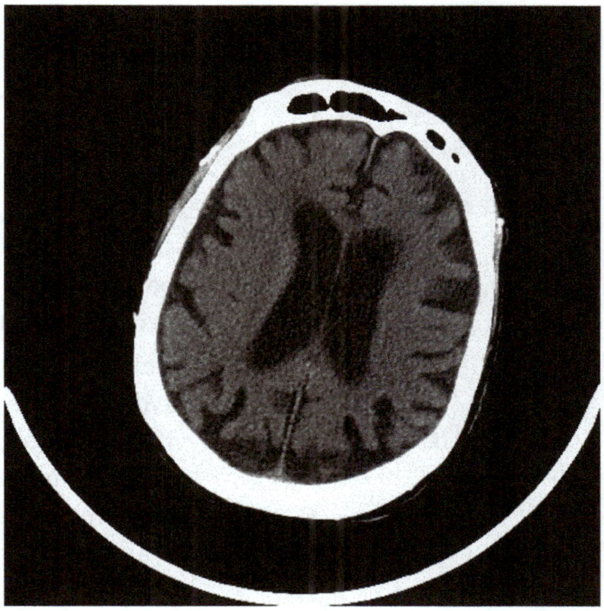

FIGURE 27.3 Noncontrast CT brain shows involutional and chronic ischemic changes: global parenchymal volume loss, enlarged ventricles, and white matter hypoattenuation. Courtesy of Jose Ribas, MD.

KEY POINT

The neuropathologic hallmarks of AD are extracellular accumulation of amyloid plaques (i.e., neuritic plaques) and intracellular accumulation of neurofibrillary tangles (NFTs). The plaques are composed of Aβ peptide and the NFTs of hyperphosphorylated protein-tau (p-tau). These deposits first occur in the hippocampus and then spread to neocortical areas. They lead to loss of synapses and neurons and result in prominent cholinergic deficits.

Clinical Manifestations

Dementia causes a slow but steady decline in neurocognitive functioning. More acute changes can be precipitated by triggers, such as pain, infections, medication side effects, fatigue, change in environment, and any worsening of medical conditions. Behavioral and psychological disturbances (BPSD) occur in five out of every six patients with dementia at some point in their illness. BPSDs, such as depression, agitation, delusions, hallucinations, and apathy, increase caregiver burden and are strong predictors for poor quality of life and nursing home admission (APA, 2013; Elahi & Miller, 2017; Hugo & Ganguli, 2014; Nowrangi, 2011).

CLINICAL TIP

Dementia causes a slow but steady decline in neurocognitive functioning. More acute changes can be precipitated by triggers, such as pain, infections, medication side effects, fatigue, change in environment, and any worsening of medical conditions. Behavioral and psychological disturbances (BPSD) occur in five out of every six patients with dementia at some point in their illness.

CLINICAL TIP

Vascular dementia symptoms vary, depending on the location and size of the stroke. The progression can be in an acute stepwise pattern following each major stroke or show a more gradual pattern in the case of progressive microvascular deterioration.

CLINICAL TIP

Lewy body dementia symptoms include parkinsonism, recurrent visual hallucinations, and fluctuating cognition. In DLB, cognitive impairment occurs before motor symptoms, whereas in Parkinson's disease, the cognitive impairment occurs in the context of established Parkinson's disease.

- Alzheimer's disease is typically diagnosed around age 80 or 90. Presentation is slow and progressive. Short-term memory and the learning of new information are predominantly impaired. It also impacts executive functioning.
- The clinical symptoms of vascular dementia vary, depending on the location and size of the stroke. The progression can be in an acute stepwise pattern following each major stroke or show a more gradual pattern in the case of progressive microvascular deterioration. Executive function is commonly affected.
- Symptoms of LBD usually progress gradually after the age of 60. Core symptoms are parkinsonism, recurrent visual hallucinations, and fluctuating cognition. In DLB, cognitive impairment occurs before motor symptoms, whereas in Parkinson's disease, the cognitive impairment occurs in the context of established Parkinson's disease.
- FTLD is divided into two categories, depending on which group of symptoms is most prominent: The behavioral variant (bvFTD) accounts for 50% of presentations and is characterized by early behavioral disinhibition and socially inappropriate behavior, apathy, loss of empathy, and perseverative or compulsive behavior. The temporal variant, also known as semantic dementia (SD), is characterized by a gradual loss of knowledge and word comprehension but intact verbal fluency, while the progressive nonfluent aphasia subtype (PNFA) presents with early speech impairments, including with loss of fluency, anomia, and agrammatism.
- NCD caused by prion disease is rapidly progressive with a survival of less than a year. It combines rapid cognitive decline and motor symptoms, such as myoclonus and ataxia.

Diagnosis

Dementia is diagnosed when cognitive impairment has become severe enough to compromise social and/or occupational functioning. Once the criteria for major NCD are met, etiologic subtypes can be attributed. Probable and possible categories should also be specified when there is not enough available data to clearly link an etiology to the deficits (e.g., possible Alzheimer's disease in a patient with memory deficits but no evidence of the mutation by genetic testing or family history). It is also important to remember several types of dementia can coexist, such as AD and vascular, and the most common subtype diagnosed in the United States is dementia not otherwise specified (92.9% prevalence; APA, 2013).

According to the *DSM*, the diagnosis of major NCD requires the presence of significant cognitive decline in one or more cognitive domains (e.g., complex attention, executive function, learning and memory, language, perceptual-motor, or social cognition). The decline could be reported by the individual, a knowledgeable informant, or the clinician and should also be demonstrated by a substantially impaired performance on an objective cognitive measure. The cognitive deficits *must* interfere with independence in everyday activities. Neurocognitive testing is the best way to establish a diagnosis. However, a full neuropsychological evaluation should be used to better assess the pattern of cognitive loss in an individual suspected of having FTD and to help rule out psychiatric etiologies for an individual's symptoms. Screening neuropsychological testing takes several hours and is done by a neuropsychologist or sometimes under the direction of a neuropsychology technician. This provides additional supportive evidence for the FTD diagnosis, keeping in mind that some patients perform within normal limits when features are mild. When primary progressive aphasia (PPA) is suspected, a comprehensive evaluation by a speech/language pathologist is warranted. Finally, the deficit should not occur exclusively in the context of delirium. Since underlying dementia is a major vulnerability for the development of delirium, it is not uncommon to find acute delirium superimposed (APA, 2013; Sachdev et al., 2014). Several considerations apply to the diagnosis of dementia, including:

- AD requires a decline in at least two cognitive domains, one of which should be learning and memory. Insidious onset and gradual progression of symptoms increase the diagnostic certainty to probable. Causative mutation is found in *APP, PSEN1,* or *PSEN2* genes. Biomarkers of AD, such as abnormal glucose metabolism and accumulation of amyloid and tau seen in positron emission tomography (PET) are currently used in research but have not been validated for clinical use.
- The diagnosis of probable vascular dementia is made if the clinical syndrome follows a documented cerebrovascular event or enough evidence of cerebrovascular disease to account for the neurocognitive deficits. Evidence may be obtained from history, physical examination, and/or neuroimaging showing white matter changes and lacunar infarcts (APA, 2013).
- Frontotemporal degeneration is probable when a causative genetic mutation or neuroimaging evidence of disproportionate frontal and/or temporal lobe involvement is present. Glucose PET scans (F-FDG PET/CT) can be useful in differentiating FTD from other dementias;

CLINICAL TIP

The clinical symptoms of vascular dementia vary, depending on the location and size of the stroke. The progression can be in an acute stepwise pattern following each major stroke or show a more gradual pattern in the case of progressive microvascular deterioration.

it reveals decreased metabolism in frontal and temporal cortices. A number of causative mutations have been identified in familial cases (*C9ORF72*), and in genes coding for microtubule-associated protein tau (*MAPT*), granulins (*GRN*), TAR DNA-binding protein 43 (*TDP-43*), transitional endoplasmic reticulum ATPase (*VCP*), charged multivesicular body protein 2b (*CHMP2B*), and FUS protein (*FUS*; Elahi & Miller, 2017).

- NCD with Lewy bodies requires at least two core features (fluctuating cognition, recurrent visual hallucinations, and spontaneous parkinsonism occurring at least a year after cognitive decline) or at least one suggestive feature (REM sleep behavior disorder or severe neuroleptic sensitivity) with at least one core feature present. DaTscan, a specific type of photon emission computed tomography (SPECT), helps visualize dopamine transporter levels in the brain. Low dopamine transporter uptake is consistent with PD and PDD diagnosis.
- In prion disease, frequent periodic sharp-wave complexes (1–2 Hz) with occasional triphasic morphology on EEG are supportive of a CJD diagnosis. Classical MRI findings include T2 hyperintensity along the cerebral cortex (cortical ribboning) and hyperintense pulvinar and dorsomedial thalamus (hockey stick sign). CSF biomarkers show high concentration of proteins 14-3-3 and S100 (Elahi & Miller, 2017).

KEY POINT

Creutzfeldt–Jakob disease has characteristic EEG findings, which include frequent periodic sharp-wave complexes (1–2 Hz) with occasional triphasic morphology.

Treatment

There are currently no disease-modifying therapies available for cognitive deficits caused by dementia. Three cholinesterase inhibitors (donepezil, rivastigmine, and galantamine) are approved for use in mild to moderate AD. Donepezil and an NMDA antagonist (memantine) are approved for moderate to severe AD. While not approved by the U.S. Food and Drug Administration (FDA) for this use, cholinesterase inhibitors and memantine could be slightly beneficial in some patients who have vascular dementia. Controlling the underlying pathology of VaD was found to be more helpful for cognitive dysfunction than antipsychotics and cognitive enhancers (Abraha et al., 2017; Dyer et al., 2018; Perng et al., 2018).

QUICK POINT

Three cholinesterase inhibitors (donepezil, rivastigmine, and galantamine) are approved for use in mild to moderate AD. Donepezil and an NMDA antagonist (memantine) are approved for moderate to severe AD.

Anticholinesterase inhibitors remain the treatment of choice for DLB. Rivastigmine has a higher level of evidence (RCT) for safety and effectiveness in treating cognitive and noncognitive symptoms in DLB and PPD. There is currently no cure for prion diseases. Some recent studies suggest that genetically targeted drugs designed to lower the brain's prion protein levels might be promising.

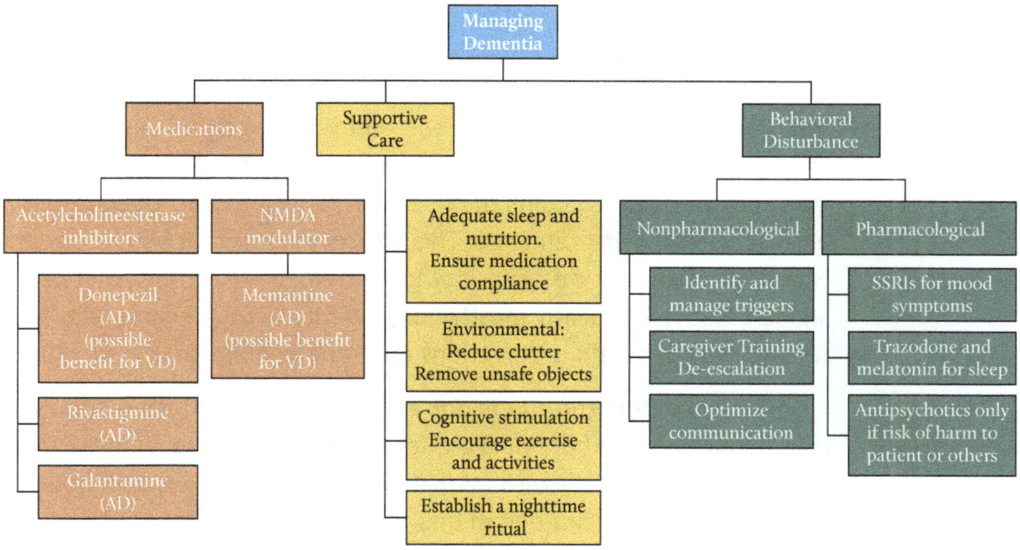

FIGURE 27.4 Overview of management of dementia.

Neuropsychiatric Symptoms (NPS)

Nonpharmacologic treatment should be implemented as first-line management of NPS. When they fail or the NPS are causing severe distress and significant risk to patients or others, pharmacological approaches can be tried (Reus et al., 2016).

Depression is the most common NPS in dementia. The evidence for the use of antidepressants is not robust. A trial of a low-dose SSRI should be attempted, whereas tricyclic antidepressants and other agents with significant anticholinergic effects should be avoided.

> **CLINICAL TIP**
>
> Depression is the most common neuropsychiatric symptom in dementia. The evidence for the use of antidepressants is not robust. A trial of a low-dose SSRI should be attempted, whereas tricyclic antidepressants and other agents with significant anticholinergic effects should be avoided.

When the implementation of sleep hygiene is not sufficient, pharmacologic interventions can be tried. Cholinesterase inhibitors at bedtime can improve sleep latency. If they fail, low-dose trazodone has been shown to be helpful. Melatonin in doses up to 10 mg were not found to be effective (Phan et al., 2019; Ringman & Schneider, 2019). Due to the increased risk of falls and worsening cognition, benzodiazepines and benzodiazepine receptor agonists (zolpidem and zopiclone) should be avoided.

Psychotic symptoms in dementia, such as delusions and hallucinations, do not always require treatment. In cases of DLB, donepezil can improve psychotic symptoms. Psychosis is common in PDD, where dopamine replacement therapy plays a key role in its development. Appropriate management of psychosis should begin with an evaluation of existing PD medications and withdrawal of offending agents when possible. The APA recommends nonemergency antipsychotic medication to be used only for the treatment of agitation or psychosis in patients with dementia when symptoms are severe, are dangerous, and/or cause significant distress to the patient. In April 2005, the FDA issued an advisory and subsequent black-box warning regarding the risks of atypical antipsychotic use among elderly patients with dementia. This advisory warns that elderly patients with dementia-related psychosis who are treated with antipsychotics face an increased risk of death, mostly due to cardiovascular events (e.g., heart failure, sudden death) or infections (e.g., pneumonia; Reus et al., 2016).

CLINICAL TIP

Pharmacologic treatment for aggression and agitation should be considered when the behaviors are severe and attempts to remove triggers have failed.

Pharmacologic treatment for aggression and agitation should be considered when the behaviors are severe and attempts to remove triggers have failed. In patients with milder cognitive impairment and moderate agitation, low-dose citalopram might be potentially beneficial and safe. Antipsychotics can be helpful but should only be tried if there is a risk of harm to patient or others, as discussed. The data for antiepileptic drugs is mixed and limited. Depakote has been shown to have little impact and significant side effects. Carbamazepine might be more beneficial, but a slower titration is recommended. There is little evidence for chronic benzodiazepine use, and it has a clear association with falls and cognitive decline. There is good evidence that cholinesterase inhibitors can reduce apathy and agitation in patients who have dementia. There is no evidence that memantine is a beneficial treatment for agitation in patients with dementia. Trazodone is usually well tolerated, and its sedative effect can be used to treat agitation, whether sundowning or as a PRN for acute agitation (Phan et al., 2019; Reus et al., 2016; Ringman & Schneider, 2019).

Psychotherapy, including cognitive- and emotion-oriented interventions, have been studied. Cognitive stimulation sessions occur in small groups of four to five, are led by trained providers, and include activities, such as word games, puzzles, music, cooking, gardening, and discussing past and present events. Reminiscence therapy aims to help people share and value their experiences by talking about past events and memories. Validation therapy's goal is encouraging the expression of feelings to help patients resolve unfinished conflicts. Video/audiotapes made by family members containing scripted telephone conversations about cherished memories have been used in simulated presence therapy (SPT). Interactive computerized cognitive interventions, such as computer exercises, computer games, mobile devices, gaming consoles, and virtual reality, have not been found to be helpful in enhancing cognitive function (Abraha et al., 2017).

Other Treatments

A systematic review looking at sensory stimulation interventions found music therapy to be the only effective treatment for the reduction of agitation and aggression, and possibly anxiety, in dementia. The effectiveness of aromatherapy and massage therapy is nonconclusive (Livingston et al., 2014).

Behavioral management techniques, including behavioral or cognitive behavioral therapy, functional analysis of specific behavior, individualized behavioral reinforcement strategies, and communication training were studied in a family care setting, assisted living setting, and residential setting. Formal caregiver training and dementia mapping (a formal tool for staff observation of patients) provided in residential care were found to be effective at reducing agitation.

There is some evidence that multicomponent interventions that use a comprehensive, integrated, multidisciplinary approach combining medical, psychiatric, and nursing interventions can reduce severe behavioral problems in nursing home patients. Many nonpharmacological approaches require additional research to enable adequate evidence for the assessment of their effectiveness as alternative treatments.

SUMMARY

Delirium and dementia are the most prevalent psychiatric illnesses in the elderly. There is usually significant overlap in hospital settings, and it is often impossible to clarify the diagnosis without collateral information from family and caregivers. Early detection and management of delirium is crucial for good clinical outcomes. Untreated delirium can lead to complications, which result in loss of function and nursing home placement. Management of dementia focuses on helping patients retain function and independence for as long as possible. As life expectancy has advanced in the past century, the number of older adults is increasing at a faster pace than ever before. This will present a challenge to the existing health and economic systems and an urgent need for increased public awareness and public health policies that will help safely and humanely care for patients with these conditions.

MEMORY TIP

Useful mnemonic for distinguishing between delirium and dementia: CAD BAD MASCOT.

		Delirium	Dementia
C	Consciousness	Altered; fluctuates; either decreased (clouded) or hyperalert	Not altered; alert
A	Alertness	Disturbed	Generally intact
D	Diurnal variation	Fluctuates through the day	Steady
B	Bp and vitals	Fluctuate in some etiologies	Steady
A	Attention	Impaired	Generally intact until later stages
D	Delusion	Acute and fluctuating	More fixed and gradual
M	Memory	Poor-working immediate and short-term memory	Poor short- to long-term memory
A	Age	Any	Late adulthood to elderly population
S	Sleep disturbance	Fragmented sleep–wake pattern; disrupted circadian rhythm	Sleep–wake diurnal pattern changes
C	Course	Waxing and waning (comes and goes)	Steady decline
O	Onset	Acute or subacute	Chronic or gradual
T	Treatment course	Treatment of underlying cause(s) resolves symptoms	Treatments may slow progression or symptoms

Created by Edore Onigu-Otite

RESOURCES

1 Cognitive Health and Older Adults | National Institute on Aging (nih.gov)

2 Promoting Health for Older Adults | CDC

3 Alzheimer's and Dementia Resources for Professionals | National Institute on Aging (nih.gov)

4 Alzheimer's Disease and Healthy Aging | CDC

5 American Delirium Society Home | American Delirium Society

REFERENCES

Abraha, I., Rimland, J. M., Trotta, F. M., Dell'Aquila, G., Cruz-Jentoft, A., Petrovic, M., Gudmundsson, A., Soiza, R., O'Mahony, D., Guaita, A., & Cherubini, A. (2017). Systematic review of systematic reviews of non-pharmacological interventions to treat behavioural disturbances in older patients with dementia: The SENATOR-OnTop series. *BMJ Open, 7*(3), e012759. https://doi.org/10.1136/bmjopen-2016-012759

Alzheimer's Disease International. (n.d.). *Dementia statistics.* https://www.alzint.org/about/dementia-facts-figures/dementia-statistics/

American Psychiatric Association. (2013). Diagnostic and statistical manual of mental disorders (5th ed.).

Dyer, S. M., Harrison, S. L., Laver, K., Whitehead, C., & Crotty, M. (2018). An overview of systematic reviews of pharmacological and non-pharmacological interventions for the treatment of behavioral and psychological symptoms of dementia. *International Psychogeriatrics, 30*(3), 295–309. http://dx.doi.org/10.1017/S1041610217002344

Elahi, F., & Miller, B. (2017). A clinicopathological approach to the diagnosis of dementia. A clinicopathological approach to the diagnosis of dementia, *13*, 457–476. https://doi.org/10.1038/nrneurol.2017.96

Francis, J., Jr., & Young, B. G. (n.d.). *Diagnosis of delirium and confusional states.* https://www.uptodate.com/contents/diagnosis-of-delirium-and-confusional-states

Goodman, R. A., Lochner, K. A., Thambisetty, M., Wingo, T. S., Posner, S. F., & Ling, S. M. (2017). Prevalence of dementia subtypes in United States Medicare fee-for-service beneficiaries, 2011–2013. *Alzheimer's & Dementia: The Journal of the Alzheimer's Association, 13*(1), 28–37. https://doi.org/10.1016/j.jalz.2016.04.002

Hugo, J., & Ganguli, M. (2014). Dementia and cognitive impairment: epidemiology, diagnosis, and treatment. *Clinics in Geriatric Medicine, 30*(3), 421–442. https://doi.org/10.1016/j.cger.2014.04.001

Inouye, S. K., van Dyck, C. H., Alessi, C. A., Balkin, S., Siegal, A. P., & Horwitz, R. I. (1990). Clarifying confusion: The confusion assessment method: A new method for detection of delirium. *Annals of Internal Medicine, 113*(12), 941–948. https://doi.org/10.7326/0003-4819-113-12-9416

Inouye, S. K., Westendorp, R. G., & Saczynski, J. S. (2014). Delirium in elderly people. *Lancet, 383*(9920), 911–922. https://doi.org/10.1016/S0140-6736(13)60688-1

Kishi, T., Hirota, T., Matsunaga, S., & Iwata, N. (2016). Antipsychotic medications for the treatment of delirium: A systematic review and meta-analysis of randomised controlled trials. *Journal of Neurology, Neurosurgery, and Psychiatry, 87*(7), 767–774. https://doi.org/10.1136/jnnp-2015-311049

Livingston, G., Kelly, L., Lewis-Holmes, E., Baio, G., Morris, S., Patel, N., Omar, R. Z., Katona, C., & Cooper, C. (2014). A systematic review of the clinical effectiveness and cost-effectiveness of sensory, psychological and behavioural interventions for managing agitation in older adults with dementia. *Health Technology Assessment, 18*(39). https://doi.org/10.3310/hta18390

Marcantonio E. R. (2017). Delirium in hospitalized older adults. *The New England Journal of Medicine, 377*(15), 1456–1466. https://doi.org/10.1056/NEJMcp1605501

Nikooie, R., Neufeld, K. J., Oh, E. S., Wilson, L. M., Zhang, A., Robinson, K. A., Needham, D. M. (2019). Antipsychotics for treating delirium in hospitalized adults: A systematic review. *Annals of Internal Medicine, 171*(7), 485–495. https://doi.org/10.7326/M19-1860

Nowrangi, M. A., Rao, V., & Lyketsos, C. G. (2011). Epidemiology, assessment, and treatment of dementia. *The Psychiatric Clinics of North America, 34*(2), 275–294. https://doi.org/10.1016/j.psc.2011.02.004

Oh, E. S., Fong, T. G., Hshieh, T. T., & Inouye, S. K. (2017). Delirium in older persons: Advances in diagnosis and treatment. *JAMA, 318*(12), 1161–1174. https://doi.org/10.1001/jama.2017.12067

Perng, C., Chang, Y. & Tzang, R. (2018). The treatment of cognitive dysfunction in dementia: A multiple treatments meta-analysis. *Psychopharmacology, 235*, 1571–1580. https://doi.org/10.1007/s00213-018-4867-y

Phan, S. V., Osae, S., Morgan, J. C., Inyang, M., & Fagan, S. C. (2019). Neuropsychiatric symptoms in Dementia: Considerations for pharmacotherapy in the USA. *Drugs in R&D, 19*(2), 93–115. https://doi.org/ 10.1007/s40268-019-0272-1

Reus, V. I., Fochtmann, L. J., Eyler, A. E., Hilty, D. M., Horvitz-Lennon, M., Jibson, M. D., Lopez, O. L., Mahoney, J., Pasic, J., Tan, Z. S., Wills, C. D., Rhoads, R., & Yager, J. (2016). The American Psychiatric Association practice guideline on the use of antipsychotics to treat agitation or psychosis in patients with dementia. *The American Journal of Psychiatry, 173*(5), 543–546. https://doi.org/10.1176/appi.ajp.2015.173501

Ringman, J. M., & Schneider, L. (2019). Treatment options for agitation in dementia. *Current Treatment Options in Neurology, 21*(7), 30. https://doi.org/10.1007/s11940-019-0572-3

Sachdev, P. S., Blacker, D., Blazer, D. G., Ganguli, M., Jeste, D. V., Paulsen, J. S., & Petersen, R. C. (2014). Classifying neurocognitive disorders: The DSM-5 approach. *Nature Reviews: Neurology, 10*(11), 634–642. https://doi.org/10.1038/nrneurol.2014.181

CHAPTER 28

Personality Disorders[1]

Erik W. Larsson, M.D.

"I do not want people to be very agreeable, as it saves me the trouble of liking them a great deal."

— Jane Austen.

OBJECTIVES

At the end of this chapter, students will be able to do the following:

- describe personality
- distinguish between categorical and dimensional models of personality
- discuss types of personality disorders

CASE VIGNETTE

Ms. J is a 35-year-old female psychiatry patient, who is currently admitted to the psychiatry unit. This is her third admission this year for a suicide overdose. A review of her early childhood shows that when Ms. J was 4, her parents got divorced. Within a year, her mother remarried and left the country to start a new life. Although she lived with her father, who did the best he could to make her happy, Jane felt abandoned. Over the next few years, unknown to her father, she was sexually abused by several relatives. She did not disclose this to anyone. Through high school and college, she had multiple partners. Her relationships were dramatic but followed a pattern. At first, she fell head over heels in love with her partner, showered them with gifts, and idolized them. This was usually short-lived before she invariably began tearing and wearing them down with her words and intense

(*continued*)

1 Readers may also see "Defense Mechanisms: The Hidden Gymnastics of Protecting the Self" (Chapter 14) for related material.

emotional swings. They ended up excusing themselves from the relationship and leaving. In times of stress, she often decompensated and resorted to binge eating and binge drinking alcohol. She often made suicidal gestures, including cutting her wrists.

Over the years, she was treated by several psychiatrists and therapists. Some providers experienced countertransference toward her. She made several suicide attempts and was a frequent patient of the local ER. She had several inpatient psychiatric hospitalizations. During hospitalization, Jane manifested a maladaptive coping strategy called splitting. She berated the nurses to the psychiatrist, whom she adulated. After discharge, she was engaged with a therapist who provided dialectic behavior therapy. With this, Ms. J learned the skills to manage her emotions and prevent the downward spiral that previously led her to self-harm. She also saw a psychiatrist in the same facility and was treated for the accompanying depression and anxiety, which often co-occur with borderline personality disorder.

DEFINITIONS AND KEY CONCEPTS

KEY POINT

Personality disorders are "an enduring pattern of inner experience and behavior that deviates markedly from the expectation of the individual's culture" (APA, 2013). A personality disorder occurs when behaviors, cognitions, and emotional patterns become pathological and inflexible to such a degree that they impair functioning or causes distress.

The word *personality* derives from the Latin word *persona*. In ancient Roman culture, a *persona* was a mask worn by a stage actor. Such a mask was commonly used to project some particular quality of the character in question, such as evil or kindness. Today, we use the word *personality* to define human beings based on specific combinations of behaviors, cognitions, and emotional patterns (Corr & Matthews, 2009). Such patterns can be measured and construed in a variety of ways, using different conceptual tools. A *personality disorder* is what happens when these patterns become pathological and inflexible to such a degree that they impair functioning or causes distress. Personality disorders have traditionally been regarded as fixed and stable over time, although some studies have questioned this assumption (Durbin & Klein, 2006). An important distinction of personality pathology is that it tends to be in sync with the self-image of the individual, or *ego-syntonic*. As the pathology fits with the individual's self-image, the individual will often see nothing wrong with their behavior and disposition. This fact alone makes personality disorders very difficult to treat. Another problem with the concept of personality pathology is that it depends, at least to some degree, on prevailing social and cultural norms (Jane et al., 2007). For this reason, and others, personality pathology is regarded by many as one of the most controversial areas of psychiatry (Arntz, 1999).

INTRODUCTION

The topic of personality disorders (PDs) is often a source of frustration, particularly for medical students. The diagnostic definitions tend to be vague and hard to tell apart. There are no FDA-approved medications for treating the disorders. And with the notable exception of *borderline personality disorder*, these diagnoses are almost never the cause for a hospital admission, or even a visit to a doctor's office. The obvious question arises: What is the point of PDs as a diagnostic category?

The question has many answers. First, PDs are everywhere. All of us have at some point—either in our personal or professional lives—encountered people with PDs. Second, personality pathology is associated with significant, and often dire, personal consequences. Third, well-defined diagnostic categories and distinct terminology are important tools that may help us recognize pathological tendencies in others, as well as ourselves.

Although difficult to treat directly, the presence of a PD in a patient may also impact our choice of treatment for comorbid psychiatric conditions. As a general rule, psychiatric patients with underlying PDs tend to be more difficult to treat, and the overall prognosis of such patients tends to be worse in comparison to patients without PDs. For example, the presence of a comorbid PD may make a depressed patient less likely to respond to electroconvulsive treatment (Lee et al., 2019)—a method used to treat refractory depression.

CATEGORIES VERSUS DIMENSIONS

There are essentially two different models for studying personality: a *categorical* model and a *dimensional* model. In this chapter, we will largely focus on the categorical model, as this is the model currently used in psychiatry and endorsed by the *DSM-5*. The categorical model assumes that each PD is a separate and distinct entity, defined by a particular set of criteria. For example, to be diagnosed with *schizotypal personality disorder*, an individual would have to fulfill at least five out of a list of nine criteria. The categorical model has some obvious benefits in that it is fairly uncomplicated and user friendly. Unfortunately, it also has some problems associated with it. There is, for example, a high degree of overlap of PDs with each other and other mental disorders. An individual who meets the diagnostic criteria for one PD may sometimes meet the criteria for another. The validity and reliability of the categorical model are also considered to be fairly limited for most disorders (Zachar & Kreuger, 2016). In other words, the simplicity and neatness of the categorical model come at the expense of accuracy.

In contrast, dimensional models are more subtle and allow for varying degrees of impairment or severity. The most commonly used dimensional tool for measuring personality traits is the so-called *five-factor model* (Table 28.1). This model identifies five basic factors that make up an individual's personality: *openness to experience*, *conscientiousness*, *extraversion*,

KEY POINT

Five basic factors that make up an individual's personality: *openness to experience, conscientiousness, extraversion, agreeableness,* and *neuroticism.*

agreeableness, and *neuroticism*. These traits are quantified on a scale from 1 to 100, usually on the basis of self-report.

TABLE 28.1 Five-Factor Model Traits and Their Characteristics

Dimension	High	Low
Openness to experience	Creative, prefers variety, open to new ideas	Conventional, concrete, traditional
Conscientiousness	Well organized, thoughtful, reliable	Careless, undisciplined, easy-going
Extraversion	Assertive, sociable, optimistic	Reserved, aloof, pessimistic
Agreeableness	Trusting, kind, affectionate	Difficult, competitive, mistrustful
Neuroticism	Nervous, moody, prone to depression	Secure, calm, emotionally stable

In general, PDs tend to be associated with high levels of neuroticism, low levels of agreeableness, and low levels of conscientiousness. However, there are many exceptions to this rule. Although the validity and reliability of the five-factor model are generally regarded as superior to the *DSM-5* categorical model (Lynam & Widiger, 2001), it has not yet been adopted by the psychiatric community. There are several reasons for this. Some have argued that personality dimensions are simply too complex to be clinically useful. For all their faults, the categorical diagnoses are at least comprehensible to most clinicians and confer some practical utility. However, few clinicians would know how to interpret a set of numerical scores about a patient's personality and may find it cumbersome. Others have pointed out that the *egosyntonic* nature of PDs makes them hard to reliably diagnose based on self-report (Shedler et al., 2011). For these and other reasons, the categorical model of PDs remains the more commonly used model.

QUICK POINT

Estimates show that about 6% to 10% of the general population has a personality disorder. Personality disorders were previously considered to be a fixed problem that would define a person for life. Current research shows that personality disorders can improve with treatment. With treatment, individuals with personality disorders can live wholesome lives.

EPIDEMIOLOGY

The prevalence of PD is a topic of some controversy and differs widely between studies. However, an estimated range of 6% to 10% of people in the community are considered to have a PD (Samuels, 2011). The disorders are not equally common in all settings. For example, in samples consisting of psychiatric patients, the prevalence is thought to be well over 50% in outpatients and 20% in inpatients with *borderline PD* accounting for the majority of cases (Zimmerman, 2005; Chapman, 2021). An estimated half of prison inmates are also deemed to fulfill criteria for antisocial PD, whereas the schizophrenia-like cluster A personality disorders have been found to be widespread among homeless people (Connolly, 2008).

The prevalence of PDs tends to be higher among people who are separated, divorced, unemployed, or have psychiatric comorbidities. People with PDs are more likely to have a history of substance abuse, interpersonal violence, and suicidal behavior. They are also more likely to use medical services and have worse health outcomes compared to the general population (Samuels, 2011). For these reasons, personality pathology is regarded by many in the field as a serious public health concern (Lenzenweger, 2008).

SIGNS AND SYMPTOMS

Personality disorders are grouped into three clusters on the basis of descriptive similarities (Table 28.2). The cluster A personality disorders are often referred to as the "odd or eccentric" disorders and share some general features with schizophrenia-type illnesses. Cluster B disorders are called the "emotional or erratic" disorders and are characterized by emotional dysregulation, impulsivity, and frequent interpersonal conflicts. Finally, cluster C disorders are known as the "anxious or fearful" disorders and are associated with intense anxiety and negative emotion.

MEMORY TIP

Personality disorders are grouped into three clusters:

- *Cluster A*—the "odd or eccentric"
- *Cluster B*—the "emotional or erratic"
- *Cluster C*—the "anxious or fearful"

TABLE 28.2 Personality Disorders in the *DSM-5*

Cluster A	Cluster B	Cluster C
Schizotypal	Borderline	Avoidant
Schizoid	Antisocial	Dependent
Paranoid	Narcissistic	Obsessive-compulsive
	Histrionic	

THE CLUSTER A DISORDERS

As its name implies, *schizotypal personality disorder (STPD)* bears a close resemblance to schizophrenia, to the point of being considered a schizophrenia spectrum disorder, with schizotypal PD viewed as less severe than schizophrenia. Studies have shown a significant degree of genetic overlap between STPD and manifest schizophrenia (Ettinger et al., 2014). Patients with STPD are often seen as odd or eccentric by people around them. They tend to harbor unconventional, or even paranoid, beliefs and often display peculiar speech mannerisms and odd modes of dress. Patients with STPD generally present with a blunt affect and tend to feel and appear awkward in social situations. For this reason, STPD is often associated with significant social anxiety. Although they are sometimes confused with schizophrenia patients, people with STPD never develop full-blown psychosis or experience hallucinations. Instead, their signs and symptoms remain fixed at a stage that is similar to the prodrome of schizophrenia. STPD is more common in males than females.

Individuals with *schizoid personality disorder (SzPD)* display a strong tendency toward isolation, a lack of interest in social relationships, emotional coldness, and detachment. Although seemingly apathetic toward the world around them, patients with SzPD will often possess a rich but completely internal, fantasy life. For obvious reasons, the schizotypal and schizoid PDs are easily confused with one another. One way of keeping them separate is to think of how they each relate to schizophrenia. The symptoms associated with schizophrenia have historically been divided into *positive* and *negative* ones. Positive symptoms are things that *happen*, such as auditory hallucinations, delusions, and strange experiences. Negative symptoms can be thought of things that *don't happen* and include symptoms such as apathy, anhedonia, and social withdrawal. While schizotypal patients often incline toward positive symptoms, schizoid patients can be seen as a mild manifestation of the *negative symptoms* of schizophrenia. Patients with schizoid tendencies can be difficult to engage in treatment and will often fail to see the point of maintaining a psychotherapeutic relationship. SzPD is more common in males than females. In the five-factor model, SzPD is strongly associated with low levels of extraversion.

Paranoid personality disorder (PPD) describes a kind of chronic suspiciousness and generalized mistrust of others that never quite amounts to a fixed and stated delusion. Whereas frankly delusional patients will often present with one overarching delusion, patients with PPD tend to harbor a myriad of minor paranoid delusions, none of which are completely dominant. Individuals with PPD are prone to bearing grudges, interpreting others' actions as hostile, and taking things personally. In medical settings, they will often file complaints against caregivers and generally feel mistreated or neglected. PPD is more common in males than females.

THE CLUSTER B DISORDERS

Individuals with *borderline personality disorders* (BPD) display a "pattern of instability in interpersonal relationships, self-image and affects, and marked impulsivity" (APA, 2013, p. 663). It is by far the most commonly diagnosed

MEMORY TIP

Schizotypal Personality Disorder, *useful mnemonic*

ME PECULIAR

M—Magical thinking
E—Experiences unusual perceptions
P—Paranoid ideation
E—Eccentric behavior or appearance
C—Constricted or inappropriate affect
U—Unusual thinking or speech
L—Lacks close friends
I— Ideas of reference
A—Anxiety in social situations
R—Rule out psychotic or pervasive developmental disorders

(Pinkofsky, 1997)

MEMORY TIP

Schizoid Personality Disorder, *useful mnemonic*

DISTANT

D—Detached or flattened affect
I— Indifferent to criticism or praise
S—Sexual experiences of little interest
T—Tasks done solitarily
A—Absence of close friends
N—Neither desires nor enjoys close relationships
T—Takes pleasure in few activities

(Pinkofsky, 1997)

and clinically prevalent of all PDs. Patients with BPD are perhaps most well known for their tendencies toward self-harm, most typically cutting. Such behaviors often stem from a need to "feel something," as compared to feeling numb or nothingness, and these people want to escape the "chronic sense of emptiness" that is often associated with BPD (Miller et al., 2020). Patients with BPD are more often female than male by a ratio of about 3 to 1. The majority of individuals with BPD have a history of some childhood trauma or neglect, and many abuse drugs or alcohol. As many have noted, the signs and symptoms of BPD overlap considerably with those of posttraumatic stress disorder (PTSD), particularly in cases of prolonged and repeated trauma (Gunderson, 2009). Both BPD and PTSD are associated with overall emotional instability or hyperreactivity, suicidal thoughts and gestures, episodes of dissociation (a sense of unreality), anxiety, and depression. In their relationships with other people, patients with BPD will often manifest *splitting*. Splitting is a psychological defense mechanism that allows the person to tolerate difficult and overwhelming emotions by viewing someone as entirely good or entirely bad—idealized or devalued. Such designations can sometimes shift rapidly to the great frustration of both caregivers and loved ones. BPD patients are highly sensitive to feelings of abandonment and will often respond to such feelings by lashing out toward themselves or others. These feelings and behaviors are believed to stem from the BPD patient's difficulty establishing stable and trusting relationships. In the five-factor model, BPD is associated with high levels of *neuroticism* and low levels of *agreeableness*. *DEAR MAN* (Figure 28.1) is an acronym that helps people with BPD develop their interpersonal skills. It is often taught as part of psychotherapy for such patients.

Individuals with *antisocial personality disorder (ASPD)* display a pervasive and persistent disregard for social norms, morals, and the rights and feelings of others. Patients with ASPD are sometimes referred to as *psychopaths* or *sociopaths*, although these terms are generally avoided by clinicians. When diagnosed in children under the age of 18, clinicians will use the less stigmatizing term *conduct disorder* to describe these patients. Patients with ASPD tend to be male. However, although much fewer, female patients with ASPD exist. Many individuals with ASPD have a history of childhood trauma, neglect, or poverty. ASPD and BPD patients have some features in common, such as impulsivity and a lack of empathy for others. Some scholars have even argued that ASPD is the male manifestation and BPD the female manifestation of the same underlying disorder (Paris, 1997). Individuals with ASPD are vastly overrepresented among substance abusers and within the prison population. ASPD is very difficult to treat and is rarely

MEMORY TIP

Paranoid Personality Disorder, *useful mnemonic*

SUSPECT

S—Spousal infidelity suspected
U—Unforgiving (bears grudges)
S—Suspicious
P—Perceives attacks (and reacts quickly)
E—Enemy or friend? (Suspects associates and friends)
C—Confiding in others is feared
T—Threats perceived in benign events

(Pinkofsky, 1997)

MEMORY TIP

Borderline Personality Disorder, *useful mnemonic*

DESPAIRER

D—Disturbance of identity
E—Emotionally labile
S—Suicidal behavior
P—Paranoia or dissociation
A—Abandonment (fear of)
I— Impulsive
R—Relationships unstable
E—Emptiness (feelings of)
R—Rage (inappropriate)

(Caplan, 2008)

D	• Describe
E	• Express
A	• Assert
R	• Reinforce
M	• Mindful
A	• Appear Confident
N	• Negotiate

FIGURE 28.1 DEAR MAN acronym used to help individuals with borderline personality disorder develop interpersonal skills.

considered a viable target for psychiatric intervention. In the five-factor model, ASPD is associated with very low levels of *agreeableness*.

Narcissistic personality disorder (NPD) is characterized by exaggerated feelings of self-importance and an incessant craving for admiration. Individuals with NPD often appear grandiose, arrogant, and lacking in empathy for other people. Some critics have argued that NPD does not constitute a distinct disorder but is rather a milder, nonviolent form of antisocial PD (Alarcón & Sarabia, 2012). Patients with NPD can at times be difficult to distinguish from those with bipolar mania, as both conditions can present with a grandiose demeanor. A good rule of thumb is therefore to never diagnose NPD until mania has been ruled out and the patient has been stabilized. NPD is more common, and sometimes more obvious, in males than females. In the five-factor model, NPD is associated with a high degree of extraversion as well as low degrees of *agreeableness*.

Histrionic personality disorder (HPD) is characterized by an excessive need to be the center of attention and to win the approval of others. To achieve these goals, patients with HPD will sometimes act in a seductive manner or wear sexually provocative clothing. Individuals with HPD are often accused of being dramatic and overly emotional. HPD and NPD share a lot of features, and, as with borderline and antisocial disorders, show a significant gender divide. Whereas narcissists tend to be male, patients with histrionic PD tend to be female. The controversial origin of the term *histrionic* (a derivative of the old concept *hysteria*) has caused some critics to question its place in the *DSM* (Gould, 2011). In the five-factor model, HPD is associated with high levels of extraversion as well as neuroticism.

MEMORY TIP

Antisocial Personality Disorder, *useful mnemonic*

CORRUPT
C—Cannot conform to law
O—Obligations ignored
R—Reckless disregard for safety
R—Remorseless
U—Underhanded (deceitful)
P—Planning insufficient (impulsive)
T—Temper (irritable and aggressive)

(Pinkofsky, 1997)

MEMORY TIP

Narcissistc Personality Disorder, *useful mnemonic*

GRANDIOSE
G—Grandiose
R—Requires attention
A—Arrogant
N—Needs to be special
D—Dreams of success and power
I— Interpersonally exploitative
O—Others (unable to recognize feelings or needs of)
S—Sense of entitlement
E—Envious

(Senger, 1997)

THE CLUSTER C DISORDERS

Although not uncommon in the population, cluster C personality disorders are rarely diagnosed. This is largely due to their apparent similarity to more common conditions associated with negative emotional states. A good example of this is the diagnosis of *avoidant personality disorder* (APD), which implies an "enduring pattern of feelings of inadequacy, hypersensitivity to being negatively evaluated by others, and extreme shyness" (APA, 2013, p. 672). A patient with these symptoms can be quite difficult to distinguish from one with generalized or social anxiety disorder—at least on an initial exam. Given the stigma associated with personality pathology, many clinicians will favor an anxiety diagnosis over one related to personality for these patients. APD is more common in females than males. In the five-factor model, APD is associated with high degrees of *agreeableness* and *neuroticism* and a low degree of *extraversion*.

Dependent personality disorder (DPD) is characterized by a pervasive and excessive need to be taken care of that leads to submissive and clingy behavior. As with APD, this diagnosis is associated with a great deal of anxiety and a lack of self-confidence. DPD is most commonly seen in women and is associated with an increased risk of domestic abuse (Loas, 2011). It shares some features with borderline PD in that both conditions are associated with a chronic fear of abandonment. However, individuals with DPD do not display the impulsivity and lack of empathy that are typical of BPD. In the five-factor model, HPD is associated with high degrees of *agreeableness* and *neuroticism*.

Finally, *obsessive-compulsive personality disorder (OCPD)* is characterized by an *excessive* need for orderliness, neatness, and perfectionism. It is often confused with obsessive-compulsive disorder but differs from this condition in important ways. Whereas OCD is generally associated with subjective distress, individuals with OCPD do not believe that there is anything abnormal about their excessive need for orderliness. Stated differently, OCPD is *ego-syntonic*, whereas OCD is *ego-dystonic*. OCPD shows a high degree of comorbidity with autism spectrum disorders, although OCPD alone does not imply any significant cognitive or emotional deficits. OCPD is more common in males than females. Among the personality disorders, OCPD is the only one that is associated with high levels of *conscientiousness*.

ETIOLOGY

Personality disorders are generally thought to be caused by a combination of genetic and environmental factors. Persons with PDs are more likely to have experienced abuse or neglect as children or to have grown up in poverty or with a relative lack of resources. Such childhood factors are considered most

MEMORY TIP

Histrionic Personality Disorder, *useful mnemonic*

ACTRESS

A—Appearance focused
C—Center of attention
T—Theatrical
R—Relationships (believed to be more intimate than they are)
E—Easily influenced
S—Seductive behavior
S—Shallow emotions
S—Speech (impressionistic and vague)

(Caplan, 2008)

MEMORY TIP

Avoidant Personality Disorder, *useful mnemonic*

CRINGES

C—Criticism or rejection preoccupies thoughts in social situations
R—Restraint in relationships due to fear of shame
I—Inhibited in new relationships
N—Needs to be sure of being liked before engaging socially
G—Gets around occupational activities that require interpersonal contact
E—Embarrassment prevents new activity or taking risks
S—Self-viewed as unappealing or inferior

(Pinkofsky, 1997)

MEMORY TIP

Dependent Personality Disorder, useful mnemonic

RELIANCE

R—Reassurance required
E—Expressing disagreement difficult
L—Life responsibilities assumed by others
I— Initiating projects difficult
A—Alone (feels helpless and uncomfortable when alone)
N—Nurturance (goes to excessive lengths to obtain)
C—Companionship sought urgently when a relationship ends
E—Exaggerated fears of being left to care for self

(Pinkofsky, 1997)

MEMORY TIP

Obsessive- Compulsive Personality Disorder, *useful mnemonic*

SCRIMPER

S— Stubborn
C— Cannot discard worthless objects
R— Rule obsessed
I— Inflexible
M—Miserly
P— Perfectionistic
E— Excludes leisure due to devotion to work
R— Reluctant to delegate to others

(Caplan, 2008)

important for conditions associated with a high degree of impulsivity, such as borderline and antisocial PDs. Whereas dimensional personality traits are heritable at a rate of 40–60%, the genetics of PDs are less clear (Power & Pluess, 2015). However, studies have indicated that these conditions are modestly to moderately heritable (Reichborn-Kjennerud, 2010).

On the neuropathology of PDs, most research has focused on patients with borderline PD. Neuroimaging studies on individuals with BPD have shown reductions in brain regions involved in the regulation of stress responses and emotion, including the hippocampus, amygdala, and prefrontal cortex (O'Neill & Frodl, 2012). Structural and functional deficits in the prefrontal cortex—a brain area involved in empathy—have been demonstrated among individuals with antisocial PD (Yang & Raine, 2009). Brain imaging of individuals with schizotypal traits have uncovered patterns of grey matter attenuation similar to those associated with schizophrenia (Wiebels et al., 2016). However, neuroimaging is not routinely used for the purpose of diagnosing PDs.

DIAGNOSIS

Personality disorders are most commonly diagnosed on the basis of the patient history and clinical exam. Psychometric tests, such as the Minnesota Multiphasic Personality Inventory (MMPI) or the Structured Clinical Interview for *DSM-5* Personality Disorders (SCID-5-PD), are sometimes used, especially for forensic purposes. Although each PD has its own set of diagnostic descriptors, the most important, overarching criterion for diagnosing personality pathology includes long-term deviation from cultural expectations that leads to significant distress or functional impairment. These patterns should be stable across different settings and their onset traced back at least to adolescence or early adulthood. They should not be better explained as a manifestation of another mental disorder nor attributable to the effects of illicit substances, medications, or other medical conditions (such as head trauma or neurological illnesses; APA, 2013). As with other psychiatric illnesses, PDs are not reliably or consistently associated with any particular lab findings or biomarkers (Figure 28.2).

TREATMENT

For a variety of reasons, personality disorders are challenging to treat. Given the ego-syntonic nature of PDs, patients and clinicians sometimes disagree about the nature of the disorder and may not share the same goals for treatment. Nevertheless, when patients with PDs do engage effectively in treatment, the results can be life transforming. Importantly, treating comorbid symptoms and disorders can also result in symptom relief and improved functioning in patients with PDs.

CLINICAL TIP

Patients with personality disorders are challenging to engage in treatment because they lack insight. To them, their perception is egosyntonic (fits comfortably with the individual's self-concept). Due to this, they often do not see the need for treatment, even though those around them can see the need.

Psychopharmacology

Research on treatments for personality disorders is beset with challenges. The patient population is extremely heterogeneous, and clinicians often diagnose the same patient with different disorders. Regarding pharmacotherapy, there are currently no FDA-approved treatments for any of the PDs. Notably, smaller studies of individual disorders have yielded positive results, although risk to benefit ratios remain unclear. For example, some patients with schizotypal PD have experienced overall improvement from treatment with antipsychotics (Bateman et al., 2015). However, no such data currently exist in regard to the paranoid and schizotypal PDs. Although not generally recommended by clinical guidelines, patients with severe BPD are often prescribed mood stabilizers and atypical antipsychotics to mitigate impulsivity. Regarding cluster C disorders, treatment data is very sparse, although some studies indicate that antidepressants can be effective in patients with avoidant PD (Bateman et al., 2015).

Psychotherapy

A variety of psychotherapeutic modalities have been researched and provide evidence-based therapies for patients with PDs (Gabbard, 2000). These include mindfulness-based therapies, psychodynamic-oriented therapies, cognitive behavioral therapy, exposure therapies, and supportive therapies. Research on psychotherapy has largely focused on the treatment of borderline PDs. *Dialectical behavior therapy (DBT)*, a form of mindfulness-based therapy developed by psychologist and BPD sufferer Marsha Linehan, is an evidence-based psychosocial treatment that helps alleviate symptoms and mitigate impulsivity and self-harm in patients with BPD. *Mentalization-based therapy* (MBT; Bateman & Fonagy, 2010) is a form of structured psychodynamic psychotherapy that helps patients with BPD differentiate their own thoughts and feelings from those of people around them. *Cognitive behavior therapy* (CBT), systematic desensitization, graduated exposure, and social skills training have been shown to be effective in the treatment of patients with avoidant personality disorder (Alden, 1989). Brief forms of psychotherapy have been shown to be cost effective in psychiatric inpatients with PDs (Gabbard 2000).

CLINICAL TIP

Several types of psychotherapy have been found to be effective in reducing symptoms and improving functioning of patients with personality disorders. These include *dialectical behavior therapy* (DBT) for borderline personality disorder, mentalization-based therapy, cognitive behavior therapy, systemic desensitization, graded exposure, and social skills training.

SUMMARY

Personality disorders are a group of psychiatric conditions characterized by enduring and maladaptive patterns of behavior, cognition, emotions, and inner experiences that differ markedly from the cultural norm and cause distress and disability. They are generally diagnosed on the basis of clinical exam and patient history. There are no imaging procedures or lab tests that can determine who has a PD. Perhaps not surprisingly, clinicians sometimes disagree on which patient has what PD.

Nevertheless, PDs are associated with a negative outcomes, such as unemployment, divorce, homelessness, criminality, substance abuse, mental illness, and suicide. The 10 PDs listed in the *DSM-5* cover a wide variety of behaviors and symptoms—from the strange and erratic to the anxious and obsessive. People with PDs generally have poor insight into their pathology and are often unmotivated to start or stick with psychiatric treatment. This often makes them challenging for clinicians to work with.

Treatments for PDs can be effective when patients engage in treatment. Medications may help associated symptoms. Psychotherapy, although challenging to initiate and maintain over time, can result in substantial progress and improved quality of life for the patient. Also, many patients benefit from psychotherapeutic treatment for related problems and comorbidities. It is worth noting that what we call personality disorders merely reflect the great complexity and diversity that constitute the human condition. While helping patients adjust to the norms of society is a worthwhile and noble cause, we should also remember that such norms are often fluid and subject to change. In our efforts to help our patients, we should remain curious about their world, bear in mind the limits of our knowledge, and not allow for psychiatric diagnoses to become instruments of intolerance.

RESOURCES

1 The Big Five Personality Traits (simplypsychology.org)

2 Gabbard GO. Mind, brain, and personality disorders. Am J Psychiatry. 2005 Apr;162(4):648-55. doi: 10.1176/appi.ajp.162.4.648. PMID: 15800133. appi.ajp.162.4.648 (psychiatryonline.org)

3 Personality Disorder
Personality Disorder | Mental Health America (mhanational.org)

REFERENCES

Alarcón, R. D., & Sarabia, S. (2012). Debates on the narcissism conundrum: Trait, domain, dimension, type, or disorder? *The Journal of Nervous and Mental Diseases*, *200*(1), 16–25.

American Psychiatric Association. (2013). *Diagnostic and statistical manual of mental disorders* (5th ed.).

Arntz, A. (1999). Do personality disorders exist? On the validity of the concept and its cognitive-behavioral formulation and treatment. *Behaviour research and therapy*, , *37*(1), S97–134. https://doi.org/10.1016/s0005-7967(99)00052-2

Bateman, A., & Fonagy, P. (2010). Mentalization based treatment for borderline personality disorder. *World psychiatry: Official journal of the World Psychiatric Association (WPA)*, *9*(1), 11–15. https://doi.org/10.1002/j.2051-5545.2010.tb00255.x

Bateman, A. W., Gunderson, J., & Mulder, R. (2015). Treatment of personality disorder. *Lancet, 385*(9969), 735–743.

Caplan J. P., & Stern, T. A. (2008) Mnemonics in a nutshell: 32 AIDS to psychiatric diagnosis. *Current Psychiatry, 7*, 27–33.

Chapman, J., Jamil, R. T., Fleisher, C. (2021). *Borderline personality disorder.* StatPearls.

Connolly, A. J. (2008). Personality disorders in homeless drop-in center clients. *Journal of Personality Disorders, 22*(6), 573–588.

Corr, P. J., & Matthews, G. (2009). *The Cambridge handbook of personality psychology.* Cambridge University Press.

Durbin, C. E., & Klein, D. N. (2006). Ten-year stability of personality disorders among outpatients with mood disorders. *Journal of Abnormal Psychology, 115*(1), 75–84. https://doi.org/10.1037/0021-843X.115.1.75

Ettinger, U., Meyhöfer, I., Steffens, M., Wagner, M., & Koutsouleris, N. (2014). Genetics, cognition, and neurobiology of schizotypal personality: A review of the overlap with schizophrenia. *Frontiers in Psychiatry, 5*, 18.

Gabbard G. O. (2000). Psychotherapy of personality disorders. *The Journal of Psychotherapy Ppractice and Research, 9*(1), 1–6.

Gould, C. S. (2011). Why the histrionic personality disorder should not be in the DSM: A new taxonomic and moral analysis. *International Journal of Feminist Approaches to Bioethics, 4*(1), 26–40.

Gunderson, J. G. (2009). *Borderline personality disorder: A clinical guide.* American Psychiatric Publishing.

Jane, J. S., Oltmanns, T. F., South, S. C., & Turkheimer, E. (2007). Gender bias in diagnostic criteria for personality disorders: An item response theory analysis. *Journal of Abnormal Psychology, 116*(1), 166–175.

Lee, J. H., Kung, S., Rasmussen, K. G., & Palmer, B. A. (2019). Effectiveness of electroconvulsive therapy in patients with major depressive disorder and comorbid borderline personality disorder. *The Journal of ECT, 35*(1), 44–47.

Lenzenweger, M. F. (2008). Epidemiology of personality disorders. *Psychiatric Clinics of North America, 31*(3), 395–403.

Loas, G., Cormier, J., & Perez-Diaz, F. (2011). Dependent personality disorder and physical abuse. *Psychiatry Research, 185*(1–2), 167–170.

Lynam, D. R., & Widiger, T. A. (2001). Using the five-factor model to represent the DSM-IV personality disorders: An expert consensus approach. *Journal of Abnormal Psychology, 110*(3), 401–412. https://doi.org/10.1037//0021-843x.110.3.401

Miller, C. E., Townsend, M. L., Day, N. J. S., & Grenyer, B. F. S. (2020). Measuring the shadows: A systematic review of chronic emptiness in borderline personality disorder. *PLoS One, 15*(7), e0233970.

O'Neill, A., & Frodl, T. (2012). Brain structure and function in borderline personality disorder. *Brain Structure & Function, 217*, 767–782.

Paris, J. (1997). Antisocial and borderline personality disorders: Two separate diagnoses or two aspects of the same psychopathology? *Comprehensive Psychiatry, 38*(4), 237–242.

Pinkofsky H. B. (1997). Mnemonics for DSM-IV personality disorders. Mnemonics for DSM-IV personality disorders, *48*(9), 1197–8.

Power, R. A., & Pluess, M. (2015). Heritability estimates of the big five personality traits based on common genetic variants. *Translational Psychiatry, 5*(7), e604.

Reichborn-Kjennerud, T. (2010). The genetic epidemiology of personality disorders. *Dialogues in Clinical Neuroscience, 12*(1), 103–114.

Samuels J. (2011). Personality disorders: Epidemiology and public health issues. *International Review of Psychiatry (Abingdon, England), 23*(3), 223–233. https://doi.org/10.3109/09540261.2011.588200

Senger H. L. (1997). Borderline mnemonic. *The American Journal of Psychiatry, 154*(9), 1321. https://doi.org/10.1176/ajp.154.9.1321b

Wiebels, K., Waldie, K. E., Roberts, R. P., & Park, H. R. (2016). Identifying grey matter changes in schizotypy using partial least squares correlation. *Cortex, 81*, 137–150.

Yang, Y., & Raine, A. (2009). Prefrontal structural and functional brain imaging findings in antisocial, violent, and psychopathic individuals: a meta-analysis. *Psychiatry Research: Neuroimaging, 174*(2), 81–88.

Zachar, P., Krueger, R. F., & Kendler, K. S. (2016). Personality disorder in DSM-5: An oral history. *Psychological Medicine, 46*(1), 1–10. https://doi.org/10.1017/S0033291715001543

Zimmerman, M., Rothschild, L., & Chelminski, I. (2005). The prevalence of DSM-IV personality disorders in psychiatric outpatients. *The American Journal of Psychiatry, 162*(10), 1911–1918. https://doi.org/10.1176/appi.ajp.162.10.1911

CHAPTER 29

Addiction and Substance Use Disorders[1]

Edore Onigu-Otite, M.D.; Benjamin Li, M.D.;

Daryl Shorter, M.D.; and Thomas R. Kosten, M.D.

> *"Every form of addiction is bad, no matter whether the narcotic be alcohol or morphine or idealism"*
>
> — Carl Jung

OBJECTIVES

After reading this chapter, students will be able to do the following:

- define addictive disorders
- describe the biopsychosocial approach to conceptualization and treatment of addictive disorders
- understand the neurobiology of addiction
- discuss the psychopharmacological effects of major categories of drugs of abuse
- review evidence-based treatment for addictive disorders

CASE VIGNETTE

JR is a 32-year-old male with substance use disorder. He has a history of daily use of alcohol and opioids. He occasionally uses benzodiazepines to calm his nerves. He also has a history of cocaine and cannabis abuse. While naturally very shy, JR finds drinking

1 Readers may also see "Prescription Drug Misuse and Abuse: Opioids, Stimulants, and Sedative–Hypnotics" (Chapter 30), "Psychopharmacology" (Chapter 31) and "Psychiatric Emergencies" (Chapter 38) for related material.

alcohol makes him social. JR has been to rehab numerous times. Upon discharge, he does well for short periods—only to relapse again.

A look into JR's early development showed that he was a quiet kid and had an early diagnosis of ADHD and Asperger's syndrome in elementary school. At age 9, his parents divorced. This was a difficult time, and he sought comfort in playing video games. During childhood, he received treatment for depression, social anxiety, and ADHD but was never consistent with treatment with long lapses in his clinic attendance. His family struggled financially, and this contributed to his lack of attendance at appointments. He played video games, sometimes without pausing for up to 36 hours at a stretch. Because JR stayed up at night playing video games, he was too sleepy to attend school during the day. Over the next few years, JR was placed on probation for truancy. He began binge drinking alcohol. Each year, he had the opportunity to attend summer school to get promoted to the next grade but was unable to comply, particularly because of the extent of his gaming. He eventually dropped out of school with plans to get his GED instead.

At age 18, now a young adult, he began attending parties where he used illegal substances, including cocaine, cannabis (illegal in his state), and methamphetamine in addition to alcohol. His drinking increased. He drank daily and engaged in other high-risk behaviors. JR said that at parties, whenever he saw a male he liked, he could not stop at just talking to them; he "had to" go all the way and usually ended up sleeping with them. He kept multiple sexual partners. He developed a sexually transmitted disease and his PCP prescribed HIV-prophylaxis. He began gambling and quickly got into debt. He was involved in a motor vehicle accident, sustained a back injury, and was prescribed pain medications. In addition to the pain pills prescribed by his doctor, he obtained opioids illegally. This progressed to his injecting heroin. He had multiple visits to the emergency room for near overdose situations, several of which were actual suicide attempts. He had several inpatient psychiatry admissions. He engaged fleetingly in follow-up treatment. His medical care was obtained through crises when he presented in the ER. Social workers in the ER provided him with resources, but there was little follow-through as he returned to drug use. Upon discharge from one of his hospitalizations, JR's family loaned him money to get an apartment, but JR gambled the money away over the course of a week, which only added to his gambling debt.

JR was homeless for several years, living with drug-using friends. He engaged in illegal activities to support his habit and was always uncomfortable when he saw police officers. JR's family was often unaware of his whereabouts. A family member reached out to him through social media and convinced him to come home. JR agreed to seek treatment while living with his family. He began attending a local alcoholics anonymous (AA) meeting and obtained a sponsor. With support, JR now attends a comprehensive drug program. He receives monthly injections of vivitrol (for alcohol and opioid use), an SSRI for depression and anxiety, weekly individual therapy, and group therapy. He continues to attend daily AA meetings and report to his sponsor. His medical symptoms are also closely monitored and treated. Through this program, he has secured work at a local community center. He has been abstinent for 2 years so

(continued)

far. He still gambles occasionally, but now he has one bank account, dual signatures are required from him and a designated cosigner for check withdrawals, and there is a limit on how much he can withdraw within a specific time period.

CASE COMMENTARY

From an early age, JR manifested compulsive gaming behaviors as a child and gambled as an adult. In his teens he binge drank alcohol and began using substances as a young adult. He self-medicated his anxiety in party settings with alcohol, which disinhibited him, increasing his engagement in compulsive high-risk behaviors, including promiscuity. This in turn led to sexually transmitted infections and a host of medical problems. With the help of treatment, by the end of the vignette, JR had achieved 2 years of sobriety and met criteria for alcohol use disorder, severe, in full sustained remission and opioid use disorder, severe, in full sustained remission. He placed financial restrictions to limit his gambling activities and prevent against further financial losses.

DEFINITIONS AND KEY CONCEPTS

The word *addiction* comes from the Latin word *addicere*. This was originally a commercial term used for goods and originally meant "to hand over." Succinctly, addiction can be seen to mean "to hand over" one's resources (including one's thoughts, actions, time, and energy) to an item of addiction. In a peculiar way, individuals with addiction are devoted to their object of addiction—be it a substance or a behavioral addiction.

KEY POINT

Addiction is a chronic medical and mental health disorder with biological, psychological, social, and environmental factors influencing its onset, development, intermission, and maintenance. Addiction is a complex condition, a chronic brain disease characterized by compulsive drug-seeking/taking behavior, despite harmful consequences.

Addiction is a chronic medical and mental health disorder with biological, psychological, social, and environmental factors influencing its onset, development, intermission, and maintenance. Addiction is a complex condition, a chronic brain disease characterized by compulsive drug-seeking/taking behavior, despite harmful consequences (National Institute of Drug Abuse [NIDA], 2020b). Addiction is characterized by an inability to consistently abstain, impairment in behavioral control, craving, diminished recognition of significant problems with one's behaviors and interpersonal relationships, and a dysfunctional emotional response (American Society of Addiction Medicine [ASAM], 2011). This is reflected in an individual pathologically pursuing reward and relief by substance use and other behaviors. "Like other chronic medical diseases, addiction often involves cycles of relapse and remission. Without treatment or engagement in recovery activities, addiction is progressive and can result in disability or premature death" (ASAM, 2011). Addiction is considered the most severe form of a full spectrum of substance use disorders and is a medical illness caused by repeated misuse of a substance or substances (NIDA, 2020). In the *Diagnostic and Statistical Manual*, 5th edition (*DSM-5*), nomenclature, the diagnosis is substance use disorder with the particular substance usually specified, rather than the term *addiction.*

The individual with an addiction is exceedingly focused on their item of addition, be it a substance or a behavior. They lack the ability to prevent themselves from moving toward, using, or engaging in activities leading to using their item of addiction. Related to their item of addiction, the individual has a strong "go button" and an absent (or far weaker) "no go" (or stop) button. In a sense, the individual with an addictive disorder is *unable to stop going* toward their item of addiction. This causes them to use compulsively, devoting most of their thoughts, plans, and behavior to their item of addiction. This, in turn, causes neglect to other activities, causing significant psychological and social problems in other areas of their life with a significant impact on their families and society.

KEY POINT

Medication-assisted treatment (MAT) is the use of medications in combination with counseling and behavioral therapies to provide a whole-patient approach to the treatment of SUDs.

Drugs of abuse refer to drugs that are taken for their mind-altering effects. This term relates more specifically to illegal drugs, which are sometimes referred to as street drugs. The classification of cannabis is often controversial, given that medical marijuana is legal in some states in the United States. For the purpose of this text, due to its psychoactive properties, nonmedical marijuana, including recreational use of cannabis, is included as a drug of abuse. Common socially accepted substances, such as nicotine/tobacco and caffeine, have mind-altering properties, albeit to a milder degree than illegal drugs. They are also included in the *DSM-5* because they can lead to addiction with significant health consequences.

KEY POINT

Dual diagnosis refers to the co-occurrence of a substance use disorder with a mental health disorder. Co-occurring mental health conditions are the norm in patients with SUDs. As such, the dual diagnosis approach is a useful approach to diagnosis and treatment which improves treatment outcomes for patients with addiction.

Medication-assisted treatment (MAT) is the use of medications in combination with counseling and behavioral therapies to provide a whole-patient approach to the treatment of SUDs (SAMHSA, 2021). MAT is associated with improved patient outcomes, including improved patient survival, increased engagement, and retention in treatment, decreased illicit drug use, and decreased criminality among individuals with SUDs. MAT improves the patient's ability to obtain and maintain employment. For pregnant patients with SUD, MAT improved birth outcomes and reduces the occurrence and effects of intrauterine drug exposure.

Dual diagnosis refers to the co-occurrence of a substance use disorder with a mental health disorder. Co-occurring mental health conditions are the norm in patients with SUDs. As such, the dual diagnosis approach is a useful approach to diagnosis and treatment which improves treatment outcomes for patients with addiction.

INTRODUCTION

Addiction is an aspect of psychiatry that shows up in every facet of the medical field. Addiction is a treatable chronic medical disease involving complex interactions among brain circuits, genetics, the environment, and an individual's life experiences (ASAM, 2019). Addiction is a compulsive pattern of behavior where acquiring and using a drug, or engaging in certain behaviors, becomes the most important preoccupation and activity in an individual's life. People with addiction use substances or engage in behaviors that become compulsive and often continue despite harmful consequences (ASAM, 2011, 2019). At the core of addiction is a loss of control. Compulsive behaviors can include using substances (e.g., drugs of abuse, nonmedical use of prescription medications) and nonsubstance-related behaviors (behavioral addictions with gambling are officially recognized in the *DSM-5*). Addictive disorders can affect the very young, including young preschoolers who can get addicted to electronic devices, school-aged children with gaming addictions, preteens vaping compulsively, adolescents with substance use or gaming addictions, adult substance users, gamblers, and elderly individuals with substance use disorders. Figure 29.1 provides an overview of addictive disorders in the *DSM-5*.

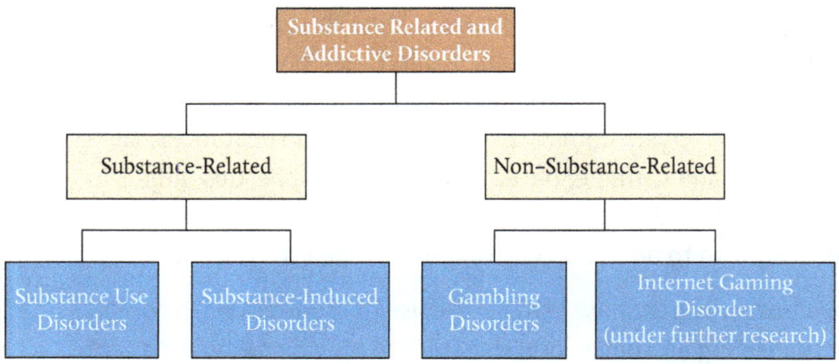

FIGURE 29.1 Overview of substance-related and addictive disorders.

Substance use disorders (SUD), including drugs of abuse and nonmedical use of prescription medications, are aspects of psychiatry that show up in every facet of the medical field. The effects of substance use may result in medical consequences in or across organ systems. Individuals with addictive disorders can neglect their basic living needs and conditions, mental and physical health, and often have concurrent disease states. As patients, individuals with addictive disorders can provoke strong negative reactions (including countertransference) in their treatment providers. In some cases, these feelings within clinicians can harm the working relationship and create conflict or distance between patients and providers. As a result, patient outcomes are affected, and there may be premature termination of the encounter, including being discharged prematurely or against medical advice. Without adequate treatment, individuals with addictive disorders are likely to return for repeat admission, further increasing health care utilization and costs. As such, increasing knowledge and awareness of SUD symptoms and the various states can robustly boost a provider's ability to manage the challenges associated with patients with addictive disorders and their families, while more effectively shifting the patient toward favorable patient outcomes.

KEY POINT

Substance use disorders (SUD), including drugs of abuse and nonmedical use of prescription medications, are aspects of psychiatry that show up in every facet of the medical field. The effects of substance use often result in medical consequences in or across organ systems. Individuals with addictive disorders can neglect their basic living needs and conditions, mental health, and physical health, which worsens their overall health conditions.

Individuals of all ages suffer the effects of addiction. Babies who are exposed to drugs in utero are born prematurely, underweight, and with persisting developmental problems. Adolescents who use drugs are at risk of delinquency, while young adults who use drugs are at risk of dropping out of school or college with poorer social outcomes. Adults with substance use disorders suffer significant mental health and psychosocial problems. There is an increasing number of adults initiating drug use in their elderly years. Individuals with addiction begin their use of substances for a variety of reasons. For children and adolescents, the presence of substances in their environment may lead to experimentation. There is a belief that the recreational use of substances can be enjoyable and fun and is not harmful. Many individuals with addictive disorders may initially begin using substances recreationally—others begin using in a quest to solve a problem and often to, unknowingly, self-treat underlying psychiatric symptoms. Once substance use has been initiated, however, a set of neurobiochemical processes are triggered downstream, resulting in chronic changes within the brain. These alterations are the underlying basis of the symptoms of addictive disorders, including craving and physiologic dependence, manifested as tolerance and withdrawal in some cases.

Addiction does not discriminate between individuals, cultures, or social groups. The manifestation of addiction may vary based on social encounters. While those in a lower socioeconomic bracket may be more susceptible to negative consequences, such as policing or limited access to health care or social support resources, those in a higher socioeconomic bracket may have more resources at their disposal to conceal the problem and its effects. Regardless of these apparent differences, addiction remains a potentially fatal disease.

CLINICAL TIP

SUD is common, co-occurs with a range of mental health disorders, and often goes untreated. Co-occurrence of SUD and mental health conditions is the norm rather than the exception. Identifying and treating both SUD and the mental health condition, the dual diagnosis and treatment approach results in improved patient outcomes.

EPIDEMIOLOGY

Substance-related and addictive disorders are a major public health problem worldwide. It is estimated that a total of 246 million people, or 1 out of 20 people between the ages of 15 and 64 years, used an illicit drug in 2013 (United Nations Office of Drugs and Crime, UNODC, 2015). Based on

QUICK POINT

Addiction can be a severe and sometimes fatal disease, but recognizing this is obstructed by several stereotypes. Stereotypes are unhelpful and can be dangerous because, while providing unproven reasons for the addictive behaviors (the presumed "why" the behaviors are happening), it neglects the dangers of the behaviors (the actual "what" is happening). The major impediment is that **stereotypes cause distraction and delay** in identifying treatment need, accessing treatment resources, providing those resources, and engaging the patients in productive escapes from addictions.

national surveys, an estimated 23 million adults in the United States have struggled with problematic drug use (National Institute of Mental Health [NIMH], 2015). National studies have found that SUD is common, co-occurs with a range of mental health disorders, and often goes untreated. In 2014, about 20.2 million adults in the United States had a SUD, and 7.9 million had both a SUD and another mental illness. About 10% of adults have had a drug use disorder at some time in their lives, yet up to 75% report not receiving any form of treatment (NIMH, 2015). About 11.2% of persons aged 12 years and over had used an illicit drug use in the past month, while about 2.2% had nonmedical use of a psychotherapeutic (Centers of Disease Control and Prevention [CDC], 2018). Opioid-related overdoses have a disproportionately high impact on national fatalities, surpassing motor vehicle accidents and firearms as a leading cause of death (National Safety Council, 2019).

The economic cost of substance use is staggering. Substance use, including abuse of tobacco, alcohol, and abuse drugs, cost the United States over $740 billion annually in health care costs, productivity loss, and crime (NIDA, 2020). Tobacco alone is estimated to cost $130 billion in health care dollars and $295 billion to the economy. Alcohol use costs at least $25 billion in health care dollars and about $225 billion in total economic cost. The bill for drugs of abuse is estimated to be $193 billion, which includes at least $11 billion in health care and other expenses related to loss of productivity and prison costs (NIDA, 2020).

THE PROBLEM WITH STEREOTYPES IN ADDICTION

Addiction can be a fatal disease, but recognizing this serious consequence suffers from several stereotypes. These stereotypes surround individuals with addictive disorders and often impede treatment. Among these stereotypes about individuals with addictive disorders are beliefs about characterological flaws, faulty socialization, and lack of spirituality. Such stereotypes accept the individual's symptoms as untreatable, and the individuals are sometimes viewed as manipulative, self-centered, and persistently in need of others' help. They are sometimes seen as making repeated poor decisions, which are the primary causes of their problems, and, as such, they "deserve" their negative life consequences, ranging from homelessness to incarceration. In others, the impact of their addiction is downplayed, and they are presented as functioning addicts.

Stereotypes are unhelpful and can be dangerous because, while providing unproven reasons for the addictive behaviors (the presumed "why" the behaviors are happening), it neglects the dangers of the behaviors (the actual "what" is happening). The major impediment is that *stereotypes cause distraction and delay* in identifying treatment need, accessing treatment resources, providing those resources, and engaging the patients in productive escapes from addictions. Sometimes this delay in accessing, providing, or engaging the patient in treatment is fatal. For the pregnant woman struggling with an addiction, delaying treatment could have permanent adverse outcomes on the unborn child. In the young, the delay in treatment comes at the cost of continued damage to the developing brain, significantly impacting the individual's life and developmental trajectory. It is crucial to be mindful of the potential for implicit bias when encountering individuals with addictive disorders. In this case, implicit bias refers to unconscious perceptions and attitudes that affect our understanding, actions, and decisions regarding individuals with addictive disorders. The more effective clinical view is to regard the patient as "a person with an addictive disorder" and then identify their symptoms and work to decrease or eliminate those symptoms. Increased focus on the importance of delivering care to patients, especially during pregnancy, improves health care and health service utilization outcomes for all, including the unborn child.

MODELS OF ADDICTION

A model is a way to conceptualize a disease. In the field of addiction, various models exist for understanding the origins, development, presentation, and treatment of addictive disorders. This section focuses on the more common models—the core features of which are summarized in Table 29.1. The biopsychosocial approach is a functional approach to understanding the origins, development, presentation, and treatment of addictive disorders.

TABLE 29.1 Models of Drug Addiction

Model	Moral model	Social learning model	Psychodynamic model	Disease model	Brain disease model of addiction (BDMA)
Description of viewpoint	• Drug addiction is caused by a moral or character flaw. • Drug addiction is immoral or illegal.	• Drug addiction is a learned behavior and the result of the conditioning and modeling of drug use.	• Drug addiction is the result of unaddressed childhood trauma. • Drug use may be an unconscious response to difficulties stemming from unaddressed childhood trauma.	• Drug addiction is a disease that originates from within the individual themselves. • Sees addiction as a disease that does not exist on a continuum; it is either present or absent ("once an addict, always an addict").	• Drug addiction is a brain disease. • Drug addiction is caused by brain changes in response to the presence of drugs.
Advantages	• Highlights the importance of spirituality, which is a positive treatment factor in many patients	• Highlights the importance of social environment in exposure to, initiation of, promotion of, and risk perception of drug use	• Highlights the importance of assessing, identifying, and treating (usually through psychotherapy) for adverse childhood experiences and other childhood trauma	• Highlights addiction as a health issue • Provides a framework for patients to understand their behavior, which in turn removes some of the sense of shame often experience	• Corrects (or attempts to correct) underlying brain malfunction
Disadvantages	• Assumes patients are patients because they are of weaker characters • Encourages public disregard • Encourages punishment over treatment of the patient • Misdirects resources from treatment to other sources (e.g., incarceration) • Stereotypical and promotes implicit bias	• Discourages engagement in treatment • Focuses on the environment (patients sometimes are not able to control or influence this) • Increases the sense of inevitability of the patient's symptoms • Stereotypical and promotes implicit bias	• Focus on historical experiences	• Encourages engagement in treatment (correcting a pivotal underlying problem) • Sees addiction as irreversible and incurable (patients are labeled for life) • Removes responsibility from the patient to control their behavior • Reduced clinical utility due to the removal of symptom severity (e.g., drinking 1 drink is almost as bad as drinking 20 drinks) • Offers only one course of treatment, total abstinence	• Often criticized for its seemingly narrow focus on neurobiology

Model	Moral model	Social learning model	Psychodynamic model	Disease model	Brain disease model of addiction (BDMA)
Resolution of symptoms	• Attaining optimal spirituality. • Spiritual direction through a spiritual organization.	• The patient arrives at their personal decision that risks of drug use outweigh the benefit.	• Addresses childhood trauma and coping strategies.	• Total abstinence.	• Correction of neurobiology through psychopharmacological treatment.
Problems in treatment	• Discourages engagement in treatment	• Discourages engagement in treatment	• Relies on memory recall (memory is sometimes affected by drug use)	• Discourages the belief that a patient can change • Limits help (or support and treatment) to the few who can achieve total abstinence, while leaving the others without help	• Apparent narrow focus (addiction is more than a brain disease; it manifests in psychological and social spheres); however, BDMA does not exclude the inclusion of other psychosocial aspects of treatment
Evidence-base (when used alone)	• No evidence	• No evidence	• Limited evidence	• Limited evidence • Alcoholics Anonymous (AA) is based on the disease model	• Greatest body of evidence supporting efficacy of treatment

The Brain Disease Model of Addiction

Substance use often results in neuroadaptive changes that initiate, promote, and maintain addiction's compulsive behaviors. The brain disease model of addiction (BDMA) asserts that addiction-related behavior results from biological factors stemming from an organ, in this case the brain, and is a consequence of physical or organic alterations or disruptions in brain structures, neurotransmitters, and epigenetics following chronic substance use. Other bodily systems, such as the endocrine system (e.g., hypothalamic–pituitary–adrenal [HPA] axis), are also implicated in the manifestation of addiction. At its core, the BDMA defines addiction as a chronic brain illness with biological, neurological, genetic, and psychological correlations. These neurobiological factors are also influenced by social forces, which serve as potential antecedents and perpetuate the consequences. Addiction is a chronic disease like other chronic diseases, such as type 2 diabetes, cancer, and cardiovascular disease. Like other chronic diseases, addictive disorders often result from a combination of factors, including genetic predisposition,

KEY POINT

Substance use often results in neuroadaptive changes that initiate, promote, and maintain addiction's compulsive behaviors. The brain disease model of addiction (BDMA) asserts that addiction-related behavior results from biological factors stemming from an organ, in this case the brain, and is a consequence of physical or organic alterations or disruptions in brain structures, neurotransmitters, and epigenetics following chronic substance use.

early childhood factors, stress, mental health symptoms, and exposure (see Figure 29.2). These all play a part in the onset of the disease of addiction.

> **KEY POINT**
>
> The biopsychosocial systems approach to addiction allows for comprehensive conceptualization of addiction as a multifactorial condition. This includes genetic, epigenetic, and biological factors; psychological factors; and sociocultural factors, which all contribute to the initiation, development, and manifestation of addictive disorders and their treatment. In this model, psychosocial factors complement and interact with neurogenetics.

Biopsychosocial Approach to Addiction

The biopsychosocial systems approach to addiction allows for comprehensive conceptualization of addiction as a multifactorial condition (Buchman et al., 2010). This includes genetic, epigenetic, and biological factors; psychological factors; and sociocultural factors, which all contribute to the initiation, development, and manifestation of addictive disorders and their treatment. In this model, psychosocial factors complement and interact with neurogenetics. Due to its utility, coherence, and efficacy in medicine, the biopsychosocial model is perhaps the best comprehensive model to guide the field of addiction. Figure 29.2 depicts factors within the biopsychosocial systems approach.

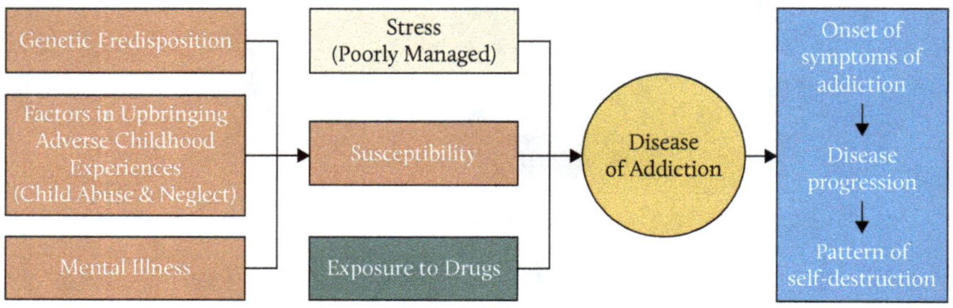

FIGURE 29.2 Biopsychosocial factors related to addictive disorders.

> **KEY POINT**
>
> The neurobiology of addictive disorders is believed to be rooted in the disruption of our natural reward system. This involves the mesolimbic dopaminergic system, a collection of brain structures referred to as the brain reward circuit, which is responsible for memory related to pleasurable (or rewarding) activities and their motivating behaviors.

NEUROBIOLOGY OF ADDICTION

Addiction is a brain-based disease with ramifications in the psychological and social realms. Often, what first gains attention are the social consequences experienced by the individual, including school, work, legal, and family problems. The neurobiology of addictive disorders is believed to be rooted in the disruption of our natural reward system. This involves the mesolimbic dopaminergic system, which is a collection of brain structures referred to as the brain reward circuit that is responsible for memory related to pleasurable (or rewarding) activities and their motivating behaviors. In this way, the brain reward circuit regulates actions around behaviors by causing pleasurable (or rewarding) effects. The brain structures in the reward circuit include the nucleus accumbens (NA), ventral tegmental area (VTA), the prefrontal cortex (PFC), and the limbic system, which handles feelings and emotions (Figure 29.3).

Several neurochemical systems are involved in addiction. These include the catecholamines (dopamine, norepinephrine, and serotonin); endogenous opioids; gamma-aminobutyric acid (GABA); and glutamate, acetylcholine, and endocannabinoid systems. Dopamine is the neurochemical most strongly and consistently associated with addictive disorders, and dopamine release is the final common pathway that precipitates and perpetuates reward-seeking behavior.

Natural rewards, such as food and sex, lead to dopamine release, causing "natural highs" (feel-good experiences), reinforcing the behaviors necessary for propagating the species. Most substances of abuse have the potential to increase dopamine levels rapidly and for longer durations than foods or activities that cause natural highs. In effect, they usurp the reward center, causing it to activate intensely around the perceived reward. This causes brain disruption and depletion of certain neurochemical stores. Of note, some substances, including hallucinogens, cannabis, and anabolic steroids, have additional mechanisms of action, which are less directly linked to the reward system.

KEY POINT

Most substances of abuse have the potential to increase dopamine levels rapidly and for longer durations than foods or activities that cause natural highs. In effect, they take over the reward center, causing it to activate intensely around the perceived reward—in this case, the drug.

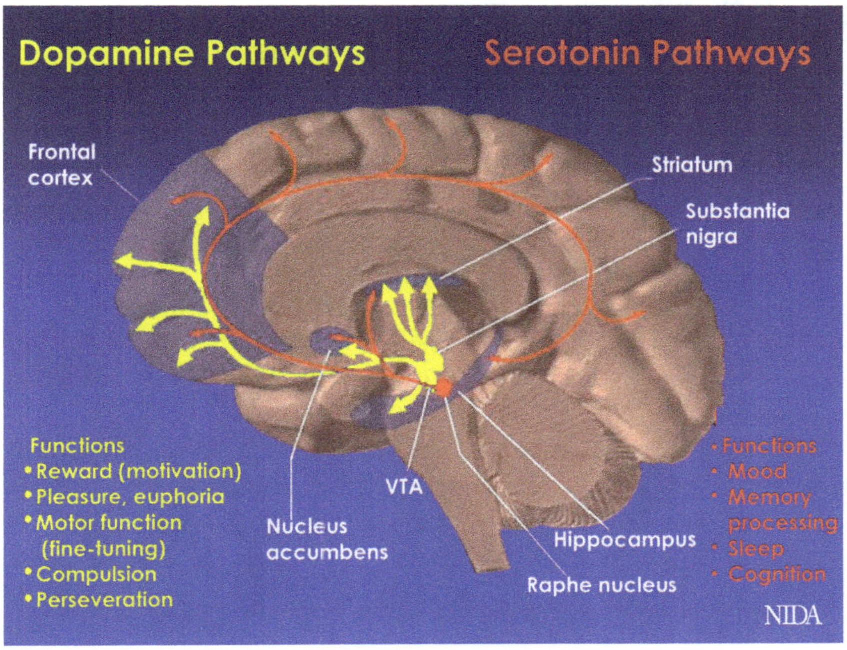

FIGURE 29.3 The neuroanatomy of the human reward system. Image courtesy of National Institute on Drug Abuse.

Source: https://commons.wikimedia.org/wiki/File:Brain_Pathways_DA_5HT.jpg.

ADDICTION AS A DEVELOPMENTAL PROCESS

QUICK POINT

Addiction is a developmental disease. Symptoms of addiction most often begin in youth. Without early identification and intervention, symptoms progressively worsen into adulthood often with great mental health and psychosocial consequences.

Addictive disorders begin early in life. Over 90% of adults with SUD report beginning to use in adolescence. Compulsive gaming behaviors are often present in school-aged children and sometimes as early as preschool. Some were exposed to drugs in utero, some experienced adverse childhood experiences (ACEs) in early childhood, and others were raised in environments where drug use was witnessed and normalized and risk perception was lowered. Nevertheless, it is becoming increasingly common to find individuals with no known family history of addiction or trauma presenting with addictive disorders.

Individuals who progress to develop addictive disorders in adulthood often show certain behavioral traits early in life. They are often thrill seekers, reward sensitive, and described as impulsive. Sensation seeking (also called thrill seeking or excitement seeking) is the tendency to seek and pursue new or novel and different sensations, feelings, and experiences. From the neurocognitive viewpoint, impulsivity is the inability to inhibit behavioral impulses and thoughts. They often manifest high reward sensitivity, high risk-taking, or low harm avoidance. Reward-sensitivity is the tendency to detect, pursue, learn from, and derive pleasure from positive stimuli. A disproportionate number of individuals with ADHD go on to develop addictive disorders. The age of onset is delayed, the risk of addictive disorders decreases, and the severity of symptoms of addictive disorders are reduced with optimal treatment of this underlying neurodevelopmental disorder. Other disorders that increase the risk of addictive disorders include mood and anxiety disorders. Childhood trauma and different adverse childhood experiences are strongly linked to substance use disorders.

The disease of addiction hardly ever begins suddenly. Although it can develop within a short period of time, it is more often a more insidious process. Recognizing addiction as a process provides the opportunity for intervention. Symptoms begin and worsen over time, sometimes taking years before the treatment need is identified. Early identification of the need for treatment, and provision of this treatment, interrupts the progression of the disease process.

Adolescent Addiction

Addiction is a disorder that often begins in adolescence. Over 90% of adults with addictive disorders, including substance and nonsubstance related, had the onset of their symptoms in adolescence. Drug exposure, even with experimentation, in youth may result in different neuroadaptive changes than those seen in adults. This is in part due to the accelerated neurodevelopmental changes occurring during adolescence. Adolescents often use multiple substances simultaneously, including over-the-counter (OTC) medications.

Monitoring the Future (MTF), a yearly survey that measures drug and alcohol use and related attitudes among adolescent students nationwide, provides an overview of drug use trends among teens in the United States. The most common substances used by adolescents include alcohol, nicotine, and cannabis. The 2020 MTF survey showed the level of vaping of cannabis and nicotine in teens remains high. Opioid use, addiction, and overdose deaths in adolescents and young adults, including heroin and nonmedical use of prescription opioids, is a public health problem of epidemic proportions (Fishman, 2020; Levy, 2019; Gandhi, 2006; Sharma, 2016; NIDA, 2020a). Alcohol remains the most commonly used substance in adolescence. Nearly 10% of adolescents report drinking and driving. Approximately 40% of adolescent drug-related visits to the emergency room involve alcohol (Grigsby et al., 2016). Adolescents with substance use have unique treatment needs that adult-based treatment types do not always meet. Family pressure and consequential legal interventions can play a central role in getting adolescents to enter, stay in, and complete treatment—all of which could be critical in the youth's life.

QUICK POINT

Drug exposure, even with experimentation, in youth may result in different neuroadaptive changes than those seen in adults. This is in part due to the accelerated neurodevelopmental changes occurring during adolescence. Adolescents often use multiple substances simultaneously, including over-the-counter (OTC) medications.

CLINICAL TIP

In adolescents, working with the family is central to preventing and treating substance use. Specifically, the development of trust, rapport, and communication within the family sets the standard for preventing adolescent substance use.

Adult Addiction

Adults may have a different profile of substance use compared to adolescents. Of lifetime illicit drug use in persons aged 18 or older, about half used cannabis and about one in six persons have tried cocaine or hallucinogens. Most addiction research and treatment has been done in adults. Within the adult population, specific populations with SUD, including pregnant women; incarcerated persons; persons living with HIV or hepatitis; physicians; and members of the lesbian, gay, bisexual, transgender, queer (LGBTQ+) community require carefully tailored care to provide effective treatment.

Geriatric Addiction

In the geriatric population (age 65 years or older), problematic drinking and alcohol use disorder is the leading SUD, followed by prescription drug use disorder. Prescription drug use commonly involves either or both prescription opioids and benzodiazepines. SUDs may be more difficult to recognize in older adults due to medical comorbidities and neurocognitive

QUICK POINT

In the geriatric population (age 65 years or older), problematic drinking and alcohol use disorder is the leading SUD, followed by prescription drug use disorder. Prescription drug use commonly involves either, or both, prescription opioids or benzodiazepines. SUDs may be more difficult to recognize in older adults due to medical comorbidities and neurocognitive impairment, which mask symptoms and alter behaviors.

impairment, which mask symptoms and alter behaviors (Seim et al., 2020). Geriatric persons are also particularly at risk, since aging is associated with a decrease in lean muscle mass, in total body water, and in hepatic metabolism of alcohol and medications or drugs. Altogether, these factors make older individuals more vulnerable to both the intoxicating and chronic physiological effects of alcohol. Benzodiazepines with a long half-life may cause sedation. Older adults are more likely to experience cognitive and psychomotor sequelae related to benzodiazepine and alcohol use. It is sometimes challenging to recognize when an elderly person has problematic drug use or meets the criteria for substance use disorder. The natural alteration tolerance and decreased participation in life activities, which may naturally occur with aging, are also cardinal symptoms of SUD. The criteria that most successfully identify alcohol use disorder in older adults include unsuccessful efforts to cut back alcohol use, withdrawal symptoms, and social or interpersonal problems (Kuerbis et al., 2014). Several factors complicate SUD treatment in older adults, including social isolation, grief and bereavement, depression, guardianship or capacity issues, and limited transportation.

ADDICTION IN PREGNANCY

As a subpopulation of patients with addiction, pregnant women and their offspring do not receive adequate treatment. This is often due to poor recognition of the need for treatment and lack of treatment facilities suited to their needs. Due to the nature of addiction symptoms and accompanying inattention to body signs, some pregnant women, left on their own, do not even realize they are pregnant. Nevertheless, increased attention to the critical importance of delivering care to mothers mitigates adverse maternal and fetal outcomes.

In pregnant women, substance use can have significant adverse effects on both the fetus and mother. Fetal alcohol spectrum disorder (FASD) is a leading cause of preventable congenital defects and the leading preventable cause of intellectual disability with both increasing the risk of adverse life outcomes in offspring (Streissguth et al., 2004). The use of opioids during pregnancy poses a challenge to health care delivery. In 2019, about 7% of women reported prescription opioid use during pregnancy. One in five of these pregnant women obtained these medications from a source other than a health care provider, over a quarter wanted or needed to cut down or stop using, and one third (31.9%) reported not receiving counseling on how opioid pain medications could affect their baby (Ko et al., 2020). Opioid use disorder in pregnancy can result in a withdrawal syndrome in newborns called neonatal abstinence syndrome or neonatal opioid withdrawal syndrome (NAS/NOWS). This causes extended hospital stays, poor feeding, irritability, failure to thrive, and other developmental problems. It is estimated that about every 15 minutes a baby is born with NAS/NOWS (Ko et al., 2020).

The American College of Obstetricians and Gynecologists (2017) and the American Academy of Pediatrics (AAP) recommend refraining from marijuana use during pregnancy and lactation (Ryan & O'Conner, 2017). However, almost 10% (9.8%) of women self-reported marijuana use before pregnancy, 4.2% during pregnancy, and 5.5% after pregnancy. During pregnancy, the most common reasons for cannabis use were to relieve stress or anxiety, nausea or vomiting, and pain (Ko, Coy, et al., 2020).

KEY POINT

Alcohol exposure during pregnancy can be harmful to the brain of a developing baby and may result in fetal alcohol spectrum disorders (FASDs). Fetal alcohol spectrum disorder (FASD) is a leading cause of preventable congenital defects and the leading preventable cause of intellectual disability with both increasing the risk of adverse life outcomes in offspring (Streissguth et al., 2004).

ADDICTION AMONG PHYSICIANS

Though they are considered healers of others, physicians and other health workers are also prone to developing SUDs with some specialties at higher risk. Although overall rates among U.S. physicians are similar to rates in the general population, anesthesiologists and emergency medicine physicians at greater risk for developing SUDs,. Among the drugs abused, emergency medicine physicians tend to use more illicit drugs, anesthesiologists tend to use opioids, and psychiatrists are more prone to use benzodiazepines. Fortunately, physician health monitoring programs are in place to provide treatment to physicians with SUDs, so they can remain in medical practice (Galanter, 2008).

DRUGS OF ABUSE

There are 10 classes of substances listed in the *DSM* and International classification of disease (ICD; Table 29.2). Beyond this list, other substances, including drugs and medications, have the potential for abuse or psychological or physiologic dependence. The Drug Enforcement Agency (DEA) maintains a separate classification of substances, drugs, and medications, based on their potential to cause addiction (Table 29.3). Some substances, although with less abuse potential, such as cannabis, have a relatively high potential to cause addiction.

TABLE 29.2 *DSM-5* Classes of Substances of Abuse

	Substance
1.	Alcohol
2.	Caffeine
3.	Cannabis
4.	Hallucinogens
5.	Inhalants
6.	Nicotine/tobacco
7.	Phencyclidine (commonly known as PCP)
8.	Opioids
9.	Sedatives, hypnotics, and anxiolytics
10.	Other (or unknown)

TABLE 29.3 DEA Schedules for Drugs

Schedule	Drugs
Schedule I	Substances considered to have no currently accepted medical use. This includes substances considered most dangerous with a high potential for abuse and severe psychological or physiological dependence, such as heroin, lysergic acid diethylamide, 3,4-methylenedioxymethamphetamine (ecstasy), methaqualone, peyote, synthetic cannabis, and organic cannabis.
Schedule II	Drugs for medical use but with a high potential for abuse or severe psychological or physiological dependence with currently accepted dependence. These include opioid combination products (< 15 mg of hydrocodone, Vicodin), hydromorphone (Dilaudid), meperidine (Demerol), oxycodone (Oxycontin), fentanyl, cocaine, methamphetamine, methadone, amphetamines (Dexedrine and Adderall), and methylphenidates (Ritalin).
Schedule III	Drugs with currently accepted medical use but with a moderate to low potential for abuse or severe psychological or physiological dependence. These include buprenorphine, opioid combination products (< 90 mg of codeine/dosage unit; e.g., Tylenol and codeine), ketamine, anabolic steroids, and testosterone.
Schedule IV	Drugs with currently accepted medical use but with a low potential for abuse and low risk of dependence. These include benzodiazepines; sedatives and hypnotics, such as lorazepam (Ativan); alprazolam (Xanax); diazepam (Valium); zolpidem (Ambien); carisoprodol (Soma); opioids; pentazocine/naloxone (Talwin); and tramadol (Ultram).
Schedule V	Drugs with lower potential for abuse or severe psychological or physiological dependence than schedule IV. These include preparations containing limited quantities of certain narcotics, including antidiarrheal, antitussive, and analgesic medications, such as cough preparations (with < 200 mg of codeine or per 100 milliliters [Robitussin]), diphenoxylate/atropine (Lomotil), defenoxin/atropine (Motofen), and pregabaline (Lyrica),

New Psychoactive and Emerging Substances

Beyond the relatively well-known substances, many new psychoactive substances (NPS) and new emerging drugs (NEDs) continue to make their debut on the market. These are often synthetic drugs made to mimic established drugs of abuse, while evading detection and legal problems. In the past decade, about 750 different psychoactive substances from various classes were reported worldwide with at least 80 new substances identified worldwide per year (UNDOC, 2017). Some of these emerge quickly and disappear, while others become more established with little to no regulation. Some examples include spice (synthetic cannabinoids), khat, salvia, and kratom, which is linked to hepatotoxicity and severe neurologic complications, including life-threatening encephalopathy and seizures (National Institute of Diabetes and Digestive and Kidney Diseases, 2012; Pantano et al., 2016).

SUBSTANCE-INDUCED DISORDERS

Substance use, intoxication, and withdrawal states cause neuropsychiatric and other physical symptoms. Each substance induces unique symptoms based on its psychopharmacologic properties. Several substance-induced states and disorders are identified. They are intoxication, withdrawal, delirium and dementia, amnestic disorder, psychotic disorder, mood disorder, anxiety disorder, sexual dysfunction, and sleep disorders. To meet criteria for substance-induced disorders, the symptoms need to match specific criteria as outlined in the *DSM-5*.

> **CLINICAL TIP**
>
> Individuals with SUDs often have mental health conditions occurring alongside their SUDs. This often presents a treatment challenge in patients with SUD. Clinical symptoms of both SUD and mental health present in a myriad of ways including preceding, consequent to, influencing, or worsening the ongoing substance use and mental health symptoms. The dual diagnosis approach, where both conditions are diagnosed and treated fully, is a more effective strategy for diagnosis and treatment which improves treatment outcomes in patients with SUD.

CLINICAL FEATURES

Due to their compulsive behaviors, patients with addictive disorders are often preoccupied with seeking, obtaining, using, and recovering from their drugs of abuse. This causes them to neglect other duties and facets of life. This comes at a great cost to themselves and their families, who often experience neglect and abuse, including offspring. People who drink alcohol engage in high-risk sexual behaviors, increasing their risk of infectious diseases. Individuals who use substances by intravenous routes of administration are at risk for infectious diseases, such as HIV and hepatitis, due to the sharing of dirty syringes. Abscesses and cellulitis may occur at local areas of injection, and systemic spread can produce more severe complications, such as endocarditis. The use of cocaine and methamphetamine has been associated with medical problems, including myocardial infarction, seizures, psychosis, pulmonary edema, skin ulcers, dental problems, significant weight loss, and rhabdomyolysis. These problems have ramifications for society, making drug abuse a significant public health concern (Schwetz et al., 2019).

Different classes of substances produce different effects through their interaction with different neurochemical systems. The following table highlights the different classes of drugs and medications more commonly associated with abuse and addiction. It distinguishes them based on the affected biological receptors, acute symptoms, withdrawal states, unique associated characteristics of chronic use, and effects when used with alcohol.

ALCOHOL

KEY POINT

For the same amount of alcohol, women experience more effects than men. This is because women have lower levels of enzymes that metabolize alcohol and a smaller distribution volume.

Alcohol, often referred to as ethanol, is one of the oldest and most common recreational substances. Alcohol stimulates gamma-aminobutyric acid (GABA-A) receptors and inhibits excitatory glutamatergic neurotransmission, leading to a compensatory down regulation of receptor-mediated inhibitory neural tone with chronic drinking. In the short term, alcohol can produce a sense of relaxation, decreased anxiety, increased sociability, and euphoria. It is a CNS depressant and can cause disinhibition; sedation; and impairment of cognitive memory, sensory, and motor functions. Quantifying the amount of alcohol consumed by a patient is often a challenge. In the United States, one standard drink (one alcoholic drink equivalent) contains roughly 14 grams of pure alcohol. Figure 29.4 shows standard drink measurements. Figure 29.5 depicts the acute effects of alcohol on brain function based on the number of drinks. With chronic use, tolerance develops. When alcohol is stopped or reduced, inhibition decreases, and excitation increases, leading to the clinical presentation of alcohol withdrawal.

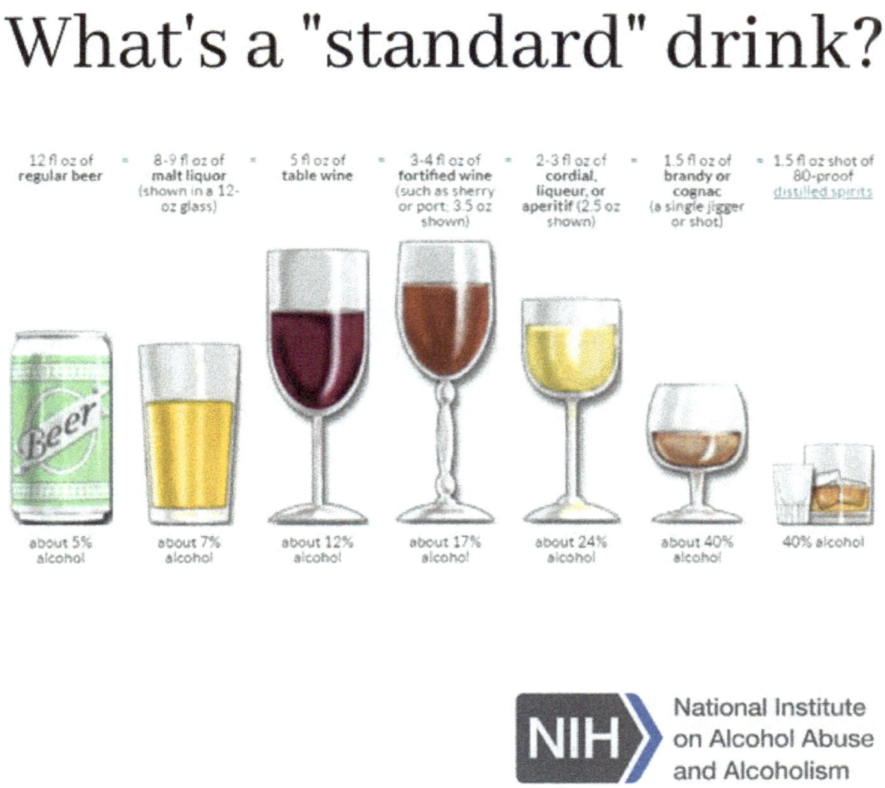
What's a "standard" drink?
12 fl oz of regular beer
8-9 fl oz of malt liquor (shown in a 12-oz glass)
5 fl oz of table wine
3-4 fl oz of fortified wine (such as sherry or port; 3.5 oz shown)
2-3 fl oz of cordial, liqueur, or aperitif (2.5 oz shown)
1.5 fl oz of brandy or cognac (a single jigger or shot)
1.5 fl oz shot of 80-proof distilled spirits
Beer
about 5% alcohol
about 7% alcohol
about 12% alcohol
about 17% alcohol
about 24% alcohol
about 40% alcohol
40% alcohol
NIH
National Institute on Alcohol Abuse and Alcoholism

FIGURE 29.4 Quantifying alcohol consumption: What is a standard drink?

Source: https://www.rethinkingdrinking.niaaa.nih.gov/How-much-is-too-much/What-counts-as-a-drink/Whats-A-Standard-Drink.aspx.

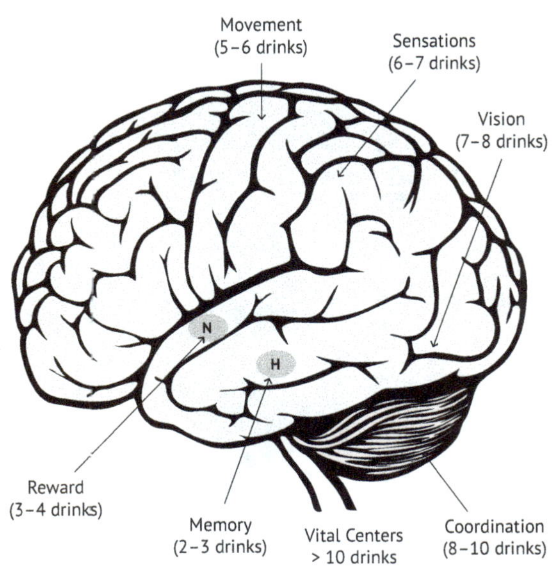

FIGURE 29.5 Number of drinks and effect of alcohol on brain function. N = Nucleus accumbens; H = Hippocampus.

Adapted from Copyright © 2013 Depositphotos/spirit-alex.

QUICK POINT

Alcohol consumption is associated with short- and long-term health risks, including motor vehicle accidence, violence, sexual risk behaviors, and a variety of medical problems. Epidemiologic data show an increase in morbidity when daily consumption exceeds two drinks for men and one for women.

CLINICAL TIP

The 2020–2025 dietary guidelines for Americans recommends that adults can choose not to drink or to drink in moderation by limiting intake to *two drinks or less in a day for men or one drink or less in a day for women* on days when alcohol is consumed (U.S. Department of Agriculture and U.S. Department of Health and Human Services, 2020).

Patterns of Drinking

Alcohol is most often consumed recreationally and in small amounts, which is generally socially acceptable. The National Institute of Alcohol Abuse and Alcoholism (NIAAA) recommends a maximum of one alcohol drink (for women) or two drinks (for men) a day or less than seven drinks (for women) or 14 drinks (for men) in a week.

Binge drinking, consuming alcohol in large amounts within a short period, is the most common pattern of excessive alcohol consumption in the United States. Binge drinking is defined as a drinking pattern that brings an individual's BAC to ⩾ 0.08 g % (80mg/dL) or higher. Such drinking and rises in BAC often occur within about 2 hours for adults, but the BAC rises can be much faster for adolescents. Most binge drinkers do not consider themselves to have a problem with alcohol. Table 29.4 summarizes the approximate number of drinks that raise a BAC above 80 mg/dL according to age and gender. High-intensity drinking is defined as consuming 10 or more drinks in a row. This occurs in a subset of binge drinkers, including youth out of high school who do not live with their parents. High-intensity drinking often occurs within the context of celebratory occasions, such as parties, birthdays, or sleepovers. Moreover, this drinking pattern is associated with severe social outcomes, including motor vehicle accidents and engagement in high-risk behaviors. Heavy alcohol use is defined as consuming more than four drinks on any day for men or more than three drinks for women. Chronic alcohol use, sometimes called alcoholism, is a drinking pattern that occurs over many years, often with repeated episodes of intoxication and withdrawal states.

TABLE 29.4 Binge Drinking: Approximate Number of Drinks That Raise a BAC above 80 mg/dL

Category	Age (years)	Number of drinks in a row
Men	⩾ 18	⩾ 5
Women	⩾ 18	⩾ 4
Boys	16–17	5
	14–15	4
	9–13	3
Girls	9–17	3

TABLE 29.5 BAL and corresponding symptoms in patients without tolerance

Blood alcohol concentration(BAC) mg/dl	Symptoms
50–80	Decreased anxiety, relaxation, increased socialization
80–100	Impaired judgement, impaired (slowed) reflexes
100–150	Clumsiness, ataxia, forgetfulness
150–200	Drowsiness, anterograde amnesia
300–400	Amnesia, severe dysarthria, hypothermia
400–600	Coma
> 600	Fatality

Alcohol Intoxication and Withdrawal

Alcohol intoxication is an acute clinical condition associated with drinking too much alcohol in a short amount of time. Alcohol intoxication can be fatal. Signs of alcohol intoxication include slurred speech, incoordination, unsteady gait, nystagmus, impaired attention or memory, and stupor or coma, which may occur during or shortly after alcohol use. Alcohol intoxication is sometimes associated with blackouts. An alcohol-induced blackout is an amnesia for the events of any part of a drinking episode without loss of consciousness (Lee et al., 2009). It is characterized by memory impairment during intoxication in the relative absence of other skill deficits. During blackouts, individuals continue to engage in purposeful and often complex actions, such as interacting with others, driving, selling, and purchasing items for which they have no recollection later. Alcohol is metabolized by zero-order kinetics, which means only a specific amount can be metabolized within a given time. With the body's continuous metabolization of alcohol, the BAC reduces by about 20 mg/dl per hour with levels gradually reducing over hours to days, depending on the amount of alcohol consumed. Intoxicated patients should be monitored in an emergency room to ensure protection of their airway, breathing, and circulation (the ABCs). The necessary laboratory tests should be ordered, including a BAL; complete blood count and differential, comprehensive metabolic panel; and urinalysis. Adequate fluids should be maintained parenterally. Many individuals with alcohol use disorder often suffer nutritional deficits and should be given thiamine before glucose. This is to avoid precipitating an acute encephalopathic condition known as Wernicke's encephalopathy.

KEY POINT

Clinical signs of alcohol intoxication vary depending on tolerance. Generally, signs of alcohol intoxication start to become obvious at blood alcohol levels between 100–150 mg/dL. Drowsiness is more prevalent at BACs of 150–200 mg/dL. Alcoholic coma can occur at BACs of 400–600 mg/dL BACs can be fatal over 600 mg/dL. Important to note is that signs of alcohol intoxication vary depending on individual levels of tolerance. Individuals who have developed high levels of tolerance to alcohol may not show signs of intoxication at BACs that could cause coma in other individuals.

CLINICAL TIP

When an intoxicated patient presents to an emergency department, management consists of monitoring airway, breathing, and circulation (the ABCs); ordering laboratory studies; and hydrating the patient with fluids and replenishing vitamins, such as thiamine, magnesium, and folic acid, which are at risk of being deficient in people with chronic alcohol use. To prevent precipitating encephalopathy, thiamine is given before glucose-containing IV fluids.

KEY POINT

When treating patients with alcohol intoxication, thiamine should be given before glucose. This avoids precipitating Wernicke's encephalopathy.

Alcohol Withdrawal Syndrome (AWS)

Alcohol withdrawal syndrome (AWS), a well-known condition precipitated by the intentional or unintentional abrupt cessation of constant heavy drinking, occurs in about 8% of hospitalized AUD inpatients. Approximately 15–30% of patients admitted to intensive care units (ICU) have an AUD and are at risk for developing AWS (Perry, 2014). AWS is characterized by two or more of the following, which develop within several hours or days after the cessation or reduction of alcohol: autonomic hyperactivity (manifested as hypertension, tachyarrhythmias, diaphoresis, peripheral vasoconstriction, and hyperthermia), increased hand tremor, insomnia, nausea or vomiting, transient hallucinations, psychomotor agitation, anxiety, or generalized tonic–clonic seizures. It is important to note that alcohol withdrawal does not occur exclusively in the context of complete cessation and can also occur with reduced intake. Alcohol withdrawal seizures occur in about 15% of patients, and they are typically of the grand mal type. Of significant concern is a severe and later stage of alcohol withdrawal called delirium tremens (DTs). DTs is a life-threatening condition that occurs in about 15% of patients. As its name may imply, it is characterized by agitation, tremulousness, autonomic instability (manifested as hypo- or hypertension, hypo- or hyperthermia, tachy- or bradycardia, hyper- or hypohidrosis, fevers, auditory and visual hallucinations, and disorientation). Three risk factors that may place a patient at increased risk of DTs are elevated systolic blood pressure, medical comorbidity, and prior complicated alcohol withdrawal syndromes. Prompt treatment must be provided for DTs, as the mortality rate can be as high as 20% (Galanter, 2008).

The gold-standard treatment of alcohol withdrawal includes the use of a benzodiazepine, as they are cross tolerant. Cross tolerance is when tolerance to one drug produces tolerance to another drug. In this case, both drugs stimulate the GABA-A receptors. Benzodiazepines reduce withdrawal severity and incidence of seizures and DTs. The choice of benzodiazepine used for management of alcohol withdrawal may rely on several factors, such as the half-life of the drug, liver function, and, in some cases, abuse potential. Two methods of alcohol detoxification utilizing benzodiazepines exist: fixed tapering dose regimen (FTDR) and symptom triggered regimen (STR). In FTDR, fixed doses of benzodiazepines are administered in a tapered pattern over scheduled intervals. In STR, the scheduled doses are not fixed, and doses are given only in response to symptom severity based on the scores of withdrawal scales that are administered at fixed intervals. One favorable outcome of STR is that, compared to FTDR, it may require a shorter duration of treatment and lower total doses of medication (Sachdeva et al., 2015) but requires keen attention to the patient's symptoms.

KEY POINT

Cross tolerance is when tolerance to one drug produces tolerance to another drug. The gold-standard treatment of alcohol withdrawal includes the use of a benzodiazepine, as they are cross tolerant.

Monitoring Patients With Alcohol Use Disorders

As patients with significant alcohol intake may tend to minimize or underreport the amount of drinking, one must remain vigilant of any findings on a routine or more specialized lab work. Carbohydrate-deficient transferrin (CDT) with high specificity may detect excessive alcohol intake of greater 50–80 g ethanol per day for at least 1 to 2 weeks. A panel of other more available and less costly tests, such as mean corpuscular volume, gamma-glutamyl transferase, aspartate transferase (AST or SGOT), and alanine transferase (ALT or SGPT) may also be helpful, but they are not as specific as CDT. These tests, on their own, are nonspecific. A combination of markers of elevated CDT, MCV, and GGT may provide greater sensitivity and specificity of 88% and 95%, respectively. Other measures that provide a longer window of detection than breath alcohol levels are sweat patches, and urine or other tissues for ethyl glucuronide, which remain in the human body for up to 3 days after consumption of alcohol and, therefore, is a useful method for monitoring abstinence and identifying relapse to heavy drinking. There is also a flexible wearable sensor that can accurately measure a person's blood alcohol level from sweat and transmit the data wirelessly to a laptop, smartphone, or other mobile device.

Because the liver metabolizes alcohol, the hepatic status of patients with heavy alcohol consumption must be monitored carefully. About 20% of individuals with AUD develop fatty liver disease, which can be reversed if consumption is stopped. Alcoholic hepatitis occurs when there are inflammatory changes, liver degeneration, and fibrosis of liver cells. About 40% of the cases develop into cirrhosis. In cirrhosis, scar tissue replaces normal liver tissue, and in later stages, jaundice and gastrointestinal disease may occur (Andresen-Streichert et al., 2018).

MEMORY TIP

Useful mnemonic for Wernicke-Korsakoff syndrome.

Wernicke-Korsakoff syndrome: COAT RACK
Wernicke's encephalopathy (acute phase)
C—Confusion
O—Ophthalmoplegia
A—Ataxia
T—Thiamine deficiency

Korsakoff's Amnestic syndrome (chronic phase): RACK
R—Retrograde amnesia
A—Anterograde amnesia
C—Confabulation
K—Korsakoff psychosis

Alcohol Use Disorders and Neurologic Complications

Wernicke's encephalopathy is a thiamine deficiency–associated neuropsychiatric condition leading to signs of ophthalmoplegia, nystagmus, ataxia, and inability to concentrate. Persons with AUD are at risk for thiamine deficiency due to poor diet and reduced thiamine absorption secondary to alcohol. Findings can be seen in the gray matter of mammillary bodies, thalamus, and periventricular gray (Sullivan, 2009).

Korsakoff syndrome may develop without further treatment. This syndrome is characterized by anterograde and retrograde memory deficits with the former being more prominent than the latter. Confabulation, filling memory gaps with made-up stories, may also exist.

MEMORY TIP

Wernicke-Korsakoff's triad: Alcoholics drink CANs of beer

C—Confusion
A—Ataxia
N—Nystagmus

CANNABIS

> **QUICK POINT**
>
> From 9% to 30% of those who use cannabis may develop some degree of cannabis use disorder. Individuals who begin using cannabis before age 18 are four to seven times more likely than adults to develop a marijuana use disorder (Hasin, 2015; Winters 2008).

Cannabis is a greenish-gray mixture of the dried flowers of the family of *Cannabaceae* plants. It occurs worldwide and goes by other names, including *weed*, *herb*, *pot*, *grass*, *bud*, and *ganja*. In humans, it exerts its effects through the endocannabinoid system. The endocannabinoid system (ECS) modulates several functions, including cognition, memory, attention and focus, sleep, appetite, mood, stress, fear, anxiety, and pain. It includes two main cannabinoid receptors, CB1 and CB2, which in addition to the brain are found in other body cells, including the immune, reproductive, respiratory, and gastrointestinal systems. The rewarding and positive reinforcing effects of the primary psychoactive component of cannabis is delta-9-tetrahydrocannabinol (THC), which exerts its effect mainly through the cannabinoid CB1 receptors in the brain, resulting in an increased risk of compulsive behaviors of addiction and produces a wide range of biological and behavioral responses. THC and other CB1 agonists activate the mesolimbic dopamine system and mediate cannabinoid dependence and expression of withdrawal upon cessation of drug administration. Different strains contain different levels of THC. The potency of cannabis has steadily risen in THC concentration over the past few decades. The plant also contains more than 500 other chemicals, including more than 100 compounds that are chemically related to THC, called *cannabinoids*. Dronabinol, a cannabinoid medication, is approved for the treatment of anorexia and chemotherapy-induced nausea and vomiting. Cannabidiol, commonly known as CBD oil, is one of the cannabinoids that has recently been explored for use in medical treatment. In 2018, the Federal Drug Administration approved a CBD-based medication, Epidiolex, for the treatment of seizures associated with Lennox–Gastaut syndrome (LGS), Dravet syndrome (DS), or tuberous sclerosis complex (TSC) in patients 1 year of age and older.

> **QUICK POINT**
>
> Cannabis significantly impairs judgment, reaction time, and motor coordination. Studies have found a direct relationship between blood THC concentration and impaired driving ability. Drivers with THC in their blood were found to be twice or more as likely to be involved in fatal motor vehicle accidents when compared to drivers who had not used drugs or alcohol (Biecheler, 2008, Asbridge, 2012, Preuss, 2021).

In the United States, Cannabis is most commonly smoked in hand-rolled cigarettes (*joints*), hand-rolled cigar wraps (*blunts*), or water pipes (*bongs*). It is ingested orally and brewed in teas or mixed into food, such as brownies, cookies, or candies. More recently, cannabis increasingly is vaporized through vaping devices in the form of oils or wax. Effects of cannabis are summarized in Table 29.6.

TABLE 29.6 Cannabis, Receptor Targets, and Effects

Substance group	Substance name	Neurochemistry	Acute	Long term	With alcohol	Withdrawal symptoms	Special populations	Medical-related problems or syndromes
Cannabinoids	Cannabis	Cannabis > 66 cannabinoids (∂-9-THC main active ingredient); acts on CB1 (brain, gut, and spinal cord); CB2 receptors (brain, gut, and immune system) and other receptors involved in the endocannabinoid system	Heightened sensory perception; euphoria followed by drowsiness/ relaxation; impaired short-term memory, attention, judgment, and other cognitive functions; impaired coordination and balance; increased heart rate; anxiety; paranoia; psychosis; persistent (lasting longer than intoxication but may not be permanent); impaired learning and coordination; sleep problems; depression	Potential for addiction: increased risk of cannabis and other drug and alcohol use disorders; cognitive (may be permanent); impairments in attention, learning and memory, and potential loss of IQ; increased risk of psychosis (including subclinical); increased risk of schizophrenia in people with genetic vulnerability	Magnified tachycardia and effect on blood pressure; intensified cognitive impairment, impaired psychomotor function, and impaired driving performance	Irritability, difficulty sleeping, strange nightmares, cravings, and anxiety	Adolescents: adolescent males with a history of cannabis use may develop subclinical psychosis, which remains present even after 1 year of abstinence	Lung disease, including chronic cough, bronchitis, electronic vaping–assisted lung injury (EVALI), and lung cancer; cannabis hyperemesis syndrome

KEY POINT

Cannabis intoxication symptoms include mood changes (euphoria and anxiety), cognitive changes (perception of slowed time), impaired judgement, impaired motor coordination, increased appetite, and withdrawal from social interaction. Signs of cannabis intoxication include conjunctival injections and tachycardia.

KEY POINT

Cannabis withdrawal symptoms include mood changes (irritability, anxiety, and depression), concentration problems, sleep disturbance, headache, nausea, diarrhea, decreased appetite, weight loss, and cravings. Signs of cannabis withdrawal include restlessness, tremor, sweating, fever, and chills.

Cannabis Intoxication and Withdrawal

To meet criteria for cannabis intoxication, a patient must experience two (or more) of the following symptoms within recent use of cannabis: impaired motor coordination, euphoria, anxiety, a sensation of slowed time, impaired judgment, and social withdrawal. In addition, two (or more) of the following must develop within 2 hours of use: conjunctival injection, increased appetite, dry mouth, and tachycardia. Cannabis withdrawal is characterized by three or more of the following symptoms within 1 week of cessation: irritability, anxiety, insomnia, decreased appetite or weight loss, restlessness, depressed mood, and physical symptoms (abdominal pain, tremor, sweating, fever, chills, or headache).

Cannabis Hyperemesis Syndrome

Chronic use of cannabis may result in cannabis hyperemesis syndrome, characterized by severe nausea and vomiting, abdominal pain, and the unique quality of having symptom relief with compulsive hot baths. This was first described in 2004 and is thought to be mediated via CB1 receptors in the gastrointestinal tract. Episodes of vomiting may return every few weeks or months. Patients tend to take frequent hot showers and baths. They often seek treatment in emergency settings and remain underdiagnosed. Their presentation is sometimes confounded by the fact that the same patients sometimes use cannabis to suppress nausea and vomiting. Figure 29.6 depicts the clinical stages of cannabis hyperemesis syndrome.

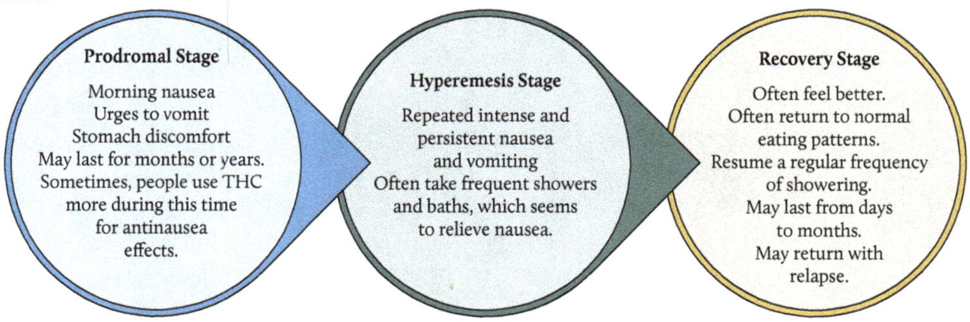

FIGURE 29.6 Stages of cannabis hyperemesis syndrome.

There are no clear clinical guidelines for its treatment and management. Supportive treatment, such as preventing dehydration (IV if patient cannot tolerate oral fluids), pain relievers if abdominal pain is present, antacids, and antiemetics, may be useful. Decreasing or stopping cannabis use often leads to symptom resolution. Symptoms tend to disappear with abstinence and return with relapse.

HALLUCINOGENS AND DISSOCIATIVE ANESTHETICS

Hallucinogens exert their effect primarily through serotonergic receptors. LSD has a chemical structure similar to serotonin. To meet criteria for hallucinogen intoxication (other than PCP), a patient must exhibit signs of behavioral changes, perceptual changes, and physical effects. Behavioral changes include anxiety or depression, fear of "losing one's mind," paranoia, and impaired judgment. Perceptual changes include depersonalization, derealization, illusions, hallucinations, and synesthesia. Physical symptoms include pupillary dilation, tachycardia, sweating, palpitations, blurry vision, tremors, and incoordination. Of note, contrary to most other drug classes, there is no withdrawal syndrome related to hallucinogens. However, a unique residual effect from hallucinogen use called hallucinogen persisting perception disorder (HPPD) may affect a percentage of patients. HPPD occurs even after there has been cessation of the drug and is marked by reexperiencing, primarily visual, disturbances, such as geometric hallucinations, flashes of color, trails of images of moving objects, afterimages, and halos around objects. These disturbances may last for years. Although patients may experience these hallucinations, they may not have a primary psychotic disorder.

PCP, previously used as a dissociative analgesic, is a hallucinogenic drug. It is an NMDA receptor antagonist and exerts its effect through glutamate. PCP intoxication includes clinically significant behavioral changes, such as belligerence, assaults, impulsiveness, unpredictability, psychomotor agitation, and impaired judgement. In addition, two or more of the following must be present: vertical or horizontal nystagmus; hypertension or tachycardia; numbness or diminished responsiveness to pain; ataxia; dysarthria; muscle rigidity; seizures or coma; and hyperacusis. No withdrawal syndrome exists. Other dissociative anesthetics include ketamine. At high doses, dextromethorphan is classified as a dissociative general anesthetic and hallucinogen. Dextromethorphan is often misused by teens, sometimes in conjunction with alcohol, which can cause more impairment and severe CNS depression. Effects of hallucinogens and dissociative anesthetics are summarized in Table 29.7.

CLINICAL TIP

A residual effect of hallucinogen use is hallucinogen persisting perception disorder (HPPD). HPPD occurs even after full abstinence. HPPD is characterized by reexperiencing, primarily visual, disturbances, such as geometric hallucinations, flashes of color, trails of images of moving objects, afterimages, and halos around objects. These disturbances may last for years. Although patients may experience these hallucinations, they may not have a primary psychotic disorder.

TABLE 29.7 Hallucinogens and Dissociative Anesthetics, Receptor Targets, and Effects

Substance group	Substance name	Neuro-chemistry	Acute	Long term	With alcohol	Withdrawal symptoms	Special populations	Medical-related problems or syndromes
Hallucinogens and dissociative drugs	Lysergic acid diethylamide (LSD)	Serotonin increase	Alters a user's mood, thoughts or perceptions; frightening flashbacks; dry mouth; sweating; elevated blood pressure; rapid mood swings; panic; fear; hostility; and aggression	Hallucinogen persisting perception disorder (HPPD); low addictive potential; and tolerance does develop	May drink to reduce unpleasant aftereffects of LSD; LSD may lead to reduction in perceived effects of alcohol, making it more likely to drink greater amounts of alcohol	Subjective (objective physical symptoms are rare)	Often used in parties and dubbed a "club" or "party" drug	Stroke
	Psilocybin (mushrooms)	Relaxation and altered sensory perception	Increased energy and heart rate; decreased appetite, nausea, yawning, feeling relaxed, and lack of coordination; distorted sense of time, place, and reality; introspective experience; anxiety; paranoia; panic; and hallucinations	Low addictive potential but may produce tolerance	Nausea, vomiting, drowsiness, panic, hallucination, and impaired self-awareness can contribute to alcohol poisoning	Subjective (objective physical symptoms are rare)	Often used in parties and dubbed a "club" or "party" drug for its hallucinogenic properties	Nausea and vomiting
Dissociative Anesthetics	Phencyclidine (PCP)	NMDA receptor antagonist (low doses)	Shallow, rapid breathing; tachycardia; high blood pressure; numbness; disorientation; confusion; muscle contractions; analgesia; altered perceptions; and feeling separated from body	Anxiety; depression; suicidal ideation; and low addictive potential but may produce tolerance	Sedative effects enhanced with alcohol; impaired self-awareness can contribute to alcohol poisoning	Muscle twitching; tremors, irritability; agitation; aggression; sweating; hyperthermia; and rotatory nystagmus	Often used in parties and dubbed a "club" or "party" drug	Catatonia; acidosis; vertigo; vomiting; and malnutrition

Substance group	Substance name	Neuro-chemistry	Acute	Long term	With alcohol	Withdrawal symptoms	Special populations	Medical-related problems or syndromes
		NMDA receptor antagonist (high doses)	Feelings of invincibility; markedly increased physical strength; seizures; coma; and hyperthermia					
	Ketamine	NMDA modulation (high doses)	Anxiety; agitation; insomnia; euphoria; slurred speech; blurred vision; arrhythmias; low body temperature; clammy skin; and bradycardia	Low addictive potential but may produce tolerance	Increased risk of memory loss; slow breathing; coma; and death	Depression; anxiety; insomnia; diplopia; tachycardia; and tachypnea	Often used in parties and dubbed a "club" or "party" drug for its hallucinogenic properties; appropriately used as an anesthetic gas and for treatment-resistant depression (both with FDA approval)	Slow breathing; coma; death; urinary problems, including increased frequency and pain on micturition; blood in urine; and abdominal pain
		NMDA modulation (low doses)	Sedation; analgesia; and impaired attention; memory; and motor function					
		NMDA modulation (high doses)	Immobility; distortions of auditory and visual perceptions; feelings of being separated from one's body and environment; hallucinations; memory problems; and refractory pain					
OTC and cough syrups	Dextromethorphan	NMDA receptor antagonists	Euphoria; dissociative effects; and hallucinations	Repeatedly seeking to experience that feeling may result in addiction	Drowsiness; slow or slurred speech	Depression	Often abused by teens	

INHALANTS

CLINICAL TIP

Sudden sniffing death is a complication of inhalant use, which results in acute and fatal heart failure within minutes of prolonged sniffing.

Inhalants only have an intoxication syndrome and not a withdrawal syndrome. This includes intended or unintended inhalation of a volatile hydrocarbon, which may include glues, fuels, or paints/solvents. There must be clinically problematic behavioral changes, such as belligerence, assaults, apathy, and impaired judgment. Two or more of the following symptoms develop with use: dizziness, nystagmus, incoordination, slurred speech, unsteady gait, lethargy, depressed reflexes, psychomotor retardation, tremor, generalized muscle weakness, blurred vision, stupor or coma, and euphoria. Death can also occur from a single episode of inhalant use in a healthy person by asphyxia. Sudden sniffing death occurs when chemicals in solvents can lead to fatal heart failure within minutes of prolonged sniffing. Effects of inhalants are summarized in Table 29.8.

STEROIDS

QUICK POINT

Athletes use some substances, including steroids, at substantially higher rates than nonathletes. Despite this, athletes' rates of addiction may be lower than nonathletes (McDuff & Baron, 2005).

Steroids are often used with the intention of increasing muscle mass and athletic performance enhancement. They are most often abused in the sports world. Most effects caused by anabolic steroids are reversible; however, some are semipermanent or permanent. Serious and life-threatening adverse effects are underreported due to other ongoing drug use. A variety of side effects can occur when anabolic steroids are misused, ranging from mild effects to ones that are harmful or even life-threatening. Steroid use is associated with multiple medical changes including high blood pressure, atherosclerosis, dyslipidemia, myocardial infarctions, and stroke. Steroid misuse can cause acne, hair loss on the head, cysts, and oily hair and skin. Steroid use causes hormonal imbalance resulting in hypogonadism and testicular atrophy. In men, irreversible male-pattern baldness and gynecomastia can occur. In women, masculinization can occur with breast atrophy, growth of body hair, voice deepening, and enlargement of the clitoris. In children or adolescents, steroid use can result in premature fusion of the growth plates resulting in stunted growth. Effects of steroids are summarized in Table 29.9.

TABLE 29.8 Inhalants, Receptor Targets, and Effects

Substnace group	Substance name	Neurochemistry	Acute	Long term	With alcohol	Withdrawal symptoms	Special populations	Medical-related problems or syndromes
Inhalants	Inhalants	GABA-mediated responses (like anesthetics)	Euphoria; slurred/altered speech; poor coordination; hallucination, delusions; dizziness; loss of consciousness; and reduced inhibition	Myelin breakdown can lead to muscle spasms; tremors; permanent neurological impairment; and liver or kidney damage. Addiction in a minority (report needing to continue using, despite severe adverse consequences)	Slow or slurred speech; slow muscle movements; slow reflexes; nausea; vomiting; extreme headaches; hallucinations; and erratic behavior	Mild withdrawal syndrome (e.g., irritability, restlessness, insomnia, headaches, poor concentration) can occur with long-term inhalant abuse	Abused mostly by younger rather than older teens	Dramatic weight loss; fatal cardiac arrhythmia; sudden sniffing death; long-term use with white matter changes

TABLE 29.9 Steroids, Receptor Targets, and Effects

Substance Group	Neurochemistry	Acute	Long term	With alcohol	Withdrawal symptoms	Special populations	Medical-related problems or syndromes
Steroids	Chemically related to testosterone	Paranoia; extreme irritability or aggression (e.g., "road rage"); irritability; and aggression	Mania; irritability; aggression	May be synergistic in precipitating impulsive violent behavior	Mood swings; fatigue; restlessness; loss of appetite; insomnia; reduced sex drive; steroid cravings; depression; and sometimes leads to suicide attempts	Adolescents may experience stunted growth; premature skeletal maturation; and accelerated puberty changes	Elevated blood pressure; blood clots; strokes; and artery damage Males experience shrunken testicles; decreased sperm count; infertility; baldness; gynecomastia; and an increased risk of prostate cancer Females experience facial hair growth; male-pattern baldness; menstrual changes/cessation; enlargement of the clitoris; and a deepened voice

OPIOIDS

Opioids are a potent group of pain-relieving substances with both pain-relieving properties and the potential for addiction. Patients with OUDs constitute a unique patient population in addiction and require specialized treatment to engage, manage, and treat. For additional information, see Chapter 30, "Prescription Drug Abuse: Opioids, Stimulants and Sedative-Hypnotics."

SEDATIVES, HYPNOTICS, OR ANXIOLYTICS

Sedatives, hypnotics, and anxiolytics are a group of substances that include prescription medications, which have multiple uses in psychiatry and medicine. For additional information, see Chapter 30, "Prescription Drug Abuse: Opioids, Stimulants and Sedative-Hypnotics."

STIMULANTS

Stimulants are a class of drugs that include amphetamines (including methamphetamine and amphetamine, whether prescribed or illegal) and cocaine. Criteria for stimulant intoxication includes behavioral changes, such as euphoria, changes in sociability, hypervigilance, interpersonal sensitivity, anxiety, tension, or anger; stereotyped behaviors; and impaired judgment. In addition, two or more of the following symptoms are required: tachycardia or bradycardia, pupillary dilation, elevated or lowered blood pressure; perspiration or chills; nausea or vomiting; weight loss; psychomotor agitation or retardation; muscular weakness, respiratory depression, chest pain, or cardiac arrhythmias; and confusion, seizures, dyskinesias, dystonia, or coma (APA, 2013). Stimulant withdrawal is characterized by dysphoric mood and two or more of the following: fatigue; vivid and unpleasant dreams; insomnia or hypersomnia; increased appetite; and psychomotor retardation or agitation (APA, 2013). Effects of stimulants are summarized in Table 29.10.

CLINICAL TIP

Stimulant withdrawal symptoms include dysphoric mood, fatigue, increased appetite, psychomotor retardation or agitation, insomnia or hypersomnia, and vivid or unpleasant dreams.

KEY POINT

Cocaethylene is cardiotoxic compound resulting from the concomitant use of cocaine and alcohol.

TABLE 29.10 Stimulants, Receptor Targets, and Effects

Substance group	Substance name	Neurochemistry	Acute	Long term	With alcohol	Withdrawal symptoms	Special populations	Medical-related problems or syndromes
Stimulants	Cocaine	DA in mesolimbic pathway (addictive); TRI (triple reuptake inhibitor on DA, NE, and 5HT); sodium channel blocker (anesthetic/ sudden cardiac death)	Dilated pupils; increased body temperature, heart rate, and blood pressure; nausea; increased energy and alertness; euphoria; decreased appetite and sleep; and, in high doses, erratic and violent behavior and panic attacks	Addiction; restlessness; anxiety; irritability; paranoia; panic attacks; mood disturbances; insomnia; nasal damage; difficulty swallowing (from snorting); GI problems; and HIV	Greater risk of overdose and sudden death than either drug alone; combining cocaine with alcohol produces cocaethylene (a cardiotoxic chemical)	Depression; fatigue; increased appetite; insomnia or hypersomnia; vivid, unpleasant dreams; psychomotor retardation; and agitation	Pregnant patients may experience premature delivery; low birth weights; and small for gestational age	Cocaethylene is cardiotoxic (EKG changes); myocardial infarction; seizures; psychosis; pulmonary edema; skin ulcers; dental problems; significant weight loss; and rhabdomyolysis
	MDMA (ecstasy/ molly)—a synthetic psychoactive substance similar to both a stimulant (amphetamine) and hallucinogen (mescaline)	Serotonin–norepinephrine–Dopamine-releasing agent and reuptake inhibitor	Euphoria; increased energy; alertness; tactile sensitivity; empathy; decreased fear; anxiety; increased or irregular heartbeat; dehydration; chills; sweating; impaired cognition and motor function; reduced appetite; muscle cramping; teeth grinding or clenching; and, in rare cases, hyperthermia, rhabdomyolysis, and death	Impulsiveness; irritability; sleep disturbances; anxiety; and addiction	Disinhibition and aggressive behavior	Irritability and aggression	Often used by youth at parties	Elevated blood pressure and pulse; muscle spasms; myocardial infarction; and seizures

Substance group	Substance name	Neurochemistry	Acute	Long term	With alcohol	Withdrawal symptoms	Special populations	Medical-related problems or syndromes
	Meth-amphetamine	Serotonin–norepinephrine–Dopamine-releasing agent and reuptake inhibitor	Increased wakefulness; increased physical activity; decreased appetite; tachypnea; tachyarrhymias; elevated blood pressure; increased body temperature; paranoia; hallucinations; and violent behavior	Sleep disturbance; memory and cognitive problems; anxiety; and paranoia	Disinhibition; aggressive behavior; and violent behavior	Depression; lethargy; anxiety; increased appetite; muscle pain and spasms; and psychosis	HIV-positive individuals may show worsening progression of HIV/AIDS; HIV causes more nerve damage and cognitive problems in HIV patients who use meth-amphetamine compared to those who do not	Dehydration; extreme weight loss; infectious disease (e.g., HIV, hepatitis B, and hepatitis C); severe dental problems ("meth mouth"); skin lesions from intense skin itching; strokes; and myocardial infarction
	Synthetic cathinones ("bath salts")	Monoamine–serotonin–norepinephrine–dopamine increase	Euphoria; paranoia; delusions; increased friendliness; increased sex drive; sweating; elevated blood pressure; increased body temperature	High addictive potential	Markedly aggressive behavior	Depression; anxiety; sleep problems; and tremors	Labels often read, "not for human consumption"	Neuroleptic malignant syndrome; excited delirium; catatonic states; dehydration; rhabdomyolysis; kidney failure; tachyarrhythmias; chest pain; death

TOBACCO AND NICOTINE

KEY POINT

Nicotine is highly addictive due to its effects on the dopaminergic pathway and short half-life. The rewarding effects of nicotine include improved attention, decreased lethargy or increased energy, faster reaction time, and improved or elevated mood. Nicotine also causes physical symptoms including increased heart rate and blood pressure, vasoconstriction, increased cerebral flow, decreased appetite, and relaxation of skeletal muscle.

Tobacco is prepared from the leaves of the tobacco plant by curing (drying to remove chlorophyll). Tobacco contains nicotine. Nicotine is an alkaloid with stimulant properties, which raises levels of physiological activity in the body. Tobacco was first discovered in America, where indigenous peoples used it in spiritual ceremonies, social ceremonies, and in the treatment of ailments, such as toothaches, cuts and wounds, and the common cold. With exportation, use spread to other continents. In 1563, a Swiss physician, Conrad Gesner, first described its psychoactive properties. He found that chewing or smoking a tobacco leaf had the effect of producing a calming effect. Nicotine was first isolated from the tobacco plant in 1828 by chemists in Germany. Currently, about 6.7 million tons of tobacco are produced worldwide each year. Tobacco is consumed in many forms, including smoking (via cigars, cigarettes, and pipe tobacco) and smokeless tobacco (via chewing, snuff, snus, and dipping). In modern times, tobacco's psychoactive component, nicotine, has been synthesized and is vaporized using electronic vaping atomizers.

About 37.8 million adults (15.5% of all adults in the United States), 17.5% of males, and 13.5% of females are cigarette smokers. Tobacco accounts for about 480,000 deaths per year from smoking-related medical illnesses such as lung cancer, chronic obstructive pulmonary disease (COPD), cardiovascular disease, and cerebrovascular accident (CVA) or stroke. This amounts to about one in five deaths, making it the leading cause of preventable death. Tobacco alone costs the United States over $300 billion each year, yet thousands of young people start smoking cigarettes every day, while many adult cigarette smokers want to quit smoking.

The nicotine content of cigarettes varies from 6 to 24 mg, depending on the strength, with the average cigarette containing about 12 mg of nicotine. Traditional cigarettes contain over 7,000 chemicals, out of which at least 70 are carcinogenic. Similarly, e-cigarettes and other vaping devices expose the lungs to various chemicals, including those added to e-liquids and other chemicals produced during the heating or vaporizing process.

Nicotine and Mental Health Illness

Nicotine has mood-altering effects that can temporarily mask the negative symptoms of mental illness, putting people with mental illness at higher risk for cigarette use and nicotine addiction. Although often overlooked, tobacco smoke can interact with and inhibit the effectiveness of certain medications taken by mental health and substance abuse patients. Individuals with mental illness smoke more than those without mental illness. More than one in three adults (36%) with mental illness smoke cigarettes, compared with about one in five adults (21%) with no mental illness. Compared to 15–20% of the general population who smoke, about 80% of patients with schizophrenia and 60–70% with bipolar disorder smoke. Patients with ADHD are more likely to smoke and are more likely to become addicted to nicotine than the general population. People with mental illness or SUDs are less likely to stop smoking than those without mental illness. They also die about 5 years earlier than those without these disorders. Many of these deaths are caused by smoking cigarettes. It is essential to note that although working with smokers may be challenging, many smokers, including those with mental illness, want to quit.

QUICK POINT

More than one in three adults (36%) with mental illness smoke cigarettes, compared with about one in five adults (21%) with no mental illness. Compared to 15–20% of the general population who smoke, about 80% of patients with schizophrenia and 60–70% with bipolar disorder smoke. Patients with ADHD are more likely to smoke and are more likely to become addicted to nicotine than the general population.

Nicotine Withdrawal

Nicotine has a half-life of 1–2 hours, while cotinine, the metabolite of nicotine, has a half-life of 18–20 hours. Symptoms of nicotine withdrawal typically peak within 2 to 3 days. This is often experienced as flu-like symptoms, lethargy, difficulty concentrating, restlessness, mood changes (irritability, depression, anxiety), insomnia, weight gain, and cravings. This can be an unpleasant experience.

KEY POINT

Nicotine's half-life is about 2 hours. Nicotine withdrawal symptoms include mood changes (irritability, anxiety, and depression), restlessness, difficulty maintaining alertness and focus, insomnia, increased appetite, weight gain, and cravings. Nicotine withdrawal symptoms can last weeks to months.

SCREENING

There are several evidence-based screening tools for alcohol and drug abuse. Table 29.11 summarizes components of the most commonly used screeners, including the AUDIT (alcohol use disorders identification test; Babor et al., 2001), CAGE (Ewing, 1984), and CRAFFT (Knight et al., 2002).

TABLE 29.11 Commonly Used Screening Tools for Alcohol and Drug Use

Acronym	Validated for use in	Questions	Scoring	Positive screen
AUDIT	Adults	10-item screening questionnaire with three questions on the amount and frequency of drinking, three questions on alcohol dependence, and four questions on problems caused by alcohol	Varies with question item	⩾ 8 indicates harmful or hazardous drinking
AUDIT-C	Adults	1. How often do you have a drink containing alcohol? 2. How many standard drinks containing alcohol do you drink in a typical day? 3. How often do you have six or more drinks on one occasion?	Each item scored 0 or 4	⩾ 3 in women ⩾ 4 in men
CAGE	Adults	1. Have you ever felt you should *cut down* on your drinking? 2. Have you ever ridden in a *car* driven by someone (including yourself) who was "high" or had been using alcohol or drugs? 3. Have people *annoyed* you by criticizing your drinking? 4. Have you ever felt bad or *guilty* about your drinking? 5. Have you ever had a drink first thing in the morning to steady your nerves or to get rid of a hangover (i.e., an *eye opener*)?	Each item scored 0 or 1; a higher score is an indication of alcohol problems	⩾ 2 positive answers
CRAFFT	Adolescents	1. Have you ever ridden in a *car* driven by someone (including yourself) who was "high" or had been using alcohol or drugs? 2. Do you ever use alcohol or drugs to *relax*, feel better about yourself, or fit in? 3. Do you ever use alcohol or drugs while you are by yourself or *alone*? 4. Do you ever *forget* things you did while using alcohol or drugs? 5. Do your family or friends ever tell you that you should *cut down* on your drinking or drug use? 6. Have you ever gotten into *trouble* while you were using alcohol or drugs?	Each item scored 0 or 1; a higher score is an indication of alcohol problems	⩾ 2 positive answers; even those teens who deny using any drugs or alcohol should still be asked the CRAFFT "car" question.

DRUG TESTING

Drug testing can be used in cases of suspected drug use, preemployment tests, and postaccident tests. Drug testing can be used to detect, deter, or delay drug use. Drug tests, preferably random drug testing, help detect the presence of substances. It is most useful in monitoring patients and measuring treatment outcomes. Nevertheless, drug testing has some limitations. A negative drug test does not preclude that the patient is using drugs. A positive drug test does not measure the severity of disease or establish the diagnosis of a SUD.

DIAGNOSIS

Addictive disorders are viewed along a continuum based on the severity of the current and recent symptoms. As such, a person with an addictive disorder can be free of symptoms for several years, but due to the underlying changes in brain structure and function resulting from chronic use, symptoms of substance use disorder could return if not actively prevented. The *DSM-5* defines an addictive disorder as a problematic pattern of using an intoxicating substance, leading to clinically significant impairment or distress, as manifested by at least two symptoms occurring within a 12-month period. The symptoms associated with SUD fall into four major groups: impaired control, social impairment, risky use, and physiologic criteria (see Table 29.12).

TABLE 29.12 Diagnostic Criteria for a SUD (APA, 2013)

Category	Symptoms
Impaired control	1. The substance is often taken in larger amounts or over a longer period than was intended.
	2. There is a persistent desire or unsuccessful effort to cut down or control use of the substance.
	3. A great deal of time is spent in activities necessary to obtain the substance, use the substance, or recover from its effects.
Social impairment	4. Recurrent use of the substance resulting in a failure to fulfill major role obligations at work, school, or home.
	5. Continued use of the substance despite persistent or recurrent social or interpersonal problems caused or exacerbated caused by the use of, or recovery from, effects of the substance.
	6. Important social, occupational, or recreational activities are given up or reduced because of use of the substance.
Risky use	7. Recurrent use of the substance in situations in which it is physically hazardous.
	8. Use of the substance is continued, despite knowledge of having a persistent or recurrent physical or psychological problem that is likely to have been caused or exacerbated by the substance.
Physiologic	9. A craving, strong desire, or urge to use the substance.[a]
	10. Tolerance: A need for markedly increased amounts to achieve intoxication or desired effect or markedly diminished effect with continued use of the same amount.[b]
	11. Withdrawal: A characteristic syndrome caused by cessation or significant reduction in the amount of the substance consumed or the substance is used to avoid withdrawal.[b]

[a] *Craving is thought to be due to a change in brain state and may remain present for years well beyond active substance use. As such, it is the only symptom that does not imply the lack of remission if present.*

[b] *Tolerance and withdrawal (two pharmacological criteria) are not considered to be met for individuals taking opioids solely under appropriate medical supervision.*

> **MEMORY TIP**
>
> **Substance Use History**, *useful mnemonic*
>
> **TRAPPED**
> **T**—Treatment history (e.g., detoxification, treatment programs, medications, and 12-step programs)
> **R**—Route of administration (e.g., smoked, orally ingested, snorted, inhaled/"huffed," or injected IV/IM/SC)
> **A**—Amount (e.g., money spent, "pills," "bags," "vials," grams, ounces per bottle, and frequency)
> **P**—Pattern of use (e.g., binge, daily, solitary, and period of heaviest use)
> **P**—Prior abstinence (e.g., duration and what has helped in past, both in and out of a controlled environment)
> **E**—Effects (e.g., direct and indirect, adverse, physical, social, legal, positive, and withdrawal)
> **D**—Duration of use (e.g., age of first use and most recent use)
>
> *(Welsh, 2014)*

In addition to the severity of symptoms, certain specifiers apply to substance use disorders specifically, and these include the following:

1. Physiological dependence
    a. With physiological dependence: evidence of tolerance or withdrawal
    b. Without physiological dependence: no evidence of tolerance or withdrawal
2. Remission:
    a. Early: 3–12 months (except craving)
    b. Sustained: Greater than 12 months (except craving)
3. In a controlled environment (where access to substance use is restricted)
4. On maintenance therapy (if taking prescribed meds for maintenance treatment)
5. Unspecified category

TREATMENT

The goals of treatment are to eliminate the symptoms (abstinence) or to decrease the symptoms (harm reduction). While total abstinence is often a primary goal, harm reduction can sometimes be the initial or secondary goal while working progressively toward the primary goal of abstinence. Regardless, an excellent clinical goal is to engage the patient in treatment, help them identify their goals, and work with them toward achieving their health goals.

Biological Treatments

Medication-assisted treatment (MAT) is the use of medications, in combination counseling and behavioral therapies, to the treatment of substance use disorders. Medications approved by the FDA to treat addictive disorders and prevent relapse to SUD are currently available for nicotine, alcohol, and opioid use disorders. Some of these medications are sometimes used "off-label" in older adolescents. Other medications specifically target with withdrawal syndromes from alcohol and opioids such as benzodiazepines for alcohol and lofexidine for opioids. There are no FDA-approved medications to treat cocaine, amphetamine, cannabis, benzodiazepine, hallucinogen, or inhalant use disorders; however, many off-label options have been investigated with limited efficacy at best. Tables 29.13 and 29.14 summarize medications currently used for SUD treatment.

TABLE 29.13 Medications for Alcohol Use Disorders

Drug Information	Naltrexone	Disulfiram	Acamprosate
Mechanism	• Opioid receptor antagonist • Blocks μ-opioid receptor (associated with pleasurable effects)	• Inhibition of aldehyde dehydrogenase, causing a buildup of alcohol acetaldehyde with consequent unpleasant effects	• Glutaminergic effect
Formulation	• Oral, daily (naltrexone, Revia) • IM Depot, every 28 days (Vivitrol)	• Oral tab	• Oral tab
Contraindications	• Active opioid use • Liver failure • Naltrexone sensitivity		• Hypersensitivity to acamprosate • Severe renal impairment
Pregnancy	• Relatively contraindicated	• Insufficient studies	• Insufficient studies
Office-based	• Yes	• Yes	• Yes
Other comments	• Daily compliance required (for oral).	• Daily compliance required. • Unpleasant experience on consumption of alcohol may not deter severe alcoholics.	• Does not cause alcohol aversion (like disulfiram) or decreased pleasurable effect (like naltrexone in some alcoholics). Does not reduce occurrence of episodic or binge drinking.

MEMORY TIP

Addictive Disorder Symptoms, *useful mnemonic*

ADDICTeD

A—Activities are given up or reduced
D—Dependence, physical: tolerance
D—Dependence, physical: withdrawal
I—Intrapersonal (Internal) consequences, physical or psychological
C—Can't cut down or control use
T—Time-consuming
D—Duration or amount of use is greater than intended

(Bogenschutz & Quinn, 2001)

TABLE 29.14 Medications for Nicotine Use Disorders

Drug Information	Nicotine replacement	Bupropion	Varenicline
Mechanism	• Binds to nicotine receptors, reducing withdrawal symptoms	• Norepinephrine–dopamine reuptake inhibitor	• Partial agonist
Formulation	• Gum • Inhaler • Lozenge • Patch • Spray	• Oral (IR, SR, XL)	• Oral
Contraindications		• Seizure disorder	
Pregnancy	• Possibly safe	• Insufficient studies	• Insufficient studies
Office-based	• Yes	• Yes	• Yes
Other comments	• Low rate of cessation when used alone		• Strongest single agent

SCREENING, BRIEF INTERVENTION, AND REFERRAL TO TREATMENT (SBIRT)

SBIRT is an approach to the delivery of early intervention and treatment to people with substance use disorders and those at risk of developing these disorders. It involves screening to assess the severity of substance use, brief intervention and referral to treatment, based on the identified treatment needs (SAMHSA).

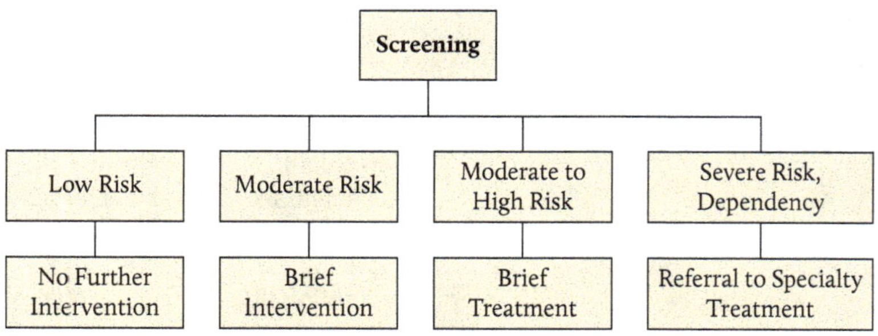

FIGURE 29.7 Flow chart for SBIRT process.

Psychosocial Treatments

Providers may adopt different approaches to working with patients with SUDs. While some may tend to be more directive or giving advice, others may utilize motivational interviewing (MI) techniques. However, evidence suggests that even with the best intentions, advice-giving alone is largely ineffective and may cause resistance from the patient. The use of MI is a patient-centered approach that can best be described as a "collaborative conversation style for strengthening a person's motivation and commitment to change" (Miller, 2013). Since giving direct advice may naturally lead to resistance from the patient, utilizing MI techniques may lead a patient who is ambivalent to changing substance use to explore and reflect on reasons to change the status quo. Motivational interviewing has been found to be helpful, even in brief encounters of 15 minutes, where 64% of studies show an effect (Rubak et al., 2005). Cognitive behavioral therapy (CBT) is widely used in various mental health disorders, including addiction.

Self-help groups occur within the community and are lead and attended by those in recovery. In some, to join, the individual does not have to already be abstinent; simply having a desire to "be sober" is sufficient. These groups' advantage is that they are nearly ubiquitous and held in person, in online in chat rooms, and virtually via video (including during community shutdowns, such as during the COVID-19 pandemic).

Twelve-step groups are composed of recovering addicts and offer help and support on how to achieve and maintain sobriety. There are specific groups for specific substance use, such as AA (Alcoholics Anonymous), NA (Narcotics Anonymous), CA (Cocaine Anonymous), MA (Marijuana Anonymous). Twelve-step groups, such as AA and NA, are associated with greater abstinence likelihood, often for prolonged periods up to 16 years. In addition, frequent, consistent, and early attendance is associated with better outcomes. However, the level of involvement (such as doing service at meetings, reading literature, doing step work, and getting a sponsor) may be a better predictor of abstinence than merely attending meetings. The 12-step approach has been expanded to behavioral additions, such as GA (Gamblers Anonymous) and SLAA (Sex and Love Addiction Anonymous), to name a few. These groups can pose a challenge for some patients because of their emphasis on spirituality and/or their conflict with psychiatric or psychological treatments.

Twelve-step facilitation is a professionally led therapy that is widely employed in residential treatment programs, which promotes active engagement. The efficacy of 12-step programs (and 12-step facilitation) in treating alcohol dependence has been established and appears promising for other forms of substance use. Relapse prevention (RP) involves learning certain skills, such as identifying triggers and high-risk situations for use (such as "people, places, and things."). Ultimately, if treatment does not work adequately in an outpatient setting, then residential treatment may be recommended.

STAGES OF CHANGE

The transtheoretical model of behavior change describes the process of intentional behavior change. Using this model, patients go through five stages of change where they are at baseline (no intent to change), then begin to conceptualize, prepare for, engage in, and maintain the desired behavior changes. Notably, the process is bidirectional and can work in reverse with previously abstinent patients beginning to contemplate a return to substance use (Prochaska & DiClemente, 1983; Prochaska et al., 1992). This model has also been used in other chronic medical disease for which behavioral and lifestyle changes optimize treatment outcomes (Figure 29.6). Notably, relapse is a factor in the action or maintenance stages of change. Ideally, relapse should be anticipated, identified early, and the process of relapse should be interrupted. For a variety of reasons, people who have previously successfully changed their behavior may reinitiate drug use or return to previous patterns of behavior. Understanding the process of relapse for the particular patient and taking the necessary steps to identify early and interrupt the process are pivotal to successful treatment.

TABLE 29.15 Stages of Change in the Transtheoretical Model

Stage of change	Description (related to change)	Provider tasks	Goal or outcome (for patient)
Precontemplation	• Not ready	• Provide facts and information around SUD	• Interested, concerned, and willing to consider
Contemplation	• Getting ready Considering change • Getting mindset ready	• Risk–reward analysis	• Decision-making
Preparation	• Ready • Preparing	• Creating a plan that is effective/acceptable	• Commitment to the plan
Action	• Initial change	• Implementing the plan	• Review and revise as needed
Maintenance	• Sustained change	• Consolidating change into lifestyle	• New established lifestyle

Adapted from DiClemente, 2003.

NONSUBSTANCE-RELATED (BEHAVIORAL) ADDICTIONS

The behavioral addictions, sometimes called process addictions, are considered by some to be the "pure" and "hidden" addictions—pure because they are not caused by the intake of addicting substances and hidden because they are extensions of common, socially accepted behavior, making detection more challenging. The *DSM-5* has two conditions in this category: gambling and internet gaming disorder, which is listed under conditions for further research. The behavioral addictions resemble substance addictions in many ways, including their phenomenology, adverse consequences, overlapping genetic contribution, neurobiological mechanisms, comorbidity, development of tolerance, and response to treatment. Both show natural histories of chronicity with periods of abstinence and relapsing patterns. Both individuals with behavioral addictions and those with substance use disorders score high on impulsivity and sensation-seeking measures and generally low on measures of harm avoidance. As in substance use disorders, social, financial, and marital problems are common in behavioral addictions. Like individuals with substance use disorders, those with addictions will often engage in illegal acts, including stealing, online credit card fraud, misappropriation, and embezzlement of family and company funds, either to fund their addictive behavior in an attempt to recover from their losses or to cope with the consequences of the behavior (Grant et al., 2010). Table 29.16 contrasts substance and nonsubstance-related disorders.

QUICK POINT

The behavioral addictions, sometimes called process addictions, are considered by some to be the "pure" and "hidden" addictions. They are called pure because, unlike substances, they are not caused by exogenous chemicals disrupting the brain. They are called hidden because they are extensions of common, socially accepted behavior, making detection even more challenging.

TABLE 29.16 Contrasting Substance- and Nonsubstance-Related Addictions

Aspect of item of addiction	Nonsubstance related	Substance related
Age of initiation (first use)	• Early onset (school age or earlier)	• Adolescence or young adulthood
Availability	• Available in most settings (e.g., electronic devices available in most homes, schools, and public settings)	• Not available in most settings • Not available in most homes, schools, or public settings • Available in localized places
Acceptability	• Activities acceptable in most settings	• Activities not accepted in most settings
Ease of detection	• Less readily detectable • (hidden within normal daily activities and most physical locations)	• More readily detectable • (more difficult to hide within normal daily activities or most physical locations)
Ability to restrict access (or attain abstinence)	• Comparatively less feasible • Often a major challenge • May be nonpractical, irrespective of setting	• Comparatively more feasible • Often a challenge • May attain remission in controlled setting (e.g., hospital, jail, etc.)
Detection	• No laboratory test	• Drug testing available
Behavior type	• Comparatively less openly disruptive	• Comparatively more openly disruptive behavior (including from tolerance, intoxication, and withdrawal from substances)

KEY POINT

Gambling is the wagering of money or some item(s) of value (referred to as "the stakes") on an event with an uncertain outcome with the primary intent of winning money or material goods.

Gambling

Gambling is the wagering of money or some item(s) of value (referred to as "the stakes") on an event with an uncertain outcome with the primary intent of winning money or material goods. It involves three elements, including the consideration (a promise of something of value given by someone in exchange for something of value given by a promise); the risk (making a bet on an uncertain outcome); and the prize (usually money or property). People gamble in various ways and places, including in arcades, bingo halls, casinos, lotteries, electronic devices, and online. Gambling disorder includes symptoms of preoccupation with present, future, or past gambling activities; tolerance (gambling with increased amounts of money); withdrawal; loss of control; lying; stealing; and engaging in illegal acts at significant risk to the individual's family, job, or education.

Gambling activities range from recreational gambling to gambling addiction. Social gamblers occasionally gamble for fun and stick to the limits (time and money). Serious gamblers gamble regularly as a hobby and usually stick to the limits. Although rare, professional gamblers gamble as a job to make money. Some individuals with antisocial personality disorder gamble as a manifestation of their personality. Gambling becomes problematic when it causes repeated dysfunction in the individual's life. Major life problems due to gambling can have significant consequences on individual and family savings and plans.

QUICK POINT

An electronic game is an electronically interactive platform through which a player influences outcomes, usually visually represented on a screen. They are played on various platforms, such as Xbox, PlayStation, and Nintendo consoles; computers; and smartphones. They are played online or offline, alone, with friends, or in competitions. Electronic sports (esports) have transformed online gaming into a spectator sport in which competitors compete for large prizes.

In general, there are two major types of gamblers: the action and the escape gamblers. Action gamblers tend to be of early onset, male, and narcissistic and view gambling as a game of skill. They gamble for competition or power, to obtain a rush (or high), and to seek to win. This is also associated with major depressive episodes. On the other hand, escape gamblers tend to be of later onset and female and use gambling as a means of relief or dissociation from problems. They tend to use more slot machines. There is no winning phase. This has been associated with persistent depressive disorder (dysthymia) and cluster C and A personality types. Gambling activities can go in phases, including the winning, losing, desperation, and hopelessness phases. After the winning phase, burrowing begins through credit cards, legal loans from friends and families, and illegal money sources. Bailouts received from any source lead to an upsurge of omnipotence but also a loss of personal control. Desperation causes individuals to cross the legal line. Individuals with gambling disorders have high rates of co-occurrence of substance use disorders, including nicotine dependence and alcohol use disorders. Some studies have found problem gamblers to be a high-risk group for suicidality with an odds ratio of suicidality up to 5.3 times higher than the general population. This risk is partly mediated by depression, anxiety, ADHD, and co-occurring substance use disorders (Wardle et al., 2020).

Gaming

Both the ICD-11 and DSM-5 acknowledge gaming disorder, with internet gaming disorder listed in section III of the *DSM-5* under conditions for further research, and this includes non-internet gaming. Electronics use has become a daily tool for communication, entertainment, and education. Its pivotal importance only increased with the recent COVID-19 global pandemic and shift to online education, entertainment, and socially distanced media communication.

> **CLINICAL TIP**
>
> Symptoms of internet gaming disorder include preoccupation (e.g., reliving the past or future and obsession with watching others play, including virtually); tolerance; withdrawal symptoms (e.g., irritability, anxiety, or sadness when unable to play); unsuccessful attempts to control participation; loss of interest in previous hobbies and entertainment; continued excessive use, despite knowledge of psychosocial problems; use to escape or relieve negative mood states; jeopardizing significant relationships, jobs, education, or career opportunities; and deception of family members, therapists, or others on amount of gaming. The symptoms can be mild, moderate, or severe, based on the disruption of normal or expected activities.

An electronic game is an electronically interactive platform through which a player influences outcomes, usually visually represented on a screen. They are played on platforms, such as Microsoft's Xbox consoles, Sony's PlayStation consoles, and Nintendo's consoles; computers; and smartphones. In research, inconsistencies in measurement of disordered use cause difficulty accurately assessing the prevalence of this disorder. Symptoms of internet gaming disorder include preoccupation (e.g., reliving the past or future and obsession with watching others play, including virtually); tolerance; withdrawal symptoms (e.g., irritability, anxiety, or sadness when unable to play); unsuccessful attempts to control participation; loss of interest in previous hobbies and entertainment; continued excessive use, despite knowledge of psychosocial problems; use to escape or relieve negative mood states; jeopardizing significant relationships, jobs, education, or career opportunities; and deception of family members, therapists, or others on amount of gaming. The symptoms can be mild, moderate, or severe, based on the disruption of normal or expected activities.

Like gambling, gaming activities range from recreational gaming to severe gaming addiction. Most individuals occasionally game, for fun, and stick to the limits (time and money). Serious gamers game regularly, as a hobby. Although less commonly, professional gamers compete for a win, sometimes in national and international competitions, with millions of dollars as the prize.

Gaming becomes problematic when it causes repeated dysfunction in an individual's life. Children as young as preschool can experience disruption. This includes disturbances in sleep, appetite, and using the bathroom. Social skills development is sometimes neglected. Adolescents with gaming disorders sometimes miss out on real-life peer group relationships. For others, their online gaming friends may provide a source of support, particularly during periods of stress. Individuals with mental health conditions who spend more time on electronic media activities are more likely to play violent electronic games. Comorbid conditions include ADHD, depression, social anxiety, and Asperger's syndrome (often seen as high-functioning autism). Behavioral traits associated with gaming addiction include hostility, lower social competence, and narcissistic personality traits. Table 29.17 summarizes symptoms and signs of gaming disorders.

TABLE 29.17 Gaming Disorder Symptoms

Biological	Psychological	Social
• Mood changes o Anxiety over future playing o Irritability, anger outbursts, or aggression when asked to stop playing o Bouts of depression when unable to play	• Loss of control o Spends more time than promised o Unable to quit even when trying o Time spent is excessive	• Conduct-type symptoms o Chatting about or watching others play video games excessively o Lying, manipulating, o Stealing (e.g., charging up parents' credit cards)
• Self-care o Gaming interferes with eating o Gaming interferes with sleep o Lack of personal care	• Defense mechanisms o Minimalizing o Denial o Anger o Bargaining o Threatening o Providing "logical" reasons to play	• Social interests o Shrunken social interests o Decreased social interaction o Declining grades or work performance
• Physical symptoms o Headaches o Visual problems o The Tetris effect* o Muscle, back pains o Seizures	• Dreams or uncontrollable thoughts (obsessions) about gaming	• Peers o Contracted peer group o Online friends

** Tetris effect or syndrome is a condition where, due to time devoted to gaming, gaming images begin to pattern an individual's thoughts, mental images, and dreams.*

Treatment of Behavioral Addictions

The biopsychosocial treatment approach provides the most comprehensive treatment for patients with behavioral addictions. Identifying and optimally treating underlying conditions, such as ADHD, depression, anxiety, or other SUDs, improves treatment outcomes. Psychosocial interventions help reduce symptoms. Treatment is most successful when family members are involved. Currently, no pharmacotherapies have FDA approval for treatment of behavioral addictions.

SUMMARY

Addictive disorders are manifested by behaviors that reveal an individual's compulsive use of substances or other objects (s) of addiction. They include substance and nonsubstance related disorders. Addiction is a chronic medical disease best viewed, assessed, and treated within a biopsychosocial framework. Several effective treatments exist. Pharmacological agents provide the highest, most reliable, and most consistent efficacy of the available treatment options. Psychosocial interventions are essential in treating addictive disorders. Addictive disorders continue to place a heavy medical, emotional, and financial toll on individuals, families, and society. Preventive strategies help mitigate this disease, especially in youth. Comprehensive programs that target addiction at all stages of development are needed.

RESOURCES

1 https://www.youtube.com/watch?v=-w8n9UOiBxE

2 https://nida.nih.gov

3 Drugs of Abuse (2017 Edition) (dea.gov)

4 Home - American Academy of Addiction Psychiatry (aaap.org)

5 Home - American Academy of Addiction Psychiatry (aaap.org)

6 www.monitoringthefuture.org

REFERENCES

American College of Obstetricians and Gynecologists. (2017). *Marijuana use during pregnancy and lactation. Committee Opinion* (no. 722).

American Psychiatric Association. (2013). *Diagnostic and statistical manual of mental disorders* (5th ed.).

American Society of Addiction Medicine. (2011). *ASAM releases new definition of addiction* [Press release]. https://www.asam.org/docs/default-source/publications/asam-news-archives/vol26-3.pdf?sfvrsn=0

American Society of Addiction Medicine. (2019). *Definition of addiction*. https://www.asam.org/Quality-Science/definition-of-addiction

Andresen-Streichert, H., Müller, A., Glahn, A., Skopp, G., & Sterneck, M. (2018). Alcohol biomarkers in clinical and forensic contexts. *Deutsches Arzteblatt International, 115*(18), 309–315. https://doi.org/10.3238/arztebl.2018.0309

Asbridge M., Hayden J. A., Cartwright J. L. (2012). Acute cannabis consumption and motor vehicle collision risk: Systematic review of observational studies and meta-analysis. *BMJ, 344*:e536. https://www.doi.org/10.1136/bmj.e5367

Babor, T. F., Saunders, J., & Grant, M. (2001). *AUDIT. The Alcohol Use Disorders Identification Test Guidelines for use in primary care.* http://whqlibdoc.who.int/hq/2001/WHO_MSD_MSB_01.6a.pdf

Biecheler M-B, Peytavin J-F, Sam Group, Facy F., & Martineau H. (2008). SAM survey on "drugs and fatal accidents": search of substances consumed and comparison between drivers involved under the influence of alcohol or cannabis. *Traffic Injury Prevention, 9*(1):11–21. https://www.doi.org/10.1080/15389580701737561

Bogenschutz M. P., Quinn D. K.. (2001). Acronyms for substance use disorders. *The Journal of Clinical Psychiatry, 62*(6), 474–5.

Buchman, D. Z., Skinner, W., & Illes, J. (2010). Negotiating the relationship between addiction, ethics, and brain science. *AJOB Neuroscience, 1*(1), 36–45. https://doi.org/10.1080/21507740903508609

Bush, K., Kivlahan, D. R., McDonell, M. B., Fihn, S. D., & Bradley, K. A. (1998). The AUDIT alcohol consumption questions (AUDIT-C): An effective brief screening test for problem drinking. Ambulatory Care Quality Improvement Project (ACQUIP). Alcohol Use Disorders Identification Test. *Archives of Internal Medicine, 158*(16), 1789–1795. https://doi.org/10.1001/archinte.158.16.1789

Centers for Disease Control and Prevention. (2018). Illicit drug use. https://www.cdc.gov/nchs/fastats/drug-use-illicit.htm

DiClemente, C. C. (2003). *Addiction and change: How addictions develop and addicted people recover.* Guilford.

Ewing, J. A. (1984). Detecting alcoholism: The CAGE Questionnaire. *JAMA, 252*(14), 1905–1907. https://doi.org/10.1001/jama.1984.03350140051025

Fishman, M., Wenzel, K., Scodes, J., Pavlicova, M., Lee, J. D., Rotrosen, J., & Nunes, E. (2020). Young adults have worse outcomes than older adults: Secondary analysis of a medication trial for opioid use disorder. *The Journal of Adolescent Health: Official Publication of the Society for Adolescent Medicine, 67*(6), 778–785. https://doi.org/10.1016/j.jadohealth.2020.07.038

Galanter, M. K. H. (2008). *Textbook of substance abuse treatment (4th ed.).* American Psychiatric Publishing.

Gandhi, D. H., Kavanagh, G. J., & Jaffe, J. H. (2006). Young heroin users in Baltimore: A qualitative study. *The American journal of drug and alcohol abuse, 32*(2), 177–188. https://doi.org/10.1080/00952990500479290

Grant, J. E., Potenza, M. N., Weinstein, A., & Gorelick, D. A. (2010). Introduction to behavioral addictions. *The American Journal of Drug and Alcohol Abuse, 36*(5), 233–241. https://doi.org/10.3109/00952990.2010.491884

Grigsby, T. J., Forster, M., Unger, J. B., & Sussman, S. (2016). Predictors of alcohol-related negative consequences in adolescents: A systematic review of the literature and implications for future research. *Journal of Adolescence, 48*, 18–35. https://doi.org/10.1016/j.adolescence.2016.01.006

Hasin D. S., Saha T. D., Kerridge B. T. Goldstein, R. B., Chou, S. P., Zhang, H., Jung, J., Pickering, R. P., Ruan, W. J., Smith, S. M., Huang, B., & Grant, B. F. (2015). Prevalence of Marijuana Use Disorders in the United States Between 2001-2002 and 2012–2013. *JAMA Psychiatry, 72*(12), 1235–1242. https://www.doi.org/10.1001/jamapsychiatry.2015.1858.

Knight, J. R., Sherritt, L., Shrier, L. A., Harris, S. K., & Chang, G. (2002). Validity of the CRAFFT substance abuse screening test among adolescent clinic patients. *Archives of Pediatrics & Adolescent Medicine, 156*(6), 607–614.

Ko, J. Y., Coy, K. C., Haight, S. C., Haegerich, T. M., Williams, L., Cox, S., Njai, R., & Grant, A. M. (2020). Characteristics of marijuana use during pregnancy - eight states, pregnancy risk assessment monitoring system, 2017. *MMWR. Morbidity and Mortality Weekly Report, 69*(32), 1058–1063. https://doi.org/10.15585/mmwr.mm6932a2

Ko, J. Y., D'Angelo, D. V., Haight, S. C., Morrow, B., Cox, S., Salvesen von Essen, B., Strahan, A. E., Harrison, L., Tevendale, H. D., Warner, L., Kroelinger, C. D., & Barfield, W. D. (2020). Vital signs: Prescription opioid pain reliever use during pregnancy - 34 U.S. jurisdictions, 2019. *Morbidity and Mortality Weekly Report, 69*(28), 897–903. https://doi.org/10.15585/mmwr.mm6928a1

Kuerbis, A., Sacco, P., Blazer, D. G., & Moore, A. A. (2014). Substance abuse among older adults. *Clinics in Geriatric Medicine, 30*(3), 629–654. https://doi.org/10.1016/j.cger.2014.04.008

Lee, H., Roh, S., & Kim, D. J. (2009). Alcohol-induced blackout. *International Journal of Environmental Research and Public Health, 6*(11), 2783–2792. https://doi.org/10.3390/ijerph6112783

Levy S. (2019). Youth and the Opioid Epidemic. *Pediatrics, 143*(2), e20182752. https://doi.org/10.1542/peds.2018-2752

Miller, W. R. R (2013). *Motivational interviewing: Helping people to change* (3rd ed). Guilford.

McDuff, D. R., & Baron, D. (2005). Substance use in athletics: A sports psychiatry perspective. *Clinics in Sports Medicine, 24*(4), 885–897. https://doi.org/10.1016/j.csm.2005.06.004

National Institute of Diabetes and Digestive and Kidney Diseases. (2012). *Kratom.*

National Institute on Drug Abuse. (2020a). *Drug use trends among U.S. teens: Monitoring the Future 2020 Survey results.* https://www.drugabuse.gov/drug-topics/related-topics/trends-statistics/infographics/monitoring-future-2020-survey-results

National Institute on Drug Abuse. (2020b). *The science of drug use and addiction: The basics.*

National Institute on Alcohol Abuse and Alcoholism. (2021). *Rethinking drinking: Alcohol & your health.* https://www.rethinkingdrinking.niaaa.nih.gov/Default.aspx

National Institute on Drug Abuse. (2020). *Costs of substance abuse.* https://www.drugabuse.gov/drug-topics/trends-statistics/costs-substance-abuse

National Institute of Mental Health. (2015). *Ten percent of US adults have drug use disorder at some point in their lives* [Press release]. https://www.nih.gov/news-events/news-releases/10-percent-us-adults-have-drug-use-disorder-some-point-their-lives

National Safety Council. (2019). *For the first time, we're more likely to die from accidental opioid overdose than motor vehicle crash* [Press release]. https://www.nsc.org/newsroom/for-the-first-time,-were-more-likely-to-die-from

Pantano, F., Tittarelli, R., Mannocchi, G., Zaami, S., Ricci, S., Giorgetti, R., Terranova, D., Busardò, F. P., & Marinelli, E. (2016). Hepatotoxicity Induced by "the 3 Ks": Kava, kratom and khat. *International Journal of Molecular Sciences, 17(*4), 580–580. https://doi.org/10.3390/ijms17040580

Perry, E. C. (2014). Inpatient management of acute alcohol withdrawal syndrome. *CNS Drugs, 28*(5), 401–410. https://doi.org/10.1007/s40263-014-0163-5

Preuss, U. W., Huestis, M. A., Schneider, M., Hermann, D., Lutz, B., Hasan, A., Kambeitz, J., Wong, J., & Hoch, E. (2021). Cannabis Use and Car Crashes: A Review. *Frontiers in Psychiatry, 12*, 643315. https://doi.org/10.3389/fpsyt.2021.643315

Prochaska, J. O., & DiClemente, C. C. (1983). Stages and processes of self-change of smoking: Toward an integrative model of change. *Journal of Consulting and Clinical Psychology, 51*(3), 390–395. https://doi.org/10.1037//0022-006x.51.3.390

Prochaska, J. O., Velicer, W. F., Rossi, J. S., Goldstein, M. G., Marcus, B. H., Rakowski, W., Fiore, C., Harlow, L. L., Redding, C. A., & Rosenbloom, D. (1994). Stages of change and decisional balance for 12 problem behaviors. *Health Psychology, 13*(1), 39–46. https://doi.org/10.1037//0278-6133.13.1.39

Rubak, S., Sandbaek, A., Lauritzen, T., & Christensen, B. (2005). Motivational interviewing: A systematic review and meta-analysis. *The British Journal of General Practice: The Journal of the Royal College of General Practitioners, 55*(513), 305–312.

Ryan, S. A., & O'Connor, M. E. (2017). Marijuana use during pregnancy and breastfeeding: Implications for neonatal and childhood outcomes. *Pediatrics, 142(3),* e20181889.

Sachdeva, A., Choudhary, M., & Chandra, M. (2015). Alcohol withdrawal syndrome: Benzodiazepines and beyond. *Journal of Clinical and Diagnostic Research, 9*(9), VE01–VE07. https://doi.org/10.7860/JCDR/2015/13407.6538

Schwetz, T. A., Calder, T., Rosenthal, E., Kattakuzhy, S., & Fauci, A. S. (2019). Opioids and infectious diseases: A converging public health crisis. *The Journal of Infectious Diseases, 220*(3), 346–349. https://doi.org/10.1093/infdis/jiz133

Seim, L., Vijapura, P., Pagali, S., & Burton, M. C. (2020). Common substance use disorders in older adults. *Hospital Practice (1995), 48*(1), 48–55. https://doi.org/10.1080/21548331.2020.1733287

Sharma, B., Bruner, A., Barnett, G., & Fishman, M. (2016). Opioid Use Disorders. *Child and adolescent psychiatric clinics of North America, 25*(3), 473–487. https://doi.org/10.1016/j.chc.2016.03.002.

Streissguth, A. P., Bookstein, F. L., Barr, H. M., Sampson, P. D., O'Malley, K., & Young, J. K. (2004). Risk factors for adverse life outcomes in fetal alcohol syndrome and fetal alcohol effects. *Journal of Developmental and Behavioral Pediatrics, 25*(4), 228–238. https://doi.org/10.1097/00004703-200408000-00002

Substance Abuse and Mental Health Services Administration. (n.d.). Medication-assisted treatment (MAT). Retrieved December 04, 2021, from https://www.samhsa.gov/medication-assisted-treatment

Sullivan, E. V., & Pfefferbaum, A. (2009). Neuroimaging of the Wernicke-Korsakoff syndrome. *Alcohol and Alcoholism, 44*(2), 155–165. https://doi.org/10.1093/alcalc/agn103

United Nations Office on Drugs and Crime. (2015). *World Drug Report 2015.* https://www.unodc.org/documents/wdr2015/WDR15_Drug_use_health_consequences.pdf

United Nations Office on Drugs and Crime. (2017). *World Drug Report 2017.*

U.S. Department of Agriculture and U.S. Department of Health and Human Services. (2020). *Dietary guidelines for Americans, 2020–2025* (9th ed.). https://www.dietaryguidelines.gov

Wardle, H., John, A., Dymond, S., & McManus, S. (2020). Problem gambling and suicidality in England: Secondary analysis of a representative cross-sectional survey. *Public Health, 184*, 11–16. https://doi.org/10.1016/j.puhe.2020.03.024

Welsh, C. J. (2003). "Trapped": A Mnemonic for Taking a Substance Use History. *Academic Psychiatry : The Journal of the American Association of Directors of Psychiatric Residency Training and the Association for Academic Psychiatry, 27*, 289. https://doi.org/10.1176/appi.ap.27.4.289

Winters K. C., Lee C-YS. (2008). Likelihood of developing an alcohol and cannabis use disorder during youth: Association with recent use and age. *Drug and Alcohol Dependence, 92*(1–3), 23–247. https://www.doi.org/10.1016/j.drugalcdep.2007.08.005.

CHAPTER 30

Prescription Drug Misuse and Abuse

Opioids, Stimulants, and Sedative–Hypnotics[1]

Edore Onigu-Otite, M.D.; Benjamin Li, M.D.; Daryl Shorter, M.D.; and Thomas R. Kosten, M.D.

> *"The person who takes medicine must recover twice, once from the disease and once from the medicine."*
>
> — William Osler, MD.

OBJECTIVES

After reading this chapter, students will be able to do the following:

- understand the neurobiological effects of prescription opioids, stimulants, and sedative hypnotics
- summarize medications used in opioid and sedative–hypnotic use disorders
- define prescription drug use, misuse, and abuse
- recognize patient behaviors related to prescription drug misuse and abuse
- describe good physician prescription practice
- discuss ways to address drug misuse or abuse in the physician's office

1 Readers may also see "Addiction and Substance Use Disorders" (Chapter 29), "Psychopharmacology" (Chapter 31), and "Psychiatric Emergencies" (Chapter 38) for related material.

CASE VIGNETTE

Anthony is a 14-year-old male who lives with his parents and 9-year-old sister. He presented to his primary care provider (PCP) on the advice of his school. He was a shy kid, who was slightly overweight and loved by his teachers. Since his elementary school years, he had a history of inattention but was smart and made good grades until this year—his first in high school. He was failing some of his classes. Based on the clinical assessment and corroborative information via forms completed by several teachers and his parents, his PCP diagnosed him with attention-deficit disorder and prescribed stimulant medications. He tries a few with varying results until his symptoms respond to an amphetamine preparation. Anthony made remarkable progress in school and at home, and things were stable for about a year.

One week, his parents went out of town. Anthony "accidentally" took two pills instead of one. He felt good, had decreased appetite, and found he did not need to bother eating lunch or dinner. Without his parent's knowledge, Anthony double-dosed on his medications several times over the next few weeks. He lost a few pounds and liked that more girls now wanted to be in his company. He skipped taking meds over the weekends so that he could double-dose during the week. Anthony began to get asked out to parties, which were usually held on weekends. At one of the parties, he was offered pain pills, which he impulsively accepted. He began to seek out parties, including now on school nights to get these pills. He was often sleepy during school hours. In school, his class participation dropped, as did his grades due to projects and assignments he never even started. At home, he interacted little with family members, totally forgot his sister's birthday, and failed to do his chores—all of which were unusual for him. Anthony had always been a rule follower. He knew the way he was taking the medication (both prescribed and nonprescribed) was wrong and possibly dangerous. He tried to stop but instead found himself taking even more pills and more frequently. He was a good student and knew he was now struggling in his classes because of his drug use.

At his next clinic appointment, as usual, he was screened for drug use. He self-reported his double and triple-dosing on his medications and his now regular use of pain pills, which he used twice or thrice a week, often taken from relatives or obtained from friends. Contrary to expectation, his urine drug screen that day in the clinic was negative. Anthony had been aware of the date of this appointment and had stayed off the pain pills for 3 days. Anthony's doctor counseled him and his parents and recommended he attend a program specialized in treating teens with drug use. Anthony declined to go. He said he saw nothing wrong or dangerous with what he was doing and felt he wanted to continue using. Nevertheless, his parents began inquiring and making plans to get Anthony into a program.

Later that week, a friend texted Anthony's parents to check up on him. During school, he had asked his friend for pills which worried the friend. The same friend had seen Anthony buying something after school which he was trying to hide. Later that day, his friend texted Anthony, but there was no response. Anthony's friend texted his parents who came home immediately but to a silent house. They expected Anthony to be home from school. They knew he was home because, as usual, he texted to let them know he was at home. He was not in his bedroom. They called his phone several times, but there was no answer.

They searched the house. They found Anthony in the basement, unconscious and stiff, with a small open pill container on the floor. His phone lay beside him with multiple missed calls from his parents and friends. His last text to a friend read, "Flunked a test. Feel down in the dumps. Pills make me feel good!" Unfortunately, this time, he had bought pills laced with fentanyl. Anthony had died of an accidental overdose. There were no family members at home at the time who could have intervened. His family was distraught.

ANTHONY'S DIAGNOSIS

Anthony began by misusing his prescribed medication (taking a higher dose), and this progressed to abusing his medication (taking a medication for a reason other than prescribed). He was introduced to nonprescribed pain pills on which he quickly became addicted.

Given his symptoms, Anthony met criteria for opioid use disorder, moderate severity, based on the following specific criteria:

- The substance is often taken in larger amounts or over a longer period than was intended.
  - Anthony increased the frequency of taking nonprescribed medications (pain pills).
- There is a persistent desire or unsuccessful effort to cut down or control use of the substance.
  - He tried to stop, but instead he found himself taking even more pills more frequently.
- Use of the substance is continued despite knowledge of having a persistent or recurrent physical or psychological problem that is likely to have been caused or exacerbated by the substance.
  - Anthony knew the way he was taking the medications (both prescribed and nonprescribed) was wrong and possibly dangerous. He was a good student and knew he was now struggling in his classes because of his drug use.
- Recurrent use of the substance resulting in a failure to fulfill major role obligations at work, school, or home.
  - Anthony's participation in class decreased. He did not even start his class projects. He did not fulfill expected social obligations at home, including remembering his only sister's birthday and failing to do his chores—both of which were unusual for him.
- A great deal of time is spent in activities necessary to obtain the substance, use the substance, or recover from its effects.
  - He began to want to go to parties, including on school nights, to get these pills. He was often sleepy during school hours.

Given his symptoms, Anthony met criteria for stimulant use disorder, mild severity, based on the following specific criteria:

- The substance is often taken in larger amounts or over a longer period than was intended.
  - Anthony took increased doses of his prescribed medication (prescription stimulant).
- There is a persistent desire or unsuccessful effort to cut down or control use of the substance.

(*continued*)

- He tried to stop, but instead he found himself taking even more pills more frequently.
- Use of the substance is continued, despite knowledge of having a persistent or recurrent physical or psychological problem that is likely to have been caused or exacerbated by the substance.
  - Anthony knew the way he was taking the medications (both prescribed and nonprescribed) was wrong and possibly dangerous.

DEFINITIONS AND KEY CONCEPTS

Medical use of prescription medications is taking a medication as prescribed, including for the reason, the dose, duration, and according to the dosing schedule, it was prescribed. *Nonmedical use of prescription medications (NUPM)* is the use of a prescription medication in a manner or for a reason that was not prescribed. This includes the use of a prescription medication by a person for whom the medication was not prescribed, or the use of a prescription medication by the person for whom it was prescribed but for a reason, at a dose, dosing schedule, or duration other than prescribed. This could be even if the prescription medication is taken for a legitimate medical complaint such as pain; or to feel euphoria (i.e., to get high) (National Institute of Drug Abuse, 2020b). NUPM includes prescription drug misuse and abuse. *Prescription drug misuse* is taking a medication at a dose or dosing schedule other than as prescribed. *Prescription drug abuse* is taking a medication for a reason other than as prescribed, such as to alter one's emotional or behavioral state. In the more severe cases, it includes having an extreme desire to obtain and use the drug, using greater amounts than prescribed, and developing clinically significant impairment or distress. *Prescription drug diversion* is the unlawful channeling of regulated pharmaceuticals from legal sources to the illicit marketplace. This includes transferring medications to people for whom they were not prescribed. Drug diversion has serious social and legal consequences. *Medication-assisted treatment (MAT)* is the use of medications, alongside counseling and behavioral therapies, to provide a whole-patient approach to the treatment of substance use disorders.

KEY POINT

Many legally prescribed medications, and some over-the-counter (OTC) medications, have psychoactive properties with the potential to alter an individual's experience, including their emotions, behavior, and how they perceive their internal state or external surroundings. Some prescription medications, related to their potential for abuse, are often diverted and used by persons other than for whom the medications were prescribed.

INTRODUCTION

Prescription medications are consumed for different reasons and in different ways. Many legally prescribed medications, and some over-the-counter (OTC) medications, have psychoactive properties with the potential to alter an individual's experience, including their emotions, behavior, and how they perceive their internal state or external surroundings. Some prescription medications, related to their potential for abuse, are often diverted and used by persons other than for whom the medications were prescribed. These prescription medications are known to have "street value."

The three most misused, abused, and diverted prescription medication classes are opioids (prescribed for pain); central nervous system depressants, including sedatives, hypnotics, and tranquilizers (prescribed to treat anxiety and sleep disorders); and prescription stimulant medications, such as amphetamine salts methylphenidate (prescribed to treat ADHD; NIDA, 2020). Of these, NMU of opioids have gained attention due to the opioid epidemic associated with a sharp rise in drug overdose, including among youth (Fishman, 2020; Levy, 2019; Gandhi, 2006; Sharma, 2016). NMU of prescription medications often occurs within the context of other substance use. National surveys show that the majority of NMU opioid users report using other drugs, including cigarettes, alcohol, marijuana, or hard drugs (e.g., cocaine, methamphetamine, etc.) They were also at increased risk of having underlying mental health conditions, including suicidal ideations and major depressive episodes (Grigsby & Howard, 2019). This highlights the need to assess patients for underlying mental and medical health conditions and treat them optimally.

QUICK POINT

The three most misused, abused, and diverted prescription medication classes are opioids (prescribed for pain); central nervous system depressants, including sedatives, hypnotics, and tranquilizers (prescribed to treat anxiety and sleep disorders); and prescription stimulant medications, such as amphetamine salts, methylphenidate (prescribed to treat ADHD; NIDA, 2020).

Unintentional drug poisoning, which includes fatal drug overdose, is the leading cause of accidental death in the United States. Each year, drugs of abuse, nonmedical prescription drug use, and alcohol contribute to over 90,000 deaths per year. Drug overdose deaths rose from 38,329 in 2010 to 70,237 in 2017. In 2017, about 68% of the 70,237 U.S. drug overdose deaths involved an opioid (Wilson et al., 2020). In 2018, more than 67,300 Americans died from drug-involved overdoses, including from illicit drugs and prescription opioids (NIDA, 2019), causing opioid-related overdoses to surpass motor vehicle accidents and firearms as a leading cause of injury in the United States (National Safety Council, 2019). According to recent provisional data from the Centers for Disease Control and Prevention (2020), in a 12-month period ending in May 2020, drug overdose deaths increased to 81,000, the highest number of overdose deaths ever recorded in a 12-month period, and reflected the challenges individuals struggling with addictions, including opioid use disorders (OUDs), faced during the COVID-19 pandemic.

QUICK POINT

Opioids are responsible for over 70% of all overdose deaths in the United States (Wilson et al., 2020). In 2019, more than 70,000 drug overdose deaths occurred—over half of which were caused by synthetic opioids, particularly fentanyl. Cocaine overdose deaths were driven by opioids (Mattson, 2021). Early in the COVID-19 pandemic, provisional data indicates this rose to over 100,000 drug overdose deaths in the 12-month period ending in April 2021 (CDC, 2021). This reflected an almost 30% increase over the same time in the preceding year.

Among deaths attributed to drugs, the most common categories are cocaine, heroin, and prescription opioids. Among suicide drug overdose attempts, 19.6 to 22.5% involved benzodiazepines and 15.4 to 17.3% involved opioids. The risk that an overdose will be fatal is highest if an opioid or barbiturate is involved (Miller et al., 2020). OUD has a stronger relationship with suicide than other substance use disorders. Past-year and weekly or more frequent prescription opioid misuse is associated with suicidal ideation, suicide planning, and suicide attempts (Bohnert et al., 2017). Suicides involving opioids accounted for more than 40% of suicide and overdose deaths in 2017 (Braden et al., 2017). Even then, this is likely to be an underreported. Figure 30.1 shows the national trends in overdose in the United States over the past two decades.

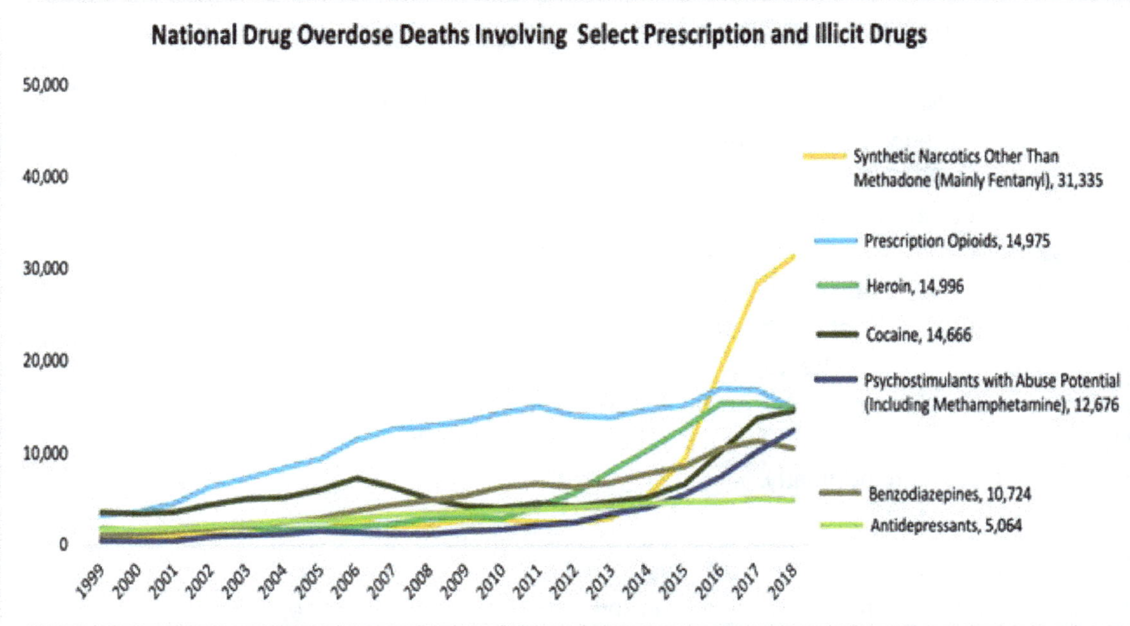

FIGURE 30.1 National trends in drug overdose deaths involving select prescription and illicit drugs.

Source: https://www.drugabuse.gov/drug-topics/trends-statistics/overdose-death-rates.

This chapter is focused on the prescription drugs most frequently misused and diverted. This includes three major drug classes: opioids, stimulants, and sedative hypnotics. Table 30.1 summarizes the properties of the three classes of medications most commonly involved in prescription drug misuse, abuse, and diversion.

OPIOIDS

Opioids are a class of potent pain-relieving drugs. They and derivatives of the naturally occurring opiates found in the opium poppy plant. They include synthetic or semisynthetic derivates, such as heroin, fentanyl, and prescription pain medications, including morphine, hydrocodone (Vicodin), oxycodone (OxyContin), and codeine. Opioids have potent pain-relieving properties. They include morphine, methadone, fentanyl, tramadol (Ultram), Meperidine

(Demerol), oxycodone (OxyContin), hydrocodone (Vicodin), and codeine (contained in various cough syrups). Different opioids have different potencies and durations of action and are indicated for pain conditions based on severity. For example, fentanyl is used in severe pain conditions, such as in cancer patients. Fentanyl is 50 to 100 times more potent than morphine and can cause fatal overdose if not used appropriately. Opioids are often manufactured illegally, including potent opioids like fentanyl. This is a significant contributing factor to OUD and illicit and prescription drug overdoses worldwide.

Apart from their helpful pain-reducing properties, opioids can also cause euphoria, which increases their potential for addiction and diversion. Opioids also fatally suppress respiration when taken in excess of what the body can tolerate. Tolerance develops with opioids. This tolerance decreases and is sometimes lost when the use of opioids is discontinued.

Opioid Intoxication

Opioid intoxication can be fatal if not reversed within minutes. It includes behavioral changes, including euphoria, dysphoria, psychomotor agitation or retardation, and impaired judgment. In addition, pupillary constriction must occur, along with one of the following: drowsiness or coma, slurred speech, and impairment in memory or attention (*DSM-5*). If a patient is experiencing respiratory depression or is even in stupor or unresponsive, emergency treatment using the opioid antagonist naloxone is given to reverse the potential for death from overdose. Naloxone is available by auto-injection (Evzio) and with much less expensive manual injection devices, which are often carried by patients and family members to prevent fatalities from opioid use.

KEY POINT

Opioid intoxication triad:

- decreased level of consciousness
- respiratory depression
- miosis (pinpoint pupils)

Opioid Withdrawal

Opioid withdrawal, while not typically fatal, can be extremely uncomfortable to experience and often leads back to using opioid agonists to relieve withdrawal symptoms. These symptoms include dysphoric mood; nausea or vomiting; muscle aches; lacrimation or rhinorrhea; pupillary dilation, piloerection, or sweating; diarrhea; yawning; fever; and insomnia (*DSM-5*).

KEY POINT

Symptoms of opioid withdrawal include irritability, diaphoresis, nausea, diarrhea, muscle aches, piloerection, and yawning.

Medication-Assisted Treatment (MAT)

Medication-assisted treatment (MAT) is the use of medications in combination with counseling and behavioral therapies to provide a whole-patient approach to the treatment of SUDs. MAT is associated with improved patient outcomes, including improved patient survival; increased engagement and

KEY POINT

For opioids, suboxone is an effective office-based treatment, while methadone is delivered within specialized treatment programs.

retention in treatment; decreased illicit opioid use; and decreased criminality among individuals with SUDs. MAT improves the patient's ability to obtain and maintain employment. For pregnant patients with SUD, MAT improves birth outcomes and reduces the occurrence and effects of intrauterine drug exposure. Table 30.2 provides information on medications used in Opioid use disorders, including intoxication, withdrawal, and MAT.

TABLE 30.1 Opioids, Receptor Targets, and Effects

Substance category	Neuro-chemistry	Acute	Long term	With alcohol	Withdrawal symptoms	Special populations	Medical-related problems or syndromes
Prescription opioids (morphine, hydrocodone, oxycodone, and codeine)	Opioid receptors (μ, κ, δ, and noc) in brain, spinal cord, and gut Mainly inhibitory, hyperpolarization/ decreased neuronal excitability	Pain relief, drowsiness, nausea, constipation, and euphoria—in some When taken by routes other than as prescribed (e.g., snorted, injected), increased risk of depressed respiration, leading to coma or death	Tolerance and addiction Opioid-induced hyperalgesia	Dangerous slowing of heart rate and respiration, coma, or death	Restlessness, muscle and bone pain, insomnia, diarrhea, vomiting, cold flashes with goosebumps ("cold turkey"), and leg movements	Youth can develop genuine pain conditions (e.g., cancer, post-op, sickle cell disease, etc.); 8–10% of high school seniors have used Vicodin nonmedically in the past year; spontaneous abortions as well as low birth weights are possible among pregnant patients; among adults, there is a higher prevalence of pain and a greater number of prescriptions for opioid pan meds	May initially cause aversive symptoms, including nausea, vomiting, constipation, pruritus, dizziness, dry mouth, and sedation—feelings of euphoria may develop thereafter; respiratory overdose—fatal if not reversed within minutes

Treatment

As part of SUD in general, the psychosocial aspects of OUD treatment are covered in general in Chapter 29. Table 30.2 summarizes medications currently FDA approved for treating OUD.

TABLE 30.2 Medications for Opioid Use Disorders

Drug information	Naltrexone	Buprenorphine	Methadone	Naloxone
Mechanism	• Opioid receptor antagonist • Blocks μ-opioid receptor (associated with pleasurable effects)	• Partial agonist/ antagonist • Agonist (partial) at мu receptors • Agonist at δelta • Antagonist at κappa receptors	• Full agonist	• Potent antagonist at R мu receptor • Reverses opioid use
Formulation	• Oral tablet (naltrexone, Revia) • Intramuscular depot every 28 days (Vivitrol)	• Combination drug (plus naloxone; sublingual tab, sublingual film, or trans-dermal patch) • Standalone (Buprenex: IM, IV) • Combination with naloxone (Suboxone) • Implant (Probuphine)	• Oral (syrup or tablet)	• Auto-injectable (Evzio) • Injectable • Nasal spray
Contraindica-tions/cautions	• Active opioid use • Liver failure • Naltrexone sensitivity	• Buprenex/Buprenorphine sensitivity • Risk of diversion	• Risk of addiction (significant) • Risk of diversion	
Pregnancy	• Relatively contraindicated • Category C	• Yes • Category C	• Yes • Category C	• Category C
Neonates abstinence/ withdrawal syndrome	• N/A	• N/A	• Yes	• Yes
Office based	• Yes	• Yes	• No • Requires special treatment program with close monitoring	• Emergencies or overdose situations
Other comments	• Can precipitate withdrawal (if given in active/ recent use)	• Suboxone: sublingual (reduces diversion) • Subutex: IM form (used in pregnancy) • Naloxone: to deter diversion (precipitates withdrawal if injected)		• Auto-injectable (Evzio) can be used in home or other settings by family members

PRESCRIPTION STIMULANTS

Prescription stimulants are a class of medications that increase the brain's level of attention. They include methylphenidates (e.g., Concerta, Methylin, Metadate, Quillivant ER, and Daytrana), dexmethylphenidates (e.g., Focalin), mixed amphetamines (e.g., Adderall, Adzenys, and Mydayis), and dextro-amphetamines (e.g., Dexedrine, Procentra, and Vyvanse). Prescription stimulants are the first line of medications used in treating attention deficit and related disorders. They are also sometimes prescribed as adjunctive agents in depression. In addition to increasing the brain's level of activity, they raise the body's level of activity and can cause elevated pulse and blood pressure. They have the potential to lower the seizure threshold and can lead to seizure activity, especially in overdose situations

NMU of stimulant medications is common in college students. Most are associated with minor or no medical effects when taken orally. However, adverse medical outcomes, including death, occur in some individuals, especially when taken by nonoral routes. The most common reason for stimulant NMU is the hope that it will improve performance. However, evidence is lacking regarding the effects on persons without ADHD (Faraone et al., 2020). Effects of prescription stimulants are shown in Table 30.3.

TABLE 30.3 Prescription Stimulants, Receptor Targets, and Effects

Substance category	Neuro-chemistry	Acute	Long term	With alcohol	Withdrawal symptoms	Special populations	Medical-related problems or syndromes
Prescription stimulants (mixed amphetamine salts and methylphenidates)	Increases dopamine and norepinephrine in the prefrontal cortex (improved alertness)	Increased alertness, attention, and energy; irregular heartbeat; dangerously high body temperature; potential for cardiovascular failure or seizures	High doses, especially, or alternate routes of administration (e.g., snorting and injecting) can lead to anxiety; hostility; paranoia; psychosis; and addiction	Masks depressant action of alcohol; increases risk of alcohol overdose; and may increase BP	Depression; fatigue; increased appetite; insomnia or hypersomnia; vivid unpleasant dreams; psychomotor retardation; and agitation	Used equally or in greater amounts by young females versus males to stay awake to study or perform better on exams and to lose weight	May be misused/ abused for weight loss

SEDATIVES AND HYPNOTICS

Sedatives, hypnotics, and anxiolytics exert their activity on the GABA-a receptor, much like alcohol. This group of substances include benzodiazepines and less commonly barbiturates. Thus, intoxication and withdrawal criteria are virtually identical (see the section on clinical features of alcohol; APA, 2013). As seen with discontinuation of alcohol consumption, withdrawal from benzodiazepines is potentially fatal and must be monitored closely. Typically, detoxification following chronic benzodiazepine use requires a gradual tapering process with a longer-acting benzodiazepine to reduce the risk of breakthrough withdrawal symptoms. Different benzodiazepines have different pharmacokinetic properties, which influence their clinical use. Table 30.4 shows a comparison of commonly used benzodiazepines. In overdose situations, flumazenil, a competitive benzodiazepine receptor antagonist, reverses the effects of benzodiazepines. Flumazenil has a short duration of action of about 30 to 60 minutes. Due to this, with single doses, sedation and respiratory depression can recur if the duration of the benzodiazepine exceeds that of flumazenil. In such situations, repeated doses of flumazenil will be needed. Effects of sedative hypnotics are shown in Table 30.5.

CLINICAL TIP

Flumazenil is a benzodiazepine receptor antagonist that is effective at reversing symptoms of benzodiazepine overdose. Flumazenil has a short duration of action of 30 to 60 minutes. With single doses of flumazenil, symptoms of intoxication, such as sedation and respiratory depression, may recur. Repeated doses may be needed in cases in which the overdose includes intermediate to long-acting benzodiazepines.

TABLE 30.4 Sedative Hypnotics, Receptor Targets, and Effects

Substance category	Neuro-chemistry	Acute	Long term	With alcohol	Withdrawal symptoms	Special populations	Medical-related problems or syndromes
Sedative hypnotics	GABA-A receptors	Drowsiness; relaxation; respiratory depression; and overdose	Tolerance; physical dependence; addiction; and amnesia and dementia	Slows both heart rate and respiration, which can be fatal	Discontinuing prolonged use absent a physician's guidance can lead to serious withdrawal symptoms, including seizures. For barbiturates, abrupt cessation can be life threatening	Used in treatment of anxiety disorders, trauma- and stress-related disorders; sleep disorders	Long-term use association with dementia

TABLE 30.5 Comparison Chart for Benzodiazepines

Name	FDA-approved uses	Onset of action	Time to peak (hours)	Half-life (hours)	Duration of action	Metabolites	Formulations
Alprazolam (Xanax)	• Anxiety • Panic disorder	• Fast	• 1–2	• 6–12	• Short-acting	• Weaker metabolites 4-hydroxyalprazolam and α-hydroxyalprazolam.	• Oral
Clonazepam (Klonopin®)	• Panic disorder • Seizure disorder	• Intermediate	• 1–4	• 18–50	• Long-acting	• Inactive	• Oral
Chlordiazepoxide (Librium®)	• Anxiety • Preoperative sedation • Alcohol withdrawal (off-label)	• Intermediate	• 1–4	• 6–25		• Active metabolites (including oxazepam)	• Oral, IM, and IV
Diazepam (Valium®)	• Anxiety • Alcohol withdrawal • Sedation (preoperative, ICU) • Muscle spasms • Seizure disorder • Status epilepticus	• Fast	• 1–2	• 20–70	• Long acting • Duration is variable, depending on dose and dosing frequency	• Active metabolites (including desmethyldiazepam and oxazepam)	• Oral, IM, IV, and rectal
Lorazepam (Ativan®)	• Anxiety disorders • Insomnia (short term) • Preoperative sedation • Status epilepticus • Anxiolytic/sedation (off-label)	• Intermediate	• 1–4	• 8–10	• Intermediate acting	• Inactive	• Oral, IM, and IV
Oxazepam (Serax®)	• Anxiety • Agitation • Alcohol withdrawal	• Slow	• 3	• 3–8	• Short acting	• No active metabolites	• Oral

DRUG DIVERSION

Diverted drugs are most often sourced from a family member or friend but can also be sourced online, from pharmacies or laboratories outside of the country, or bought from drug dealers. Diversion of prescription drugs can happen at any point along the supply chain. However, the most common point is at or beyond the point of the provider–patient interface. Primary health care, emergency room visits, and hospital discharges are known points of diversion. National surveys show that most are obtained from friends/relatives for free and the health care system (Hudgins et al., 2019; Park & Wu, 2020). In teens, significantly more females than males report using any prescription opioid (Park & Wu, 2020). The primary sources of prescription drugs on the street include patients with chronic pain and older adults. Unfortunately, health care workers are sometimes involved in prescription drug diversion, which is associated with profound professional risks. Table 30.6 shows commonly diverted drugs.

TABLE 30.6 Commonly Diverted Drugs

Class	Drugs
Antipsychotics	• Olanzapine • Quetiapine
Anesthetic drugs	• Ketamine • Propofol
Benzodiazepines	• All
GABA agonists	• Gabapentin • Pregabalin
Opioids	• All
Stimulants	• Mixed amphetamines • Dextroamphetamine • Pseudoephedrine • Methylphenidate

CLINICAL FEATURES

Behaviors around prescription medications vary. Paying keen attention to a patient's behavior around prescription medications, including their compliance with doses and dosing schedules, as well as their reasons for taking and requesting medication refills or changes, is a key part of good clinical practice. It is important to be aware that a patient may misuse or abuse a medication at any time. For example, a patient may abuse a medication as simple as OTC melatonin, which has low or no addictive potential. They may double or triple their usual nighttime dose to avoid being woken up by an angry spouse or may halve the dose but take this during the day with the intent of providing a light sense of sedation to numb their stressful home, work, or school environment. As such, with medication misuse or abuse, it is the behavior that is the focus, not the medicinal properties of the medication. If a person has a problematic behavior around taking medications, they increase their risk of engaging in the same problem behavior with more dangerous medications. In some cases, even a single prescription medication misuse incident can be fatal, while prescription drug addiction can become chronic, worsening over months or years. For example, a single misuse of prescription pain medication, such as taking a higher than prescribed dose of OxyContin, may lead to fatal overdose. Problem behaviors associated with prescription medications are depicted in Figure 30.2. The main difference between misuse and abuse depends on the patient's intent which often impacts their symptom-reporting. A useful chart to help check for prescription medication misuse, abuse, or addiction appears in Table 30.7.

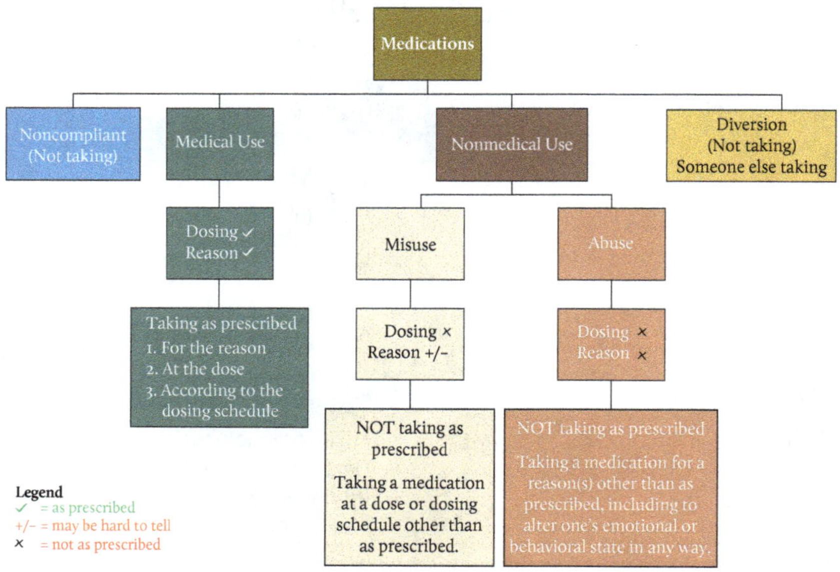

FIGURE 30.2 Behaviors around medications: What does the patient do with the medication?

CLINICAL TIP

Appropriate medication use is when a person takes a medication:

- for the reason it was prescribed
- at the dose it was prescribed
- according to the dosing schedule it was prescribed.

Inappropriate medication use occurs when a person takes a medication under any of the following circumstances:

1. not for the reason it was prescribed
2. not at the dose it was prescribed
3. not according to the dosing schedule it was prescribed

CLINICAL TIP

Nonmedical Use of Prescription Medications (NMUP): Medications are tools intended to promote health and healing. Misusing a tool can result in harm. Similarly, misusing medications can result in harm. The main difference between medication misuse and abuse lies in the patient's intent. A patient may misuse their pain medication by not taking it as prescribed (e.g., by taking more frequent or higher doses) intending to reduce their pain. A patient may abuse their pain medication by taking it for reasons not prescribed (e.g., intending to alter their emotional experience, such as to feel calm or high). Both scenarios present a challenge for the prescriber because it is sometimes difficult to accurately determine the reasons for NMUP. NMUP can be dangerous and cause significant functional impairment with possible fatality regardless of the reason.

TABLE 30.7 Prescription Medication Misuse to Addiction

Category of use	Takes meds as prescribed[1]	Takes meds for reason prescribed[2]	Patient's intent	Secondary gain[3]	Addictive behavior
Use	Yes	Yes	• Intends to use for reason prescribed • To reduce/remove symptoms	May be absent	May be absent
Misuse	No	Yes	• Intends to use for reason prescribed • To reduce/remove symptoms	May be present[4]	May be absent
Abuse	No	No	• Intends to use for reason other than prescribed • May report increased symptoms to obtain more meds	Present	May be present
Addiction	No	No	• Intends to use for reason other than prescribed • May report increased symptoms to obtain more meds • May generate extra reasons for symptoms to obtain more meds	Present	Present[5]

[1]*According to dosing strength and dosing schedule*

[2]*For symptoms or disorder*

[3]*Using medication for reasons other than prescribed)*

[4]*Patient may still take meds for reason prescribed. They may also take medications for additional reasons not prescribed. Both can occur concurrently.*

[5]*Addictive behavior is present and worsening due to loss of control at the core of the patient's addiction, usually a consequence of physiological changes secondary to repeated presence of the drug(s).*

GOOD PRESCRIBING PRACTICE

Good prescribing includes prescribing the right medication for the right disease condition at the right dose and dosing schedule and providing appropriate refills. Problematic prescribing comes in several forms, including underprescribing, overprescribing, inappropriate prescribing, irrational prescribing, prescribing errors, and providing inappropriate refills (Aronson, 2006). Such problems in prescribing can have serious consequences, including precipitating or promoting addiction and drug diversion.

The Science and Art of Prescribing

The word *prescribe* comes from a Latin word that means "to write in advance." In medicine, the actual writing of a prescription is the end of a series of steps (Figure 29.3). These include the following:

1. *Clinical assessment*—First, a clinical assessment that results in an accurate diagnosis based on the patient's symptomatology and the provider's understanding of the disorder's basic pathophysiology is essential. If a medication does not match the symptoms, disorder, or pathophysiology of the patient's condition, it is a wrong prescription.
2. *Risk-benefit analysis*—This includes weighing the risks and benefits of having the patient take the medication and not having the patient take the medication. Assessing the balance of benefit to the harm of a medication or treatment is important in deciding whether to treat at all. If the benefits of taking the medication outweigh the risks, then it could be a safe medication choice for the patient. If the risks of taking the medication outweigh the benefits, including precipitating, perpetuating, or in any way promoting addiction or diversion, then the medication may be a risky or even dangerous medication choice for the patient.
3. *Practical considerations*—These include the form of the medication to be prescribed (e.g., syrups for young children who have trouble swallowing pills, intramuscular depot shots for chronic schizophrenics who are noncompliant, buprenorphine for adult patients with OUD in full sustained remission who hold busy jobs, or methadone for adult patients with severe OUD who need daily engagement in specialized treatment programs).
4. *Obtain informed consent*—Discussing the potential risks and benefits with the patient, including potential beneficial effects and adverse effects, should be discussed. The patient should be made aware of alternative options to make an informed choice.
5. *Discuss expectations*—These expectations include expected, acceptable, and nonacceptable or problem patient behaviors around medication consumption. This should include an agreement that the patient will take the medication as prescribed by the doctor and inform the doctor of any concerns or unwanted effects.
6. *Prescribe*—Prescribe an appropriate medication for the patient's condition at an appropriate dose and dosing schedule. It is often better for medications with known potential for addiction to provide an initial prescription, then follow up with the patient and check their prescription use behavior before providing further refills.
7. *Monitor patients' behaviors around medication use*—This should be done periodically. Check periodically with the patient what exactly they are taking and when. This should be done especially for medications that could precipitate or promote addictive behaviors or propagate diversion.

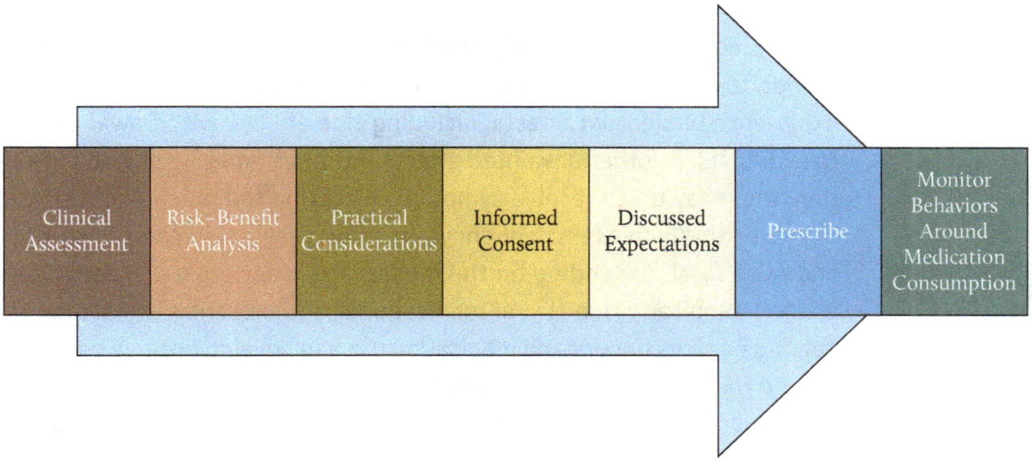

FIGURE 30.3 Good prescribing practice.

8. *Detect early signs of misuse, abuse, or diversion*—Providers should be alert to patients' behaviors, such as switching from appropriate use (use as prescribed) to inappropriate use (use not as prescribed). This could include a patient using a higher dose, a usual dose but more frequently, requesting refills too early, providing seemingly rational reasons to obtain additional scripts (e.g., lost scripts/meds that cannot be accounted for), and so on.

Addressing Patient Behaviors Around Medications

Medications including psychopharmacologic medications are tools for wellness that we give our patients. Patients have different expectations and experiences around such medications. This includes the expected, actual, and side effects of medications. Their experience with medications also includes their thoughts and feelings around taking medications. Some patients resist the idea of medications because they want to try on their own (e.g., to overcome depression) and may feel they have "lost the battle" if they "give in" to medications.

Providing psychoeducation about the medication is part of informed consent. Education around medications should include what the medication is prescribed for and what effect it is anticipated to have on the target symptoms it is being prescribed for. Specifically, discuss the benefits of taking the medications as prescribed and the risks and the dangers of not doing so. It is essential to document this discussion, including what was discussed.

CLINICAL TIP

Patients have different expectations and experiences about such medications. This includes the expected, actual, and side effects of medications. Their experience with medications also includes their thoughts and feelings around taking medications. Creating the space for patient to discuss their thoughts and feelings around the medications they are prescribed can facilitate treatment engagement.

For a variety of reasons, our patients may or may not take medications as we prescribed them. It helps to discuss with them their reasons for, or for not, taking their medications as prescribed. Sometimes, they genuinely experience unpleasant effects, including side effects, withdrawal effects, toxic effects, or other unwanted effects. At other times, with good intention, they may try to resolve symptoms by taking too much (higher dose) or too often (increased frequency). In some cases, this can be harmful, and even fatal, depending on the medication. Knowing the medication's pharmacological properties of medication(s) you prescribe is essential for helping patients understand medication use and develop positive behaviors around medications. It can also help interrupt negative behaviors around medications, which can cause the patient serious side effects or even fatality.

KEY POINT

Providing psychoeducation about the psychotropic medication is part of informed consent. Information provided to the patient should include what the medication is prescribed for and what effect it is anticipated to have on the target symptoms it is being prescribed for. Specifically, discuss the benefits of taking the medications as prescribed and the risks and the dangers of not doing so. It is essential to document this discussion, including what was discussed.

10 TIPS FOR CREATING SPACE TO DISCUSS PATIENTS' MEDICATION EXPERIENCES

It is good practice to periodically take the time to have discussions with your patients about their experience on medications. This is also helpful in building the doctor–patient relationship. Simple steps that can be taken include:

1. *Prepare for the discussion*—Most conversations are easy and go well. Sometimes, this can be difficult to have with some patients, especially if it uncovers problem behaviors around medications.
2. *Ask how they are taking their medications*—Ask about what medication is being taken, dosage, and frequency.
3. *Check if they are taking the medications as it is prescribed*—Address any discrepancies if they are present.
4. *Ask if they miss doses*—If yes, how often? For example, ask how many times a day or week they miss doses.
5. *Ask if they take extra doses*—If yes, how often? For example, ask how many times a day or week they take extra doses.
6. *Validate patients for adherence*—This helps them maintain positive behaviors around medications and increases the likelihood of positive patient outcomes.
7. *Discuss the benefits (and risks) of taking the medications as prescribed*—This discussion is important when indicated (e.g., if the patient is not taking medications as prescribed).

a. *Discuss the patient's perspective*—Discuss the benefits as seen by the patient *and* any risks, if present.

b. Discuss the risks of *not* taking the medications as prescribed

c. Discuss the benefits of taking the medications as prescribed.

8. *Take the nonjudgmental stance*—It may help to remember that you are there to treat—not to judge. Check to see whether your patient's symptoms are adequately treated. (The agreement between doctors and patients on adequate treatment can sometimes be a sticking point). Nevertheless, check if you need to adjust your prescription based on your patient's experience. Your patient's symptoms may genuinely be suboptimally treated. On the other hand, their symptoms may not match up with a genuine illness in some cases. The latter occurs less frequently and may be an assessment of exclusion.
9. *Practical considerations*—Consider alternative forms of medications if the patient is having trouble taking the medications (e.g., such as syrups for young children who have trouble swallowing pills and intramuscular injections for repeated poor adherence).
10. *Discuss expectations*—This should include the expected effects and the medication's utility as well as its limitations for treating mental health problems.

Psychopharmacologic medications are a key tool within the collection of tools used to treat mental health conditions. Patients often need to attend psychotherapy and engage in other social activities without which an overreliance on medications may repeatedly fall short of expectations.

SUMMARY

Opioids are potent pain medications that also have a strong potential to cause addiction. Effective treatments are available for OUDs. NMU has a disproportionately high impact on fatalities nationwide. Alertness to behaviors suggestive of misuse or abuse of medications is clinically helpful. Good prescribing practices and systems can prevent the development of drug misuse or abuse. Prescription monitoring programs that monitor medications' prescribing and dispensing can mitigate drug diversion, particularly for controlled substances.

RESOURCES

1 *Instructional video: Infomercial: Prescription Opioids: Even When Prescribed by a Doctor. Video Courtesy of Center for Disease Control; US Department of Health and Human Services. Running Time: 1:30mins Video is in the public domain: https://youtu.be/EsAgnVMWxBc.*

2 https://www.youtube.com/watch?v=16YhXNlC414

3 https://www.youtube.com/watch?v=Jv-mqsYytoA

4 https://www.cms.gov/files/document/opioids022316pdf

5 Opioid Overdose Reversal with Naloxone. https://www.drugabuse.gov/drug-topics/opioids/opioid-overdose-reversal-naloxone-narcan-evzio

REFERENCES

American Psychiatric Association. (2013). *Diagnostic and statistical manual of mental disorders* (5th ed.). https://doi.org/10.1176/appi.books.9780890425596

Aronson, J. K. (2006). A prescription for better prescribing. *British Journal of Clinical Pharmacology, 61*(5), 487–491. https://doi.org/10.1111/j.1365-2125.2006.02649.x

Bohnert, K. M., Ilgen, M. A., Louzon, S., McCarthy, J. F., & Katz, I. R. (2017). Substance use disorders and the risk of suicide mortality among men and women in the US Veterans Health Administration. *Addiction, 112*(7), 1193–1201. https://doi.org/10.1111/add.13774

Braden, J. B., Edlund, M. J., & Sullivan, M. D. (2017). Suicide deaths with opioid poisoning in the United States: 1999–2014. *American Journal of Public Health, 107*(3), 421–426. https://doi.org/10.2105/AJPH.2016.303591

Centers for Diseases and Control. (2020). *Overdose deaths accelerating during COVID-19* [Press release]. https://www.cdc.gov/media/releases/2020/p1218-overdose-deaths-covid-19.html

Center for Disease Control and Prevention. (2021). Drug overdose deaths in the U.S. top 100,000 annually. Retrieved February 12, 2022, from https://www.cdc.gov/nchs/pressroom/nchs_press_releases/2021/20211117

Faraone, S. V., Rostain, A. L., Montano, C. B., Mason, O., Antshel, K. M., & Newcorn, J. H. (2020). Systematic review: Nonmedical use of prescription stimulants: Risk factors, outcomes, and risk reduction strategies. *Journal of the American Academy of Child & Adolescent Psychiatry, 59*(1), 100–112. https://doi.org/10.1016/j.jaac.2019.06.012

Fishman, M., Wenzel, K., Scodes, J., Pavlicova, M., Lee, J. D., Rotrosen, J., & Nunes, E. (2020). Young Adults Have Worse Outcomes Than Older Adults: Secondary Analysis of a Medication Trial for Opioid Use Disorder. *The Journal of Adolescent Health: Official Publication of the Society for Adolescent Medicine, 67*(6), 778–785. https://doi.org/10.1016/j.jadohealth.2020.07.038

Gandhi, D. H., Kavanagh, G. J., & Jaffe, J. H. (2006). Young heroin users in Baltimore: A qualitative study. *The American Journal of Drug and Alcohol Abuse, 32*(2), 177–188. https://doi.org/10.1080/00952990500479290

Grant, J. E., Potenza, M. N., Weinstein, A., & Gorelick, D. A. (2010). Introduction to behavioral addictions. *The American Journal of Drug and Alcohol Abuse, 36*(5), 233–241. https://doi.org/10.3109/00952990.2010.491884

Grigsby, T. J., & Howard, J. T. (2019). Prescription opioid misuse and comorbid substance use: Past 30-day prevalence, correlates and co-occurring behavioral indicators in the 2016 National Survey on Drug Use and Health. *The American Journal on Addictions, 28*(2), 111–118. https://doi.org/10.1111/ajad.12866

Hudgins, J. D., Porter, J. J., Monuteaux, M. C., & Bourgeois, F. T. (2019). Prescription opioid use and misuse among adolescents and young adults in the United States: A national survey study. *PLoS medicine, 16*(11), e1002922. https://doi.org/10.1371/journal.pmed.1002922

Mattson, C. L., Tanz, L. J., Quinn, K., Kariisa, M., Patel, P., Davis, N. L. (2021). Trends and geographic patterns in drug and synthetic opioid overdose deaths—United States, 2013–2019. Morbidity Mortality Weekly Report (MMWR). 70, 202–207.

Miller, T. R., Swedler, D. I., Lawrence, B. A., Ali, B., Rockett, I. R. H., Carlson, N. N., & Leonardo, J. (2020). Incidence and lethality of suicidal overdoses by drug class. *JAMA Network Open, 3*(3), e200607–e200607. https://doi.org/10.1001/jamanetworkopen.2020.0607

National Institute on Drug Abuse. (2020a). *Drug use trends among U.S. teens. Monitoring the future 2020 survey results.* https://www.drugabuse.gov/drug-topics/related-topics/trends-statistics/infographics/monitoring-future-2020-survey-results

National Institute of Drug Abuse. (2019). *Trends & statistics.* https://www.drugabuse.gov/drug-topics/trends-statistics

National Institute of Drug Abuse. (2020b). *Misuse of prescription drugs research report, overview.* https://www.drugabuse.gov/publications/research-reports/misuse-prescription-drugs/overview

National Safety Council. (2019). *For the first time, we're more likely to die from accidental opioid overdose than motor vehicle crash* [Press release]. https://www.nsc.org/newsroom/for-the-first-time,-were-more-likely-to-die-from

Park, J. Y., & Wu, L. T. (2020). Sources of misused prescription opioids and their association with prescription opioid use disorder in the United States: Sex and age differences. *Substance use & misuse, 55*(6), 928–936. https://doi.org/10.1080/10826084.2020.1713818

Sharma, B., Bruner, A., Barnett, G., & Fishman, M. (2016). Opioid use disorders. *Child and Adolescent Psychiatric Clinics of North America, 25*(3), 473–487. https://doi.org/10.1016/j.chc.2016.03.002.

Wilson, N., Kariisa, M., Seth, P., Smith, H. t., & Davis, N. L. (2020). Drug and opioid-involved overdose deaths—United States, 2017–2018. *MMWR Morbidity and Mortality Weekly Report, 69*(11), 290–297. https://doi.org/10.15585/mmwr.mm6911a4

UNIT IV

TREATMENT OF PSYCHIATRIC DISORDERS

Unit IV discusses the various treatment modalities currently used in psychiatry. Psychotherapy was one of the earliest treatment modalities, and it is incorporated in most psychiatry treatment plans today. The psychotherapy chapter provides a brief history of psychotherapy and an understanding of the field today and how it has developed to include many evidence-based treatments for specific disorders and their use in other medical fields. The chapter on psychopharmacology covers major psychiatric medications, their mechanisms of action, side effects, and known medication syndromes associated with different medication classes. More advanced neuropsychiatry treatments, including electroconvulsive therapy, transcranial magnetic stimulation, light therapy, and, the more recently approved, ketamine treatment for depression are covered in the chapter on neuromodulation. Each chapter contains a case vignette that portrays the journey of a patient through their disorder and treatment.

CHAPTER 31

Psychopharmacology[1]

Sarah Shafer, M.D.; Sindhu Idicula, M.D.;

and Edore Onigu-Otite, M.D.

"Follow your heart, but take your brain with you."

— Alfred Adler

OBJECTIVES

After reading this chapter, students will be able to do the following:

- discuss mechanisms of action of major psychiatric medications
- review the effects and side effects of common psychiatric medications
- describe common medical syndromes associated with psychotropic medication use

CASE VIGNETTE

A 21-year-old college student presents to the ER. Her roommate brought her in because she seemed confused and dazed and was not acting herself. Her past psychiatry history reveals she has an anxiety disorder, which has responded well to sertraline. Her past medical history shows she has a history of migraines. About 2 weeks ago, she was started on a new medication for her worsening migraines. Three days ago, she developed a cough and had been taking over-the-counter cough syrup that contains dextromethorphan. She looks quite anxious. On examination, her skin is hot, sweaty, and has goosebumps. Her pupils look dilated. She is becoming more agitated. Her limbs jerk with any little contact.

(*continued*)

1 Readers may also see "Addiction and Substance Use Disorders " (Chapter 29), "Prescription Drug Misuse and Abuse: Opioids, Stimulants, and Sedative-Hypnotics" (Chapter 30), and "Psychiatric Emergencies" (Chapter 38) for related material.

You review her active medication list and discover she was recently started on sumatriptan for her migraine. Given this information and presentation, what is the likely condition?

A. Hypertensive crisis
B. Serotonin discontinuation syndrome
C. Neuroleptic malignant syndrome
D. **Serotonin syndrome**

DEFINITIONS AND KEY CONCEPTS

Psychopharmacologic agents are medications capable of affecting the mind, emotions, and behavior. Psychopharmacologic medications are sometimes called psychotropics or psychoactive medications.

INTRODUCTION

Psychiatric diseases can have complex etiologies with contributions from genetic factors, life experience, structural brain changes, neurotransmitter dysfunction, and xenobiotic effects. Successful management usually involves a combination of medications and psychotherapy. This chapter will focus on the biological contributors to schizophrenia, depression, anxiety disorders, mood disorder, attention- deficit/hyperactivity disorder, and substance use disorder, particularly underlying neurotransmitter dysfunction, since these are often the target of pharmaceutical treatments.

QUICK POINT

Regardless of their specialty, most providers will likely prescribe psychopharmacologic medications at various times. About 75% of retail psychotropic prescriptions in the United States are written by nonpsychiatrists (Mark et al., 2009).

It is crucial to keep in mind that nonpsychiatrists prescribe most psychopharmacologic medications. About 75% of retail psychotropic prescriptions in the United States are written by nonpsychiatrists (Mark et al., 2009). Almost all specialties prescribe psychopharmacologic medications. Regardless of their specialty, most providers will encounter psychoactive drug abuse or drug overdose situations in some form. A summary of medications used in major psychiatric disorders are shown in Figure 31.1. A summary of common neuroreceptors and neurochemical systems involved in exerting the effects and side effects of psychotropics is shown in Table 31.1.

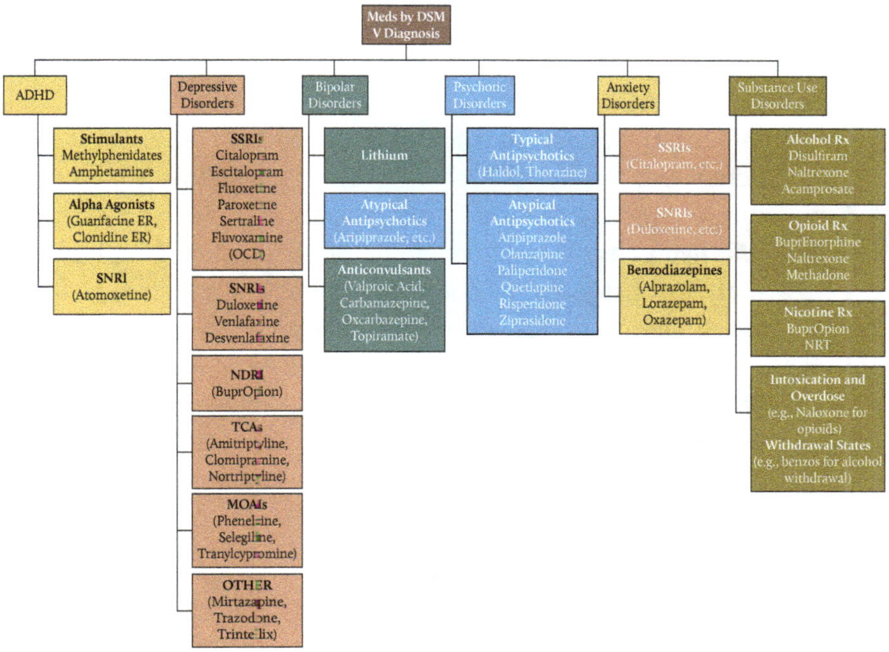

FIGURE 31.1 Overview of medications used in major psychiatry disorders.

TABLE 31.1 Summary of Effects and Side Effects of Psychotropics on Various Receptors

Receptor	Symptoms affected	Side effects (usually dose-dependent)
Dopamine	• Positive symptoms in schizophrenia	• Acute dystonic reactions • Extrapyramidal side effects (pseudo parkinsonism) • Tardive dyskinesia • Hyperprolactinemia
Serotonin	• Depression • Anxiety • Negative symptoms in schizophrenia	• Serotonin syndrome (serotonin toxicity) • Serotonin discontinuation syndrome (serotonin withdrawal)
Histamine	• Sleep • Anxiety • Appetite	• Sedation • Appetite increase • Weight gain
Alpha-1	• Blood pressure	• Orthostatic hypotension
Muscarinic (acetylcholine)	• Cholinergic symptoms	• Blurred vision • Dry mouth • Urinary retention • Constipation

SCHIZOPHRENIA

Neuropathology

In 1967, the dopamine hypothesis theorized that excessive dopamine action was responsible for the positive symptoms (e.g., paranoia, hallucinations, and delusions) of schizophrenia (Seeman & Kapur, 2000). This hypothesis was derived from the observation that dopamine-stimulating substances (e.g., amphetamines and cocaine) elicited similar symptoms in patients who were not diagnosed with schizophrenia, while dopamine antagonists, such as antipsychotic medications, decreased these symptoms (Kapur & Mamo, 2003; Meltzer et al., 2003; Seeman et al., 1996). Later, studies confirmed the correlation between excessive dopamine activity and patients who develop symptoms of schizophrenia (Abi-Dargham et al., 2000).

KEY POINT

In schizophrenia, there is a disturbance of the brain's dopaminergic system:

- Hyperactivation of the D_2 dopamine receptors in the mesolimbic pathways leads to positive symptoms, such as hallucinations and delusions.
- Hypoactivation of the D2 receptors in the mesocortical pathway leads to negative symptoms, such as poor motivation and organization.

Schizophrenia involves both increased and decreased activation of the dopamine receptors in different brain regions. The four major dopamine pathways affected by schizophrenia or treatment of schizophrenia are as follows:

- Mesolimbic
- Mesocortical
- Nigrostriatal
- Tuberoinfundibular

KEY POINT

The four major pathways relevant to the pharmacology of antipsychotics in schizophrenia are:

- Mesolimbic pathway (associated with positive symptoms)
- Mesocortical pathway (associated with negative symptoms)
- Nigrostriatal pathway (associated with movement disorders, such as acute dystonia, extrapyramidal side effects, and tardive dyskinesia)
- Tuberoinfundibular pathway (associated with prolactin release)

For example, excessive activation of the D_2 dopamine receptors in the mesolimbic pathways leads to positive symptoms, such as hallucinations and delusions (Meltzer & Stahl, 1976; Seeman & Kapur, 2000). Hypoactivation of the D_2 receptors in the mesocortical pathway leads to negative symptoms, such as poor motivation and organization (Meltzer et al., 2003). Antipsychotics work by decreasing the action of dopamine at the D_2 receptor, which helps attenuate the positive symptoms in the mesolimbic pathway. However, all four pathways are affected, leading to some of the common side effects of antipsychotic medications. Decreased D_2 activity in the mesocortical pathway leads to the worsening of negative symptoms. Decreased D_2 activity in the nigrostriatal pathway leads to movement disorders (Trosch, 2004), while decreased hypothalamic D_2 activity leads to excessive prolactin release, which causes gynecomastia and galactorrhea (Meltzer & Stahl, 1976). Decreased D_2 activity in the chemoreceptor trigger zone decreases nausea and vomiting, which allows us to use some antipsychotics as antiemetic medications. Of note, such antiemetics, including promethazine

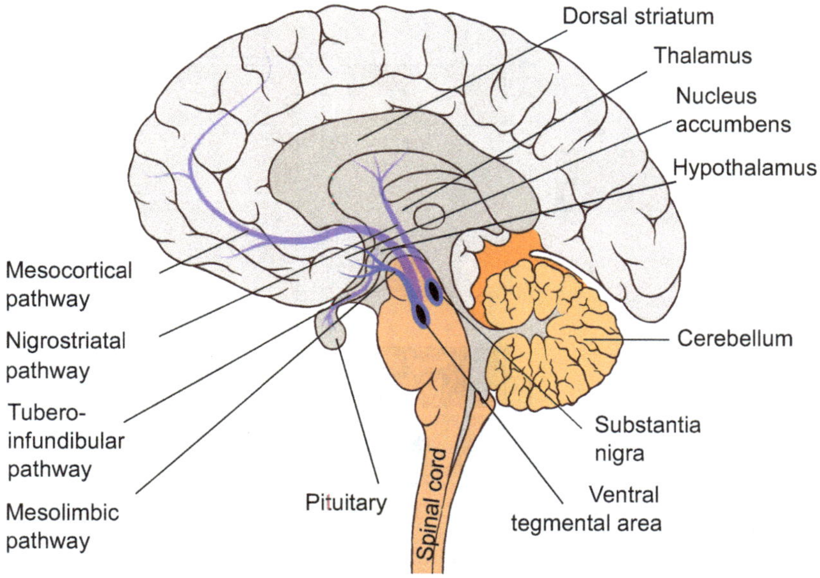

FIGURE 31.2 Four main dopamine pathways affected in schizophrenia and treatment.

Copyright © by Slashme (CC BY-SA 4.0) at https://commons.wikimedia.org/wiki/File:Mesolimbic_pathway.svg.

(Phenergan), metoclorpramide (Reglan), and droperidol (Inapsine) have the potential to cause side effects associated with antipsychotics, including dystonic reactions and dyskinesias.

Antipsychotics also affect several other receptors, which vary from medication to medication. Antimuscarinic effects can produce mild anticholinergic effects at therapeutic doses and serious anticholinergic symptoms in the setting of overdose. Alpha-1 antagonism can lead to orthostatic hypotension that can become significant hypotension during an overdose. Antipsychotics also have varying action at myocardial voltage-gated fast sodium channels, which becomes significant in the setting of overdose and can lead to impaired cardiac function. They also affect delayed-rectifier potassium channels, which are responsible for the QT interval–prolonging effect of many antipsychotic medications.

CLINICAL TIP

Antiemetics, including promethazine (Phenergan), metoclopramide (Reglan), and droperidol (Inapsine) have the potential to cause side effects associated with antipsychotics, including dystonic reactions and dyskinesias.

Typical Antipsychotics

Typical antipsychotics can be divided into two major categories based on their affinity for the D2 receptor: high potency (e.g., haloperidol, perphenazine, and fluphenazine) and low potency (e.g., chlorpromazine and thioridazine; Table 31.2). High-potency antipsychotics have a greater

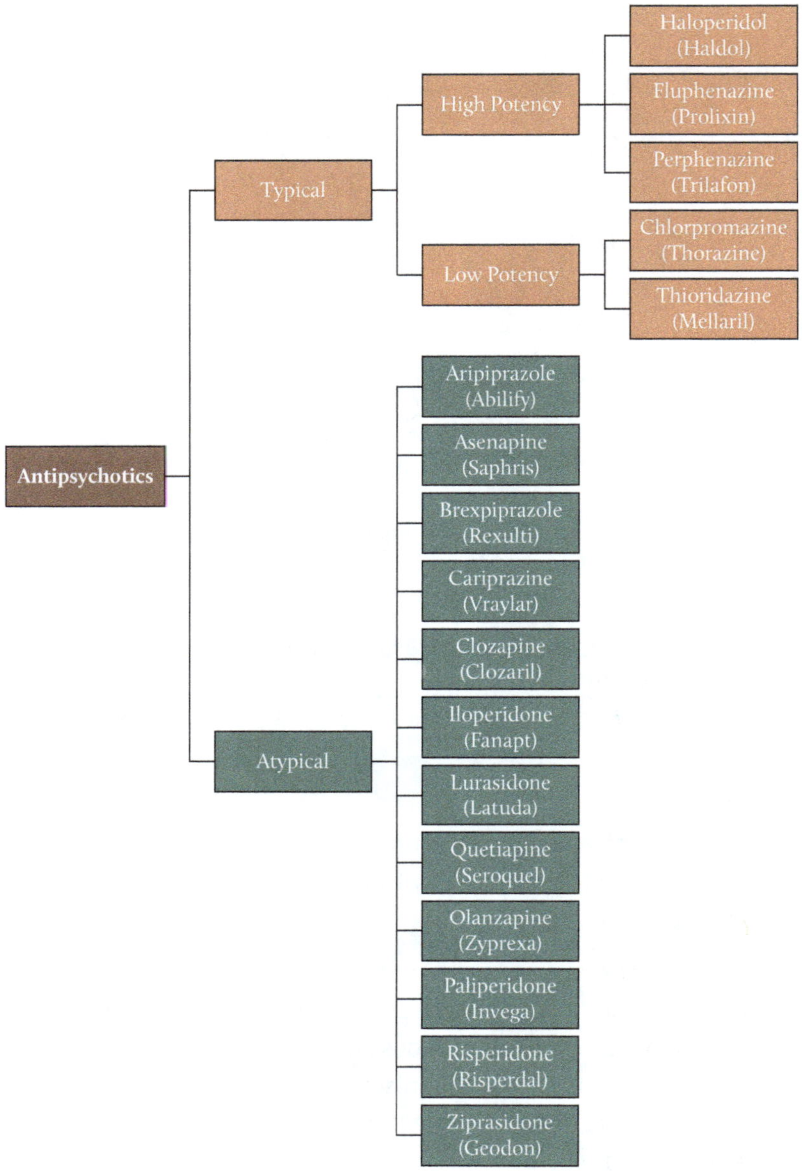

FIGURE 31.3 Antipsychotics used in psychotic disorders (FDA approved).

affinity for the D2 receptor and have a greater risk of extrapyramidal symptoms (EPS), which consists of neuromuscular symptoms, such as dystonia, akathisia, and tardive dyskinesia. Low-potency antipsychotics have less risk of EPS, although they may have more side effects due to their antihistaminergic, anticholinergic, and alpha-blocking effects.

Typical antipsychotics are effective at treating the positive symptoms of schizophrenia (e.g., hallucinations, delusions, paranoia, and disorganized thoughts), although they are less effective at treating the negative symptoms (e.g., flat affect, social withdrawal, and low motivation). Because of this and their side effect profile, their use has declined in favor of atypical antipsychotics. The most commonly prescribed typical antipsychotic is haloperidol (ClinCalc, 2020).

TABLE 31.2 Antipsychotic Comparison by Class

	Antipsychotic classes	
	Typical	Atypical
Potency	High	Low
Dosage	Lower	Higher
D2 antagonism	Potent D2	Less potent
Anticholinergic side effect	Lower	Significant
Risk of EPS	Higher	Lower
Risk of TD	Higher	Lower
Risk of NMS	Higher	Lower

Legend: D2 = dopamine 2 receptors; EPS = extrapyramidal side effects; TD = tardive dyskinesia; and NMS = neuroleptic malignant syndrome.

Atypical Antipsychotics

Atypical antipsychotics have become favored over typical antipsychotics because they are more successful in treating both the positive and negative symptoms of schizophrenia and because they are less likely to cause EPS (Burns, 2001; Table 31.3). Compared to typical antipsychotics, atypical antipsychotics bind to the D2 receptor with a lower affinity and shorter binding time, which leads to decreased development of EPS and TD (Burns, 2001). They also have serotonin antagonism at the $5HT_{2A}$ receptor, which allows more dopamine to function in areas where it is relatively deficient. This allows atypical antipsychotics to be more potent at lower doses, decrease the risk of causing EPS, and have more success at managing the negative symptoms of schizophrenia (Burns, 2001).

However, atypical antipsychotics are more likely to cause metabolic side effects, such as weight gain, insulin resistance, dyslipidemia, and diabetes (Leucht et al., 2009). They are also more associated with QT prolongation (Burns, 2001). The side effect profiles of the various atypical agents can have wide variation between the individual drugs in the class, so treatment decisions should consider individual drug effects. The most commonly prescribed typical antipsychotics in descending order are quetiapine, aripiprazole, risperidone, olanzapine, and ziprasidone (ClinCalc, 2020).

Clinical Syndromes

Antipsychotics carry different risks and benefits, often depending on their class, as summarized in Table 31.3. Beyond this, several clinical syndromes are associated with antipsychotics medications.

TABLE 31.3 Comparison of Typical and Atypical Antipsychotics Side Effects Profile

	Typical antipsychotic	Atypical antipsychotic
Symptoms	Strong effect on positive symptoms (e.g., reduced hallucinations and disorganization)	Strong effect on negative symptoms (e.g., improved motivation and attention) and strong effect on positive symptoms
Dosage	Lower mg doses	Variable
D2 blockade	Potent D_2 antagonism	Shorter D_2 binding
Cholinergic blockade	Lower anticholinergic SE	Variable
Serotonin antagonism	Lower	Stronger $5HT_{2A}$ blockade
Histaminic	Lower	Lower
EPS	Higher	Lower
NMS	Higher	Lower
Insulin resistance	Lower	Higher
Dyslipidemia	Lower	Higher
Weight gain	Lower	Higher

Legend: D2 = dopamine 2 receptors; EPS = extrapyramidal side effects; TD = tardive dyskinesia; and NMS = neuroleptic malignant syndrome.

Dystonia

Acute dystonia occurs within hours or days of starting therapy. It is a movement disorder characterized by involuntary movements of the head and neck, face, eyes, and extremities, which may include torticollis, acute laryngospasm, or oculogyric crisis. Patients may appear to be having seizures while awake and demonstrate a high level of distress due to the involuntary movements, although the condition is not medically serious except in the rare case of acute laryngospasm. Dystonia is associated with antipsychotic medications, although it can also be associated with other medications, such as metoclopramide, antidepressant medications, and cocaine. It improves over days if the offending medication is stopped. However, episodes of acute dystonia respond well to treatment with benztropine or diphenhydramine.

Akathisia

Akathisia is a term that describes a sense of restlessness, and patients may appear uncomfortable due to their inability to sit still. It appears to be dose-related and can manifest days to weeks after initiation of therapy (Trosch, 2004). Decreasing the antipsychotic dose or switching to an atypical antipsychotic may relieve symptoms. Patients may also get temporary relief from treatment with benztropine, benzodiazepines, or propranolol.

Parkinsonism

Parkinsonism is an adverse effect of antipsychotic therapy that looks clinically similar to Parkinson's disease. Patients present with limb rigidity, bradykinesia, and shuffling gait several weeks after starting therapy. Symptoms generally resolve after a few weeks after medication discontinuation (Trosch, 2004). Some patients may respond to treatment with benztropine or amantadine.

Tardive Dyskinesia

Tardive dyskinesia is a distinctive, repetitive, involuntary movement of the mouth or face that occurs after long-term treatment with antipsychotics. Most cases present after months to years of therapy. Symptoms may persist even after medication discontinuation, and tardive dyskinesia is historically known to be resistant to medical therapy. In 2017, the FDA approved two new medications for the treatment of tardive dyskinesia called valbenazine and deutetrabenazine. They are the first medications designed for the treatment of tardive dyskinesia. They are both vesicular monoamine transporter type 2 (VMAT-2) antagonists, resulting in decreased dopamine release into the synapse (Touma & Scarff, 2018). Further data is needed to determine long-term efficacy and safety information about these new medications.

Neuroleptic Malignant Syndrome

Neuroleptic malignant syndrome (NMS) is a serious, life-threatening adverse effect of antipsychotic therapy. Patients classically present with hyperthermia, lead-pipe rigidity, altered mental status, and autonomic dysfunction. They may also present with lab findings of rhabdomyolysis, lactic acidosis, and leukocytosis. It is associated with both typical antipsychotics and atypical antipsychotics, although some data suggest that patients who take atypical antipsychotics are less likely to present with rigidity or EPS symptoms (Trollor et al. 2012). Atypical antipsychotics are also associated with lower mortality from NMS than typical antipsychotics

MEMORY TIP

- D_2 blockage in the nigrostriatal pathway
  - → ↑ movement disorder/symptoms (such as acute dystonia, akathisia, extrapyramidal side effects, tardive dyskinesia)
- D_2 blockade in the tuberoinfundibular pathway
  - → ↑ prolactin release (causing galactorrhea)

MEMORY TIP

Neuroleptic Malignant Syndrome (NMS), *useful mnemonic*

FEVER
F—Fever
E—Encephalopathy
V—Vital sign instability
E—Enzyme elevation—CPK
R—Rigidity

(Christensen, 2005)

(Trollor et al., 2012). Patients are at increased risk for developing NMS if they have received multiple types of antipsychotics in a short period of time, escalating doses, intentional overdose, or concurrent lithium therapy. However, most cases of NMS occur during normal therapeutic use and progress over a period of days to weeks (Strawn et al., 2007).

NMS is thought to occur due to low levels of central dopaminergic activity, leading to alterations in thermoregulation and autonomic dysfunction. Patients with dopamine withdrawal, usually due to an abrupt change or interruption in dopamine-agonist therapy, can also present with symptoms of NMS despite never being prescribed antipsychotic medication, which further lends support to the theory that NMS is caused by a low level of central dopaminergic activity.

NMS is a challenging diagnosis because patients may not present with classic signs of NMS, and if they are altered, they may be unable to provide a history of antipsychotic exposure. It is ultimately a diagnosis of exclusion, so clinicians must maintain a high level of suspicion while ruling out other potential causes for the patient's presentation. Patients should receive supportive care with aggressive management of hyperthermia with cooling measures and agitation with benzodiazepines. All patients suspected of NMS should be taken off of antipsychotic medications. Patients presenting with NMS due to dopamine withdrawal should be restarted on their dopamine agonist as soon as possible. Patients with antipsychotic-related NMS can be started on bromocriptine—a centrally acting dopamine agonist.

DEPRESSION

Neuropathology

Medical treatment for depression has largely followed the tenets of the "monoamine hypothesis," which hypothesizes that depression is a result of monoamine (e.g., serotonin, norepinephrine, and dopamine) deficiency in the brain. Monoamine oxidase inhibitors (MAOIs) were the first major class of drugs used as first-line therapy for depression. Monoamine oxidase was responsible for the presynaptic breakdown of monoamine neurotransmitters, which also includes tyramine. By inhibiting monoamine oxidase, presynaptic levels of serotonin, norepinephrine, and dopamine increase, treating the symptoms of depression. However, presynaptic levels of tyramine levels also increased, which leads to a tyramine reaction if a patient ingested tyramine-containing food.

Because of the undesirable side effects of MAOI, tricyclic antidepressants (TCA) became the mainstay of therapy for depression starting in the 1970s. Their primary therapeutic effect comes from inhibition of norepinephrine and serotonin reuptake, which increases concentrations in the synapse (Hillhouse & Porter, 2015). They also inhibit histamine, muscarinic, and alpha-1 adrenergic receptors, which can lead to side effects of drowsiness, weight gain, tachycardia, dizziness, and orthostatic hypotension. Not only do their side effect profile make them difficult to tolerate, but TCAs can also cause severe cardiovascular toxicity, seizure, and death in overdose. Because of these considerations, the development of selective serotonin reuptake inhibitors (SSRIs) with similar efficacy, less severe side effects, and better safety in overdose started replacing TCAs in the 1980s.

Typical and atypical antidepressant medications have become the mainstay of modern pharmaceutical management of depression, largely replacing the use of MAOIs and TCAs. These therapies continue to target the monoamine neurotransmitters. However, there are new areas of research into the role of the glutamatergic system dysfunction in depression that suggest the monoamine hypothesis does not fully explain the neuropathology of depression. There is evidence that monoamine targeting therapies also have a modulating effect on the glutamatergic system (Hillhouse & Porter, 2015). There are ongoing investigations into medications that specifically target the glutamatergic system, particularly with medications that interact with the NMDA receptor, such as ketamine (Hillhouse & Porter, 2015).

Typical Antidepressants

Typical antidepressants, which include selective serotonin reuptake inhibitors (SSRI) and serotonin-norepinephrine reuptake inhibitors (SNRI), are serotonin-modulating medications that are typically prescribed for the treatment of depression. However, they have broad application not only for the management of mood disorders but also for various neurologic complaints. SSRIs, which include paroxetine, sertraline, fluoxetine, citalopram, and escitalopram, are associated with fewer side effects than their MAOI and TCA predecessors. However, they are associated with increased risk of falls, GI bleed, SIADH, and sexual dysfunction (De Picker et al., 2014). They are also associated with the risk of serotonin syndrome. Citalopram and escitalopram carry an additional risk of QT prolongation with therapeutic use, and in overdose they can cause seizures. SNRIs, which include venlafaxine, desvenlafaxine, and duloxetine, prevent reuptake of both serotonin and norepinephrine. They have similar side effects as SSRIs with the addition of side effects associated with elevated norepinephrine levels, such as hypertension and tachycardia.

Atypical Antidepressants

Atypical antidepressants include antidepressants with different mechanisms than SSRIs and SNRIs. Bupropion is a dopamine and norepinephrine reuptake inhibitor with strong sympathomimetic effects compared to its effects on serotonin. It lowers the seizure threshold even with therapeutic use, and there is a strong risk of seizure in overdose. Bupropion is less associated with the sexual side effects and weight gain associated with SSRIs and SNRIs. Mirtazapine is an alpha-2 antagonist that has a mechanism of action that results in increased serotonin activity. Its antihistamine effects lead to sedation and weight gain. Trazodone is a serotonin reuptake inhibitor and an alpha-1 adrenergic antagonist that commonly causes sedation. It is also associated with an increased risk of priapism, which requires emergent management.

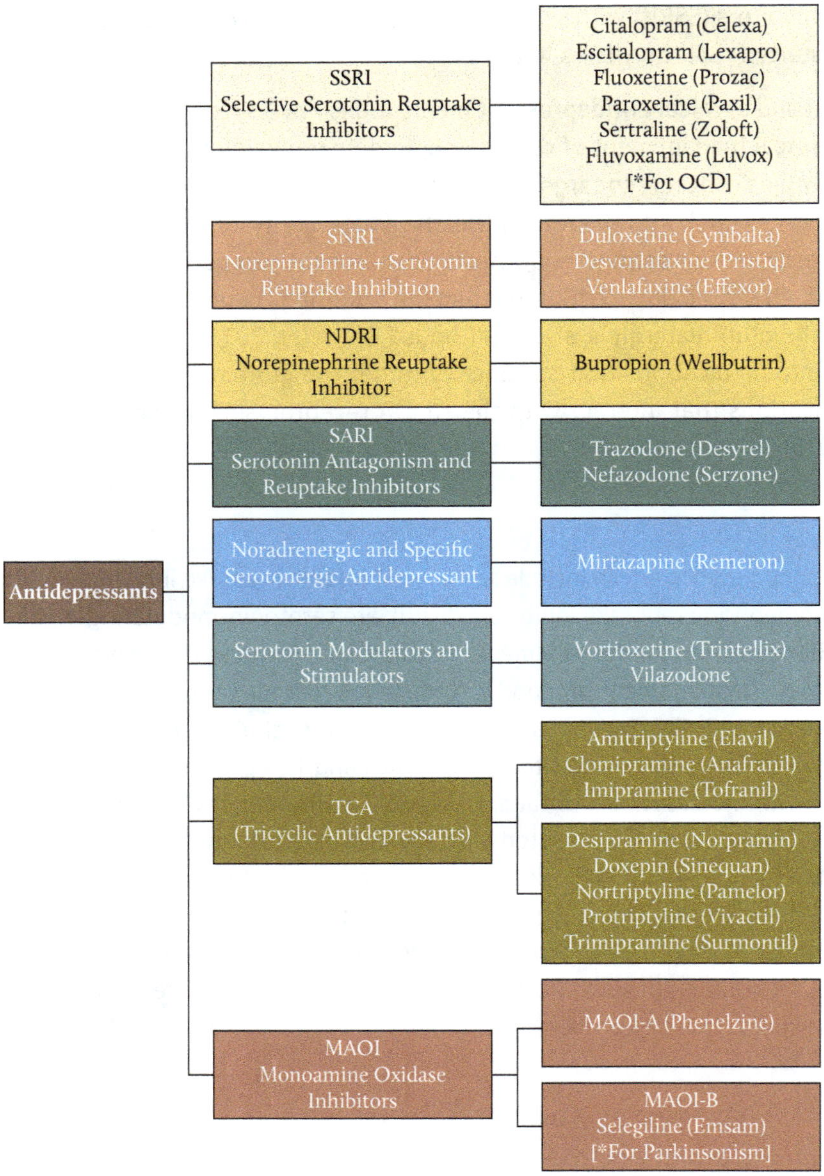

FIGURE 31.4 Antidepressants used in depressive disorders (FDA approved). *Although classified as an antidepressant, this medication is FDA approved for treating another condition and not for treating depression.

Monoamine Oxidase Inhibitors (MAOIs)

MAOIs, including phenelzine, isocarboxazid, and tranylcypromine, are irreversible, nonspecific inhibitors of monoamine oxidase (Fiedorowicz & Swartz, 2004). Selegeline is a type B monoamine oxidase inhibitor and is mostly prescribed for management of Parkinson's disease. MAOIs have largely fallen out of favor for management of depression due to their side effects, including the risk of hypertensive crisis. Because MAOIs prescribed for depression are irreversible inhibitors, a 14-day wash-out period is required to avoid drug interactions when patients are switched from MAOI to a new class of medication. MAOIs may also cause serotonin syndrome, so they should not be used in combination with other serotonergic medications (Fiedorowicz & Swartz, 2004).

Tricyclic Antidepressants (TCAs)

Tricyclic antidepressants inhibit reuptake of sodium and norepinephrine, which accounts for their antidepressant properties. However, they are associated with a larger side effect profile than other antidepressants because of their antihistamine, antimuscarinic, and anti-alpha-1 adrenergic effects. TCAs include amitriptyline, imipramine, nortriptyline, clomipramine, and doxepine. They have fallen out of favor as treatment for depression because of their side effect profile and significant toxicity in overdose. TCAs are also used for bipolar disorder, headache prophylaxis, and chronic pain management.

KEY POINT

Medication dosing, additive effects, interactions with drugs, and, in some cases, interaction with food can result in clinical syndromes—these range in severity from unpleasant and uncomfortable to dangerous and potentially lethal.

Clinical Syndromes

Medication dosing, additive effects, interactions with drugs, and, in some cases, interaction with food can result in clinical syndromes—these range in severity from unpleasant and uncomfortable to dangerous and potentially lethal. Drugs, including those used outside of psychiatry, often have effects that vary based on their metabolism and how that is affected by other drugs' metabolisms. It is wisest to perform a drug-to-drug interaction check whenever adjusting medications. Table 31.5 summarizes the findings in the major syndromes.

MEMORY TIP

Useful mnemonic for Anticholinergic toxicity: Red as a beet, blind as a bat, dry as a bone, mad as a hatter, hot as a hare, full as a flask, mad as a hatter.

- Red as a beet (flushed)
- Blind as bat (mydriasis)
- Dry as a bone (dry skin)
- Hot as a hare (hyperthermia)
- Full as a flask (urinary retention)
- Mad as a hatter (delirium)

Hypertensive Crisis

MAOIs are associated with a particular medication effect called tyramine crisis or hypertensive crisis. Ingestion of tyramine-rich foods, such as aged cheese, red wine, cured meats, and chocolate, can trigger sudden onset of a severe, pulsating headache, palpitations, diaphoresis, nausea, and elevated blood pressure (Blackwell et al., 1967). Some reactions are so severe that patients develop a stroke and have even died because of a tyramine reaction (Blackwell et al., 1967). Prior dietary restrictions were stringent due to concerns about triggering a hypertensive crisis, but now there are better guidelines regarding tyramine levels of food and how much is safe for ingestion (Fiedorowicz & Swartz, 2004).

Tricyclic Antidepressant (TCA) Toxicity

While safe for therapeutic use, TCAs are dangerous medications in overdose. They cause sodium channel blockade, which leads to cardiac arrhythmias, seizure, coma, then death. They also cause symptoms of anticholinergic toxicity in overdose, so patients may initially present with tachycardia, mydriasis, decreased bowel sounds, and delirium. The first sign of dangerous sodium channel blockade is an EKG finding of a QRS greater than 100 ms. This is associated with an increased risk of seizure, while a QRS of greater than 160 is associated with ventricular arrhythmia (Boehnert & Lovejoy, 1985). There may also be QT prolongation and signs of conduction delay on EKG. Patients with a widened QRS should be treated with sodium bicarbonate boluses to bring the QRS below 100 ms with EKG monitoring for the first 24 hours after ingestion to be able to treat any further episodes of QRS widening.

> **MEMORY TIP**
>
> ***Serotonin Syndrome***, *useful mnemonic*
>
> **SHIVERS**
>
> **S**—Shivering: neuromuscular symptom that is unique to serotonin syndrome
> **H**—Hyperreflexia and myoclonus: seen in mild to moderate cases. Most prominent in the lower extremities. This can help differentiate from neuroleptic malignant syndrome, which would present with lead-pipe rigidity.
> **I**—Increased temperature: not always present but usually observed in more severe cases
> **V**—Vital sign abnormalities: tachycardia, tachypnea, and labile blood pressure
> **E**—Encephalopathy: mental status changes, such as agitation, delirium, and confusion
> **R**—Restlessness: common due to excess serotonin activity
> **S**—Sweating: autonomic response to excess serotonin. This symptom can help differentiate from anticholinergic toxicity in which the patients would present with increased temperature but dry to the touch
>
> *(Christensen, 2006)*

Serotonin Syndrome

Serotonin syndrome is a life-threatening syndrome that occurs due to excessive serotonin activity, often triggered by a cross-reaction between two serotonergic medications. Serotonin syndrome can occur after exposure to a single serotonergic agent, especially when initiating the medication, during dose increases, or during overdose. Early signs of serotonin syndrome are tachycardia, mydriasis, bowel hyperactivity, hyperreflexia, and clonus. As the disease progresses in severity, patients develop altered mental status, agitation, hypertension, tachycardia, tremor, spontaneous clonus, ocular clonus, hyperthermia, and rigidity. The Hunter criteria is a clinical tool designed to be more sensitive in diagnosing serotonin syndrome than the more traditional Sternbach criteria (Dunkley et al., 2003; Figure 31.5). The causative medication should be immediately discontinued with careful review of the patient's medication list to see if there are other medications with serotonergic activity. Patients with hyperthermia and agitation should be aggressively managed, since these conditions are signs of severe disease. Hyperthermia can be managed by external cooling methods, and agitation is best managed using benzodiazepines and, in severe cases, neuromuscular paralytics. Cyproheptadine is a first-generation antihistamine medication that also acts as a serotonin receptor antagonist. It may help decrease the severity of symptoms, although it does not appear to shorten the duration of disease (McDaniel, 2001). Further research is needed to fully understand the benefits of cyproheptadine therapy and the optimal dosing regimen. Most patients who develop serotonin syndrome show significant improvement after the first 24 hours of supportive care and cessation of all serotonergic medication, although some people may have prolonged symptoms, depending on the formulation (immediate versus extended release), active metabolites, and drug half-life. A list of drugs that have been associated with serotonin syndrome is shown in Table 31.4.

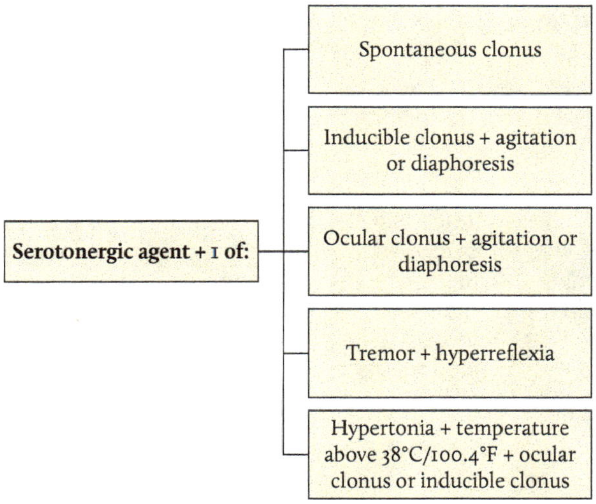

FIGURE 31.5 Hunter's criteria for serotonergic syndrome (serotonin toxicity).

MEMORY TIP

Hunter's Criteria for Serotonin Syndrome, *useful mnemonic*

MOAT-HD
M—Myoclonus (spontaneous, inducible)
O—Ocular clonus (spontaneous, inducible)
A—Agitation
T—Tremor
H—Hyper- (Hyperthermia, Hypertonia, Hyperreflexia)
D—Diaphoresis

(Created by Edore Onigu-Otite)

TABLE 31.4 Medications That Have the Potential to Cause or Contribute to the Development of Serotonergic Syndrome (Due to Additive Effect)

	Mechanism of action	*Medication class*	*Examples*
	Serotonin reuptake inhibitors	SSRIs	Citalopram, fluoxetine, fluvoxamine, and paroxetine
		SNRIs	Duloxetine, venlafaxine, and desvenlafaxine
Prescription meds		TCAs	Amitriptyline, clomipramine, and imipramine
		MAOIs	Phenelzine and selegiline
	Serotonin agonists	Triptans	Sumatriptan, zolmitriptan, naratriptan, rizatriptan, almotriptan, eletriptan, and frovartriptan
Controlled substances	Serotonin releasers	Narcortics and pain medications	Tramadol, meperidine, methadone, and fentanyl
Substances			Ecstasy (MDMA), amphetamine, cocaine, and methamphetamine
OTC meds	Serotonin precursors		L-tryptophan
			5-hydroxytryptophan
			Dextromethorphan, chlorpheniramine, brompheniramine, and St. John's wort
Miscellaneous			buspirone, metoclorpramide, carbamazepine, lithium, and valproic acid

TABLE 31.5 Summary Chart of Drug-Related Medical Syndromes in Psychiatry

	Serotonin discontinuation syndrome	Serotonergic syndrome	TCA toxicity	Hypertensive crisis	Neuroleptic malignant syndrome
Etiology	Withdrawal state due to an abrupt drop in serotonergic drug levels (e.g., SSRIs)	Serotonin toxicity (e.g., drug interactions involving SSRIs and drugs with serotonergic properties)	TCA above toxic levels (due to drug interactions, decreased elimination, etc.)	Acute severe increase in BP, often due to drug side effects or interactions (e.g., MAOIs' interaction with drug or food)	Excessive antagonism at dopamine D2 receptor site (e.g., by antipsychotics)
General	Flu-like symptoms (e.g., nausea, irritability, tearfulness, and fatigue)	Nausea and vomiting; diaphoresis; shivering; and goose bumps	Hot dry skin	Nausea and vomiting; and diaphoresis	Nausea and vomiting; diaphoresis and drooling
Vitals	Typically normal	Fever (hyperthermia = danger sign); autonomic instability (hypo- or hypertension); tachycardia; irregular pulse; and tachypnea	Fever; tachycardia; and hypotension	Elevated BP; irregular pulse; tachycardia; and tachypnea	Fever (hyperthermia = danger sign); autonomic instability (hypo- or hypertension); irregular pulse; tachycardia; and tachypnea
Psychological	Low or irritable mood	Restlessness and agitation	Restlessness and agitation	Severe anxiety and agitation	Anxiety and agitation
Central nervous system	Shock-like sensation and dizziness	Headache; blurred vision; pupillary dilatation; confusion; drowsiness; coma; and seizure	Pupillary dilatation; altered mental status; confusion; drowsiness; delirium; seizures; and coma	Severe headache; blurred vision; confusion; unresponsiveness; and seizures	Altered mental status
Cardiovascular system		Palpitations and cardiac arrhythmias	Palpitations; chest pain; and cardiac arrhythmias	Nosebleeds; palpitations; chest pain; and cardiac arrhythmias	Chest pain
Respiratory		Shortness of breath	Respiratory depression	Shortness of breath and chest pain	Difficulty breathing

	Serotonin discontinuation syndrome	Serotonergic syndrome	TCA toxicity	Hypertensive crisis	Neuroleptic malignant syndrome
Neuromuscular		Loss of muscle coordination; muscle twitching; muscle rigidity; tremors; clonus; and exaggerated reflexes			Muscle rigidity
Gastrointestinal		Diarrhea	Decreased bowel sounds		
Laboratory findings			EKG–QRS >100 ms		Elevated WBC; markedly elevated; and creatinine kinase
Severity of condition in itself	Unpleasant but not dangerous	May cause death	May cause death	May cause death or may cause permanent organ damage (e.g., stroke or cardiac or kidney failure)	May cause death or may cause permanent organ damage (e.g., stroke or cardiac or kidney failure)
Warning signs of severity		Hyperthermia; cardiac arrhythmias; drowsiness; unconsciousness; and seizures			Hyperthermia; cardiac arrhythmias; drowsiness; unconsciousness; and seizures

a Hyperthermia = very high fever of 102 to 104 degrees Fahrenheit.

ANTIANXIOLYTICS

Neuropathology

Anxiety disorders include a diverse range of diseases, including generalized anxiety disorder, social anxiety, phobias, and panic disorder. Other disorders that include some symptoms of anxiety include obsessive compulsive disorder (OCD) and posttraumatic stress disorder (PTSD). All these diseases share neurobiological dysfunction of the emotion-processing limbic system, which includes the insular cortex, cingulate cortex, hippocampus, and amygdala (Martin et al., 2010). The etiology for anxiety disorders is complex—not only involving dysfunction of serotonin, norepinephrine, and dopamine neurotransmitter systems but also the interplay between the hypothalamic–pituitary–adrenal (HPA) axis via the hippocampus, which controls our stress response and the amygdala (Martin et al., 2010; Schmidt et al., 2018). The amygdala is responsible for feelings of aggression and fear, and it also plays a role in the way we form and access memories, especially memories associated with fear. Amygdala hyperfunction, especially under triggering stimuli, may be modified by an imbalance between inhibitory γ-amino-butyric-acid (GABA) and excitatory glutamate (Martin et al., 2010) (Schmidt et al., 2018).

There is significant overlap between anxiety disorders and major depressive disorder with a comorbidity rate > 50% (Kessler et al., 1996). Functional brain studies have demonstrated that the two conditions modify each other, and both involve dysfunction of the prefrontal cortex and amygdala (Engels et al., 2010). This overlap explains why first-line therapies for anxiety disorders are the same SSRIs and SNRIs that we use to treat depression.

First-Line Therapy

First line therapy for management of anxiety-related disorders is treatment with SSRIs and SNRIs. Both medications increase the amount of serotonin in the synapse by blocking serotonin reuptake. SNRIs additionally increase norepinephrine levels in the synapse by blocking norepinephrine reuptake. The decision for which SSRI or SNRI to use for therapy will depend on patient treatment response and tolerance to medication side effects.

Benzodiazepines

Benzodiazepines are gamma-butyric acid (GABA) agonists that are frequently prescribed for anxiety disorders, although their use in anxiety disorders is controversial (Cloos & Ferreira, 2009). Both patients and clinicians report good clinical effect with a rapid response to treatment, in contrast to SSRIs that may take several weeks to reach full effect (Cloos & Ferreira, 2009). Notably, rebound anxiety and lack of efficacy in long-term anxiety management is a concern with benzodiazepine treatment. Importantly, benzodiazepine use can result in physical dependence with additional concern for abuse. The most commonly prescribed benzodiazepines in descending order are as follows: alprazolam, lorazepam, clonazepam, diazepam, and temazepam (ClinCalc, 2020). Parenterally, midazolam, diazepam, and lorazepam are commonly used in an inpatient setting. The main difference between the different types of benzodiazepines is duration of action. Short-acting benzodiazepines include midazolam, alprazolam, and oxazepam. Intermediate-acting benzodiazepines include lorazepam, temazepam, and clonazepam. Diazepam and chlordiazepoxide are long-acting benzodiazepines.

Clinical Syndromes

Sedative–Hypnotic Toxidrome

Benzodiazepines do not cause any clinical syndromes with therapeutic usage, but in overdose they can cause signs and symptoms of sedative–hypnotic toxidrome. Patients with sedative–hypnotic toxidrome present with excessive sedation, mydriasis, bradycardia, hypotension, and respiratory depression. They may appear similar to patients with opioid overdose, although with much less respiratory depression and hypoxia than is typical for opioid toxidrome. Patients with severe sedative–hypnotic toxidrome may respond to treatment with flumazenil, a GABA antagonist. However, treatment with flumazenil should only be given to patients who have no history of ethanol or benzodiazepine dependency, since it may trigger acute withdrawal with benzodiazepine-resistant seizures.

BIPOLAR DISORDER

Neuropathology

There is no clear neuropathology to explain the etiology for bipolar disorder. It is thought to be due to dysregulation of dopamine, serotonin, and norepinephrine—the same neurotransmitters implicated in the other mood disorders (Ware et al., 2016). The goal of therapy is to treat acute episodes and to prevent their reoccurrences so that patients can have an improved quality of life (Ware et al., 2016).

Lithium

Lithium is an elemental ion that is physiologically treated similarly to sodium. It has long been used for the management of bipolar disorder, although its mechanism of action is still unknown. It is used to treat acute mania and is also effective as maintenance therapy (Keck & McElroy, 2002; Ware et al., 2016). Lithium becomes widely distributed in the body once it is absorbed and is excreted by the kidneys. It has a narrow therapeutic index, and levels can be greatly affected by renal function, sodium levels, and dehydration. It is also sensitive to drug interactions, so patients should have their levels monitored when starting new medications. Signs of toxicity include tremor, ataxia, nausea, vomiting, and confusion. Chronic use can cause nephrogenic diabetes insipidus and thyroid dysfunction. It is also teratogenic and should be avoided in pregnant patients because of the risk of Ebstein's abnormality. Patients who present with elevated serum levels and signs of toxicity should be managed with sodium-containing IV fluids with immediate discontinuation of lithium. Severe cases of lithium toxicity may require dialysis, especially if renal function is impaired.

Anticonvulsants

Valproic acid, carbamazepine, oxcarbazepine, and lamotrigine are commonly used as mood stabilizers. Valproic acid has an unknown mechanism of action, although it has some GABA agonism and functions as a sodium-channel blocker. It can cause dysfunction in ammonia metabolism, and many patients have mildly elevated ammonia levels without any symptoms. Serious side effects include severely elevated ammonia levels and liver failure. Carbamazepine and oxcarbazepine (a carbamazepine

CLINICAL TIP

Sedative-hypnotic toxidrome, such as with benzodiazepines, present with drowsiness, mydriasis, bradycardia, hypotension, and respiratory depression.

This presentation is like opioid overdose but has less respiratory depression and hypoxia than is typical for opioid toxidrome. For benzodiazepine overdose, flumazenil, a GABA antagonist, is used. However, treatment with flumazenil should only be given to patients who have no history of ethanol or benzodiazepine dependency, since it may trigger acute withdrawal with benzodiazepine-resistant seizures.

KEY POINT

Lithium is used in acute mania and is also effective as maintenance therapy. Once absorbed, lithium is widely distributed in the body and is excreted by the kidneys. It has a narrow therapeutic index, and levels can be greatly affected by renal function, sodium levels, and dehydration. Signs of toxicity include tremor, ataxia, nausea, vomiting, and confusion. Severe cases of lithium toxicity may require dialysis, especially if renal function is impaired.

analogue) are both sodium channel blockers. Carbamazepine is a potent inducer of the P450 system, so initiation of therapy may cause significant drug interactions. It is associated with Stevens–Johnsons syndrome and toxic epidermal necrolysis, although occurrence is rare (Ware et al., 2016). Topiramate has an unknown mechanism of action, although, like valproic acid, it is thought to have GABA agonism and sodium-channel blocking effects (Keck & McElroy, 2002). Because of its carbonic anhydrase inhibition, it is associated with an increased risk of nephrolithiasis (Keck & McElroy, 2002).

Atypical Antipsychotics

Atypical antipsychotics are used to treat schizophrenia and other psychotic disorders; mood disorders, including bipolar disorder; and adjunctive treatment for depression. Some atypical antipsychotics are approved for treating irritability in individuals with autism.

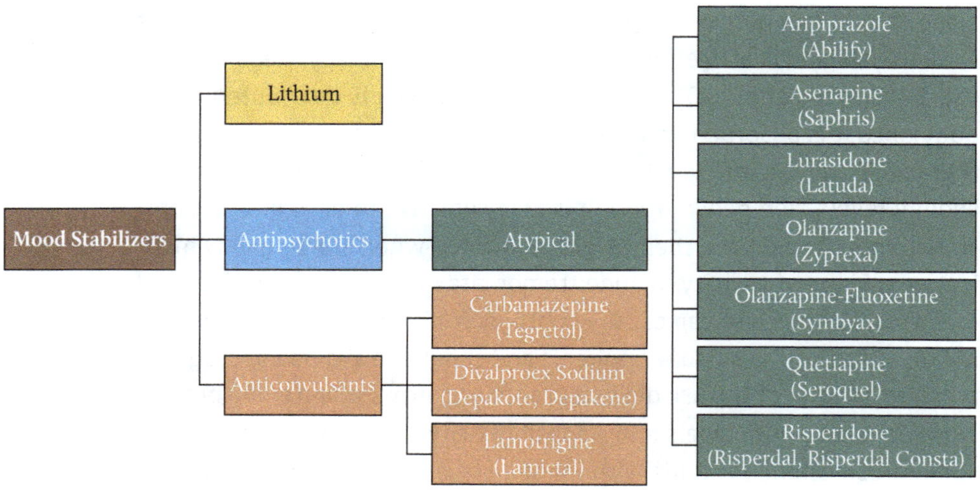

FIGURE 31.6 Mood stabilizers used in bipolar disorders (FDA approved).

ADHD

Neuropathology

Attention-deficit/hyperactivity disorder (ADHD) is a behavioral disorder that has multifactorial etiologies for its formation. Neuropathology is influenced by multiple genetic and environmental factors with ongoing studies to understand the full influence of these various components. Structural brain studies show that patients with ADHD have abnormalities in the frontostriatal network, which involves the lateral prefrontal cortex, the dorsal anterior cingulate cortex, the caudate nucleus, and putamen (Curatolo et al., 2010). ADHD is also associated with dysfunction of norepinephrine and dopamine (Pliszka, 2005), which are highly represented in the frontostriatal network (Curatolo et al., 2010). It appears that the dysfunction of norepinephrine and dopamine is not as simple as correcting deficient levels, since there is complex interplay between the two neurotransmitters, depending on what part of the brain they are located (Pliszka, 2005). Stimulant medications act on norepinephrine and dopamine systems, while nonstimulant treatment of ADHD affects the norepinephrine system (Pliszka, 2005). Treatments that only modify dopamine, or whose mechanism of action primarily affect other neurotransmitters, are found to be less effective than medications that modify dopamine and norepinephrine (Pliszka, 2005).

Stimulant Medications

Stimulant medications are considered first-line therapy for the medical treatment of ADHD due to their proven efficacy than nonstimulant medication (Southammakosane & Schmitz, 2015). They are broadly divided into two categories: methylphenidate and amphetamine salts. With all stimulant medications, patients should be screened for any personal or family history of cardiac disease, arrhythmia, or sudden death and undergo a physical exam to look for any signs of underlying cardiac disease to determine whether the patient should receive further evaluation with EKG and cardiology consult (Subcommittee on Attention-Deficit/Hyperactivity & Steering Committee on Quality Improvement and Management, 2011). However, if the patient has no known history or risk of cardiac disease, they do not require further work-up. A large, retrospective study found no increased risk of serious cardiovascular events associated with stimulant drug use for ADHD among adult patients (Habel et al., 2011). However, patients who have problems with high blood pressure or elevated heart rates should avoid stimulant medications, since they can worsen these conditions.

> **KEY POINT**
>
> Stimulant medications are considered first-line therapy for the medical treatment of ADHD. They are broadly divided into two categories: methylphenidate and amphetamine salts. Methylphenidate blocks presynaptic dopamine reuptake, increasing dopamine levels in the synapse. Amphetamine salts block dopamine and norepinephrine reuptake and promote dopamine and norepinephrine release, further increasing concentrations of dopamine and norepinephrine in the synaptic spaces.

Methylphenidate is the most commonly prescribed stimulant medication for ADHD (Greydanus et al., 2009). It blocks presynaptic dopamine reuptake, increasing dopamine levels in the synapse (Greydanus et al., 2009). It also blocks norepinephrine reuptake, increasing norepinephrine levels in the synapse (Curatolo et al., 2010). Some methylphenidate formulations only contain the dextro-enantiomer of methylphenidate, also called dexmethylphenidate. The differences between the various methylphenidate formulations mostly have to do with delivery method (pill versus wafer versus patch) and whether there is an immediate or extended release. The optimal formulation depends on individual patient needs. For example, a young patient who cannot swallow pills may benefit from a liquid formulation or a patch. Patients who have difficulty with multidose medications or who need a longer duration of effect than what they get from an immediate-release preparation, may benefit from an extended-release preparation. However, a patient who is having sleep disturbances from stimulant treatment for ADHD may benefit from an immediate-release formulation.

The other major category of stimulant medications includes amphetamine salts. Like methylphenidate, amphetamine salts block dopamine and norepinephrine reuptake. They also promote dopamine and norepinephrine release by the presynaptic cell into the synapse, further increasing concentrations of synaptic dopamine and norepinephrine (Curatolo et al., 2010). Amphetamine salt formulations are similarly divided into mixed enantiomer formulations and dextroamphetamine-only formulations (Greydanus et al., 2009). Both the mixed enantiometer and dextroamphetamine salts are further available as immediate- and extended-release formulations with prescribing decisions based on individual patient needs.

Nonstimulant Medications

KEY POINT

Nonstimulant medications for ADHD include the alpha-agonists guanfacine ER (Intuniv) and clonidine ER (Kapvay) and the norepinephrine reuptake inhibitor atomoxetine (Stratterra).

Nonstimulant medications may be indicated when patients have failed stimulant medication because of ineffective treatment response despite maximum dosages. Some patients cannot take stimulant medications due to underlying medical problems, such as cardiac disease, hypertension, hypothyroidism, or a history of psychosis. Some patients or families may have various reasons to prefer treatment with nonstimulant medication for ADHD. They may suffer from unwanted side effects that make stimulants less desirable, such as unintended weight loss, palpitations, or interrupted sleep patterns. For others, they may be concerned about the potential for abuse associated with stimulant mediations. The FDA has approved three nonstimulant medications for treatment of ADHD: clonidine, guanfacine, and atomoxetine. All three medications work by modifying norepinephrine levels at the synapse.

Both clonidine and guanfacine are alpha-2 adrenergic agonists. Their sedative and antihypertensive effects come from presynaptic alpha-2 receptor agonism. Stimulation of these presynaptic alpha-2 receptors serves to decrease norepinephrine release though a reverse feedback mechanism. However, their effect on ADHD seems to come from postsynaptic alpha-2 agonism, which has a similar effect to increasing norepinephrine levels in the synapse (Arnsten, 2000). Guanfacine seems to have less sedation and hypotension effects when compared to clonidine, so it has become more commonly prescribed for ADHD (Greydanus et al., 2009). Both medications carry the risk of rebound hypertension with the immediate release forms of the medication, so the extended-release formulations are preferred for therapy (Southammakosane & Schmitz, 2015).

Atomoxetine is a norepinephrine reuptake inhibitor, which results in the increased concentration of norepinephrine in the synapse (Greydanus et al., 2009). There is a black-box warning for atomoxetine, due to an increase in suicidality after starting the medications, so patients should be monitored for mood changes or suicidal thoughts after initiation or dosage change (Greydanus et al., 2009). There is some data that suggests atomoxetine is effective when compared to placebo (Schwartz & Correll, 2014) but still inferior to guanfacine (Signorovitch et al., 2012) .

There has also been off-label use of antidepressant medications for the management of ADHD, although these are generally considered second- or third-line agents. All patients who are started on antidepressants for ADHD should be monitored for mood changes and suicidality for several months after initiation and dosage changes. Bupropion is a dopamine and norepinephrine reuptake inhibitor with studies showing variable efficacy in treating ADHD (Buoli et al., 2016). Tricyclic antidepressants, such as nortriptyline and desipramine, have nonspecific reuptake inhibition of norepinephrine (Buoli et al., 2016). Venlafaxine blocks reuptake of serotonin and norepinephrine with weak dopamine reuptake (Greydanus et al., 2009). There is also research into the use of lithium and antipsychotic medications for the management of ADHD (Buoli et al., 2016).

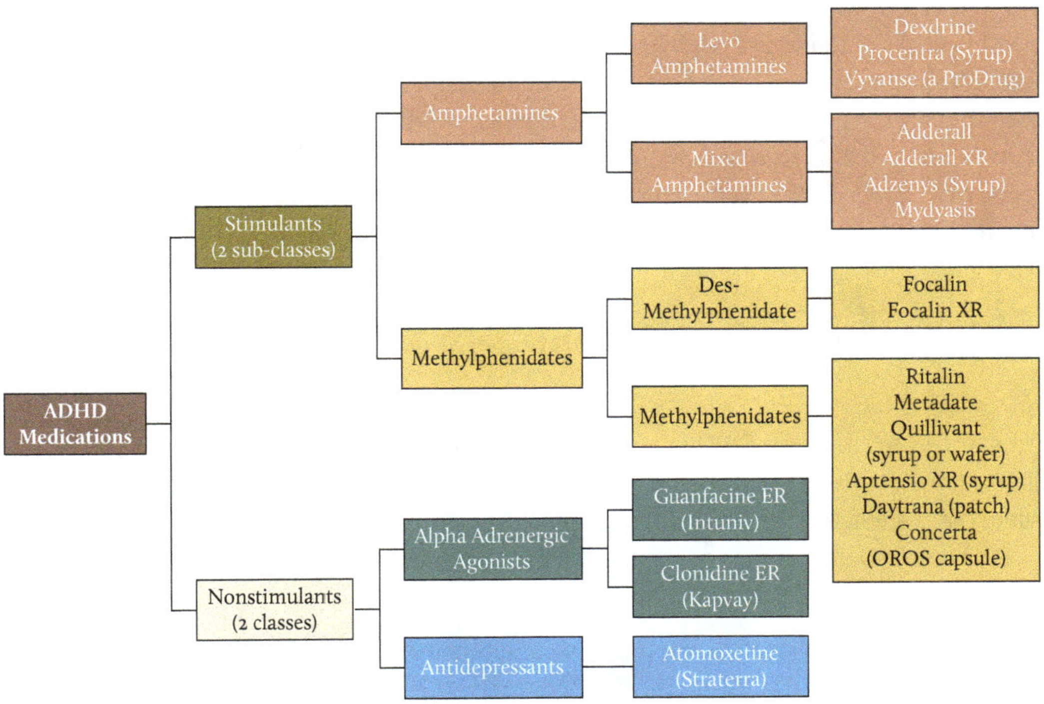

FIGURE 31.7 FDA-approved medications for treating ADHD.

Clinical Syndromes

Besides the usual medication side effects, there are no anticipated clinical syndromes associated with therapeutic use of stimulant and nonstimulant ADHD medications. However, there are distinct clinical syndromes when ADHD medications are associated with overdose.

Sympathomimetic Toxidrome

With stimulant ADHD medications, patients who overdose may present with signs of sympathomimetic toxidrome. This toxidrome is associated with any substance that mimics or promotes catecholamine action in the body, including amphetamines, cocaine, PCP, and ephedrine. Signs of sympathomimetic toxidrome include tachycardia, hypertension, agitation, mydriasis, and diaphoresis Severe sympathomimetic toxidrome may present with hyperthermia, seizure, acidosis, cardiac arrhythmia, or coma. Severely ill patients may die due to multiorgan failure and severe metabolic derangements. Treatment for sympathomimetic toxidrome involves supportive care and aggressive management for the patient's agitation with benzodiazepines, since the hypermotor activity associated with agitation drives the hyperthermia and metabolic derangements.

Alpha-2 Agonist Overdose

Patients who present with alpha-2 agonist overdose present similarly to patients who present with opioid overdose. They may both present with sedation, pinpoint pupils, bradycardia, and hypotension. It is because of the similarities between opioid toxidrome and alpha-2 agonist overdose that patients are often treated with naloxone with questionable efficacy in the setting of alpha-2 agonist overdose (Ahmad et al., 2015). While there are proponents of large doses of naloxone in the setting of alpha-2 agonist overdose (Seger & Loden, 2018), the use of naloxone remains controversial. Patients should receive supportive care with fluid and pressors as needed for hypotension. Some patients may require atropine for bradycardia. In severe cases, patients may require airway support via intubation.

SUBSTANCE USE DISORDER

Neuropathology

Substance use disorder (SUD) is a complicated disease with complex interplay between aberrant behaviors that are driven by dysfunctional neurochemical and biological processes. While there are nuances to the neuropathology of SUD, depending on the agent of addiction, all SUD involves dysfunction of the reward pathways in the brain (Gardner, 2011; Hyman et al., 2006; Koob & Le Moal, 2001).

Dopamine is the primary neurotransmitter associated with activation of reward and euphoria in the brain (Gardner, 2011; Hyman et al., 2006; Koob & Le Moal, 2001). All addicting substances enhance dopamine activity in the nucleus accumbens (Gardner, 2011; Hyman et al., 2006; Koob

& Le Moal, 2001). The nucleus accumbens is part of the mesolimbic dopamine pathway in the brain, and it is often nicknamed "the reward pathway." The mesolimbic pathway starts with dopamine-producing neurons in the ventral tegmental area (VTA) that project to the nucleus accumbens.

In addition to their effect on the mesolimbic pathway, addicting substances have a primary effect that generally occurs on the level of the synapse. Ethanol is a GABA agonist that binds to the GABA receptor and promotes the effects of GABA. Opioids are mu-receptor agonists that promote the effects of endorphins. Nicotine binds to nicotinic receptors and agonizes the effect of acetylcholine. When our cells are exposed to excessive neurotransmitter activity, they respond by desensitizing receptors or removing receptors from the cell membrane and storing them in cytoplasmic vesicles. With chronic use, they will downregulate production of the receptors. These responses lead to increased tolerance and physical dependency. With physical dependency, suddenly stopping use will lead to withdrawal symptoms. While different substances have different physical withdrawal syndromes, patients in withdrawal generally experience anhedonia, dysphoria, and cravings (Hyman et al., 2006). While it was once believed that dependence was necessary to develop addiction, we now understand that addiction can happen independently of dependence and that dependence is not always a sign of addiction (Hyman et al., 2006). We also used to believe that physical withdrawal was the motivation for relapse, but we now understand that relapse is driven by numerous complex factors (Gardner, 2011; Hyman et al., 2006). When it comes to SUD, there is no such thing as a truly curative treatment because patients remain at high risk of relapse, even if it has been many years since they ingested the drug or experienced any symptoms of withdrawal (Hyman et al., 2006).

KEY POINT

Ethanol is a GABA agonist that binds to the GABA receptor, which is a chloride ion channel. With chronic use, neurons decrease their expression of GABA receptors in anticipation of the GABA agonism of ethanol. Ethanol also inhibits N-methyl-D-aspartate (NMDA) receptors, which are excitatory receptors for glutamate, resulting in increased expression of NMDA receptors in patients with chronic use. In chronic alcohol use, the brain's homeostasis is altered. When chronic ethanol users suddenly stop drinking, their baseline cerebral functioning has been modified to overexpress excitatory systems, which is why adrenergic symptoms and seizures predominate during acute ethanol withdrawal.

Alcohol-Related Therapy

Ethanol is a GABA agonist that binds to the GABA receptor, which is a chloride ion channel. It increases GABA receptor opening, allowing more chloride to enter into the postsynaptic neuron. With chronic use, neurons decrease their expression of GABA receptors in anticipation of the GABA agonism of ethanol. Ethanol also inhibits N-methyl-D-aspartate (NMDA) receptors, which are excitatory receptors for glutamate, resulting in increased expression of NMDA receptors in patients with chronic use. When chronic ethanol users suddenly stop drinking, their baseline cerebral functioning has been modified to overexpress excitatory systems, which is why adrenergic symptoms and seizures predominate during acute ethanol withdrawal.

Initial management focuses on managing a safe withdrawal process with the use of benzodiazepines with a slow taper to allow the brain to reset the balance between excitatory and inhibitory systems. Patients who enter recovery may be placed on disulfiram as a deterrent against ethanol use. Ethanol is metabolized through a two-step process: It is metabolized into acetaldehyde by alcohol dehydrogenase. Then, acetaldehyde is metabolized into acetic acid, which is excreted. Disulfiram works by blocking the second enzyme, aldehyde dehydrogenase. This causes a buildup of acetaldehyde, which causes symptoms of flushing, tachycardia, nausea, and headache. Naltrexone is a mu-antagonist, typically associated with opioid use disorder, but it has been found to be effective at controlling cravings in patients who are in recovery from alcohol abuse (Anton, 2008). Acamprosate is another medication that can be used to reduce relapse rates, although its mechanism of action is unknown (Wright & Myrick, 2006).

Opioid-Related Therapy

Opioids are mu-receptor agonists that promote the effects of endorphins. When opioids bind the mu-receptor, which is a G-protein-linked receptor that cause potassium channel opening, the result is euphoria, sedation, and respiratory depression. Naloxone is a mu-agonist that is short acting and effective in reversal of opioid overdose symptoms. Naltrexone is a long-acting mu-agonist that can be beneficial in controlling cravings in patients who are highly motivated to be abstinent from opioids. However, recovery from opioid use disorder is generally focused on opioid maintenance therapy, where medically supervised opioids agonists are used to control the unwanted behaviors of addiction, while allowing patients to return to a functioning life. This philosophy of treatment contrasts with management of ethanol use disorder, which is focused on abstinence. Abstinence has a poor compliance rate with less than 30% of patients able to maintain abstinence after 10–30 years (Hser et al., 2015). Another study compared abstinence to treatment with buprenorphine, and at 1-year follow-up, treatment failure rate was 25% for buprenorphine and 100% for abstinence (Kakko et al., 2003).

Methadone is a long-acting synthetic opioid that is commonly used for opioid maintenance therapy. Patients usually go to daily clinics where they receive a predetermined dose of methadone. Buprenorphine is another medication that is used for opioid maintenance therapy. It is a partial mu-agonist that comes in sublingual strips that can be administered in the office or prescribed for home use in patients who have demonstrated adherence to their recovery program. Partial agonists are thought to provide some receptor activation to help manage cravings and withdrawal symptoms without utilizing full activation of the receptor.

Nicotine-Related Therapy

Nicotine binds to ion-channel nicotinic receptors, which normally respond to acetylcholine and result in sodium channel opening and sodium influx into the cell. Nicotine replacement patches and gums are meant to provide nicotine without the adverse effects associated with smoking. Patients are directed to taper the dosage of nicotine to allow for complete cessation with controlled withdrawal symptoms. Varenicline is a centrally acting partial nicotine agonist that can help control cravings and withdrawal symptoms from nicotine use. Bupropion is an antidepressant that has been found to help patients quit smoking (Hurt et al., 1997).

Clinical Syndromes

Opioid Withdrawal

Opioid withdrawal is a withdrawal process that is not life threatening and consists of symptoms of tachycardia, irritability, mydriasis, nausea, diarrhea, piloerection, and yawning. It can be quantified by the clinical opioid withdrawal scale (COWS; Wesson & Ling, 2003), which is important for buprenorphine initiation. Because buprenorphine is a partial agonist with high potency at the mu receptor, administration of buprenorphine can trigger precipitated opioid withdrawal if it is not given properly. Patients can safely be started on buprenorphine therapy if they have a COWS score of 8 or higher. Initiation of methadone will not cause precipitated withdrawal, since it is a full agonist.

> **KEY POINT**
>
> Alcohol withdrawal is a life-threatening process that requires management with GABA agonists under medical supervision. About 25% of patients will develop alcoholic hallucinations, which can be visual, tactile, or auditory. About 10% of patients develop alcohol withdrawal seizures if left untreated. Delirium tremens is the most severe form of ethanol withdrawal with symptoms starting 48–96 hours after the last drink. It is characterized by altered sensorium with typical symptoms of ethanol withdrawal, although these symptoms are usually more severe than typical withdrawal.

Ethanol Withdrawal

In contrast, ethanol withdrawal is a life-threatening process that requires management with GABA agonists under medical supervision. Patients develop autonomic instability with flushing, diaphoresis, tachycardia, hypertension, and tremors. Symptoms can begin a few hours after the patient's last drink, and patients with severe dependency can develop ethanol withdrawal, despite having serum ethanol levels that are typically associated with intoxication. About 25% of patients will develop alcoholic hallucinations, which can be visual, tactile, or auditory (Mirijello et al., 2015). About 10% of patients will develop alcohol withdrawal seizures (Mirijello et al., 2015). Patients in ethanol withdrawal may demonstrate irritability, but overall, they should have a clear sensorium. Delirium tremens is the most severe form of ethanol withdrawal with symptoms starting 48–96 hours after the last drink. It is characterized by altered sensorium with typical symptoms of ethanol withdrawal, although these symptoms are usually more severe than typical withdrawal (Mirijello et al., 2015).

CLINICAL TIP

Patients with alcohol withdrawal develop autonomic instability manifested by flushing, diaphoresis, tachycardia, hypertension, and tremors. Symptoms can begin a few hours after the patient's last drink. The management of ethanol withdrawal is treatment with GABA agonists, typically benzodiazepines.

The management of ethanol withdrawal is treatment with GABA agonists, typically benzodiazepines. Diazepam is preferred in patients with serious withdrawal symptoms, since it has rapid onset when given intravenously. Patients with benzodiazepine-resistant withdrawal, characterized by persistent, severe withdrawal, despite high doses of benzodiazepines, may respond better to phenobarbital, a barbiturate that is also a GABA agonist. Patients who require intravenous benzodiazepines should be admitted to the hospital for continued management of their withdrawal symptoms. The modified CIWA scale can be used to quantify the degree of ethanol withdrawal and the need for continued GABA agonist therapy (Sullivan et al., 1989).

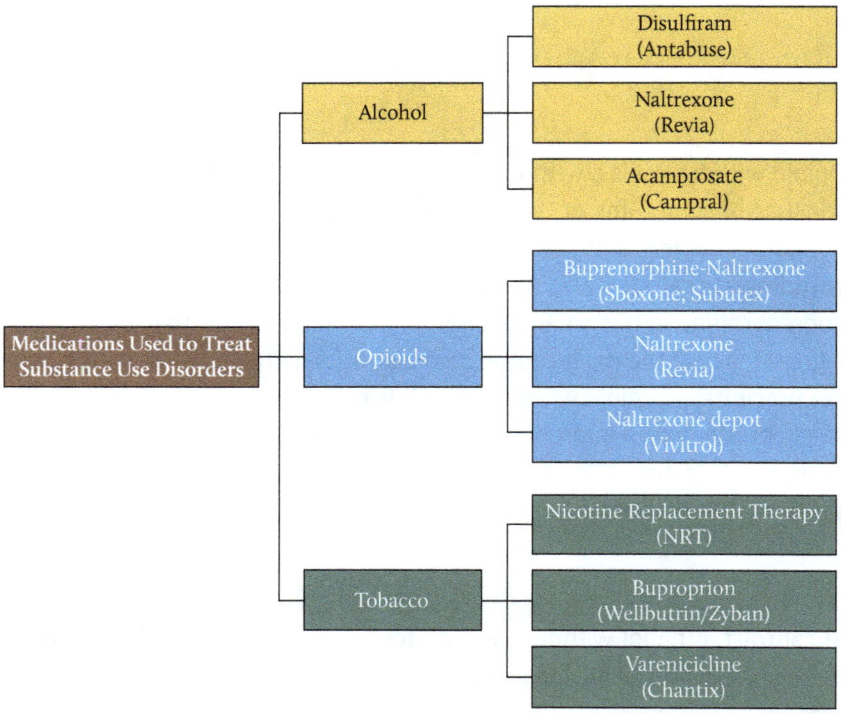

FIGURE 31.8 Medications used in substance use disorders (FDA approved).

SUMMARY

A good knowledge base of psychopharmacology is pivotal for treating mental health conditions effectively. The different classes of medications used in psychiatry have specific mechanisms of actions. Within these classes, medications are indicated for treatment of specific psychiatric disorders with newer ones developed. In psychiatry, drugs are used for known effects and sometimes for side effects that may be beneficial to patients. As in other fields, certain medications and medication classes are associated with known medical syndromes. The physician's knowledge and awareness of this increases early detection, and with appropriate treatment can reduce morbidity and mortality.

RESOURCES

1. Stahl, S. M. (2013). *Stahl's essential psychopharmacology: Neuroscientific basis and practical applications*, 4th ed. New York, NY, US: Cambridge University Press.
2. Division of Psychopharmacology and Substance Abuse, American Psychiatry Association Online Resources: Psychopharmacology and Substance Abuse (apadivisions.org)
3. American Society of Clinical Psychopharmacology
   ASCP – American Society of Clinical Psychopharmacology – Promoting Evidence-Based Psychopharmacology (ascpp.org)
   https://clincalc.com/DrugStats

REFERENCES

Abi-Dargham, A., Rodenhiser, J., Printz, D., Zea-Ponce, Y., Gil, R., Kegeles, L. S., Weiss, R., Cooper, T. B., Mann, J. J., Heertum, R. L. V., Gorman, J. M., & Laruelle, M. (2000). *Increased baseline occupancy of d2 receptors by dopamine in schizophrenia*. PNAS. https://www.pnas.org/content/97/14/8104.

Ahmad, S. A., Scolnik, D., Snehal, V., & Glatstein, M. (2015). Use of naloxone for clonidine intoxication in the pediatric age group: Case report and review of the literature. *American Journal of Therapeutics, 22*(1), e14–16. https://doi.org/10.1097/MJT.0b013e318293b0e8

Anton, R. F. (2008). Naltrexone for the management of alcohol dependence. *The New England Journal of Medicine, 359*(7), 715–721. https://doi.org/10.1056/NEJMct0801733

Arnsten, A. F. (2000). Genetics of childhood disorders: XVIII. ADHD, Part. 2: Norepinephrine has a critical modulatory influence on prefrontal cortical function. *Journal of the American Academy of Child and Adolescent Psychiatry, 39*(9), 1201–1203. https://doi.org/10.1097/00004583-200009000-00022

Blackwell, B., Marley, E., Price, J., & Taylor, D. (1967). Hypertensive interactions between monoamine oxidase inhibitors and foodstuffs. *The British Journal of Psychiatry: The Journal of Mental Science, 113*(497), 349–365. https://doi.org/10.1192/bjp.113.497.349

Boehnert, M. T., & Lovejoy, F. H., Jr. (1985). Value of the QRS duration versus the serum drug level in predicting seizures and ventricular arrhythmias after an acute overdose of tricyclic antidepressants. *The New England Journal of Medicine, 313*(8), 474–479. https://doi.org/10.1056/NEJM198508223130804

Buoli, M., Serati, M., & Cahn, W. (2016). Alternative pharmacological strategies for adult ADHD treatment: A systematic review. *Expert Review of Neurotherapeutics, , 16*(2), 131–144. https://doi.org10.1586/14737175.2016.1135735

Burns, M. J. (2001). The pharmacology and toxicology of atypical antipsychotic agents. *Journal of Toxicology. Clinical Toxicology, 39*(1), 1–14. https://doi.org/10.1081/clt-100102873

Christensen, R.C. (2005) Identify neuroleptic malignant syndrome with FEVER. *Current Psychiatry Pearls, 4*(7):102-102.

Christensen, R. C. (2006). *Get serotonin syndrome down cold with SHIVERS.* https://cdn.mdedge.com/files/s3fs-public/Document/September-2017/0502CP_Pearls2.pdf. ClinCalc. (2020). *ClinCalc DrugStats Database version 21.1*

Cloos, J. M., & Ferreira, V. (2009). Current use of benzodiazepines in anxiety disorders. *Current Opinion in Psychiatry, 22*(1), 90–95. https://doi.org/10.1097/YCO.0b013e32831a473d

Curatolo, P., D'Agati, E., & Moavero, R. (2010). The neurobiological basis of ADHD. *Italian Journal of Pediatrics, 36*(1), 79. https://doi.org/10.1186/1824-7288-36-79

De Picker, L., Van Den Eede, F., Dumont, G., Moorkens, G., & Sabbe, B. G. (2014). Antidepressants and the risk of hyponatremia: A class-by-class review of literature. *Psychosomatics, 55*(6), 536–547. https://doi.org/10.1016/j.psym.2014.01.010

Dunkley, E. J., Isbister, G. K., Sibbritt, D., Dawson, A. H., & Whyte, I. M. (2003). The Hunter serotonin toxicity criteria: Simple and accurate diagnostic decision rules for serotonin toxicity. *QJM : Monthly Journal of the Association of Physicians, 96*(9), 635–642. https://doi.org/10.1093/qjmed/hcg109

Engels, A. S., Heller, W., Spielberg, J. M., Warren, S. L., Sutton, B. P., Banich, M. T., & Miller, G. A. (2010). Co-occurring anxiety influences patterns of brain activity in depression. *Cognitive, Affective, & Behavioral Neuroscience, 10*(1), 141-156. https://www.doi.org/10.3758/CABN.10.1.141

Fiedorowicz, J. G., & Swartz, K. L. (2004). The role of monoamine oxidase inhibitors in current psychiatric practice. *Journal of Psychiatric Practice, 10*(4), 239–248. https://doi.org/10.1097/00131746-200407000-00005

Gardner, E. L. (2011). Addiction and brain reward and antireward pathways. *Advances in psychosomatic medicine, , 30*, 22–60. https://doi.org/10.1159/000324065

Greydanus, D. E., Nazeer, A., & Patel, D. R. (2009). Psychopharmacology of ADHD in pediatrics: Current advances and issues. *Neuropsychiatric Disease and Treatment, 5*, 171–181. https://doi.org/10.2147/ndt.s4075

Habel, L. A., Cooper, W. O., Sox, C. M., Chan, K. A., Fireman, B. H., Arbogast, P. G., Cheetham, T. C., Quinn, V. P., Dublin, S., Boudreau, D. M., Andrade, S. E., Pawloski, P. A., Raebel, M. A., Smith, D. H., Achacoso, N., Uratsu, C., Go, A. S., Sidney, S., Nguyen-Huynh, M. N., Ray, W. A.,Selby, J. V. (2011). ADHD medications and risk of serious cardiovascular events in young and middle-aged adults. *JAMA, 306*(24), 2673–2683. https://doi.org/10.1001/jama.2011.1830

Hillhouse, T. M., & Porter, J. H. (2015). A brief history of the development of antidepressant drugs: From monoamines to glutamate. *Experimental and Clinical and Psychopharmacology, 23*(1), 1–21. https://doi.org/10.1037/a0038550

Hser, Y. I., Evans, E., Grella, C., Ling, W., & Anglin, D. (2015). Long-term course of opioid addiction. *Harvard Review of Psychiatry, 23*(2), 76–89. https://doi.org/10.1097/HRP.0000000000000052

Hurt, R. D., Sachs, D. P., Glover, E. D., Offord, K. P., Johnston, J. A., Dale, L. C., Khayrallah, M. A., Schroeder, D. R., Glover, P. N., Sullivan, C. R., Croghan, I. T., & Sullivan, P. M. (1997). A comparison of sustained-release bupropion and placebo for smoking cessation. *The New England Journal of Medicine, 337*(17), 1195–1202. https://doi.org/10.1056/NEJM199710233371703

Hyman, S. E., Malenka, R. C., & Nestler, E. J. (2006). Neural mechanisms of addiction: The role of reward-related learning and memory. *Annual Review of Neuroscience, 29*, 565–598. https://doi.org/10.1146/annurev.neuro.29.051605.113009

Kakko, J., Svanborg, K. D., Kreek, M. J., & Heilig, M. (2003). 1-year retention and social function after buprenorphine-assisted relapse prevention treatment for heroin dependence in Sweden: A randomised, placebo-controlled trial. *Lancet, 361*(9358), 662–668. https://doi.org/10.1016/S0140-6736(03)12600-1

Kapur, S., & Mamo, D. (2003). Half a century of antipsychotics and still a central role for dopamine D2 receptors. *Progress in Neuro-Psychopharmacology & Biological Psychiatry, 27*(7), 1081–1090. https://doi.org/10.1016/j.pnpbp.2003.09.004

Keck, P. E., Jr., & McElroy, S. L. (2002). Clinical pharmacodynamics and pharmacokinetics of antimanic and mood-stabilizing medications. *The Journal of Clinical Psychiatry, 63(4)*, 3–11.

Kessler, R. C., Nelson, C. B., McGonagle, K. A., Liu, J., Swartz, M., & Blazer, D. G. (1996). Comorbidity of DSM-III-R major depressive disorder in the general population: Results from the US National Comorbidity Survey. *The British Journal of Psychiatry. Supplement, 30*, 17–30.

Koob, G. F., & Le Moal, M. (2001). Drug addiction, dysregulation of reward, and allostasis. *Neuropsychopharmacology, 24*(2), 97–129. https://doi.org/10.1016/S0893-133X(00)00195-0

Leucht, S., Corves, C., Arbter, D., Engel, R. R., Li, C., & Davis, J. M. (2009). Second-generation versus first-generation antipsychotic drugs for schizophrenia: A meta-analysis. *Lancet, 373*(9657), 31–41. https://doi.org/10.1016/S0140-6736(08)61764-X

Mark, T. L., Levit, K. R., & Buck, J. A. (2009). Datapoints: Psychotropic drug prescriptions by medical specialty. *Psychiatric Services (Washington, D.C.),60*(9), 1167. https://doi.org/10.1176/ps.2009.60.9.1167

Martin, E. I., Ressler, K. J., Binder, E., & Nemeroff, C. B. (2010). The neurobiology of anxiety disorders: Brain imaging, genetics, and psychoneuroendocrinology. *Clinics in Laboratory Medicine, 30*(4), 865–891. https://doi.org/10.1016/j.cll.2010.07.006

McDaniel, W. W. (2001). Serotonin syndrome: early management with cyproheptadine. *The Annals of Pharmacotherapy, 35*(7–8), 870–873. https://doi.org/10.1345/aph.10203

Meltzer, H. Y., Li, Z., Kaneda, Y., & Ichikawa, J. (2003). Serotonin receptors: Their key role in drugs to treat schizophrenia. *Progress in Neuro-Psychopharmacology & Biologiccal Psychiatry, 27*(7), 1159–1172. https://doi.org/10.1016/j.pnpbp.2003.09.010

Meltzer, H. Y., & Stahl, S. M. (1976). The dopamine hypothesis of schizophrenia: A review. *Schizophrenia Bulletin,2*(1), 19–76. https://doi.org/10.1093/schbul/2.1.19

Mirijello, A., D'Angelo, C., Ferrulli, A., Vassallo, G., Antonelli, M., Caputo, F.,... Addolorato, G. (2015). Identification and management of alcohol withdrawal syndrome. *Drugs, 75*(4), 353–365. https://doi.org/10.1007/s40265-015-0358-1

Pliszka, S. R. (2005). The neuropsychopharmacology of attention-deficit/hyperactivity disorder. *Biological Psychiatry, 57*(11), 1385–1390. https://doi.org/10.1016/j.biopsych.2004.08.026

Schmidt, C. K., Khalid, S., Loukas, M., & Tubbs, R. S. (2018). Neuroanatomy of anxiety: A brief review. *Cureus, 10*(1), e2055. https://doi.org/10.7759/cureus.2055

Schwartz, S., & Correll, C. U. (2014). Efficacy and safety of atomoxetine in children and adolescents with attention-deficit/hyperactivity disorder: Results from a comprehensive meta-analysis and metaregression. *Journal of the American Academy of Child and Adolescent Psychiatry,53*(2), 174–187. https://doi.org/10.1016/j.jaac.2013.11.005

Seeman, P., Corbett, R., Nam, D., & Van Tol, H. H. (1996). Dopamine and serotonin receptors: Amino acid sequences, and clinical role in neuroleptic parkinsonism. *Japanese Journal of Pharmacology, 71*(3), 187–204. https://doi.org/10.1254/jjp.71.187

Seeman, P., & Kapur, S. (2000). Schizophrenia: More dopamine, more D2 receptors. *Proceedings of the National Academy of Sciences of the United States of America, 97*(14), 7673–7675. https://doi.org/10.1073/pnas.97.14.7673

Seger, D. L., & Loden, J. K. (2018). Naloxone reversal of clonidine toxicity: Dose, dose, dose. *Clinical Toxicology (Philadelphia, Pa.), 56*(10), 873–879. https://www.doi.org/10.1080/15563650.2018.1450986

Signorovitch, J., Erder, M. H., Xie, J., Sikirica, V., Lu, M., Hodgkins, P. S., & Wu, E. Q. (2012). Comparative effectiveness research using matching-adjusted indirect comparison: An application to treatment with guanfacine extended release or atomoxetine in children with attention-deficit/hyperactivity disorder and comorbid oppositional defiant disorder. *Pharmacoepidemiology and Drug Safety, 21 Suppl 2,* 130–137. https://doi.org/10.1002/pds.3246

Southammakosane, C., & Schmitz, K. (2015). Pediatric psychopharmacology for treatment of ADHD, depression, and anxiety. *Pediatrics, 136*(2), 351–359. https://doi.org/10.1542/peds.2014-1581

Strawn, J. R., Keck, P. E., Jr., & Caroff, S. N. (2007). Neuroleptic malignant syndrome. *The Primary Care Companion fo CNS Disorders, 164*(6), 870–876. https://doi.org/10.1176/ajp.2007.164.6.870

Subcommittee on Attention-Deficit/Hyperactivity & Steering Committee on Quality Improvement and Management. (2011). ADHD: Clinical practice guideline for the diagnosis, evaluation, and treatment of attention-deficit/hyperactivity disorder in children and adolescents. *Pediatrics, 128*(5), 1007–1022. https://doi.org/10.1542/peds.2011-2654

Sullivan, J. T., Sykora, K., Schneiderman, J., Naranjo, C. A., & Sellers, E. M. (1989). Assessment of alcohol withdrawal: The revised clinical institute withdrawal assessment for alcohol scale (CIWA-Ar). *British Journal of Addiction, 84*(11), 1353–1357. https://doi.org/10.1111/j.1360-0443.1989.tb00737.x

Touma, K. T. B., & Scarff, J. R. (2018). Valbenazine and deutetrabenazine for tardive dyskinesia. *Innovations in clinical neuroscience,15*(5-6), 13–16.

Trollor, J. N., Chen, X., Chitty, K., & Sachdev, P. S. (2012). Comparison of neuroleptic malignant syndrome induced by first- and second-generation antipsychotics. *The British Journal of Psychiatry: The Journal of Mental Science, 201*(1), 52–56. https://doi.org/10.1192/bjp.bp.111.105189

Trosch, R. M. (2004). Neuroleptic-induced movement disorders: Deconstructing extrapyramidal symptoms. *J Journal of the American Geriatrics Society, 52*(12), S266–271. https://doi.org/10.1111/j.1532-5415.2004.52603.x

Ware, K., Tillery, E., & Linder, L. (2016). General pharmacokinetic/pharmacodynamic concepts of mood stabilizers in the treatment of bipolar disorder. *The Mental Health Clinician, 6*(1), 54–61. https://doi.org/10.9740/mhc.2016.01.054

Wesson, D. R., & Ling, W. (2003). The Clinical Opiate Withdrawal Scale (COWS). *Journal of Psychoactive Drugs, 35*(2), 253–259. https://doi.org/10.1080/02791072.2003.10400007

Wright, T. M., & Myrick, H. (2006). Acamprosate: A new tool in the battle against alcohol dependence. *Neuropsychiatric Disease and Treatment, 2*(4), 445–453. https://doi.org/10.2147/nedt.2006.2.4.445

CHAPTER 32

Neuromodulation Treatments in Psychiatry

Syed Z. Iqbal, M.D.; Edore Onigu-Otite, M.D.;

and Asim Shah, M.D.

> *"That is the essence of science: ask an impertinent question, and you are on the way to a pertinent answer."*
>
> — Jacob Bronowski

OBJECTIVES

After reading this chapter, students will be able to do the following:

- describe brain stimulation therapies
- summarize neurostimulation treatments, uses, indications, and side effects
- discuss catatonia

CASE VIGNETTE

James is an 84-year-old widowed man who lives with his daughter and her family. He has a diagnosis of major depressive disorder, recurrent, severe, with psychotic symptoms. He has multiple medical conditions, including hypertension, diabetes, and hyperlipidemia. Over the past 15 years, his memory has steadily deteriorated. Five years ago, he was diagnosed with Alzheimer's dementia. He sometimes becomes delirious and agitated, most often around dusk. His depressive symptoms have steadily worsened. He tried two antidepressants the past 2 years, and although he seems to improve for a while, his symptoms return. James is now very depressed, not wanting to get out of bed, not eating or drinking much, and has lost weight. He refuses to take his medications for all his medical and psychiatric conditions. He now talks about feeling he is a burden and wishing to leave this world to relieve his family. James's grandchildren are alarmed by this. His daughter scheduled an urgent appointment with a psychiatrist, who recommends electroconvulsive therapy for treatment-resistant depression. In the first week, James receives three shock treatments and then this is gradually spaced out over the next 6 months. His symptoms significantly improve; he has regained the lost weight and enjoys being with his grandchildren again and vice versa. He is now on maintenance ECT, receives shock treatments once a month, and continues to do well.

DEFINITIONS AND KEY CONCEPTS

Neuromodulation is the alteration of nerve functioning using focused delivery of external stimuli, such as electrical, magnetic, chemical, or light, to specific neurological areas. This involves a class of medical procedures used to modulate (i.e., stimulate, inhibit, or change) brain functioning to relieve neuropsychiatric symptoms. *Electroconvulsive therapy* (ECT) is the electrical induction of generalized epileptic seizures using electrodes placed on the head for a therapeutic purpose. *Transcranial magnetic stimulation* (TMS) is the use of magnetic fields to stimulate nerve cells in the brain for a therapeutic purpose. *Deep brain stimulation* (DBS) is the stimulation of nerve cells through electrodes implanted into certain brain areas. *Light therapy*, also known as phototherapy, is the use of artificial light for a therapeutic purpose. In psychiatry, it is most commonly used in seasonal affective disorders. *Ketamine*, an anesthetic gas, is an agent recently used in in treatment-resistant depression. *Catatonia* is an abnormality of movement and behavior, arising from a disturbed mental state.

KEY POINT

Neuromodulation is a class of medical procedures in which external stimuli, such as electrical, magnetic, chemical, or light, are delivered to specific neurologic areas to alter brain and nerve functioning.

INTRODUCTION

Neuropsychiatric disorders result from the interplay of biological, psychological, and social dimensions, which are all significant contributors to the pathogenesis of mental illness. Advances in neurobiology have uncovered brain-based correlates of many neuropsychiatric disorders. The biomedical model attributes the etiology of mental illnesses to abnormalities in brain functioning, often due to dysregulation in neurotransmitter systems. This has been increasingly recognized over the past few decades, leading to the development of several neuromodulating treatments.

The conventional treatment of neuropsychiatric disorders relies heavily on psychotropic medications. Psychotropic medications are some of the most prescribed medications. Antidepressants are the third most commonly prescribed class of prescription medication for those 18–44 years old in the United States (Deacon, 2013). Antipsychotics were the fifth highest revenue-generating medication class in 2011, generating $18.2 billion in sales (Deacon, 2013). Most psychiatric patients are prescribed at least two psychotropic medications, and nearly a third receive three or more (Deacon, 2013). Despite advancements in modes of delivery of psychotropic medications and their extensive use, the outcomes are only marginally improved in some patients. This highlights the importance of exploring alternate treatment modalities that work independently or in conjunction with conventional treatments.

Currently, various neuromodulation treatment modalities are used. These include brain stimulation techniques, such as transcranial magnetic stimulation, electroconvulsive therapy, vagal nerve stimulation, and deep brain stimulation. Light therapy, which influences the body's circadian rhythm, is also used in the treatment of various mental health disorders. Recently, ketamine, a well-known anesthetic agent, was FDA approved for intranasal use in conjunction with antidepressants to treat depressive disorders. This chapter focuses on neuromodulatory agents for treating neuropsychiatric disorders, elaborating on their indications, effectiveness, advantages, and disadvantages.

BRAIN STIMULATION THERAPIES

Brain stimulation therapies have an essential role in the management of neuropsychiatric conditions. They can be used to treat difficult cases of depression, mania, catatonia, obsessive compulsive disorder (OCD), and parkinsonism. These methods work by delivering electrical or magnetic impulses directly or indirectly to the brain. They are often used in conjunction with conventional treatments, such as medications and psychotherapies, when conventional treatments alone do not provide sufficient symptom relief or functional improvement. The techniques described exemplify brain stimulation therapies.

Electroconvulsive Therapy

ECT is the electrical induction of generalized epileptic seizures for a therapeutic purpose (Baghai & Moller, 2008). During a session of ECT, under anesthesia, electrodes placed on the scalp deliver a brief pulse-stimulation electric current causing a brief generalized seizure with transient muscle paralysis. During the procedure, an anesthesiologist monitors the vital signs. The electrodes are placed on specific locations on the scalp (Figure 32.1). The electric current generated travels through the brain, recruiting adjacent neurons with a lesser impact on the deep brain structures. EEG findings show the seizure is followed by 60 to 90 seconds of postictal neuronal suppression, then the return of high-voltage delta and theta waves, and finally a return to preseizure appearance within about 30 minutes. PET findings show during the seizure, cerebral blood flow and glucose metabolism increase, and there is increased permeability of the blood–brain barrier. ECT sessions are conducted in phases. In the induction phase, three ECT sessions are delivered weekly for 6 to 12 sessions to target the resolution of acute symptoms. This is followed by the maintenance phase, where the frequency of sessions varies based on the patient's symptoms and treatment needs. Generally, this varies from one session per week to one session every few months.

KEY POINT

ECT affects the brain's major neurochemical systems through neuroreceptor modulation and secondary messenger systems.

Mechanism of Action

ECT affects virtually all neurochemical systems through neuroreceptor modulation and secondary messenger systems. In the serotonergic system, various studies show ECT results in increased levels of tryptophan, serotonin's precursor, a change in presynaptic serotonin release, and an increase in postsynaptic serotonin receptors. Changes also occur in the noradrenergic and GABA systems. Elevated glutamate levels; an excitatory neurotransmitter; and changes in the endogenous endorphins, muscarinic, cholinergic and dopaminergic systems have also been found. Studies found that hippocampal volume increased (normalized), and connectivity was enhanced—a change that correlated with symptom improvement (Abbott et al., 2014). MRI studies show ECT-induced brain changes, including increases in fronto-limbic areas (Gbyl & Videbech, 2018), increased hippocampal volumes (Nordanskog et al., 2014; van Oostrom et al., 2018), and transient cortical thickness, which resolves by 6 months (Gbyl et al., 2019).

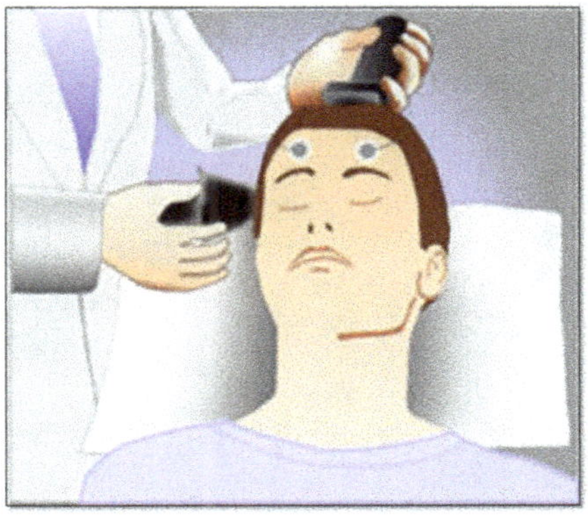

FIGURE 32.1 Electroconvulsive therapy (ECT).

Copyright © by National Institute of Mental Health (cc by-sa 4.0) at https://www.nimh.nih.gov/health/topics/brain-stimulation-therapies/brain-stimulation-therapies.shtml.

Indications

In December 2018, the Food and Drug Administration (FDA, 2018) reclassified ECT devices for use in treating specific conditions. This included catatonia, a severe major depressive episode (MDE) occurring within major depressive disorder (MDD) or bipolar disorder (BPD) in patients who are 13 or older and are either treatment resistant or who required rapid treatment response due to their psychiatric or medical condition.

KEY POINT

ECT is used in patients whose symptoms are resistant to other treatments or who require rapid response due to their psychiatric or medical condition. It is FDA-approved for treating catatonia, severe major depressive episode (MDE) occurring within major depressive disorder (MDD) or bipolar disorder (BPD).

ECT is effective in the management of treatment-resistant depression (TRD) with a response rate of 60–80% and a remission rate of 50–60% (Weiner & Reti, 2017). ECT is sometimes used as a first-line treatment in severe melancholic, catatonic, or psychotic depression, especially when there is a high suicide risk (Baghai & Moller, 2008). ECT is sometimes used as a first-line treatment in pregnancy and postpartum in patients with severe depression, psychosis, or manic symptoms, where the risks of medication use outweigh the benefits (Rose et al., 2020).

KEY POINT

Catatonia is an abnormality of movement and behavior that arises from a disturbed mental state. Catatonia is associated with severe depression. It also occurs in mania, schizophrenia, autism, acute substance use states, neuroleptic malignant syndrome, and other medical conditions. ECT has a strong anticatatonic effect, irrespective of the etiology.

Catatonia is an abnormality of movement and behavior which arises from a disturbed mental state. Catatonia can present as a psychiatric or medical urgency or emergency—the duration can range from a few hours to weeks, months, or years. Catatonia can reoccur at a variable frequency for weeks to years after the initial episode. Catatonia can be intrinsic or extrinsic, and different types of catatonia exist. These include akinetic catatonia (slow movement with the extreme of stupor with mutism), hyperkinetic catatonia (fast movement with the extreme of severe agitation associated with self-harming behavior), and malignant catatonia (hyperthermia, diaphoresis, severe tachycardia and hypertension, and delirium). Catatonia is most commonly associated with severe depressive episodes. However, it can also occur in mania, schizophrenia, autism, and other medical causes, such as acute substance use states (Mekala et al., 2020) and neuroleptic malignant syndrome (Weiner & Reti, 2017). ECT has a strong anticatatonic effect irrespective of the etiology (Lloyd et al., 2020; Sanghani et al., 2018; Weiner & Reti, 2017).

ECT is sometimes used as first-line treatment in mania, especially in patients who are resistant to mood stabilizers or who are at risk of engaging in life-threatening events resulting from mania (Weiner & Reti, 2017). ECT has been used in bipolar patients with mixed mood states with some studies showing it to be effective in as high as two thirds of the patients with severe and drug-resistant mixed states (Fountoulakis, 2020; Perugi et al., 2017). ECT has been successfully used in the treatment of other psychiatric disorders, including schizophrenia (Sanghani et al., 2018); OCD; and neuropsychiatric conditions, including dyskinesias, Tourette syndrome, and Parkinson's disease (Baghai & Moller, 2008). ECT can be particularly useful in geriatric neuropsychiatric conditions, such as agitated dementia and late-onset mania with dementia (McDonald & Thompson, 2001).

Side Effects

In the past, ECT procedures involved higher doses of electricity, which resulted in memory loss, fractured bones, and other side effects, which contributed to the stigma attached. Over the years, ECT's safety and tolerability have significantly improved with the use of modified stimulation techniques and progress in modern anesthesia. Currently, the common side effects include headache, nausea, vomiting, and muscle aches. Cognitive side effects include retrograde amnesia, short-term memory loss, or impairment, resulting in as high as 30% of treated patients. Cognitive side effects depend on the dose and positioning of the electrodes. Modified ECT techniques using either unilateral or bifrontal electrodes can reduce the cognitive side effects (Baghai & Moller, 2008). In the sessions, the patient is under anesthesia, so that aspect of the procedure is pain free. However, postseizure, muscle aches from the contraction can occur. General anesthesia carries risks of its own. Cognitive effects can be immediate (within 24 hours), short term (lasting days), or long term (lasting over a month), but they generally resolve within a few months. Cognitive side effects include impaired anterograde memory and decreases in autobiographical memory, verbal fluency, and learning verbal memory (Landry et al., 2020). With time, several studies show improvement in the cognitive side effects by the first month with a resolution of cognitive side effects by 6 months (Landry et al., 2020). In severely depressed patients, several studies have found improved cognitive functioning up to 1 to 2 years following ECT, suggesting that ECT may have unique cognitive boosting processes in the long term (Mohn & Rund, 2019). MRI studies have not supported the notion that ECT causes functional or structural brain damage (Gbyl & Videbech, 2018; Osler et al., 2018).

CLINICAL TIP

ECT's safety and tolerability in modern times has significantly improved. Common side effects include headache, nausea, vomiting, muscle aches, and cognitive side effects. Cognitive effects can be immediate (within 24 hours), short term (lasting days), or long term (lasting over a month) but generally resolve within 6 months. In severely depressed patients, several studies have found improved cognitive functioning up to 1 to 2 years following ECT.

Transcranial Magnetic Stimulation

Transcranial magnetic stimulation (TMS) is a noninvasive procedure that uses rapidly alternating magnetic fields to stimulate nerve cells in the brain. Transcranial magnetic stimulation (TMS) has emerged as a major tool used in noninvasive brain stimulation. It was developed in 1985 and approved by the FDA in 2008 to treat MDD in patients who have failed one trial of antidepressant treatment in the current episode. It is useful in treating depression, including TRD, pregnancy, and elderly patients, for whom it causes less cognitive side effects (Chail et al., 2018). Multicenter studies show that clinical outcomes compare favorably with alternative interventions for treatment-resistant depression (Sackeim et al., 2020). In 2013, TMS was approved for treating pain associated with certain migraine headaches. In August 2018, it was also approved by the FDA for the treatment of OCD. Reports have documented its use in intractable hallucinations and negative symptoms in chronic schizophrenia (Chail et al., 2018). It has been used in the treatment of migraines, anxiety disorders, and PTSD (Chail et al., 2018).

KEY POINT

TMS is indicated for the treatment of MDE with at least one previous failed treatment. It is also used for treating pain associated with certain migraine headaches, and it is approved for treating OCD.

During TMS, MRI-strength electromagnetic pulses from a coil placed over the scalp are delivered, causing the stimulation of underlying neurons (Chail et al., 2018). Depending on pulse stimulation frequency, TMS causes long-term inhibition and excitation of neurons in specific brain areas (Chail et al., 2018). A typical session lasts 30–60 minutes and does not require general anesthesia. During this time, the patient feels a slight tapping or

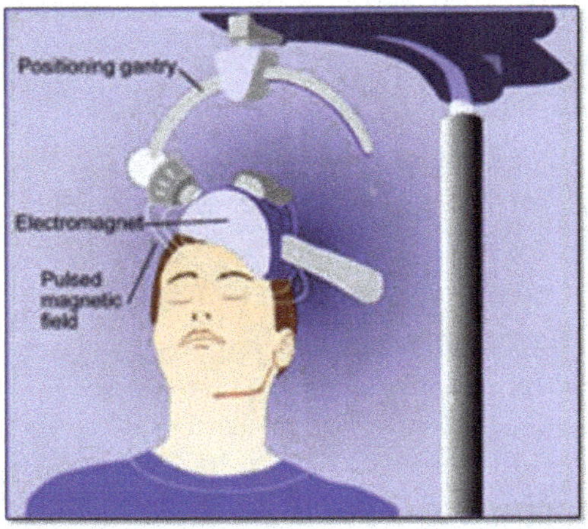

FIGURE 32.2 Transcranial magnetic stimulation (TMS) device.

Source: https://www.nimh.nih.gov/health/topics/brain-stimulation-therapies/brain-stimulation-therapies.shtml.

knocking at the site of delivery. The FDA recommends at least 20 sessions spread over 4 to 6 weeks at a frequency of five times a week.

TMS side effects are transient and generally mild to moderate. Common side effects include headache; brief lightheadedness; and tingling of the jaw, face, and scalp muscles. Transient mood or cognitive changes, syncope, and hearing loss have also been observed but are far less common. Seizure induction is a concern. Seizures are exceedingly rare and more often occur in patients on medications, potentially lowering the seizure threshold (Rossi et al., 2009).

Vagal Nerve Stimulation

Vagal nerve stimulation (VNS) was first developed as a treatment modality for epilepsy. In 2005, the FDA approved its use in TRD in adult patients with severe or recurrent depression persisting for 2 years or more with four treatment trials' failure. For TRD, studies report improved outcomes, while others show mixed results (Bottomley et al., 2019). Patients with established MDD had enhanced antidepressant effects with adjunctive VNS when compared to standard treatment (Aaronson et al., 2017). VNS also showed effectiveness in reducing suicidal ideation (Aaronson et al., 2017). The pulse generator device is surgically implanted in the upper left side of the chest and is connected via electrical lead wire to the left vagus nerve (Figure 32.3). The pulse generator is powered by a long-life battery for an average of about 10 years, and it generates 30 seconds of electrical pulses every 5 minutes, which are transmitted via the vagus nerve. These pulses modulate neurotransmitters, such as serotonin, norepinephrine, and glutamate, used in mood regulation. The side effects include hoarseness of voice, sore throat, neck pain, discomfort or tingling in areas where the device is implanted, breathing problems during exercise, difficulty swallowing, and infection at the implantation site.

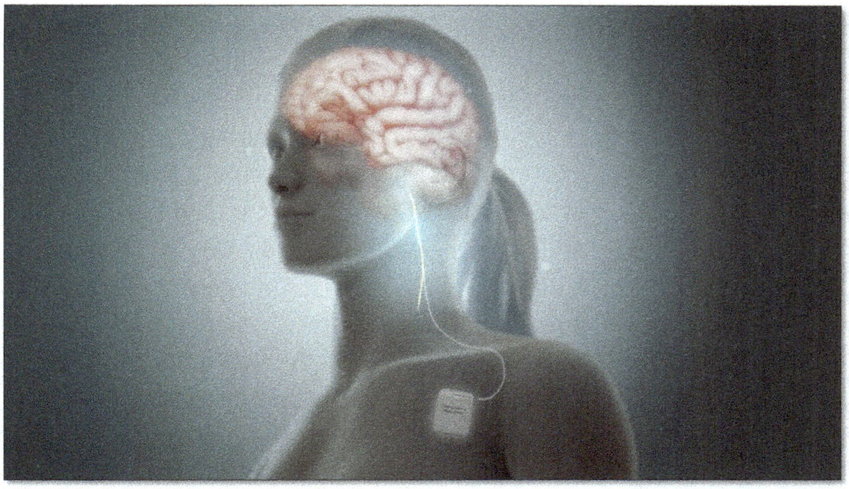

FIGURE 32.3 Vagus nerve stimulation (VNS) with the wire attached to the vagus nerve and the pulse generator, surgically implanted on the anterior chest wall.

Copyright © by Manu5 (cc by-sa 4.C) at https://commons.wikimedia.org/wiki/File:Vagus_nerve_stimulation.jpg.

Deep Brain Stimulation

Deep brain stimulation (DBS) was first used to treat Parkinson's disease to reduce tremors and uncontrolled movements. It is FDA indicated for the treatment of Parkinson disease, dystonia, essential tremors, and cases of severe epilepsy (Lozano et al., 2019). In psychiatry, it is currently used off-label for the treatment of depressive disorders and OCD. A pair of electrodes are implanted in the brain and controlled by a generator that is implanted in the chest. Brain stimulation is continuous, the frequency is customized, and it targets subcortical areas involved in depression and other mood disorders (Figure 32.4; Lozano et al., 2019). The effectiveness of DBS in the treatment of refractory cases of anorexia nervosa has been explored with some positive response (Lozano et al., 2019). This procedure has risks associated with brain surgery and can result in intracerebral bleeding, infection, disorientation, mood changes, movement disorder, lightheadedness, and symptoms of insomnia (Lozano et al., 2019).

KEY POINT

VNS is used in treatment of depression and seizures. It is indicated for treatment resistant depression in adult patients with severe or recurrent depression persisting for 2 years or more with four treatment trials' failure.

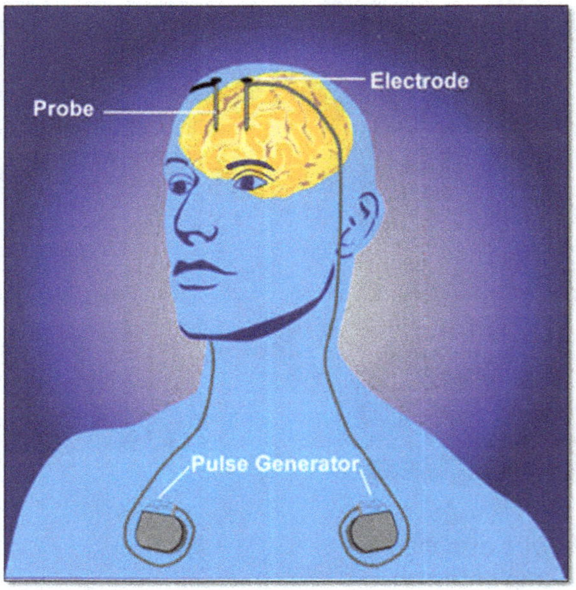

FIGURE 32.4 Deep brain stimulation (DBS).

Source: https://commons.wikimedia.org/wiki/File:Deep_brain_stimulation.jpg.

LIGHT THERAPY

Light therapy is used to treat seasonal affective disorder (SAD) and sleep disorders. It is a first-line treatment for SAD (Brouwer et al., 2017; Campbell et al., 2017). It is useful in treating both unipolar and bipolar depression, postpartum depression, neurocognitive disorders (dementia), Parkinson's disease, and fibromyalgia (Brouwer et al., 2017). Light therapy has also been effective in the treatment of antepartum depression (Campbell et al., 2017). The eyes mediate the effects of light therapy as it is relayed by the photoreceptive retinal cells via the retinal hypothalamic tract to the suprachiasmatic nucleus, which acts as a biological clock regulating the circadian rhythm located in the anterior hypothalamus (Brouwer et al., 2017; Campbell et al., 2017). This biological clock regulates daily rhythmicity by influencing melatonin and cortisol release, affecting the sleep–wake cycle (Brouwer et al., 2017). Light exposure is the most important synchronizing agent of the endogenous circadian rhythm. The effect of light therapy depends on its wavelength and duration of exposure, as previous research has shown that the blue spectrum of visible light with wavelength of 450 to 500 nm was most effective on the biological clock at controlling the circadian rhythm, as the photo receptive ganglion cells express melanopsin, which is a blue light-sensitive photopigment with peak absorption at 480 nm wave length (Brouwer et al., 2017).

> **KEY POINT**
>
> Light therapy is a first-line treatment for seasonal affective disorder. It has shown utility in treating other forms of depression and dementias.

Most of the light therapy boxes emit white fluorescent light with ultraviolet light filters at 10,000 lux measured at eye level at a specified distance from the lamp (Brouwer et al., 2017). Monochromatic green and blue light-emitting diode (LED) light boxes are also available, smaller in size, portable, and easy to use. A meta-analysis comparing the efficacy of bright light therapy (BLT) to placebo in patients with SAD showed superior efficacy of BLT versus placebo with a standardized mean difference of −0.37 (95% CI, −0.63 to −0.12) for depression rating scales (Pjrek et al., 2020). Studies have shown that 45% of patients who have received light therapy have presented with various complaints, including asthenopia, eye irritation, discomfort, burning, watery or dry eyes, photophobia, blurry vision, glare, seeing flashing lights and spots, and difficulty focusing. Studies have not shown hazardous ocular effects associated with light therapy. Patients are advised to place the light source at a 45-degree angle to the eyes to avoid the glare. Supervision with an ophthalmologist is recommended in patients who have preexisting ocular abnormalities, including diabetic retinopathy, age-related macular degeneration, and photosensitivity due to medical conditions, such as albinism or related to medication, including diuretic, antibiotics, and tricyclic antidepressant (Brouwer et al., 2017).

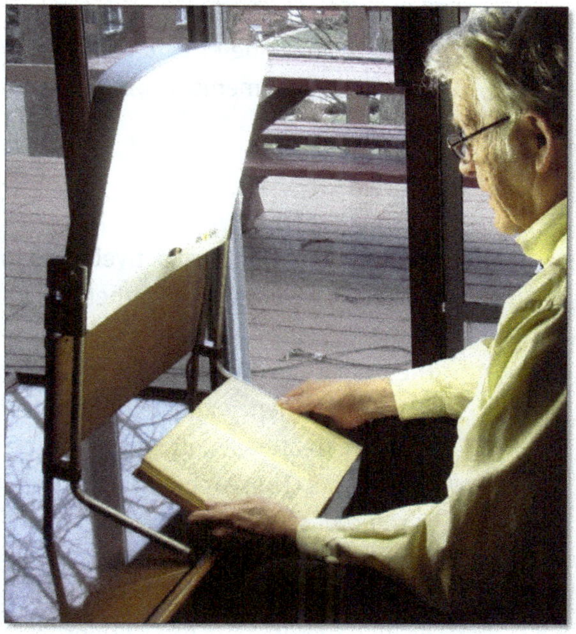

FIGURE 32.5 Light therapy.

Copyright © by Lou Sander (cc by-sa 4.0) at https://commons.wikimedia.org/wiki/File:Light_Therapy_for_SAD.jpg.

KETAMINE

Subanesthetic administration of ketamine is an emerging practice in psychiatry. In March 2019, the FDA approved intranasal ketamine, which is the S-ketamine isomer for clinical use in supervised settings as an adjunct with an antidepressant in patients with TRD and with failure to respond to two or more antidepressants. Ketamine is an NMDA receptor antagonist. It is metabolized in the liver by cytochrome enzymes to a less active metabolite called norketamine, an active NMDA receptor antagonist, but with less potency. Ketamine exerts its antidepressant effects via NMDA receptor modulation (Aleksandrova et al., 2017; Murrough et al., 2013).

> **KEY POINT**
>
> Ketamine is a dissociative anesthetic agent that exerts its antidepressant effect through NMDA receptor modulation. Ketamine has antisuicidal effects when administered at a subanesthetic dose. Studies show that ketamine restores cognitive flexibility and coping response strategy compromised by stress.

Ketamine is administered in designated facilities. Patients are required to be monitored in the facility postadministration for side effects. Ketamine is used mostly as an intravenous infusion or via the intranasal route for TRD. Systematic review articles have shown a strong ketamine effect observed within 4 hours following a single infusion, peaking at 24 hours and somewhat diminished 7 days postinfusion (Marcantoni et al., 2020). Ketamine results in a rapid onset of action, resulting in improvement in severe and chronic forms of depression (Murrough et al., 2013). Studies have shown antisuicidal effects when administered at a subanesthetic dose (Iqbal & Mathew, 2020; Price et al., 2014). Studies have shown rapid resolution in symptoms of depression within 24 hours after the administration of infusion. In some studies, ketamine has been shown to have antisuicidal effects as early as 40 minutes post-infusion (Marcantoni et al., 2020; Murrough et al., 2015; Price et al., 2014).

Longer-term studies show that ketamine restores cognitive flexibility and coping response strategies compromised by stress (Jett et al., 2015). The most common side effects include drowsiness, dizziness, poor coordination, lightheadedness, blurry vision, headache and nausea, and transient increase in blood pressure. More serious side effects include transient neurocognitive, sensorimotor, and dissociative symptoms and memory loss (Iqbal & Mathew, 2020).

SUMMARY

Neuromodulation is an actively developing field with several methods and devices at various stages of development, gathering evidence for safety and clinical utility in neuropsychiatric and other disorders. With only conventional treatment, such as medications that remain the primary neurobiological treatment modality for mental health disorders, some patients do not experience adequate symptom relief. Neuromodulation treatments offer additional effective treatment options that can be used independently or in conjunction with conventional treatments. These modalities include both invasive and noninvasive treatment options. ECT is the oldest and most studied brain stimulation therapy and carries risks associated with general anesthesia. Other noninvasive techniques, such as TMS and light therapy, have relatively fewer adverse consequences than invasive techniques like DBS and VNS, which include the risk of complications from surgery. The recent advances in the use of anesthetic agents approved for intravenous and intranasal use further improve TRD management by providing rapid resolution of depressive symptoms. Continued research is required to increase the body of research on techniques while improving safety data for their clinical use.

RESOURCES

1 https://www.youtube.com/watch?v=LPBTEHYlZK4

2 https://www.youtube.com/watch?v=L7LrovlpuE4

3 https://www.youtube.com/watch?v=nW21-AYY_fs

REFERENCES

Aaronson, S. T., Sears, P., Ruvuna, F., Bunker, M., Conway, C. R., Dougherty, D. D., Reimherr, F. W., Schwartz, T. L., & Zajecka, J. M. (2017). A 5-Year Observational Study of Patients With Treatment-Resistant Depression Treated With Vagus Nerve Stimulation or Treatment as Usual: Comparison of Response, Remission, and Suicidality. *American Journal of Psychiatry*, *174*(7), 640–648. https://doi.org/10.1176/appi.ajp.2017.16010034

Abbott, C. C., Jones, T., Lemke, N. T., Gallegos, P., McClintock, S. M., Mayer, A. R., Bustillo, J., & Calhoun, V. D. (2014). Hippocampal structural and functional changes associated with electroconvulsive therapy response. *Translational Psychiatry, 4*(11), e483. https://doi.org/10.1038/tp.2014.124

Aleksandrova, L. R., Phillips, A. G., & Wang, Y. T. (2017). Antidepressant effects of ketamine and the roles of AMPA glutamate receptors and other mechanisms beyond NMDA receptor antagonism. *Journal of Psychiatry & Neurosciience, 42*(4), 222–229. https://www.doi.org/10.1503/jpn.160175

Baghai, T. C., & Moller, H. J. (2008). Electroconvulsive therapy and its different indications. *Dialogues in Clinical Neuroscience, 10*(1), 105–117.

Bottomley, J. M., LeReun, C., Diamantopoulos, A., Mitchell, S., & Gaynes, B. N. (2019). Vagus nerve stimulation (VNS) therapy in patients with treatment resistant depression: A systematic review and meta-analysis. *Comprehensive Psychiatry, 98*, 152156. https://doi.org/10.1016/j.comppsych.2019.152156

Brouwer, A., Nguyen, H. T., Snoek, F. J., van Raalte, D. H., Beekman, A. T. F., Moll, A. C., & Bremmer, M. A. (2017). Light therapy: Is it safe for the eyes? *Acta Psychiatrica Scandinavica, 136*(6), 534–548. https://doi.org/10.1111/acps.12785

Campbell, P. D., Miller, A. M., & Woesner, M. E. (2017). Bright light therapy: Seasonal affective disorder and beyond. *The Einstein Journal of Biology and Medicine, 32*, E13–E25.

Chail, A., Saini, R. K., Bhat, P. S., Srivastava, K., & Chauhan, V. (2018). Transcranial magnetic stimulation: A review of its evolution and current applications. *Industrial Psychiatry Journal, 27*(2), 172–180. https://doi.org/10.4103/ipj.ipj_88_18

Deacon, B. J. (2013). The biomedical model of mental disorder: a critical analysis of its validity, utility, and effects on psychotherapy research. *Clinical Psychology Review, 33*(7), 846–861. https://doi.org/10.1016/j.cpr.2012.09.007

Food and Drug Administration. (2018). *Neurological devices; reclassification of electroconvulsive therapy devices; effective date of requirement for premarket approval for electroconvulsive therapy devices for certain specified intended uses* [Press release]. https://www.federalregister.gov/d/2018-27809

Fountoulakis, K. N. (2020). Neurocognitive impairment and evidence-based treatment options in bipolar disorder. *Annals of General Psychiatry, 19*, 54. https://doi.org/10.1186/s12991-020-00304-4

Gbyl, K., Rostrup, E., Raghava, J. M., Carlsen, J. F., Schmidt, L. S., Lindberg, U., Ashraf, A., Jørgensen, M. B., Larsson, H. B. W., Rosenberg, R., & Videbech, P. (2019). Cortical thickness following electroconvulsive therapy in patients with depression: A longitudinal MRI study. *Acta Psychiatrica Scandinavica, 140*(3), 205–216. https://doi.org/10.1111/acps.13068

Gbyl, K., & Videbech, P. (2018). Electroconvulsive therapy increases brain volume in major depression: A systematic review and meta-analysis. *Acta Psychiatrica Scandinavica, 138*(3), 180–195. https://doi.org/10.1111/acps.12884

Iqbal, S. Z., & Mathew, S. J. (2020). Ketamine for depression clinical issues. *Advances in Pharmacology, 89*, 131–162. https://doi.org/10.1016/bs.apha.2020.02.005

Jett, J. D., Boley, A. M., Girotti, M., Shah, A., Lodge, D. J., & Morilak, D. A. (2015). Antidepressant-like cognitive and behavioral effects of acute ketamine administration associated with plasticity in the ventral hippocampus to medial prefrontal cortex pathway. *Psychopharmacology (Berl), 232*(17), 3123–3133. https://doi.org/10.1007/s00213-015-3957-3

Landry, M., Moreno, A., Patry, S., Potvin, S., & Lemasson, M. (2020). Current practices of electroconvulsive therapy in mental disorders: A systematic review and meta-analysis of short and long-term cognitive effects. *The Journal of ECT*. https://doi.org/10.1097/YCT.0000000000000723

Lloyd, J. R., Silverman, E. R., Kugler, J. L., & Cooper, J. J. (2020). Electroconvulsive therapy for patients with catatonia: Current perspectives. *Neuropsychiatric Disease and Treatment, 16*, 2191–2208. https://doi.org/10.2147/NDT.S231573

Lozano, A. M., Lipsman, N., Bergman, H., Brown, P., Chabardes, S., Chang, J. W., Matthews, K., McIntyre, C. C., Schlaepfer, T. E., Schulder, M., Temel, Y., Volkmann, J., & Krauss, J. K. (2019). Deep brain stimulation: Current challenges and future directions. *Nature Reviews Neurology, 15*(3), 148–160. https://doi.org/10.1038/s41582-018-0128-2

Marcantoni, W. S., Akoumba, B. S., Wassef, M., Mayrand, J., Lai, H., Richard-Devantoy, S., & Beauchamp, S. (2020). A systematic review and meta-analysis of the efficacy of intravenous ketamine infusion for treatment resistant depression: January 2009–January 2019. *Journal of Affective Disorders, 277*, 831–841. https://doi.org/10.1016/j.jad.2020.09.007

McDonald, W. M., & Thompson, T. R. (2001). Treatment of mania in dementia with electroconvulsive therapy. *Psychopharmacol Bulletin, 35*(2), 72–82.

Mekala, H., Malik, Z., Lone, J., Shah, K., & Ishaq, M. (2020). Cannabis-induced catatonia: A case series. *Cureus, 12*(6), e8603. https://doi.org10.7759/cureus.8603

Mohn, C., & Rund, B. R. (2019). Neurocognitive function and symptom remission 2 years after ECT in major depressive disorders. *Journal of Affective Disorders, 246*, 368–375. https://doi.org/10.1016/j.jad.2018.12.083

Murrough, J. W., Iosifescu, D. V., Chang, L. C., Al Jurdi, R. K., Green, C. E., Perez, A. M., Iqbal, S., Pillemer, S., Foulkes, A., Shah, A., Charney, D. S., & Mathew, S. J. (2013). Antidepressant efficacy of ketamine in treatment-resistant major depression: A two-site randomized controlled trial. *The American Journal of Psychiatry, 170*(10), 1134–1142. https://doi.org/10.1176/appi.ajp.2013.13030392

Murrough, J. W., Soleimani, L., DeWilde, K. E., Collins, K. A., Lapidus, K. A., Iacoviello, B. M., Lener, M., Kautz, M., Kim, J., Stern, J. B., Price, R. B., Perez, A. M., Brallier, J. W., Rodriguez, G. J., Goodman, W. K., Iosifescu, D. V., & Charney, D. S. (2015). Ketamine for rapid reduction of suicidal ideation: a randomized controlled trial. *Psychological Medicine, 45*(16), 3571–3580. https://doi.org/10.1017/S0033291715001506

Nordanskog, P., Larsson, M. R., Larsson, E. M., & Johanson, A. (2014). Hippocampal volume in relation to clinical and cognitive outcome after electroconvulsive therapy in depression. *Acta Psychiatrica Scandinavica, 129*(4), 303–311. https://doi.org10.1111/acps.12150

Osler, M., Rozing, M. P., Christensen, G. T., Andersen, P. K., & Jørgensen, M. B. (2018). Electroconvulsive therapy and risk of dementia in patients with affective disorders: A cohort study. *Lancet Psychiatry, 5*(4), 348–356. https://doi.org/10.1016/s2215-0366(18)30056-7

Perugi, G., Medda, P., Toni, C., Mariani, M. G., Socci, C., & Mauri, M. (2017). The role of electroconvulsive therapy (ECT) in bipolar disorder: Effectiveness in 522 patients with bipolar depression, mixed-state, mania and catatonic features. *Current Neuropharmacology, 15*(3), 359–371. ttps://doi.org/10.2174/1570159X14666161017233642

Pjrek, E., Friedrich, M.-E., Cambioli, L., Dold, M., Jäger, F., Komorowski, A., Lanzenberger, R., Kasper, S., & Winkler, D. (2020). The efficacy of light therapy in the treatment of seasonal affective disorder: A meta-analysis of randomized controlled trials. *Psychotherapy and Psychosomatics, 89*(1), 17–24. https://doi.org/10.1159/000502891

Price, R. B., Iosifescu, D. V., Murrough, J. W., Chang, L. C., Al Jurdi, R. K., Iqbal, S. Z., Soleimani, L., Charney, D. S., Foulkes, A. L., & Mathew, S. J. (2014). Effects of ketamine on explicit and implicit suicidal cognition: A randomized controlled trial in treatment-resistant depression. *Depression and Anxiety, 31*(4), 335–343. https://doi.org/10.1002/da.22253

Rose, S., Dotters-Katz, S. K., & Kuller, J. A. (2020). Electroconvulsive therapy in pregnancy: Safety, best practices, and barriers to care. *Obstetrical & Gynecological Survey, 75*(3), 199–203. https://doi.org/10.1097/OGX.0000000000000763

Rossi, S., Hallett, M., Rossini, P. M., & Pascual-Leone, A. (2009). Safety, ethical considerations, and application guidelines for the use of transcranial magnetic stimulation in clinical practice and research. *Clinical Neurophysiology: The Official Journal of the International Federation of Clinical Neurophysiology,, 120*(12), 2008–2039. https://doi.org/10.1016/j.clinph.2009.08.016

Sackeim, H. A., Aaronson, S. T., Carpenter, L. L., Hutton, T. M., Mina, M., Pages, K., Verdoliva, S., & West, W. S. (2020). Clinical outcomes in a large registry of patients with major depressive disorder treated with transcranial magnetic stimulation. *Journal of Affective Disorders, 277*, 65–74. https://doi.org/10.1016/j.jad.2020.08.005

Sanghani, S. N., Petrides, G., & Kellner, C. H. (2018). Electroconvulsive therapy (ECT) in schizophrenia: A review of recent literature. *Current Opinion in Psychiatry, , 31*(3), 213–222. https:doi.org/10.1097/YCO.0000000000000418

van Oostrom, I., van Eijndhoven, P., Butterbrod, E., van Beek, M. H., Janzing, J., Donders, R., Schene, A., & Tendolkar, I. (2018). Decreased cognitive functioning after electroconvulsive therapy is related to increased hippocampal volume. *The Journal of ECT, 34*(2), 117–123. https://doi.org/10.1097/yct.0000000000000483

Weiner, R. D., & Reti, I. M. (2017). Key updates in the clinical application of electroconvulsive therapy. *International Review of Psychiatry (Abingdon, England), 29*(2), 54–62. https:doi.org/10.1080/09540261.2017.1309362

CHAPTER 33

Introduction to Psychotherapy for Medical Students[1]

M. Zachary Rosenthal, Ph.D.; Rachel Guetta, B.A.; Jacqueline Trumbull, B.A.; and Clair Cassiello-Robbins, Ph.D.

> *"In my early professional years, I was asking the question: How can I treat, or cure, or change this person? Now I would phrase the question in this way: How can I provide a relationship which this person may use for his own personal growth?"*
>
> — Carl R. Rogers

OBJECTIVES

After reading this chapter, students will be able to do the following:[1]

- describe several common factors essential to all psychotherapies
- describe several primary types of psychotherapy
- discuss some of the common challenges in learning and doing psychotherapy

CASE VIGNETTE

Yolanda came to psychotherapy to treat major depression. She is 31 years old and identifies as a biracial cisgender woman. She is married with two small children, working part-time at a grocery store, and struggling alongside her husband to pay for home and family expenses. Her primary care doctor referred to her therapy because three separate courses of antidepressants over the past year failed to remediate the symptoms or impairment associated with her depressive symptoms. Fluoxetine, venlafaxine, and paroxetine all left her feeling no better than usual and with some tolerable but unpleasant adverse side effects. These medications do not always work for the treatment of depression. For

(*continued*)

1 Readers may also see "Defence Mechanisms: The Hidden Gymnastics to Protect the Self" (Chapter 14) for related material.

Yolanda, these medications may not have worked, at least in part, because her clinical presentation extended beyond unipolar depression.

It was complicated. She was born in a foreign country where she was raised by her grandmother. At age 16 she came to the United States to live with her older brother in a rough neighborhood in New York city. After she arrived, she quickly became dependent on alcohol and used marijuana daily. She dropped out of high school, was homeless for several years, endured physical and sexual violence, and witnessed violence in her community dozens of times before she turned 21. Her substance dependence continued throughout her 20s. By the age of 25 she had been psychiatrically hospitalized twice for expressing detailed suicide plans, arrested for multiple misdemeanors related to substance use, and divorced. To be sure, Yolanda was quite depressed. She screened positive on the Personal Health Questionnaire-9 (Kroenke & Spitzer, 2002), and her Beck Depression Inventory-2 score was 35, indicating severe symptoms of depression (Beck et al., 1996). But it was more than that. To her doctors and therapist, Yolanda was a patient with a complex presentation influenced by multiple psychiatric diagnoses and a long list of past and current biopsychosocial stressors.

Yolanda had never been to therapy before, and she was both skeptical and curious. As therapy began, she asked many questions: What is therapy? How does it start? What should she talk about? What would the therapist be doing to help her? How long would it take to get better? Would it even work? And if it did, how would it help her? All of these are both good and common questions.

How can we help answer Yolanda's questions? It depends, of course, on the nature of the clinical setting (e.g., is it resourced to provide certain specific kinds of therapy?), training of the clinician (e.g., does the therapist have training or supervision in certain therapies?), and implementation of the particular therapy (e.g., what does the assessment and case conceptualization include? Are the common factors of therapy used by the therapist? Which evidence-based treatments are used?). To achieve the best outcomes, Yolanda and the therapist will need to work collaboratively within a particular therapeutic frame with a strong therapeutic alliance, careful attention to multicultural considerations, the therapist attending to common therapy processes (e.g., empathy, support, etc.), and ethical implementation of a set of treatment procedures targeting her presentation of depression and a history of substance dependence.

DEFINITIONS AND KEY CONCEPTS

Psychotherapy is the treatment of psychiatric disorders and problems in living using psychological rather than medical means. *Empathy* is the capacity to recognize, understand, and share the thoughts and feelings of another person, animal, or fictional character from within their frame of reference. *Therapeutic frame* refers to the set of norms, boundaries and expectations required for effective therapy. *Therapeutic alliance* broadly refers to the building of a working partnership toward common treatment goals between therapist and patient. Empathy (having perspective to understand what patients are communicating and affectively experiencing what patients are feeling), sympathy (sorrow or pity for patients), and apathy (lack of emotional response) are each different processes in psychotherapy. Supportive listening occurs within a safe therapeutic relationship and includes careful listening, compassion, and validation of patients. Several common types of psychotherapy include cognitive behavioral, client-centered, psychodynamic, and interpersonal psychotherapies. There are various mechanisms of change underlying why or how psychotherapies work, including common factors across therapy (e.g., therapeutic alliance, empathy, and supportive listening) and specific factors unique to certain therapeutic approaches. All therapies need to account for multicultural considerations and ethical dilemmas. For medical students and others learning about psychotherapies, it takes time and clinical supervision to learn how to implement evidence-based treatments in a flexible and creative manner across a range of medical and psychiatric clinical presentations.

KEY POINT

Psychotherapy is the treatment of psychiatric disorders and problems in living using psychological rather than medical means. Psychotherapy is an effective tool for addressing mental health disorders, adjusting to stressors and new life situations, and other problems with living.

INTRODUCTION

As medical students, psychotherapy may seem like something you have seen in the movies. You might imagine it as an abstract and unscientific process in which patients lie down on a couch or get their dreams interpreted. Or maybe you think it is something that can't change biological processes like medications can. But here is the thing: psychotherapies do change brain functioning and other biological processes, and they are backed by decades of clinical science. And, unlike what you see in the movies, they often look a bit more like training people to live their lives differently by teaching them new ways to think, feel, relate, and so on—all in the context of a safe and nonjudgmental therapeutic relationship. The time taken to truly get to know a patient (weekly appointments for up to an hour!) and the resulting reward therapists feel when they help change a patient's life can feel extraordinary, gratifying, and deeply meaningful. In this chapter, we provide a summary overview of psychotherapy with the goal of introducing medical students and other learners to some of the foundational ways to understand psychotherapy.

BRIEF HISTORY OF PSYCHOTHERAPY

Psychotherapy as we know it today is a relatively new method of helping people. Sigmund Freud's method of psychoanalysis arose in Europe in the late 1800s in the wake of Charcot, Breuer, and other physicians' use of hypnosis for what was then called hysteria. Freud's ideas took hold in the United States in the early 1900s and would, over the course of the first half of the 20th century, become the dominant psychotherapeutic approach. Freudian therapy involved various techniques intended to help address underlying unconscious problems. Free association, dream interpretation, and probing of patient responses to ambiguous stimuli were all used as ways to help patients discover and change unconscious patterns thought to be at the root of life problems. At the same time Freudian therapy was emerging, behavioral scientists were using the scientific method to understand and change human behavior. Legends, including Thorndike, Watson, and Skinner, were using empirical approaches to observe and quantify behavior change. These early scientists would soon have their work translated by psychologists and psychiatrists who brought forth alternative models of psychotherapy to rival, and ultimately eclipse, Freudian approaches.

Behavior therapy arose as a rejection of psychodynamic models of therapy that relied on theory and eschewed scientific study. In the mid and late 20th century, behavior therapists developed, manualized, tested, and began disseminating a range of treatments for many psychiatric problems. Behavior therapies, such as systematic desensitization (Wolpe, 1968), began without any emphasis on changing cognition or other unobservable phenomenon. Soon after these therapies came cognitive therapy, led by Beck, Ellis, and others, which used techniques to identify and challenge dysfunctional and irrational ways of thinking to help patients with depression, anxiety, and similar conditions. The pioneering work in cognitive therapy quickly merged with behavior therapy principles, bringing about an explosion in evidence-based treatments for psychiatric disorders and a new term: *cognitive behavioral therapy* (CBT).

But as fast as CBT was born, it would soon be challenged by what came to be called "third-wave" therapies focusing on acceptance, mindfulness, and a range of experiential change techniques deemphasizing the importance of challenging irrational thinking. Today the inclusion of behavioral, cognitive, and third-wave behavior therapies collectively comprise the broader family of cognitive behavioral therapies (CBTs). There is no such thing as one CBT treatment. Instead, just as there are classes of antidepressant medications (tricyclic antidepressants [TCAs], monoamine oxidase inhibitors [MAOIs], selective serotonin reuptake inhibitors [SSRIs], serotonin norepinephrine reuptake inhibitors [SNRIs], etc.), each with specific types, so too there are several kinds of CBTs (e.g., primarily cognitive change-focused, acceptance and mindfulness-focused, or behavior change-focused) and many specific treatment protocols.

Beyond traditional psychoanalysis and the growing family of evidence-based CBTs, there are of course many other psychotherapies. For example, supportive therapy uses common factors, such as listening, validation, and empathy. Modern psychodynamic therapies have become shorter and more evidence-based (Busch et al., 2012; Milrod et al., 2013). Interpersonal therapy focuses on roles and processes in relationships. Therapies emphasizing somatic processes have been developed. Narrative therapies use writing and storytelling techniques.

Therapists using eye movement desensitization and reprocessing (EMDR) purport to use patient's saccadic eye movements while talking about painful life events to reduce trauma-related symptoms. Marriage and family therapists use techniques to change how people relate to each other.

Therapies can occur with individuals, couples, families, or in groups across a spectrum of resource intensity—from inpatient to intensive outpatient to weekly or less often outpatient clinic visits. And of course, the rise of mobile health platforms has led to the proliferation of conventional and novel approaches to psychotherapy using remote online methods. Taken together, there are many different ways a patient like Yolanda could receive psychotherapy. To gain better perspective on how to answer Yolanda's questions about her care, we now provide more detail about the nature of psychotherapy. We review the concepts of assessment, case conceptualization, the therapeutic frame, common processes across therapies, general mechanisms of change in therapies, several common psychotherapies, challenges in learning therapies as medical students, multicultural considerations in psychotherapy, and principles used to manage ethical dilemmas in psychotherapies.

ASSESSMENTS IN PSYCHOTHERAPY

All forms of therapy typically involve three types of assessment: initial assessment, case conceptualization, and ongoing assessment of progress in treatment. The specific method of assessment may differ based on the types of therapy and the theory on which it is based. Here, we will focus on the principles relevant to assessment across psychotherapy modalities.

The Initial Assessment

The purpose of initial assessment is to understand the patient's presenting problems. In most health care settings, this assessment will focus on establishing the presence or absence of psychiatric diagnoses (e.g., Yolanda's diagnosis of major depression), as these are needed for charting and insurance purposes. This assessment process can be formal using semi-structured interviews, such as the Structured Clinical Interview for *DSM-5* (SCID-5; First, 2015) or informal without such tools. In addition to establishing the presence or absence of diagnoses, the initial assessment is also important to better understand the patient's presenting problems and primary goals for treatment. Finally, this assessment allows the clinician to gather information about contextual factors that are relevant to understanding the patient's concerns. For example, information about family structure, social support, cultural, and other contextual factors will guide the therapist's understanding of the patient.

Case Conceptualization

Most therapies also involve early and ongoing case conceptualization. This assessment is importantly different from establishing a diagnosis and refers to the process in which the therapist and patient work together to describe and explain the patient's presenting problems (Kuyken et al., 2008a). Whereas explanations for the etiology and maintenance of psychopathology differ across therapy modalities, case conceptualization typically includes an understanding of (a) how a patient's psychological problems developed (including genetic, environmental, interpersonal, and emotion-regulation processes that contributed to the development of psychological dysfunction) and (b) hypotheses about the factors maintaining the patient's difficulties (e.g., dysfunctional beliefs, engagement in ineffective behaviors, and reinforcement present in the environment). This process is important in therapy because it helps engage the patient in treatment, provides an understanding of complex problems grounded in theory, and helps the therapist select intervention components to intervene on these problems (Kuyken et al., 2008b; Pilecki & McKay, 2013). For example, when case conceptualization suggests a patient's problems are perpetuated by dysfunctional beliefs, a therapist might teach cognitive skills to challenge those beliefs and develop more flexible thinking patterns. Importantly, case conceptualization often changes over the course of the treatment as the therapist learns more about the patient and their context. Thus, this process is inherently adaptable and dynamic.

Monitoring Symptoms and Progress in Treatment

Finally, therapies commonly include routine outcome monitoring of symptoms and/or progress toward goals. This is particularly true in evidence-based psychotherapies, which are primarily CBTs, and ask patients to complete brief symptom measures at the start of each therapy session to track symptom change. Some of these evidence-based treatments also include measures to track progress toward goals on a regular basis to ensure therapy is remaining on target. For example, Yolanda's therapist might ask her to fill out a measure of depression every week to track progress in therapy. Meanwhile, other therapies include less-formal monitoring, such as weekly check-ins with patients at the start of session. However, therapists are strongly encouraged to engage in some formal routine outcome monitoring. This monitoring allows patients and therapists to identify improvements, which can increase patient motivation to continue engaging in treatment. On the other hand, this monitoring can also help identify times when therapy is not effective and allow the patient and therapist to engage in collaborative problem-solving about what changes are needed to improve the treatment (Boswell et al., 2015). Patient and therapist views of progress in treatment are inherently subjective, and thus, these measures provide a more objective metric by which progress can be measured. Taken together, there is a strong rationale for engaging in routine outcome monitoring to track symptoms, facilitate collaboration between patient and therapist, and adjust therapy as needed based on data.

Assessment starts at the beginning of the patient–therapist interaction and continues throughout treatment. Through assessment, the therapist can gain a nuanced understanding of their patient, develop hypotheses about to how to best intervene to help the patient, and track data to observe the effects of their interventions. Thus, assessment is crucial to the provision of effective treatment.

THERAPEUTIC FRAME AND RELATIONSHIP

The therapeutic frame refers to the set of boundaries and expectations required for effective therapy. This frame includes expectations set by the therapist and patient agreement about basic rules of treatment, such as confidentiality; privacy; and the setting, duration, and price of sessions (Warburton, 2014). Confidentiality requires the therapist to keep all discussions with the patient confidential, except in cases of clear risk of harm to the patient or others or when required to break confidentiality by law. These exceptions should be clearly explained to the patient at the outset in the first therapy appointment. Therapy sessions should be contained to a specific duration (commonly 45–50 minutes) with an agreed-on time, location, and fee. These expectations allow for a controlled and predictable environment in which the therapeutic relationship can develop (Warburton, 2014). The therapist is expected to provide a consistent physical environment and predictable emotional support based on mutual trust and respect, while the patient is expected to arrive on time, pay for sessions, limit communication outside of sessions, and enact any other stipulations appropriate to that particular form of therapy.

The therapeutic frame also includes expectations for the therapist's behavior. Some therapies have an expectation of anonymity, meaning that the therapist should refrain from sharing personal opinions or information. They also might expect therapists to project neutrality and avoid suggesting that any course of action or perspective is superior (Cecchin, 1987). Other therapies allow the clinician to be more self-disclosive, active, and direct. Although therapeutic frames may vary, all therapists are expected to create and nurture a relationship that is reliable, consistent, safe, and done in accordance with appropriate ethical guidelines.

THERAPEUTIC ALLIANCE

Therapeutic alliance broadly refers to the building of a working partnership toward common treatment goals between therapist and patient. This active collaboration begins in the early stages of psychotherapy and includes agreement on treatment goals and the methods by which to achieve the treatment goals (Bordin, 1994). Whereas earlier psychodynamic premises of alliance implied that the therapist activates change within the patient, more recent theories of alliance imply mutuality, transparency, and equal ownership over the therapeutic process and change. The therapist and patient create a *working* alliance that considers each patient's treatment goals in the context of the individual's capacities, expectations, and personal resources (Horvath et al., 2011).

Alliance in psychotherapy is a common psychotherapy factor in that it is not bound to any one treatment or intervention. Rather, a strong therapeutic alliance should evolve and adapt with different types and stages of therapy (Horvath et al., 2011). This working relationship, then, is fostered in conjunction with the methods and treatment targets agreed on by therapist and patient. For example, the therapist may begin a session by probing about prior difficult relationships to target distress tolerance and emotion regulation. The patient may demonstrate ambivalence discussing those relationships; the therapist may then adjust the agenda to address the ambivalence, targeting other behavioral goals of acceptance and nonjudgment. This agenda-setting and collaboration takes different forms, as treatment goals and methods shifting, both within and between sessions, is essential for successful psychotherapy. Indeed, empirical investigation has demonstrated that the strength of therapeutic alliance is a core and common factor that mediates behavioral outcomes (Gifford et al., 2011).

The finding that therapeutic alliance is a strong predictor of treatment outcome has been replicated across studies and underscored in several meta-analyses (Horvath et al., 2011; Norcross, 2011; Wampold, 2001). Of particular importance is the patients' evaluation of the quality of the alliance and the clinical recommendation to actively monitor patients' experience of the alliance. There are several well-validated instruments to measure alliance (such as the Working Alliance Inventory; Horvath & Greenberg, 1989). Tracking ratings over time and indexing alliance as a proxy for mutuality and collaboration in treatment is an effective and accessible way to attend to this important common factor.

VALIDATION AND SUPPORT IN THERAPY

Two additional common factors across psychotherapies are validation and support. Validation communicates attention, understanding, and acceptance, demonstrating to the patient that the therapist is actively listening in a nonjudgmental way (Fruzzetti & Ruork, 2018). Considered a supportive intervention in and of itself, validation promotes emotional recognition and therapeutic alliance, soothes negative emotional arousal, and ultimately paves the way for self-validation (Weinberg et al., 2011). Differentially validating healthy behaviors or vocalized beliefs can act as positive reinforcement and may be an agent of change and learning. Further, validation can be modeled in different ways depending on the patient's reaction, the treatment frame, and target behaviors. Although different types of therapy (e.g., psychodynamic, CBT) provide validation in different ways, all psychotherapies include empathetic listening and efforts to understand the patient and help the patient understand themselves.

Similarly, psychotherapists practicing different types of therapy are supportive of patients. However, the ways in which support is communicated may vary. For example, listening and being kind is supportive (i.e., social support), but so is providing active help and advice (i.e., instrumental support). Offering support as the primary intervention may be akin to the frame of client-centered therapy, whereas providing support in the context of a broader treatment frame is common to many third-wave CBTs. In addition, supportive therapy sometimes refers to a specific intervention to reduce distress and/or maladaptive symptoms and to maintain or reinforce adaptive skills, emotional well-being, and self-reliance (Pinsker, 2004). Indeed, supportive therapy is one of the areas of competence for psychiatry residents put forth by the Accreditation Council for Graduate Medical Education (ACGME, 2020). As such, support as a common factor and, as an intervention in its own right, will likely be a central training focus for medical students and psychiatry residents, in particular.

EMPATHY

Empathy is another common factor of therapy with an unequivocally important role. Recent meta-analyses suggest that empathy accounts for roughly 9% of the variance in therapy outcome (Nienhuis et al., 2018). There are at least three fundamental neural processes involved in empathy: emotional simulation, perspective-taking, and emotion regulation. The limbic system allows us to mirror the emotional experience of others to achieve emotional simulation, whereas the prefrontal cortex helps us grasp others' experiences and downregulate our own emotional response to extend help and compassion (Elliott et al., 2011). Emotion simulation is involved in affective empathy (i.e., the ability to share another's emotional experience). Perspective-taking is associated with cognitive empathy (i.e., the ability to conceptually understand the other's experience). Both forms of empathy are helpful in psychotherapy. Patients are apt to feel understood and validated when their therapists mirror affectively (e.g., facial expressions of sadness when the patient is describing feeling sad) or communicate verbally that they can understand, make sense of, or normalize patient experiences.

KEY POINT

Empathy is the capacity to recognize, understand, and share the thoughts and feelings of another person, animal, or fictional character from within one's frame of reference. There are at least three fundamental neural processes involved in empathy:

- emotional simulation
- perspective-taking
- emotion regulation

There are many factors that influence patient reports of therapists' empathy. Attentiveness, openness, and refraining from judgment are all perceived as empathetic. These qualities may be communicated through posture, vocal quality, and frequent use of emotion words; they are undermined by behavior that controls the session, such as talking too much, interrupting, or giving advice (Elliott et al., 2011). Functionally, empathy is used to reflect and expand the patient's perspective. Therapists can attempt to grasp the meaning behind the patient's words and nonverbal cues and mirror this back to them in a way that demonstrates vivid understanding and validation without simply repeating the patient's description (Elliott et al., 2011).

QUICK POINT

The limbic system allows us to mirror the emotional experience of others to achieve emotional simulation, whereas the prefrontal cortex helps us grasp others' experiences and downregulate our own emotional response to extend help and compassion (Elliott et al., 2011).

As an example, Yolanda might say, while holding back tears, "I thought this award for my work would make a huge difference in my life, but it never got any attention," to which the therapist might respond, "I see you're feeling quite sad. It's a terrible feeling to get your hopes up and dream about new possibilities only to feel like you were left on the cutting-room floor. Am I getting it?" This exchange shows the patient

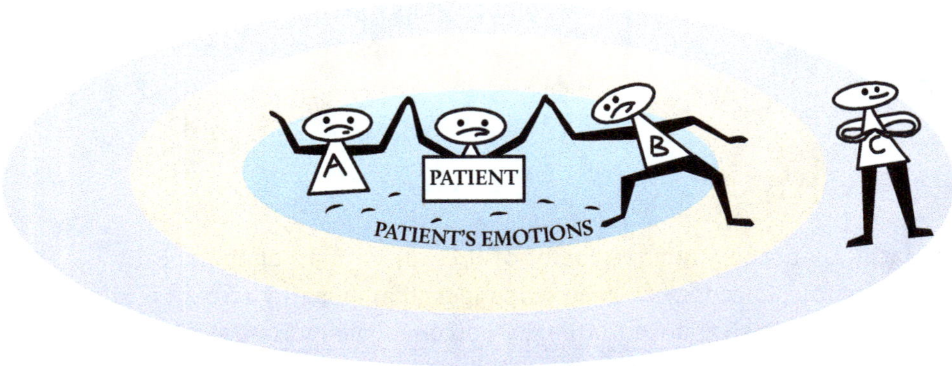

FIGURE 33.1 Provider empathy, sympathy, apathy (original drawing by authors). Sympathy (provider A): able to connect emotionally, but difficulty downregulating their emotional response. Empathy (provider B): able to connect emotionally with subsequent downregulation of their emotional response, which allows the provider help to guide the patient out of their predicament. Apathy (provider C): unable to connect emotionally (or suppression/avoidance of emotional connection). In the past, provider C might have shown the ability to emotionally connect to patients, but, often due to personal or professional experiences in their life, may now be shielding themselves from further emotional pain.

KEY POINT

Empathy is the capacity to recognize, understand, and share the thoughts and feelings of another from within their frame of reference. Empathy requires active listening to the totality of what is being communicated. Sympathy refers to feeling sorrow, pity, or a related affective state for another person's misfortunes or difficulties. Apathy refers to a lack of care, interest, or feelings.

that the therapist is attuned to their emotional cues, able to understand their experience, and open to corrective feedback. Although empathy is not a sufficient condition for successful therapy, it is a powerful factor common in all evidence-based treatments.

In contrast to empathy, sympathy refers to feeling sorrow, pity, or a related affective state for another person's misfortunes or difficulties. Sympathy is often a feeling therapists have when doing psychotherapy but can be distinguished from empathy and apathy (i.e., lack of care, interest, or feelings). Indeed, therapists do feel and communicate expressions of sympathy at times. However, most patients do not seek therapy for or benefit primarily from therapists expressing communications of sympathy. For new therapists, sometimes feelings of sympathy for patients can be overwhelming. Therapists, over time, learn to downregulate their own emotional reactions to patients to not rely on sympathy, communicating empathically while helping to facilitate therapeutic change.

COMMON PSYCHOTHERAPIES

Cognitive Behavioral Therapies

CBT refers to a skills-focused approach that helps patients learn strategies to change how they think, feel, behave, relate to themselves and others, and achieve their life goals. CBTs have evolved over time. At first, these therapies were better termed *behavior therapy* because they focused on the application of empirically supported principles of behavior change (e.g., operant conditioning) to intervene on the relationship between a stimulus and a response. For example, Wolpe is known for using reciprocal inhibition techniques in the treatment for anxiety called systematic desensitization. This process is based on the finding that one cannot feel both anxious and relaxed simultaneously. Thus, patients are exposed to feared stimuli while practicing relaxation skills, often in a hierarchically graded manner. Once patients are no longer anxious in response to a specific stimulus, they practice reciprocal inhibition with more challenging stimuli until the anxiety response is extinguished.

Over time, these treatments began to address the cognitive element of human experiences. Thus, CBTs began to target thoughts that contribute to an individual's symptoms. At this time, cognitive restructuring, a skill in which patients are taught to question their automatic thoughts, was introduced into treatment. For example, a patient with depression like Yolanda may have the thought, "I can't do anything right." Cognitive restructuring encourages patients to challenge this thought to develop a more flexible way of thinking. This patient might develop the alternative thought, "Like most people, I do some things well and not others." Currently, CBT has begun to integrate novel strategies, such as mindfulness and acceptance skills, which also help patients manage the experience of strong emotions in a way that is consistent with their long-term goals (Hofmann & Hayes, 2019). For example, mindfulness teaches patients to be present focused and nonjudgmental while experiencing strong emotions. This skill allows patients to acknowledge their feelings while continuing to engage in goal-directed behavior.

CBTs have also evolved from being diagnosis specific to being transdiagnostic. Beginning in the 1980s, these treatments were often delivered via written manuals with specific session-by-session instructions for clinicians. These manual-based treatments targeted specific diagnoses (e.g., depression and panic disorder). However, due to emerging evidence suggesting a range of diagnoses are characterized by similar psychopathological processes, transdiagnostic treatments have been

CLINICAL TIP

Most patients do not seek therapy to obtain sympathy. On the contrary, they seek treatment to manage their symptoms or problems with life better. For new providers, sometimes, feelings of sympathy for patients can be overwhelming. Over time, providers typically learn to downregulate their own emotional reactions to patients to not rely on sympathy but instead communicate empathically to facilitate therapeutic change.

KEY POINT

CBT involves a skills-focused approach to changing problematic thinking patterns to effect behavioral change toward treatment goals.

developed. These treatments target the psychological processes that are shared across diagnostic categories (e.g., Barlow et al., 2017; Hayes, 2004; Linehan et al., 2014). Like all CBTs, these treatments teach patients skills to manage the experience of strong emotions and engage in behavior that is aligned with their long-term goals but focus on processes maintaining disorders rather than disorder-specific symptoms.

CBTs are broadly considered evidence-based treatments; there is strong research supporting their ability to remediate symptoms of most common mental disorders, including mood, anxiety, obsessive compulsive, eating, sleep–wake, and trauma-related disorders (Carpenter et al., 2018; Cuijpers et al., 2013; Hofmann et al., 2012; Trauer et al., 2015). A growing literature supports the use of transdiagnostic treatments to target most common mental disorders as well (Cassiello-Robbins et al., 2020). Thus, the skills in these treatments appear to be applicable to a wide range of patients and are able to help remediate suffering. Most CBTs are relatively brief (weekly for several months), directive, and include regular home practice of cognitive and behavioral interventions. These features make CBTs commonly used in medical centers and clinical settings where resources are limited and position CBTs to be at the center of population health- and value-based care models, which use brief treatments and measurement-based approaches to help manage total health for all patients within a community.

Client-Centered Supportive Therapy

Humanistic psychology developed in the 1950s in response to the prevailing psychodynamic and behaviorist models of determinism and stimulus-response reinforcement. Carl Rogers's development of client-centered therapy offered a stark contrast, conceptualizing the person as self-determining and self-realizing (Raskin et al., 2008). Whereas psychodynamic approaches often focus on a set of defenses and subconscious processes that prevent humans from reaching their potentials, the client-centered approach elevates free will and posits that each self-realizing process can transcend circumscribed sets of defenses or sociocultural roles.

In this way, Rogers regarded self-actualization (i.e., fulfilling one's potential) as a biological motivation unique to each individual, and the way the self perceives and responds to events should direct psychotherapy. This reliance on self-potential and the individual's cognitive and emotional resources shapes the role of the therapist in client-centered supportive therapy. The common factors of empathy, authenticity, and warmth are essential in this therapy, and the role of the therapist is to reflect and amplify the patient's volition and intentions. Although Rogerian therapy is not a dominant model in today's evidence-based world of treatment, many approaches (e.g., CBTs) have integrated client-centered supportive therapy techniques into their protocols. If Yolanda received a client-centered supportive therapy, she could expect the therapist to be consistently warm and encouraging, asking a lot of open-ended questions and using listening skills, such as paraphrasing, reflecting, or summarizing back what is heard. The client-centered therapist would not be as directive as the CBT therapist and may not have a time-limited approach or use home practice and self-report measures of outcome.

Motivational interviewing (MI), similar to motivational enhancement therapy (MET), is a well-known and common brief therapy approach that has been derived in part from client-centered psychotherapy. In MI/MET, therapists use common psychotherapy listening techniques to help facilitate patient motivation to make changes in their life. Examples of these techniques include using open-ended questions (and minimizing yes/no questions), affirmations of patient capacities and expressions of desire to change, reflection, paraphrasing, and summarizing patient communications. Although these listening techniques are not unique to MI/MET, they are a core component of this approach and are critical for helping patients increase verbal expressions about making changes. MI/MET also emphasizes patient awareness and clarification of values and goals, identification of barriers to living consistently with values and attaining goals, and exploration of ways to overcome these barriers. MI/MET is an evidence-based therapy to help patients engage in treatment, remain in treatment, and make changes in their lives (Arkowitz et al., 2015; Cummings et al., 2009; Miller & Rollnick, 2012). It has been most commonly studied as a brief (e.g., one- to four-session) intervention (Rollnick et al., 1992) that can be implemented by counselors with minimal training (Daeppen et al., 2012) and can be used in combination with other psychotherapies (Arkowitz et al., 2015; Arkowitz & Miller, 2008; Moyers & Houck, 2011). Most of the research on MI/MET has been conducted with patients who struggle with substance use (Barnett et al., 2012; Carroll et al., 2006; de Gee et al., 2014) or chronic medical disease management (McKenzie et al., 2015; Moral et al., 2015), but it has been studied and used with a wide variety of patients (Arkowitz et al., 2015; McNeil et al., 2017).

Psychodynamic Therapy

Psychodynamic therapy generally aims to uncover what lies beneath the patient's conscious awareness. The therapist helps the patient to identify and change maladaptive patterns of defenses, affect regulation, and ways of relating to the self or others that are stored in implicit memory. The therapist then helps the patient translate these patterns into explicit memory—or conscious awareness—where they can be explored and changed (Gabbard, 2014). Implicit memory is involved in stimulus response and is sensory, emotional, and procedural (i.e., knowing how to walk), whereas explicit memory is organized, autobiographical, narrative, and involved in emotion regulation and identity. Our earliest childhood memories are ruled by implicit memory, as advanced brain regions, such as the hippocampus and prefrontal cortex, are undeveloped in infants (Tsujimoto, 2008). Accordingly, our earliest experiences with attachment and security are coded implicitly

KEY POINT

"MI [motivational interviewing] is a collaborative, goal-oriented style of communication with particular attention to the language of change. It is designed to strengthen personal motivation for and commitment to a specific goal by eliciting and exploring the person's own reasons for change within an atmosphere of acceptance and compassion" (Miller & Rollnick, 2013).

KEY POINT

Psychodynamic therapy aims to identify and address the foundation of problematic psychological processes to reduce symptoms and improve emotional health and well-being. Although psychological processes are employed throughout life, their foundations are often laid in early childhood.

KEY POINT

Interpersonal psychotherapy (IPT) is a form of psychotherapy that focuses on reducing symptoms by improving interpersonal functioning. It conceptualizes the patient's psychopathology as arising from four possible problem areas: grief, role disputes, role transitions, and interpersonal deficits.

(Cozolino, 2014). Bringing implicit information into explicit awareness and thereby gaining insight into these maladaptive patterns is expected to allow the patient to confront fears and help gain control over their lives (Cabaniss, 2016).

The psychodynamic therapist pays particular attention to past relationship attachments and emotionally painful memories. The patient's ineffective behavioral patterns were likely helpful in a past environment but have become harmful in new contexts. For instance, an adult who was abused as a child may have learned to be vigilant and untrusting but struggles to build secure relationships as an adult. The therapist helps the patient translate the inchoate information of implicit memory into words after which it can be stored in explicit memory and understood clearly (Cabaniss, 2016). Another way the therapist uncovers these patterns is by closely attending to the therapeutic relationship. They pay particular attention to transference, which occurs when the patient transfers implicit relational patterns onto the therapist (Cozolino, 2014). For instance, a patient may begin to reenact behaviors that existed with a certain figure from their past. If the patient had a highly critical parent, they may be particularly attuned to signs of criticism from the therapist and react similarly to when they were confronted with parental criticism. The therapist also attunes to counter-transference, which is their own emotional reaction to the patient. When the therapist notices transference or counter-transference, they can mirror this process back to the patient and help them understand how they relate to and are experienced by others.

Finally, psychodynamic therapy helps the patient relearn social and emotional development in a new, supportive context. The therapist helps the patient develop new skills for regulating their emotions as well as relating to others and managing self-esteem (Cabaniss, 2016). Because psychodynamic therapies have not been well scientifically studied compared to other psychotherapies (e.g., CBTs), are often long and expensive for patients (e.g., daily or weekly for years), and require significant resource allocation (e.g., fewer total patients can be treated than other therapeutic models), these approaches are often done in private practices and are unavailable in clinical settings that are challenged by limited resources.

Interpersonal Therapy

Interpersonal psychotherapy (IPT) is a time-limited, evidence-based treatment that intervenes on the patient's current interpersonal functioning by helping patients change the way they relate to others. Treatment focuses on the present day and the period around disorder onset with less emphasis on discussions of childhood development (Weissman et al., 2008) than in psychodynamic therapies.

During IPT, the therapist begins by collecting an interpersonal inventory from the patient. This includes a review of the patient's current relationships and awareness of relational patterns, expectations, changes, and dysfunction, particularly around the onset of the disorder (Weissman et al., 2008). The therapist then provides the interpersonal formulation of pathology and conceptualizes the patient's psychopathology as arising from four possible problem areas: grief, role disputes, role transitions, and interpersonal deficits. If the patient is experiencing grief, the therapist helps them mourn and then develop new relationships. Patients who are experiencing interpersonal conflict (role disputes) are helped to examine the relationship and either strategize resolutions or exit the dynamic. If the patient is experiencing a role transition, such as a recent breakup, move, or new role within a relationship (e.g., parenthood), the therapist helps them better understand and evaluate both the role they are assuming and the role they left behind and encourages exploration of opportunities within the new role. Finally, the patient may exhibit interpersonal deficits, which would require identification of problematic patterns and skills development. The last sessions help the patient strengthen their skills and strategize for future conflict (Weissman et al., 2008). IPT is an empirically supported treatment for use in major depression and bulimia but may not be as commonly available for patients as CBTs or client-centered therapies.

MECHANISMS OF CHANGE IN PSYCHOTHERAPY

Learning

It is often the case that changing certain patient behaviors is necessary for treatment success. Typically, a patient will have to change some of their behaviors in order for treatment to be considered successful. To effect change, therapists must understand how patients learn. There are many different models of learning used in psychotherapy that are translated from basic science. For example, using stimulus control methods drawn from classical conditioning described by Pavolv, individuals can be trained to use specific cues to develop new associations between stimuli and elicit an increased probability of an adaptive response in certain contexts. Substance users might be asked to remove cues that elicit craving and replace them with other cues in high-risk contexts for drug use. These new cues have a different learning history and can evoke a different response compared to stimuli associated with getting drunk or high. Operant conditioning (e.g., Skinner, 1965) follows the general principle (Thorndike's law of effect) that behavior followed by desirable consequences will be repeated, whereas a behavior followed by undesirable consequences will not (Thorndike, 1898, 1927). More specifically, a behavior results in the addition (positive) or removal (negative) of a stimulus, and this consequence is either reinforcing (making the behavior likely to be repeated) or punishing (making the behavior less likely to recur; Skinner 1965). For example, Yolanda might be awarded employee of the month for providing good customer service at her job. This is an example of positive reinforcement: She received the award for providing high-quality service.

Alternatively, Yolanda might find that if she gives her children a snack they stop asking her questions or behaving loudly when she is trying to focus on a household task like paying bills. This would be an example of negative reinforcement: By providing a snack, an aversive experience was taken away. If Yolanda does not pay a bill on time, she will have to pay a late fee; this is an example of a punishment. By missing the bill's deadline, Yolanda receives an aversive experience (Dixon & Rehfeldt, 2018).

To understand a patient's behavior, then, the therapist must look at its antecedents and consequences (Dixon & Rehfeldt, 2018). Take, for example, a therapist who sees a husband and wife who complain of the husband's explosive anger during shopping trips. If the therapist tracks the antecedents to the outburst, they might see that the husband makes frequent, ineffective requests to leave the store. As the husband's requests are unheeded, his anxiety rises. Once he explodes, his wife is suddenly aware and receptive to his need. They leave the store, and his behavior is temporarily rewarded. Perhaps his wife later punishes his behavior by giving him the cold shoulder. Unfortunately, behavior change becomes less likely as the duration between behavior and consequence increases (Dixon & Rehfeldt, 2018). The husband may not even realize that the cold shoulder is in response to his outburst, given how much time has elapsed. Fortunately, the therapist can help the wife to respond in a way that does not reinforce her husband's behavior. Once the positive consequences of a behavior are removed, the behavior will become less frequent in a process called extinction. The therapist can increase the likelihood of extinction by concomitantly reinforcing another behavior—perhaps by helping the husband effectively communicate his needs without anger, resulting in greater positive consequences (Dixon & Rehfeldt, 2018).

The timing and context of reinforcement can affect learning. Reinforcement can occur on a ratio or interval schedule, which can, in turn, be either fixed or variable. In a fixed ratio schedule, reinforcement occurs only after a certain number of responses, while occurring after an average number of responses in a variable ratio schedule. In an interval schedule, reinforcement occurs after either a fixed or variable period of time. Ratio schedules, particularly if reinforcing with higher frequency, result in the highest rates of responding (Skinner, 1965). The behaviors reinforced may be healthy or unhealthy. Variable ratio schedules, for instance, are responsible for the addictive nature of gambling (Rachlin, 1990). Finally, patient behavior is affected by the ability to understand which contextual factors are likely to elicit reinforcement. Phobias may develop when an individual has an aversive experience and then generalizes the conditioned response to other contexts by avoiding people, places, or things that are safe but associated with danger. For instance, a child who was tackled by a dog might later fear all dogs, including small dogs that look nothing like the one that attacked them. The therapist helps the patient learn new responses using known evidence-based principles of behavior change. For example, the therapist might help the patient discriminate between contexts and cues to learn when fear responding is and is not warranted by danger (Dixon & Rehfeldt, 2018).

Biological

Developments in neuroscience and brain imaging methodology have increased the ability to treat psychiatric disorders with pharmacology (i.e., antidepressant or antipsychotic medication), and some evidence highlights the effectiveness of dual pharmacology and psychotherapy treatments (Emslie et al., 2006; Ressler et al., 2004). Despite the broad application of both psychotherapy and medication to many psychiatric disorders, the neurobiological study of psychotherapy trails is significantly behind what we know about psychopharmacology. Much of the evidence for biological agents of change in psychotherapy has emerged from brain imaging studies comparing activity of particular brain regions pre- and posttreatment.

Early studies demonstrated that psychotherapy could produce measurable changes on brain activity. In one of the first studies of its kind, Baxter et al. (1992) demonstrated increased activity in the caudate nucleus among individuals with OCD who evidenced metabolic hypoactivation pretreatment of either SSRIs or exposure therapy. Another example can be found in depression, as psychotherapy has been shown to reverse hypoactivation of prefrontal areas with similar posttreatment effects as psychopharmacology (Brody et al., 2001; Martin et al., 2001).

Another way to bridge this gap of understanding is via pharmacological studies that can extend to psychotherapy (Etkin et al., 2005). For example, a seminal PET study for depression demonstrated that hyperactivity in the rostral anterior cingulate cortex (rACC) could predict treatment responders from nonresponders (Mayberg et al., 1997), a finding which was then replicated in EEG (Pizzagalli et al., 2001) and fMRI (Davidson et al., 2003) studies. The rACC is implicated in error detection and conflict monitoring, and individuals with depression at baseline may recruit more resources for cognitive and attentional processes needed to resolve emotionally laden conflicts. These examples of biological findings (i.e., the link between rACC activity and cognitive control) can be applied to the practice of psychotherapy (i.e., behavioral skills that target conflict perception and resolution).

Advancements in understanding the neurobiological mechanisms of change in psychotherapy may have important implications on treatment at both group and individual levels. At the group level, biological mechanisms can inform large-scale treatment design. At the idiographic level, the functional characteristics of an individual's brain could become essential to treatment matching and outcome prediction. Although there is now little dispute about the ability of psychotherapy to promote neurobiological change, future research will need to more clearly disentangle the relative contributions of medication and therapy and inform how we may apply group findings in individual psychotherapy sessions.

MULTICULTURAL CONSIDERATIONS

Attending to cultural and contextual factors in therapy is associated with lower rates of attrition, stronger therapeutic alliance, and better treatment outcomes (Hay, 2004 Lie et al., 2001; Tao et al., 2015). Thus, it is essential to consider different facets of a patient's identity when providing psychotherapy. These factors influence all parts of the therapy process, including assessment, therapeutic alliance, case conceptualization, and provision of therapy.

With regard to assessment, contextual and cultural factors influence how patients describe and understand their psychological concerns (Hinton & Patel, 2017). For example, patients from Asian backgrounds may be likely to report more physical complaints than emotional ones when experiencing depression. On the other hand, patients who have been repeatedly invalidated may overexpress their symptoms as a way to communicate their distress. With regard to Yolanda, her upbringing and life experiences will likely influence how she discusses her symptoms (e.g., she might use Venezuelan terminology). Therefore, as part of developing an accurate understanding of the patient's problems, it is necessary to consider the cultural and contextual factors that shape their experience and how they report their symptoms.

When it comes to establishing a therapeutic relationship, these factors can influence how much patients trust their therapist and the mental health care system in general. Patients from underrepresented backgrounds, such as Black or African American patients, have historically been exploited by large institutions and research studies, contributing to mistrust and ambivalence about receiving care from some clinical settings. Individuals who identify as sexual minorities may have had their sexuality pathologized or been forced into harmful treatments, such as conversion therapy. For patients who have had impactful experiences such as these, it is important to spend additional time building trust and establishing a collaborative therapeutic relationship. Beyond trust, contextual and cultural factors can affect therapist–patient interactions in other ways, including how deferential or assertive a patient is and how likely a patient is to express dissatisfaction with treatment. For example, some cultures place high status on doctors, and patients from these backgrounds may be more likely to be deferential to therapists. Other cultural backgrounds emphasize individualism and autonomy. Thus, these patients may be more likely to disagree with therapists or advocate for specific things they want.

Understanding contextual and cultural factors is crucial to case conceptualization. The process of conceptualizing a patient's presenting problems is collaborative, so it is important for the clinician not to impose their values onto the patient. Instead, the therapist can strive to be curious and nonjudgmental to get a better understanding of the patient's experiences. This process allows for collaboration and a shared understanding of the problem as well as how it will be addressed.

Because case conceptualization influences what kind of intervention will be delivered, it is important to note cultural and contextual factors may influence which types of therapy patients prefer. For example, a study of Latinx patients found these patients preferred individual therapy delivered in a primary care setting (Kaltman et al., 2014). A study of veterans found this population preferred to target sleep problems in treatments as opposed to focusing on trauma or depression (Gutner et al., 2018). Understanding these treatment preferences will influence treatment delivery. For example, treatment with some veterans could be most efficient if it begins by addressing sleep and then addresses other emotion-related concerns.

Cultural and contextual factors influence every part of the therapy process. The overarching principle of providing multiculturally conscious care is to remain curious and nonjudgmental while working to understand patients from their perspective. Doing so will allow the clinician to ask patients directly about the aspects of their identity that are most important to them, clarify cultural and contextual factors throughout treatment, and consider these factors when providing care.

CHALLENGES LEARNING PSYCHOTHERAPY

Psychotherapy is central to treating many psychiatric disorders, and psychiatry residents are often required to train in some methods of psychotherapy. All clinicians, however, could benefit from some level of psychotherapy training. Unfortunately, there are numerous challenges to learning psychotherapy within a medical training context. On a practical level, it is difficult to fit the amount of didactic and clinical hours needed to acquire skills and competency within the already saturated curriculum of medical school. The median number of hours a doctorate-level trainee has logged before applying to internship (the equivalent of a medical residency) is close to 600 hours; factoring in ample time for psychotherapy training is daunting calculus. Further, adding training modules that encompass the standards of APA competencies to the myriad existing competing demands in the medical training model likely requires significant programmatic restructuring.

A shift in focus from *what* medical students should know about psychotherapy to *how* psychotherapy can be taught and learned may be a helpful approach (Selzer et al., 2015). Integrating concepts of psychotherapy (i.e., common factors and measuring behavioral change) into preclinical curricula, didactics, and rotations can provide students with a framework and shared understanding of the dynamic relationship between psychological factors and physical health.

ETHICAL DILEMMAS AND SOLUTIONS

Ethical dilemmas abound in therapy. Fortunately, the American Psychological Association has provided an ethics code to guide clinical judgment (APA, 2017). This ethics code includes five general principles: beneficence and nonmaleficence, fidelity and responsibility, integrity, justice, and respect for people's rights and dignity. *Beneficence and nonmaleficence* asks psychologists to maximize benefit to the patient while minimizing harm. This principle requires psychologists to attend to the personal factors that may influence patient care, such as financial, social, or political conflicts of interest. *Fidelity and responsibility* requires psychologists to be responsible, professional and trustworthy colleagues and providers. *Integrity* asks psychologists to uphold accuracy and truth in clinical work and research and avoid dishonesty and corruption. *Justice* stipulates all people are entitled to quality care and that psychologists should not harm others through their limitations or biases. Finally, *respect for people's rights and dignity* means that confidentiality, privacy, and self-determination should be upheld. Clinicians should not act with prejudice or bias toward individuals on the basis of their identities and should ensure colleagues act with consideration and respect toward others (APA, 2017).

This ethical code also requires psychologists to practice according to the "scientific and professional knowledge of the discipline." Psychologists must remain up-to-date on research, communicate the effectiveness and limitations of interventions to patients, and use interventions that are professionally supported. Perhaps, a psychologist has been in private practice for 30 years and is less informed about contemporary interventions. This therapist can attend conferences and workshops and read the latest research to address this gap (Pope, 2018). Psychologists must also understand licensing requirements, laws, and regulations for their practice. Knowledge of the law guides decisions surrounding when it is necessary to break confidentiality to protect someone from harm. Another increasingly common dilemma is whether therapists can conduct sessions remotely. Perhaps, the patient requests teletherapy while they are on vacation. Legal regulations will determine whether the therapist's license extends to the patient's location and what kind of computer encryption is required (Pope, 2018). Further, it is important to understand the role of context in clinical care. Clinicians may work with patients with different social, moral, ethnic, and political backgrounds and must understand how their own beliefs affect their ability to deliver effective care to these patients (Pope, 2018). If the therapist is unable to overcome their own bias, they may seek consultation or decide to transfer the patient to a therapist who is more knowledgeable about the patient's background. Finally, psychologists must consider their own cognitive biases, as their own subjective lens can result in mistakes processing information (Pope, 2018).

Generally, when confronted with an ethical dilemma, the therapist should clearly state the dilemma, examine any factors that may bias their ability to effectively handle the problem, and determine who will be affected and consider their perspective. The therapist should review any appropriate ethical guidelines and consider consultation when determining a plan of action. They should then document the process and take responsibility for the outcome (Pope, 2018).

PSYCHOTHERAPY: ART OR SCIENCE?

Presently, the use of rigorous research methods allow us to evaluate the efficacy and effectiveness of psychotherapies. The advent and continued rise of evidence-based treatments suggests that research methods can be applied to psychotherapy in a meaningful way and produce treatments that are likely to benefit patients. As such, evidence-based treatments are firmly grounded in scientific principles.

At the level of the individual provider, there is still debate about whether psychotherapy is an art or a science. There is no doubt that empirically supported treatments or principles of change can be used in the provision of therapy. However, delivering therapy still requires flexibility and creativity that some may think of as falling more on the art side of the spectrum. For example, many therapists use metaphors in treatment to illustrate concepts. However, the metaphor used in treatment requires creativity. There are no scientific studies to indicate exactly when and how to deliver a metaphor. Thus, the therapist must rely on their own creativity and experience to choose and deliver a metaphor. As such, and in general, high-quality psychotherapy relies on both science and art to deliver effective care.

PSYCHOTHERAPY IN MEDICINE

Psychotherapies are commonly used when treating patients with medical problems. There are many reasons patients with medical disease might benefit from psychotherapy. For example, patients with diabetes may have difficulty managing health behaviors (e.g., eating, movement, tobacco, alcohol, or other substance use) that significantly impact their A1C level and associated medical complications. Patients with heart disease or cancer may have difficulties with depression and anxiety. Those with terminal illnesses may face existential questions about how to best live out the rest of their life with meaning, value, and purpose. Across medical diseases, many common mental health problems confer vulnerability for exacerbation of problems (e.g., rehospitalization after surgeries).

QUICK POINT

Psychotherapies are commonly used when treating patients with medical problems. Multiple studies report a reduction in medical costs, medical treatment utilization, and medical inpatient stays with the addition of psychotherapy when compared to medical treatment only.

Provision of medical procedures to patients with diseases may be an inadequate form of care if factors relevant to mental health are not considered. For example, patients seeking procedures such as bariatric surgery are often evaluated to ensure they are aware of the potential emotional impact of the surgery and able to implement and maintain the behavior change needed to ensure effective recovery from surgery (e.g., changes to diet and activity level). As another example, patients with HIV who experience depression are less likely to be adherent to antiretroviral treatment than those without depression (Olatunji et al., 2006). Thus, treating depression can help these patients take their medication consistently to manage their chronic illness (Olatunji et al., 2006). Because psychological and medical variables are so clearly intertwined, there is benefit to considering both when working with patients in medical settings.

SUMMARY

Psychotherapy is an effective method of treatment for psychiatric disorders, problems in living, and assisting patients through difficult or chronic medical diseases. Psychotherapy is used alone or in conjunction with other treatments (e.g., medications). There are different types of psychotherapies that are evidence-based for treating specific patient-presenting problems. Providers need to have a therapeutic framework within which the psychotherapy is conducted and a therapeutic alliance with the patients to effectively deliver care. The rise of evidence-based medicine has contributed to the prominence of CBT (and other evidence-based approaches, such as MI/MET) as a common type of psychotherapy for a wide range of problems. Across evidence-based therapies, there are known common factors that are not unique to any brand of therapy (e.g., therapeutic alliance, empathy, listening, support, and validation). Like psychotropic medications, psychotherapy is associated with neurobiological mechanisms of change. Many patients prefer psychotherapy as a treatment due to the absence of physical side effects found in psychotropic medications. The implementation of evidence-based psychotherapies in a way that carefully attends to the common factors of therapy involves creativity and flexibility as well as considering individual, cultural, and other contextual factors underlying the etiology and maintenance of patient problems.

RESOURCES

1. NIMH » Psychotherapies (nih.gov)
2. https://www.youtube.com/watch?v=vCQNtQA9Lg0
3. Psychotherapy and Genetic Neuroscience: An Emerging Dialog (nih.gov)

REFERENCES

Accreditation Council for Graduate Medical Education (ACGME). (2020). *ACGME program requirements for graduate medical education in psychiatry.* https://acgme.net/Portals/0/PFAssets/ProgramRequirements/400_Psychiatry_2020_TCC.pdf?ver=2020-06-19-123618-457.

American Psychological Association. (2017). *Ethical principles of psychologists and code of conduct.* http://www.apa.org/ethics/code/index.html

Arkowitz, H., & Miller, W. R. (2008). Learning, applying, and extending motivational interviewing. In H. Arkowitz, H. A. Westra, W. R. Miller, & S. Rollnick (Eds.), *Applications of motivational interviewing. Motivational interviewing in the treatment of psychological problems* (pp. 1–25). Guilford.

Arkowitz, H., Miller, W. R., & Rollnick, S. (Eds.). (2015). *Motivational interviewing in the treatment of psychological problems*. Guilford.

Barlow, D. H., Farchione, T. J., Bullis, J. R., Gallagher, M. W., Murray-Latin, H., Sauer-Zavala, S., Bentley, K. H., Thompson-Hollands, J., Conklin, L. R., Boswell, J. F., Ametaj, A., Carl, J. R., Boettcher, H. T., & Cassiello-Robbins, C. (2017). *The unified protocol for transdiagnostic treatment of emotional disorders compared with diagnosis-specific protocols for anxiety disorders: A randomized clinical trial. JAMA Psychiatry.* https://www.ncbi.nlm.nih.gov/pmc/articles/PMC5710228/

Barnett, E., Sussman, S., Smith, C., Rohrbach, L. A., & Spruijt-Metz, D. (2012). Motivational interviewing for adolescent substance use: A review of the literature. *Addictive Behaviors, 37*(12), 1325–1334.

Baxter, L. R., Jr, Schwartz, J. M., Bergman, K. S., Szuba, M. P., Guze, B. H., Mazziotta, J. C., Alazraki, A., Selin, C. E., Ferng, H. K., & Munford, P. (1992). Caudate glucose metabolic rate changes with both drug and behavior therapy for obsessive-compulsive disorder. *Archives of General Psychiatry, 49*(9), 681–689. https://doi.org/10.1001/archpsyc.1992.01820090009002

Beck, A. T., Steer, R. A., & Brown, G. K. (1996). *Manual for the Beck Depression Inventory-II*. Psychological Corporation.

Bentley, K. H., Boettcher, H. T., & Cassiello-Robbins, C. (2017). *Unified protocol for transdiagnostic treatment of emotional disorders: Therapist guide*. Oxford University Press.

Bordin, E. S. (1994). Theory and research on the therapeutic working alliance: New directions. *The Working Alliance: Theory, Research, and Practice, 173*, 13–37.

Boswell, J. F., Kraus, D. R., Miller, S. D., & Lambert, M. J. (2015). Implementing routine outcome monitoring in clinical practice: Benefits, challenges, and solutions. *Psychotherapy Research, 25*(1), 6–19.

Brody, A. L., Saxena, S., Stoessel, P., Gillies, L. A., Fairbanks, L. A., Alborzian, S., Phelps, M. E., Huang, S. C., Wu, H. M., Ho, M. L., Ho, M. K., Au, S. C., Maidment, K., & Baxter, L. R., Jr (2001). Regional brain metabolic changes in patients with major depression treated with either paroxetine or interpersonal therapy: Preliminary findings. *Archives of General Psychiatry, 58*(7), 631–640. https://doi.org/10.1001/archpsyc.58.7.631

Busch, F. N., Milrod, B. L., Singer, M. B., & Aronson, A. C. (2012). *Manual of panic focused psychodynamic psychotherapy–extended range* (Vol. 36). Routledge.

Cabaniss, D. L. (2016). *Psychodynamic psychotherapy: A clinical manual*. Wiley.

Carroll, K. M., Ball, S. A., Nich, C., Martino, S., Frankforter, T. L., Farentinos, C., Kunkel, L. E., Mikulich-Gilbertson, S. K., Morgenstern, J., Obert, J. L., Polcin, D., Snead, N., Woody, G. E., & National Institute on Drug Abuse Clinical Trials Network (2006). Motivational interviewing to improve treatment engagement and outcome in individuals seeking treatment for substance abuse: A multisite effectiveness study. *Drug and Alcohol Dependence*, *81*(3), 301–312. https://doi.org/10.1016/j.drugalcdep.2005.08.002

Carpenter, J. K., Andrews, L. A., Witcraft, S. M., Powers, M. B., Smits, J. A., & Hofmann, S. G. (2018). Cognitive behavioral therapy for anxiety and related disorders: A meta-analysis of randomized placebo-controlled trials. *Depression and Anxiety, 35*(6), 502–514.

Cecchin, G. (1987). Hypothesizing, circularity, and neutrality revisited: An invitation to childhood. *The Neuroscientist, 14*(4), 345–358.

Cozolino, L. (2014). *The neuroscience of human relationships: Attachment and the developing social brain*. Norton.

Cuijpers, P., Berking, M., Andersson, G., Quigley, L., Kleiboer, A., & Dobson, K. S. (2013). A meta-analysis of cognitive-behavioural therapy for adult depression, alone and in comparison with other treatments. *The Canadian Journal of Psychiatry, 58*(7), 376–385.

Cummings, S. M., Cooper, R. L., & Cassie, K. M. (2009). Motivational interviewing to affect behavioral change in older adults. *Research on Social Work Practice, 19*(2), 195–204.

Daeppen, J. B., Fortini, C., Bertholet, N., Bonvin, R., Berney, A., Michaud, P. A., Layat, C., & Gaume, J. (2012). Training medical students to conduct motivational interviewing: a randomized controlled trial. *Patient Education and Counseling, 87*(3), 313–318. https://doi.org/10.1016/j.pec.2011.12.005

Davidson, R. J., Irwin, W., Anderle, M. J., & Kalin, N. H. (2003). The neural substrates of affective processing in depressed patients treated with venlafaxine. *American Journal of Psychiatry, 160*(1), 64–75.

de Gee, E. A., Verdurmen, J. E., Bransen, E., de Jonge, J. M., & Schippers, G. M. (2014). A randomized controlled trial of a brief motivational enhancement for non-treatment-seeking adolescent cannabis users. *Journal of Substance Abuse Treatment, 47*(3), 181–188.

Dixon, M. R., & Rehfeldt, R. A. (2018). Core behavioral processes. *Process-based CBT: The science and core clinical competencies of cognitive behavioral therapy.* New Harbinger Publications.

Elliott, R., Bohart, A. C., Watson, J. C., & Greenberg, L. S. (2011). Empathy. *Psychotherapy, 48*(1), 43–49. https://doi.org/10.1037/a0022187

Emslie, G., Kratochvil, C., Vitiello, B., Silva, S., Mayes, T., McNulty, S., Weller, E., Waslick, B., Casat, C., Walkup, J., Pathak, S., Rohde, P., Posner, K., March, J., Columbia Suicidality Classification Group, & TADS Team. (2006). Treatment for Adolescents with Depression Study (TADS):Safety results. *Journal of the American Academy of Child and Adolescent Psychiatry, 45*(12), 1440–1455. https://doi.org/10.1097/01.chi.0000240840.63737.1d

Etkin, A., Pittenger, C., Polan, H. J., & Kandel, E. R. (2005). Toward a neurobiology of psychotherapy: Basic science and clinical applications. *The Journal of Neuropsychiatry and Clinical Neurosciences, 17*(2), 145–158.

First, M. B. (2014). Structured clinical interview for the DSM (SCID). *The Encyclopedia of Clinical Psychology,* 1–6.

Fruzzetti, A. E., & Ruork, A. K. (2018). Validation principles and practices in dialectical behaviour therapy. *The Oxford Handbook of Dialectical Behaviour Therapy,* 325–344.

Gabbard, G. O. (2014). *Psychodynamic psychiatry in clinical practice.* American Psychiatric Publication.

Gifford, E. V., Kohlenberg, B. S., Hayes, S. C., Pierson, H. M., Piasecki, M. P., Antonuccio, D. O., & Palm, K. M. (2011). Does acceptance and relationship focused behavior therapy contribute to bupropion outcomes? A randomized controlled trial of functional analytic psychotherapy and acceptance and commitment therapy for smoking cessation. *Behavior Therapy, 42*(4), 700–715.

Gutner, C. A., Pedersen, E. R., & Drummond, S. P. (2018). Going direct to the consumer: Examining treatment preferences for veterans with insomnia, PTSD, and depression. *Psychiatry Research, 263*, 108–114.

Hayes, S. C. (2004). Acceptance and commitment therapy, relational frame theory, and the third wave of behavioral and cognitive therapies. *Behavior Therapy, 35*(4), 639–665.

Hayes, S. C., & Hofmann, S. G. (Eds.). (2018). *Process-based CBT: The science and core clinical competencies of cognitive behavioral therapy.* New Harbinger.

Hinton, D. E., & Patel, A. (2017). Cultural adaptations of cognitive behavioral therapy. *Psychiatric Clinics, 40*(4), 701–714.

Hofmann, S. G., Asnaani, A., Vonk, I. J., Sawyer, A. T., & Fang, A. (2012). The efficacy of cognitive behavioral therapy: A review of meta-analyses. *Cognitive Therapy and Research, 36*(5), 427–440.

Hofmann, S. G., & Hayes, S. C. (2019). The future of intervention science: Process-based therapy. *Clinical Psychological Science, 7*(1), 37–50.

Horvath, A. O., Del Re, A. C., Flückiger, C., & Symonds, D. (2011). Alliance in individual psychotherapy. *Psychotherapy, 48*(1), 9.

Horvath, A. O., & Greenberg, L. S. (1989). Development and validation of the Working Alliance Inventory. *Journal of Counseling Psychology, 36*(2), 223.

Kaltman, S., Hurtado de Mendoza, A., Gonzales, F. A., & Serrano, A. (2014). Preferences for trauma-related mental health services among Latina immigrants from Central America, South America, and Mexico. *Psychological Trauma: Theory, Research, Practice, and Policy, 6*(1), 83.

Kroenke, K., & Spitzer, R. L. (2002). The PHQ-9: A new depression diagnostic and severity measure. *Psychiatric Annals, 32*(9), 509–515.

Kuyken, W., Padesky, C. A. & Dudley, R. (2008a). *Collaborative case conceptualization: Working effectively with clients in cognitive-behavioral therapy.* Guilford.

Kuyken, W., Padesky, C. A., & Dudley, R. (2008b). The science and practice of case conceptualization. *Behavioural and Cognitive Psychotherapy, 36*(6), 757.

Lie, D. A., Lee-Rey, E., Gomez, A., Bereknyei, S., & Braddock, C. H. (2011). Does cultural competency training of health professionals improve patient outcomes? A systematic review and proposed algorithm for future research. *Journal of General Internal Medicine, 26*(3), 317–325.

Linehan, M. (2014). *DBT skills training mannual* (2nd ed.). Guilford.

Martin, S. D., Martin, E., Rai, S. S., Richardson, M. A., & Royall, R. (2001). Brain blood flow changes in depressed patients treated with interpersonal psychotherapy or venlafaxine hydrochloride: Preliminary findings. *Archives of General Psychiatry, 58*(7), 641–648.

Mayberg, H. S., Brannan, S. K., Mahurin, R. K., Jerabek, P. A., Brickman, J. S., Tekell, J. L., Silva, J. A., McGinnis, S., Glass, T. G., Martin, C. C., & Fox, P. T. (1997). Cingulate function in depression: A potential predictor of treatment response. *Neuroreport, 8*(4), 1057–1061. https://doi.org/10.1097/00001756-199703030-00048

McKenzie, K. J., Pierce, D., & Gunn, J. M. (2015). A systematic review of motivational interviewing in healthcare: the potential of motivational interviewing to address the lifestyle factors relevant to multimorbidity. *Journal of Comorbidity, 5*(1), 162–174.

McNeil, D. W., Addicks, S. H., & Randall, C. L. (2017). *Motivational interviewing and motivational interactions for health behavior change and maintenance*. Oxford University Press.

Miller, W. R., & Rollnick, S. (2013). *Motivational interviewing: Helping people change* (3rd ed.). Guilford Press.

Milrod, B. (1997). *Manual of panic-focused psychodynamic psychotherapy*. American Psychiatric Publishing.

Milrod, B., Busch, F., Shapiro, T., Leon, A. C., & Aronson, A. (2013). A pilot study of psychodynamic psychotherapy in 18- to 21-year-old patients with panic disorder. *The Annals of the American Society for Adolescent Psychiatry, 29*, 289.

Moral, R. R., Torres, L. A., Ortega, L. P., Larumbe, M. C., Villalobos, A. R., García, J. A., Rejano, J. M., & Collaborative Group ATEM-AP Study (2015). Effectiveness of motivational interviewing to improve therapeutic adherence in patients over 65 years old with chronic diseases: A cluster randomized clinical trial in primary care. *Patient Education and Counseling, 98*(8), 977–983. https://doi.org/10.1016/j.pec.2015.03.008

Moyers, T. B., & Houck, J. (2011). Combining motivational interviewing with cognitive-behavioral treatments for substance abuse: Lessons from the COMBINE research project. *Cognitive and Behavioral Practice, 18*(1), 38–45.

Nienhuis, J. B., Owen, J., Valentine, J. C., Winkeljohn Black, S., Halford, T. C., Parazak, S. E., Budge, S., & Hilsenroth, M. (2018). Therapeutic alliance, empathy, and genuineness in individual adult psychotherapy: A meta-analytic review. *Psychotherapy Research: Journal of the Society for Psychotherapy Research, 28*(4), 593–605. https://doi.org/10.1080/10503307.2016.1204023

Norcross, J. C., & Lambert, M. J. (2011). *Psychotherapy relationships that work II* (vol. 48). Educational Publishing Foundation.

Olatunji, B. O., Mimiaga, M. J., O Cleirigh, C., & Safren, S. A. (2006). A review of treatment studies of depression in HIV. *Topics in HIV Medicine, 14*(3), 112.

Pilecki, B., & McKay, D. (2013). The theory-practice gap in cognitive-behavior therapy. *Behavior Therapy, 44*(4), 541–547.

Pinsker, H. (2014). *A primer of supportive psychotherapy*. Routledge.

Pizzagalli, D., Pascual-Marqui, R. D., Nitschke, J. B., Oakes, T. R., Larson, C. L., Abercrombie, H. C., Schaefer, S. M., Koger, J. V., Benca, R. M., & Davidson, R. J. (2001). Anterior cingulate activity as a predictor of degree of treatment response in major depression: evidence from brain electrical tomography analysis. *The American Journal of Psychiatry, 158*(3), 405–415. https://doi.org/10.1176/appi.ajp.158.3.405

Pope, K. S. (2018). Ethical competence in behavioral and cognitive therapies. In S. C. Hayes & S. G. Hofmann (Eds.), *Process-based CBT: The science and core clinical competencies of cognitive behavioral therapy* (pp. 83–98). New Harbinger Publications, Inc.

Rachlin, H. (1990). Why do people gamble and keep gambling despite heavy randomized placebo-controlled trials. *Depression and Anxiety, 35*, 502–514.

Raskin, N. J., Rogers, C. R., & Witty, M. C. (2008). Client-centered therapy. *Current Psychotherapies, 8*, 141–186.

Ressler, K. J., Rothbaum, B. O., Tannenbaum, L., Anderson, P., Graap, K., Zimand, E., Hodges, L., & Davis, M. (2004). Cognitive enhancers as adjuncts to psychotherapy: Use of D-cycloserine in phobic individuals to facilitate extinction of fear. *Archives of General Psychiatry, 61*(11), 1136–1144. https://doi.org/10.1001/archpsyc.61.11.1136

Rollnick, S., Heather, N., & Bell, A. (1992). Negotiating behaviour change in medical settings: The development of brief motivational interviewing. *Journal of Mental Health, 1*(1), 25–37.

Selzer, R., Ellen, S., & Adler, R. (2015). Teaching psychological processes and psychotherapy to medical students. *Australasian Psychiatry, 23*(1), 69–71.

Skinner, B. F. (1965). *Science and human behavior.* Simon and Schuster.

Tao, K. W., Owen, J., Pace, B. T., & Imel, Z. E. (2015). A meta-analysis of multicultural competencies and psychotherapy process and outcome. *Journal of Counseling Psychology, 62*(3), 337.

Thorndike, E. L. (1898). Animal intelligence: An experimental study of the associative processes in animals. *The Psychological Review: Monograph Supplements, 2*(4).

Thorndike, E. L. (1927). The law of effect. *The American Journal of Psychology, 39*(14), 212–222.

Trauer, J. M., Qian, M. Y., Doyle, J. S., Rajaratnam, S. M., & Cunnington, D. (2015). Cognitive behavioral therapy for chronic insomnia: A systematic review and meta-analysis. *Annals of Internal Medicine, 163*(3), 191–204.

Tsujimoto, S. (2008). The prefrontal cortex: Functional neural development during early childhood. *The Neuroscientist, 14*(4), 345–358.

Wampold, B. E. (2001). The great psychotherapy debate: Models. *Methods, and Findings, 62.*

Warburton, K. (2014). Establishing a therapeutic frame. In J. Lees (Ed.), *Clinical counselling in context: An introduction* (pp. 80–85). Taylor & Francis.

Weinberg, I., Ronningstam, E., Goldblatt, M. J., Schechter, M., & Maltsberger, J. T. (2011). Common factors in empirically supported treatments of borderline personality disorder. *Current Psychiatry Reports, 13*(1), 60–68.

Weissman, M. M., Markowitz, J. C., & Klerman, G. (2008). *Comprehensive guide to interpersonal psychotherapy.* Basic Books.

Wolpe, J. (1968). Psychotherapy by reciprocal inhibition. *Conditional Reflex: A Pavlovian Journal of Research & Therapy, 3*(4), 234–240.

UNIT V

SPECIAL TOPICS IN PSYCHIATRY

This unit provides complementary information, including a chapter focused on suicide, psychosomatic medicine, adverse childhood experiences and resilience, and cultural psychiatry. Mental health problems are encountered by all physicians regardless of their specialty. The chapter provides a view of mental health as encountered in other specialties, such as in the pediatrician or geriatrician's office. This is a useful perspective for medical students who may not go on to specialize in psychiatry. Lastly, research in psychiatry continues to drive understanding and effective treatments of mental health conditions. The chapter on research provides information on studies often used in psychiatry and the behavioral sciences, useful tips for interpreting study findings effectively, and classifying the quality of evidence provided by a study. This unit also provides an overview of clinical trials and the FDA drug development process, providing some understanding of use of medications on and off label in clinical care.

CHAPTER 34

Suicide[1]

Nandhini Madhanagopal, M.D. and Sindhu Idicula, M.D.

> *"Hope is a necessity for normal life and the major weapon against the suicide impulse."*
>
> — Karl A. Menninger

OBJECTIVES

After reading this chapter, students will be able to do the following:

- describe the epidemiology, risk factors, warning signs, and protective factors of suicide, suicide risk assessment, and management of suicidal patients
- review the roles of neurotransmitters, endocrine pathways, and neurotrophins in suicide
- examine the risk of suicide in patients with medical illnesses and the need for screening for suicide in the primary care physician's office

CASE VIGNETTE

Mr. A is a 68-year-old widower who currently lives alone. He is estranged from his family. He has a couple of friends with whom he spends time. He has a history of major depressive disorder, alcohol use disorder, and one suicide attempt by medication overdose during an episode of depression. He has been stable for over 8 years and discontinued medications for depression 3 years ago. Mr. A was recently diagnosed with degenerative disc disease that caused severe back pain. Although he visited the nearest emergency department for severe back pain, the prescribed pain medications did not seem to help much. He began drinking alcohol and stayed at home in his bed most of the day. His friends have been reaching out to him, but he neither attends events with them nor returns their calls. Out of concern, a friend requested a wellness check from the authorities. Mr. A was found unresponsive on his bedroom floor lying next to empty alcohol bottles and opened pain prescription bottles. An autopsy report confirmed that Mr. A had died of an overdose of prescription pain pills with alcohol intoxication.

---

1 Readers may also see "Depressive Disorders" (Chapter 20) and "Adjustment- and Grief-Related Disorders" (Chapter 22) for related material.

DEFINITIONS AND KEY CONCEPTS

Suicide is a global phenomenon and occurs throughout the life span. The word *suicide* is derived from the Latin *suicidim*: *sui*, meaning "of oneself," and *cidium* means "a killing" (Harris, 2001). Suicide is defined as "death caused by injuring oneself with intent to die," and a suicide attempt is "when someone harms themselves with to intent end their life but they do not die as a result of their actions." Suicidal ideation is the presence of thoughts regarding suicide (CDC, 2020). Nonsuicidal self-injury is defined as "direct and deliberate destruction of body tissue without any suicidal intent" (Huang et al., 2020), and it significantly increases the risk for future suicide attempt.

INTRODUCTION

Attitudes toward suicide vary with different cultures, and suicide has been viewed through the lenses of philosophy, ethics, and religion. Literature mentions suicide dating back to 500 BC in the Roman period (Harris, 2001). The Greek and Roman cultures considered suicide positively—as choosing death over disgrace. Suicide was deemed to be a sin and was penalized with the origin of Judeo-Christian ethics in 300–400 AD. A shift in thinking began in 1500 and 1800 when suicide was decriminalized and studied as a manifestation of melancholy. Researchers began studying suicide in the 19th century, and society has moved from creating laws to reduce suicide to getting medical help for those who struggle with suicidal ideations (Harris, 2001).

Historically, the discourse about suicide is fraught with pejorative language alluding to the intentions and motivations of the person dying by suicide. Recent focus on using neutral language, such as "died by suicide" and "attempted suicide," is recommended to destigmatize and encourage help seeking (Padmanathan et al., 2019).

EPIDEMIOLOGY

Every year, 800,000 people die of suicide, which translates to one person every 40 seconds (WHO, 2019). Seventy-nine percent of suicides occurred in the low- and middle-income countries (WHO, 2019). One study estimates the 12-month prevalence of suicide attempts and suicidal ideation to be 25 and 175 times the rate of suicide (Lutz et al., 2017). The rates of suicide, method of suicide, socioeconomic status of the individual, and access to health care vary based on region and country.

Age

Suicide is the second leading cause of death among 10 to 34 years old, the fourth leading cause of death among people aged 35 to 54 years, and the eighth leading cause of death among people aged 55 to 64 years old (CDC, 2020). Overall, more young people die by suicide than older individuals in terms of absolute numbers; however, rates per age group are six to eight times higher in the elderly (Bertolote & Fleischmann, 2002).

Gender

Males die of suicide almost twice as often as females, whereas females engage more frequently in suicide attempts (Freeman et al., 2017).

Socioeconomic Variables

Low income, unemployment, low education, poor social support, climate change, natural catastrophe, war, and migration are high risk factors for suicide, and they also influence suicide rates by increasing risk of psychiatric illness (Bachmann, 2018).

Special Groups

Certain groups of individuals, such as veterans, police, firefighters, first responders, minorities, refugees, and asylum seekers, are at a higher risk of suicide than the general population. Lesbian, gay, bisexual, and transgender individuals are at an elevated risk of suicide; rate of suicide attempt among transgender individuals is up to 30–50% in some countries (Bachmann, 2018).

Method of Suicide

Suicide methods vary by regions. Firearm was the most common method in the United States, whereas hanging was the most common method in Asia, Africa, Europe, Australia, and New Zealand (Bachmann, 2018).

Suicide and Mental Illness

Individuals with a psychiatric disorder had an eight-time increased risk of suicide compared to those without a psychiatric disorder (Too et al., 2019). A meta-analysis documented increased suicide risk in female anorexia nervosa patients (31-fold higher risk), patients with depression (20-fold

KEY POINT

Suicide is the second leading cause of death among 10 to 34 years old, and the leading cause of nonaccidental deaths among adolescents and young adults. In terms of absolute numbers, more young people die by suicide than older individuals. However, rates per age group are six to eight times higher in the elderly (Bertolote & Fleischmann, 2002).

QUICK POINT

Mental illness increases the risk of suicide. Individuals with a psychiatric disorder had an eight-time increased risk of suicide compared to those without a psychiatric disorder (Too et al., 2019). Up to 90% of those who die of suicide have an underlying psychiatric illness (Bertolote & Fleischmann, 2002).

higher risk), bipolar disorder (17-fold higher risk), opioid use disorder (14-fold higher risk), and schizophrenia (13-fold higher risk; Chesney et al., 2014). The 4–12 weeks following discharge from an inpatient psychiatric hospital is a highly vulnerable period for suicide, particularly among men and those with previous attempts (Bachmann, 2018).

NEUROBIOLOGY

Understanding the biological factors that underlie the psychological and behavioral changes leading up to suicide has been studied more rigorously after a recent call to action by the WHO.

Genetic Factors

The specific heritability of suicide was 17%, and for suicide attempts it was 36% after controlling for genetic transmission of psychiatric disorders (Lutz et al., 2017). Another study documented, after controlling for familial transmission of mood disorder, that the risk of suicide attempt by offspring increased five-fold when there is a history of parental suicide attempt (Brent et al., 2015).

KEY POINT

Low CSF 5HIAA (hydroxy indole acetic acid, a metabolite of serotonin) has been associated with attempted and completed suicide.

Role of Serotonin

Studies have widely documented low CSF 5HIAA (hydroxy indole acetic acid, a metabolite of serotonin) in patients who attempted suicide and in those who subsequently died of suicide (Lester, 1995). This finding is common in those with impulsive–aggressive traits, hence suicide and impulsive-aggressive traits may share serotonin regulatory pathways that are impaired with serotonin dysregulation.

Changes in Neural Circuitry

Alterations in the medial and lateral prefrontal cortex and their connections may lead to increased negative thoughts, difficulty regulating emotions, and suicidal thoughts, and disturbances in the dorsal prefrontal cortex and inferior frontal gyrus may play a role in suicide attempts. A combination of impairments in the ventral and dorsal prefrontal cortex may contribute to conversion of suicidal ideations to lethal behavior due to decreased inhibition of behavior and inflexible and maladaptive decision-making and planning (Schmaal et al., 2020).

The Hypothalamic Pituitary Adrenal Axis and Neuroinflammation

Stress is also a major risk factor for suicide. Hypothalamic–pituitary–adrenal (HPA) axis abnormalities and the presence of inflammatory cytokines in the brain are associated with suicidal vulnerability. Interestingly, such changes are also observed in patients with early life adversity, which is one of the biggest risk factors for suicide and suicide attempts.

Neurotrophins

Studies have documented decreased BDNF (brain-derived neurotrophic factor) and TrkB (a receptor for BDNF) levels in the postmortem brain of suicide victims (Dwivedi et al., 2003).

> **CLINICAL TIP**
>
> Suicide is a highly complex and multifactorial phenomenon. Suicide risk factors have been categorized as distal (indirectly contributing by increased risk), mediating, and proximal (temporally associated with suicide attempt or suicide and act as a precipitant).

CLINICAL MANIFESTATIONS

Risk Factors

Suicide is a highly complex and multifactorial phenomenon. Up to 90% of those who die of suicide have an underlying psychiatric illness (Bertolote & Fleischmann, 2002). However, many other factors, including social, cultural, economic, and individual circumstances, contribute to an increased risk of suicide. Hence, prevention of suicide involves optimal assessment and management of psychiatric illnesses and suicide risk at an individual level to addressing factors impacting the communities and populations.

Suicide is multifactorial, and there are different models that explain the events leading up to suicide. The risk factors have been categorized as distal (indirectly contributing by increased risk), mediating, and proximal (temporally associated with suicide attempt or suicide and act as precipitant). See Figure 34.1 for examples of risk factors and Figure 34.3 for a helpful mnemonic.

Warning Signs of Suicide

Educating professionals and the public increasing awareness of the warning signs of suicide is vital for early identification and intervention of individuals at risk. Rudd et al. (2006) described warning signs as the earliest detectable sign that demonstrates heightened risk for suicide in the near-term risk (e.g., minutes, hours, to a few days). Severe anxiety and extreme agitation were the most common precipitating factors for suicide in an inpatient study (see Table 34.1; Busch et al., 2003).

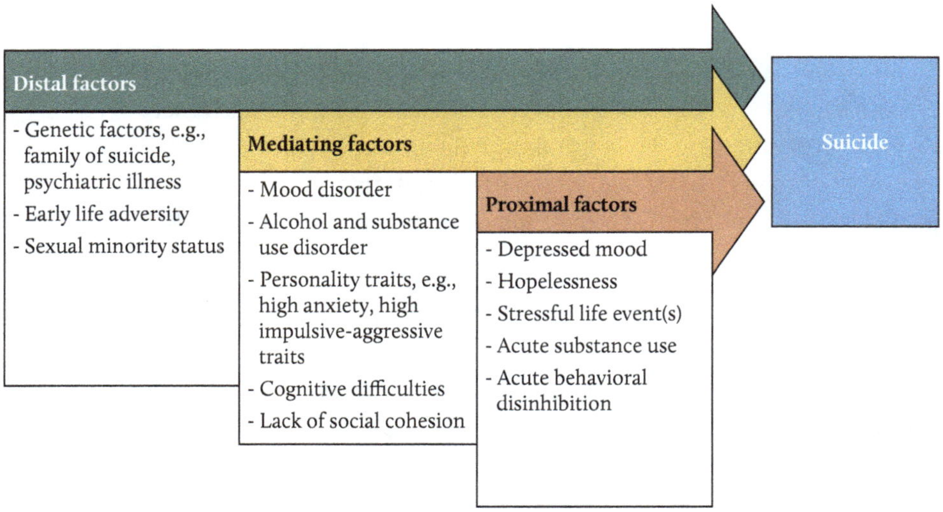

FIGURE 34.1 Risk factors for suicide.

Protective Factors

Protective factors usually mitigate risk factors, increase help-seeking behavior during stressful periods of life, and decrease suicidal behaviors. Protective factors can be divided into intrinsic factors (i.e., the person's own abilities to cope and overcome stress and adversity [self-esteem and self-efficacy]) and extrinsic factors, which include a supportive environment (family relationships and friendships). See Table 34.1 for protective factors.

BIOPSYCHOSOCIAL MODEL

Biological Factors

Biological factors that predispose an individual to suicide and suicide attempts include previous suicide attempts, diagnosis of MDD, bipolar disorder, schizophrenia, severe anxiety disorder, personality disorder, and alcohol and substance use disorder. Early-life adversity and psychosocial stress are significant risk factors for suicide and contribute to biological changes in the brain as well (Turecki & Brent, 2016).

Psychosocial Factors

According to Batty et al. (2018), the following are the most important psychosocial factors playing a role in suicide:

- *Cognitive function*—Studies indicate that impaired cognitive function is negatively associated with suicide risk (Batty et al., 2010). Children exposed to violence demonstrate lower levels of cognitive functioning. People with lower IQs may struggle with problem-solving during a crisis, whereas higher cognitive abilities are associated with greater internal locus of control and less suicide risk.

- *Early-life adversity*—Childhood adversity is associated with significant increase in self-harm, suicidal ideations, suicide attempts, and suicide. Studies found a dose–response relationship: The higher the number of adverse childhood experiences, the higher the risk of suicide is. Exposure to suicide in the family, parental psychiatric illness, and parental criminality were associated with greater risk of suicide (Björkenstam et al., 2017).
- *Personality type*—Batty et al. (2018) concluded that characteristics of empathy and cooperation, which correlate with agreeableness, are associated with lower suicide risk, whereas individuals with impulsivity and hostility typical of a neurotically prone personality are associated with a higher risk of suicide.
- *Psychosocial stress*—Acute and chronic stressors contribute to suicide attempts and suicide. Loss events, including loss of a person, health, and material possession, significantly increased the risk of suicide (Cheng et al., 2000). Stressful life events, such as financial trouble, job problems, unemployment, residence change in younger victims, and somatic illness in elderly victims, were found to be associated with suicide (Heikkinen & Lönnqvist, 1995). Low levels of communication between parents and children, family discord, loss of a romantic relationship, disciplinary trouble at school or with the law, and academic difficulties often precede adolescents' suicide (Shaffer & Pfeffer, 2001).
- *Social integration*—Social integration, in particular, marital status, social network size, and religious service attendance, offers protection against suicide (Tsai et al., 2014).

THE INTEGRATED MOTIVATIONAL–VOLITIONAL MODEL

In this model of suicide, it is proposed that defeat and entrapment lead to suicidal ideation and the presence of volitional moderators, such as access to means of suicide, exposure to suicidal behavior, fearlessness about death, and increased physical pain tolerance, impulsivity, and past suicidal behavior drive the transition from suicidal ideation to an attempt or suicide (O'Connor & Kirtley, 2018).

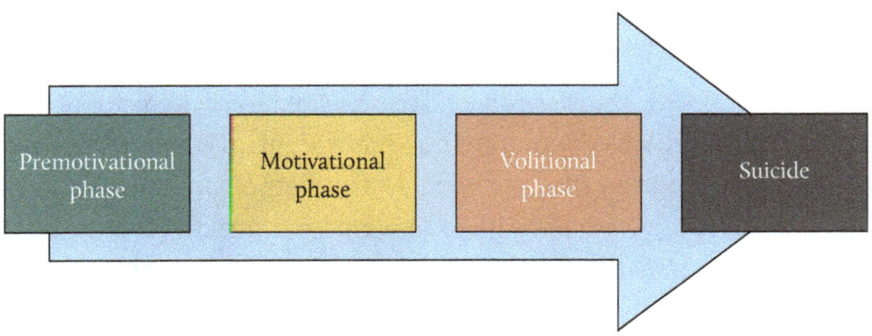

FIGURE 34.2 The integrated motivational–volitional model.

CLINICAL TIP

Suicide risk assessment is an essential and critical component of clinical practice. Of those who die by suicide, about one half had contact with a primary care professional within 1 month of their suicide, and about one in five suicide victims had visited a mental health professional within a month before their suicide (Luoma et al., 2002).

SUICIDE RISK ASSESSMENT

Suicide risk assessment is an essential and critical component of clinical practice. Of those who have died by suicide, about 1 half had contact with a primary care professional within 1 month of their suicide, and about one in five suicide victims had visited a mental health professional within a month before their suicide (Luoma et al., 2002). Hence, universal assessment and detection of patients at risk of suicide in primary care (outpatient and ED) and psychiatric care settings are vital in the prevention of suicide. However, adolescents are less likely to seek help in the last year and month before suicide, and more effective outreached programs are required in this population (Turecki & Brent, 2016).

Previous suicide attempt predicts the risk of suicide. Hopelessness, helplessness, worthlessness, and ambivalence are important indicators of elevated suicide risk. Less than one third of suicidal patients express their suicidal intent to the treating health care professional. Therefore, it is important to obtain collateral information. Mixed-state bipolar disorder and psychotic symptoms in MDD significantly increase the risk of suicide and require close monitoring (Turecki & Brent, 2016).

Scales Used for Suicide Risk Assessment

The Columbia Suicide Severity Rating Scale (C-SSRS) is a measure widely used to assess suicide risk in emergency departments, psychiatric clinics, and primary care settings. It has suicidal ideation intensity, suicidal ideation severity, and suicidal behavior subscales. The C-SSRS scale is designed to assess suicidal ideation and behavior in the past month in individuals 12 years and older. The scale also provides intervention based on the score. The authors of the scale have made different versions for use with very young children and those with cognitive impairment in English and Spanish on their Columbia Lighthouse project team website (Columbia Lighthouse Project, 2016). The short version is a six-question list that assesses for suicidal ideation severity and is used as a screening tool in primary care settings.

C-SSRS scores were found to be a significant predictor of suicidal behavior across a 6-month period in adolescents (Posner et al., 2011). Another study reported that in the adult psychiatric population with a recent episode of self-harm, C-SSRS total scores and suicidal ideation intensity scores were significant predictors of suicide attempts within 6 months (Lindh et al., 2018).

The Suicide Assessment Five-Step Evaluation and Triage (SAFE-T; Substance Abuse and Mental Health Services Administration [SAMHSA], 2009) is based on the APA practice guidelines for suicide assessment. It incorporates identifying the patient's risk and protective factors for suicide; assessing for suicidal thoughts, intents, plans, and behaviors; determining risk level; and choosing an appropriate intervention. Training the emergency department nurses to use SAFE-T-improved assessments for suicide risk and increased knowledge of identifying risk and protective factors and determining risk level and appropriate intervention (Rico, 2016).

TABLE 34.1 Warning Signs, Risks, and Protective Factors for Suicide

Risk factors for suicide	Warning signs for suicide	Protective factors for suicide
Suicidal ideation with intent and/or plan	Someone threatening to hurt or kill themselves	Someone who is hopeful or has reason to live
Past suicide attempt(s)	Someone looking for ways to kill themselves (e.g., seeking access to pills or weapons)	Responsibility for family, kids, or pets
Depressed mood (recent change in mood)	Obsessions with death or writing about death	Demonstrates adaptive coping skills and effective problem-solving
Hopelessness	One or more intense affective states	Religious faith
Acute anxiety, agitation or aggression, impulsivity, psychosis, and command hallucinations	Acting recklessly or engaging in risky behaviors	Good social support (family and friends)
Alcohol or substance intoxication or withdrawal	Feeling trapped or like there is no way out	Connected to outpatient mental health services and compliant with treatment
Stressful life event (loss or financial difficulty)	Increasing alcohol and drug use	Extraversion and optimism
Withdrawing from family and friends	No reason for living or no sense of purpose in life	Self-esteem, self-efficacy, and social skills
Poor social support (family and friends)	Sudden changes in personality, behavior, eating, or sleeping patterns	Healthy lifestyle
Family history of suicide	Decreased academic or work performance	
Recent inpatient hospital discharge and recent emergency room visit for psychiatry chief complaint		
Chronic medical illness, pain, and disability		

MANAGEMENT OF SUICIDAL PATIENTS

APA guidelines from 2003 outline the following as the most appropriate steps to take in the management of a patient with suicidality as part of their clinical picture (Jacobs et al., 2003):

1. It is important to establish and maintain a therapeutic alliance with the patient and keep in mind that the suicidal patient may not be motivated to collaborate in creating a treatment plan. Obtaining collateral information from family members is vital.
2. Prioritize patient safety during the suicide risk assessment and management process by keeping the environment (of the clinic or ED) safe and free of access to lethal means—for example, by removing the patient's belongings and any other sharps from the patient room.
3. Determine the appropriate treatment setting is based on the suicide risk assessment. Admission to inpatient psychiatry is indicated when the patient is at imminent risk of suicide. The patient may need to be admitted (ICU versus medicine floor) if the assessment was made following a suicide attempt that requires medical attention. Other treatment settings in the order of less-intense supervision include partial hospitalization, an intensive outpatient program, and regular follow-ups at the psychiatric outpatient clinic.
4. Create a treatment plan in collaboration with the patient and their family. Improve adherence to the treatment plan by regularly checking in with the patient regarding effectiveness of the treatment plan, monitoring for adverse effects of medications, and addressing the psychosocial stressors that interfere with implementing the treatment plan.
5. Periodic reassessment for suicide risk is important, as suicidality tends to wax and wane.

Psychopharmacology

A meta-analysis documented that treatment of depression with antidepressants reduced suicidal ideation in those 25 years and older. In those 24 years and younger, antidepressant treatment led to a decrease in depressive symptoms but did not always diminish suicidal ideation (Gibbons et al., 2012). Another meta-analysis reported that antidepressant treatment in those younger than 25 years old is associated with a 1%–2% risk difference in the incidence of suicidal events (new onset or worsening of suicidal ideation or suicide attempts). The study concluded that the effects of antidepressants on suicidal thought and behavior are strongly age dependent; benefits increase, and risk decreases with advancing age (Stone et al., 2009).

Lithium in drinking water may be associated with reduced suicide risk in the general population (Vita et al., 2015). A study following 51,345 bipolar patients found that the incidence of suicide-related events was down by 14% in those who were on lithium but not during valproate treatment and recommended considering lithium for bipolar disorder patients with suicidal intentions (Song et al., 2017). It is unclear how lithium leads to a decrease in suicidal behavior; it is possibly related to its mood-stabilizing effects and effects on decreasing impulsivity and aggression.

> **KEY POINT**
>
> Lithium is a medication with established antisuicidal efficacy in mood disorders. Clozapine has shown efficacy in reducing suicidal behavior in schizophrenia and schizoaffective disorders.

Clozapine is approved by the FDA for the treatment of recurrent suicidal behavior in patients with schizophrenia and schizoaffective disorder. In an international suicide prevention trial, a comparison of the risk of suicidal behavior in those treated with clozapine versus olanzapine was conducted among 980 patients with schizophrenia or schizoaffective disorder who are at risk for suicide because of current suicidal ideation or previous suicide attempts. The study concluded that clozapine demonstrated superiority in preventing suicide attempts in this high-risk population (Meltzer, 2003). A meta-analysis reported one third reduction of suicide on long-term treatment with clozapine (Hennen & Baldessarini, 2005).

Ketamine studies showed rapid onset antidepressant action and remarkable decrease in suicidal behavior in depressed patients. Preliminary studies have demonstrated a reduction in suicidal behavior following single and repeated doses of ketamine, making it a consideration for treatment of suicidal patients in the ED. These advantages must be weighed against its risks of abuse, cardiac and psychomimetic side effects, and transient response (Rajkumar et al., 2015).

Psychotherapy

Dialectical behavioral therapy (DBT) is a frequently studied psychotherapy to address recurrent suicidal behavior in patients with borderline personality disorder. DBT focuses on emotional regulation, interpersonal effectiveness, and self-efficacy and has been shown to reduce recurrences of suicidal behavior compared to community care (Stoffers-Winterling et al., 2012).

> **KEY POINT**
>
> Dialectical behavioral therapy (DBT) has been shown to reduce suicidal and nonsuicidal self-injury in patients with borderline personality disorder. Cognitive behavior therapy (CBT) has shown efficacy in suicide prevention.

Cognitive therapy for suicide prevention (CT-SP) is a well-validated suicide-specific cognitive behavioral therapy. It focuses on reducing risk factors for suicide and strengthening coping with the primary focus being elimination of suicidal behavior. A randomized controlled study concluded that cognitive therapy was effective at preventing suicide attempts in adults who recently had a suicide attempt (Brown et al., 2005).

Other Treatments

A study examined suicide, suicide attempts, and relapse rates of 519 depressed patients and documented that suicide attempts were seen less frequently in the electroconvulsive therapy (ECT) group than in the anti-depressant group (Avery & Winokur, 1978). However, ECT utilization is inhibited by fear of electricity, associated stigma, and limited availability of trained professionals and facilities (Fink et al., 2014).

Prevention of Suicide

The zero suicide initiative was implemented by National Strategy for Suicide Prevention with an objective to "transform healthcare systems to significantly reduce suicide" (Office of the Surgeon General & National Action Alliance for Suicide Prevention, 2012). This initiative recommends universal suicide risk screening of patients by health organizations at the initial and each subsequent contact.

The AIM-SP (assess, intervene, and monitor for suicide prevention) program is an operationalization of the zero-suicide initiative; the steps include the following:

1. Assessment for all patients attending the mental health clinic using the C-SSRS scale.
2. Intervention and monitoring patients on SSCP: Patients identified to be at high risk of suicide on assessment are placed on the SSCP (Suicide-Safer Care Pathway), which involves enhanced outpatient assessment and monitoring, increased intensity of clinical contact, and specialized interventions. Completing the six-step Stanley–Brown safety plan prior to the patient leaving the clinical encounter is an important component of this step.
3. Regardless of risk, all patients should be provided with information regarding crisis resources, including current clinic crisis line numbers, local crisis support services (e.g., mobile crisis teams, ED, and 911), the crisis text line (text HOME to 741741), and the National Suicide Prevention Lifeline (1-800-LIFELINE/1-800-273-8255).

> **CLINICAL TIP**
>
> Regardless of risk, all patients should be provided with information regarding crisis resources, including current clinic crisis line numbers, local crisis support services (e.g., mobile crisis teams, ED, and 911), the National crisis text line (text HOME to 741741), and the National Suicide Prevention Lifeline (1-800-LIFELINE/1-800-273-8255).

Restriction of access to lethal means is one of the few empirically supported strategies to reduce the number of deaths by suicide (Barber & Miller, 2014). This includes removing firearms and other lethal weapons, removing access to medications and sharp objects, and so on. In some public places, suicide barriers have been placed such as at the Golden Gate Bridge, Eiffel Tower, and the Empire State Building and more. An important measure to prevent suicides is to create community awareness by training non-health care professionals (e.g., teachers, clergy, and first responders) to identify and screen those individuals at high risk (Bachmann, 2018).

SUICIDE AND PHYSICAL ILLNESS

Researchers found that nine diseases were associated with increased suicide risk after adjustment for mental health and substance use diagnosis: brain injury, sleep disorders, HIV/AIDS, cancer, back pain, chronic obstructive pulmonary disease (COPD), epilepsy, migraine, and congestive heart failure (CHF). Of these, individuals with sleep disorders and HIV/AIDS had a two-fold increased risk of suicide, and those with traumatic brain injury were nine times more likely to die by suicide. The study also found back pain to be prevalent in those who die of suicide (Ahmedani et al., 2017). A study of U.S. veteran population has identified chronic back pain as a significant suicide risk factor (Ilgen et al., 2013).

The impairment of spinal cord injury and post-stroke patients increases the risk of suicide for people with these conditions. A study identified a significant increase in suicide attempts after Roux-en-Y gastric bypass for severe obesity (Backman et al., 2016). The disability, chronic pain, depression, and hopelessness during medical decline in chronic medical illness causes affective and cognitive distress, leading to an increase in suicide occurrence (Hirsch et al., 2009). Given that these physical conditions contribute frequently to physician visits, widespread suicide screening in all health care settings is warranted to prevent suicides.

SAD HARSH PLANS

S - Suicidal Ideation
A - Acute anxiety, agitation, or psychosis
D - Depressed mood

H - Hopelessness
A - Alcohol or substance use intoxication/withdrawal
R - Reliability of others is poor (poor social support)
S - Stressful life event
H - Hospitalization or emergency room visit, recent (for psych reason)

P - Plan in consideration
L - Leaving or withdrawing from family/friends
A - Attempt history
N - New, worsening, or chronic medical illness
S - Story (of family) contains suicide (family history of suicide)

FIGURE 34.3 SAD HARSH PLANS—mnemonic for suicide risk factors to look for in psychiatric emergencies.

Created by Edore Onigu-Otite

SUMMARY

Research in the past few years has led to an improved understanding and prevention of suicide. Further research is required to identify biological markers of suicide and use the latest technologies to predict and prevent suicide. Identifying suicide in subgroup populations and creating individualized treatment interventions are important steps for filling gaps in suicide prevention.

RESOURCES

1. https://www.youtube.com/watch?v=mG4y_JYdFVI https://theactionalliance.org/our-strategy/national-strategy-suicide-prevention
2. https://www.cdc.gov/violenceprevention/pdf/bullying-suicide-translation-final-a.pdf
3. https://www.mentalhealthfirstaid.org/population-focused-modules/youth/
4. Online tool for assessing suicidal ideation (safety). https://www.acep.org/patient-care/iCar2e/" https://www.acep.org/patient-care/iCar2e/

REFERENCES

Ahmedani, B. K., Peterson, E. L., Hu, Y., Rossom, R. C., Lynch, F., Lu, C. Y., Waitzfelder, B. E., Owen-Smith, A. A., Hubley, S., Prabhakar, D., Williams, L. K., Zeld, N., Mutter, E., Beck, A., Tolsma, D., & Simon, G. E. (2017). Major physical health conditions and risk of suicide. *American Journal of Preventive Medicine, 53*(3), 308–315. https://doi.org/10.1016/j.amepre.2017.04.001

Avery, D., & Winokur, G. (1978). Suicide, attempted suicide, and relapse rates in depression. *Archives of General Psychiatry, 35*(6), 749–753. https://doi.org/10.1001/archpsyc.1978.01770300091010

Bachmann, S. (2018). Epidemiology of suicide and the psychiatric perspective. *International Journal of Environmental Research and Public Health, 15*(7), 1425. https://doi.org/10.3390/ijerph15071425

Backman, O., Stockeld, D., Rasmussen, F., Näslund, E., & Marsk, R. (2016). Alcohol and substance abuse, depression and suicide attempts after Roux-en-Y gastric bypass surgery. *The British Journal of Surgery, 103*(10), 1336–1342. https://doi.org/10.1002/bjs.10258

Barber, C. W., & Miller, M. J. (2014). Reducing a suicidal person's access to lethal means of suicide: A research agenda. *American Journal of Preventive Medicine, 47*(3), S264–S272. https://doi.org/10.1016/j.amepre.2014.05.028

Batty, G. D., Kivimäki, M., Bell, S., Gale, C. R., Shipley, M., Whitley, E., & Gunnell, D. (2018). Psychosocial characteristics as potential predictors of suicide in adults: An overview of the evidence with new results from prospective cohort studies. *Translational Psychiatry, 8*(1), 1–15. https://doi.org/10.1038/s41398-017-0072-8

Batty, G. D., Whitley, E., Deary, I. J., Gale, C. R., Tynelius, P., & Rasmussen, F. (2010). Psychosis alters association between IQ and future risk of attempted suicide: Cohort study of 1,109,475 Swedish men. *BMJ (Clinical Research Ed.), 340*, c2506. https://doi.org/10.1136/bmj.c2506

Bertolote, J. M., & Fleischmann, A. (2002). Suicide and psychiatric diagnosis: A worldwide perspective. *World Psychiatry, 1*(3), 181–185.

Björkenstam, C., Kosidou, K., & Björkenstam, E. (2017). Childhood adversity and risk of suicide: Cohort study of 548,721 adolescents and young adults in Sweden. *BMJ, 357*, j1334. https://doi.org/10.1136/bmj.j1334

Brent, D. A., Melhem, N. M., Oquendo, M., Burke, A., Birmaher, B., Stanley, B., Biernesser, C., Keilp, J., Kolko, D., Ellis, S., Porta, G., Zelazny, J., Iyengar, S., & Mann, J. J. (2015). Familial pathways to early-onset suicide attempt: A 5.6-year prospective study. *JAMA Psychiatry, 72*(2), 160. https://doi.org/10.1001/jamapsychiatry.2014.2141

Brown, G. K., Ten Have, T., Henriques, G. R., Xie, S. X., Hollander, J. E., & Beck, A. T. (2005). Cognitive therapy for the prevention of suicide attempts: A randomized controlled trial. *JAMA, 294*(5), 563–570. https://doi.org/10.1001/jama.294.5.563

Busch, K. A., Fawcett, J., & Jacobs, D. G. (2003). Clinical correlates of inpatient suicide. *The Journal of Clinical Psychiatry, 64*(1), 14–19. https://doi.org/10.4088/jcp.v64n0105

Centers for Disease Control and Prevention. (2020). *Suicide fact sheet.* https://www.google.com/search?client=firefox-b-1-d&q=1.%09https%3A%2F%2Fwww.cdc.gov%2Fviolenceprevention%2Fpdf%2FSuicide-factsheet_508.pdf

Cheng, A. T. A., Chen, T. H. H., Chen, C.-C., & Jenkins, R. (2000). Psychosocial and psychiatric risk factors for suicide: Case-control psychological autopsy study. *The British Journal of Psychiatry, 177*(4), 360–365. https://doi.org/10.1192/bjp.177.4.360

Chesney, E., Goodwin, G. M., & Fazel, S. (2014). Risks of all-cause and suicide mortality in mental disorders: A meta-review. *World Psychiatry, 13*(2), 153–160. https://doi.org/10.1002/wps.20128

Columbia Lighthouse Project. (2016). *The Columbia protocol for healthcare and other community settings.* https://cssrs.columbia.edu/the-columbia-scale-c-ssrs/cssrs-for-communities-and-healthcare/

Dwivedi, Y., Rizavi, H. S., Conley, R. R., Roberts, R. C., Tamminga, C. A., & Pandey, G. N. (2003). Altered gene expression of brain-derived neurotrophic factor and receptor tyrosine kinase B in postmortem brain of suicide subjects. *Archives of General Psychiatry, 60*(8), 804–815. https://doi.org/10.1001/archpsyc.60.8.804

Fink, M., Kellner, C. H., & McCall, W. V. (2014). The role of ECT in suicide prevention. *The Journal of ECT, 30*(1), 5–9. https://doi.org/10.1097/YCT.0b013e3182a6ad0d

Freeman, A., Mergl, R., Kohls, E., Székely, A., Gusmao, R., Arensman, E., Koburger, N., Hegerl, U., & Rummel-Kluge, C. (2017). A cross-national study on gender differences in suicide intent. *BMC Psychiatry, 17*(1), 234. https://doi.org/10.1186/s12888-017-1398-8

Gibbons, R. D., Brown, C. H., Hur, K., Davis, J. M., & Mann, J. J. (2012). Suicidal thoughts and behavior with antidepressant treatment: Reanalysis of the randomized placebo-controlled studies of fluoxetine and venlafaxine. *Archives of General Psychiatry, 69*(6), 580. https://doi.org/10.1001/archgenpsychiatry.2011.2048

Harris, E. S. (2001). *The moral dimensions of properly evaluating and defining suicide.* Institute for Applied & Professional Ethics. https://www.ohio.edu/ethics/2001-conferences/the-moral-dimensions-of-properly-evaluating-and-defining-suicide/index.html

Heikkinen, M. E., & Lönnqvist, J. K. (1995). Recent life events in elderly suicide: A nationwide study in Finland. *International Psychogeriatrics, 7*(2), 287–300. https://doi.org/10.1017/S1041610295002043

Hennen, J., & Baldessarini, R. J. (2005). Suicidal risk during treatment with clozapine: A meta-analysis. *Schizophrenia Research, 73*(2), 139–145. https://doi.org/10.1016/j.schres.2004.05.015

Hirsch, J. K., Duberstein, P. R., & Unützer, J. (2009). Chronic medical problems and distressful thoughts of suicide in primary care patients: Mitigating role of happiness. *International Journal of Geriatric Psychiatry, 24*(7), 671–679. https://doi.org/10.1002/gps.2174

Huang, X., Ribeiro, J. D., & Franklin, J. C. (2020). The differences between individuals engaging in nonsuicidal self-injury and suicide attempt are complex (vs. complicated or simple). *Frontiers in Psychiatry, 11.* https://doi.org/10.3389/fpsyt.2020.00239

Ilgen, M. A., Kleinberg, F., Ignacio, R. V., Bohnert, A. S. B., Valenstein, M., McCarthy, J. F., Blow, F. C., & Katz, I. R. (2013). Noncancer pain conditions and risk of suicide. *JAMA Psychiatry, 70*(7), 692. https://doi.org/10.1001/jamapsychiatry.2013.908

Jacobs et al. (2003). Practice guideline for the assessment and treatment of patients with suicidal behaviors. *The American Journal of Psychiatry, 160*(11 Suppl), 1–60. https://pubmed.ncbi.nlm.nih.gov/14649920/

Lester, D. (1995). The concentration of neurotransmitter metabolites in the cerebrospinal fluid of suicidal individuals: A meta-analysis. *Pharmacopsychiatry, 28*(02), 45–50. https://doi.org/10.1055/s-2007-979587

Lindh, Å. U., Waern, M., Beckman, K., Renberg, E. S., Dahlin, M., & Runeson, B. (2018). Short term risk of non-fatal and fatal suicidal behaviours: The predictive validity of the Columbia-Suicide Severity Rating Scale in a Swedish adult psychiatric population with a recent episode of self-harm. *BMC Psychiatry, 18*(1), 319. https://doi.org/10.1186/s12888-018-1883-8

Luoma, J. B., Martin, C. E., & Pearson, J. L. (2002). Contact with mental health and primary care providers before suicide: A review of the evidence. *American Journal of Psychiatry, 159*(6), 909–916. https://doi.org/10.1176/appi.ajp.159.6.909

Lutz, P.-E., Mechawar, N., & Turecki, G. (2017). Neuropathology of suicide: Recent findings and future directions. *Molecular Psychiatry, 22*(10), 1395–1412. https://doi.org/10.1038/mp.2017.141

Meltzer, H. Y. (2003). Clozapine treatment for suicidality in Schizophrenia International Suicide Prevention Trial (InterSePT). *Archives of General Psychiatry, 60*(1), 82. https://doi.org/10.1001/archpsyc.60.1.82

O'Connor, R. C., & Kirtley, O. J. (2018). The integrated motivational–volitional model of suicidal behaviour. *Philosophical Transactions of the Royal Society B: Biological Sciences, 373*(1754), 20170268. https://doi.org/10.1098/rstb.2017.0268

Office of the Surgeon General & National Action Alliance for Suicide Prevention. (2012). *2012 national strategy for suicide prevention: Goals and objectives for action*. U.S. Department of Health & Human Services. http://www.ncbi.nlm.nih.gov/books/NBK109917/

Padmanathan, P., Biddle, L., Hall, K., Scowcroft, E., Nielsen, E., & Knipe, D. (2019). Language use and suicide: An online cross-sectional survey. *PLOS One, 14*(6), e0217473. https://doi.org/10.1371/journal.pone.0217473

Patterson, W. M., Dohn, H. H., Bird, J., & Patterson, G. A. (1983). Evaluation of suicidal patients: The SAD PERSONS scale. *Psychosomatics, 24*(4), 343–349. https://doi.org/10.1016/s0033-3182(83)73213-5

Posner, K., Brown, G. K., Stanley, B., Brent, D. A., Yershova, K. V., Oquendo, M. A., Currier, G. W., Melvin, G. A., Greenhill, L., Shen, S., & Mann, J. J. (2011). The Columbia–Suicide Severity Rating Scale: Initial validity and internal consistency findings from three multisite studies with adolescents and adults. *American Journal of Psychiatry, 168*(12), 1266–1277. https://doi.org/10.1176/appi.ajp.2011.10111704

Rajkumar, R., Fam, J., Yeo, E. Y. M., & Dawe, G. S. (2015). Ketamine and suicidal ideation in depression: Jumping the gun? *Pharmacological Research, 99*, 23–35. https://doi.org/10.1016/j.phrs.2015.05.003

Rico, E. (2016). Teaching and evaluation of Suicidal Assessment, Five-Step Evaluation and Triage (SAFE-T) in the emergency department. *Doctoral Projects*. https://doi.org/10.31979/etd.ecuy-p6a4

Rudd, M. D., Berman, A. L., Joiner, T. E., Nock, M. K., Silverman, M. M., Mandrusiak, M., Van Orden, K., & Witte, T. (2006). Warning signs for suicide: Theory, research, and clinical applications. *Suicide & Life-Threatening Behavior, 36*(3), 255–262. https://doi.org/10.1521/suli.2006.36.3.255

Schmaal, L., van Harmelen, A.-L., Chatzi, V., Lippard, E. T. C., Toenders, Y. J., Averill, L. A., Mazure, C. M., & Blumberg, H. P. (2020). Imaging suicidal thoughts and behaviors: A comprehensive review of 2 decades of neuroimaging studies. *Molecular Psychiatry, 25*(2), 408–427. https://doi.org/10.1038/s41380-019-0587-x

Shaffer, D., & Pfeffer, C. R. (2001). Practice parameter for the assessment and treatment of children and adolescents with suicidal behavior. *Journal of the American Academy of Child & Adolescent Psychiatry, 40*(7), 24S–51S. https://doi.org/10.1097/00004583-200107001-00003

Song, J., Sjölander, A., Joas, E., Bergen, S. E., Runeson, B., Larsson, H., Landén, M., & Lichtenstein, P. (2017). Suicidal behavior during lithium and valproate treatment: A within-individual 8-year prospective study of 50,000 patients with bipolar disorder. *The American Journal of Psychiatry, 174*(8), 795–802. https://doi.org/10.1176/appi.ajp.2017.16050542

Stoffers-Winterling, J. M., Völlm, B. A., Rücker, G., Timmer, A., Huband, N., & Lieb, K. (2012). Psychological therapies for people with borderline personality disorder. *Cochrane Database of Systematic Reviews, 8*. https://doi.org/10.1002/14651858.CD005652.pub2

Stone, M., Laughren, T., Jones, M. L., Levenson, M., Holland, P. C., Hughes, A., Hammad, T. A., Temple, R., & Rochester, G. (2009). Risk of suicidality in clinical trials of antidepressants in adults: Analysis of proprietary data submitted to US Food and Drug Administration. *BMJ, 339*, b2880. https://doi.org/10.1136/bmj.b2880

Substance Abuse and Mental Health Services Administration. (2009). *SAFE-T pocket card: Suicide assessment five-step evaluation and triage for clinicians*. https://store.samhsa.gov/product/SAFE-T-Pocket-Card-Suicide-Assessment-Five-Step-Evaluation-and-Triage-for-Clinicians/sma09-4432

Too, L. S., Spittal, M. J., Bugeja, L., Reifels, L., Butterworth, P., & Pirkis, J. (2019). The association between mental disorders and suicide: A systematic review and meta-analysis of record linkage studies. *Journal of Affective Disorders, 259*, 302–313. https://doi.org/10.1016/j.jad.2019.08.054

Tsai, A. C., Lucas, M., Sania, A., Kim, D., & Kawachi, I. (2014). Social integration and suicide mortality among men: 24-year cohort study of U.S. health professionals. *Annals of Internal Medicine, 161*(2), 85–95. https://doi.org/10.7326/M13-1291

Turecki, G., & Brent, D. A. (2016). Suicide and suicidal behaviour. *The Lancet, 387*(10024), 1227–1239. https://doi.org/10.1016/S0140-6736(15)00234-2

Vita, A., De Peri, L., & Sacchetti, E. (2015). Lithium in drinking water and suicide prevention: A review of the evidence. *International Clinical Psychopharmacology, 30*(1), 1–5. https://doi.org/10.1097/YIC.0000000000000048

World Health Organization. (2019, September 2). *Suicide*. https://www.who.int/news-room/fact-sheets/detail/suicide

CHAPTER 35

Psychosomatic Medicine[1]

Jane Gagliardi, M.D.

> *"In modern medicine, the mind and body often stay on two separate tracks in terms of treatment and health insurance reimbursement. But it's hard to maintain physical health while suffering from a psychological disorder."*
>
> — NPR

OBJECTIVES

After reading this chapter, students will be able to do the following:

- describe the psychosomatic approach to patient care (at large) as well as to consultation and liaison in psychiatry
- summarize common medical conditions with behavioral presentations or manifestations
- discuss overlapping symptoms in common medical and psychiatric conditions

CASE VIGNETTE

Ms. O is a 20-year-old woman who had no medical or mental health problems and excelled in school and sports until she was hospitalized with weight loss, abdominal pain, and shortness of breath at age 17, prompting her diagnosis with diabetic ketoacidosis and type I diabetes mellitus. Toward the end of high school, she started using drugs, escalating to injected heroin and methamphetamines; she left home and experienced various traumatic life experiences associated with obtaining and using drugs, including an unintentional overdose on heroin, requiring naloxone rescue and observation in the emergency department. She spent 2 years with poor glycemic control (with glycated

(*continued*)

1 Readers may also see "Depression in the Medically Ill" (chapter 21) for related material.

hemoglobin levels exceeding 14%) and was in and out of the hospital with multiple episodes of diabetic ketoacidosis.

A year ago, Ms. O was hospitalized involuntarily for a suicide attempt, and shortly thereafter she moved back home. Though she did not establish mental health follow-up, she has not used any drugs or alcohol, and she started seeing an endocrinologist for her diabetes mellitus. She has been taking insulin and counting carbohydrates, and her glycated hemoglobin levels have been in the range of 7–8% for the last 6 months. She is now enrolled in her local community college, where she has been earning As in challenging courses, and she has been working 40 hours per week at a job she enjoys.

Over the last month Ms. O has noticed decreased energy, severe insomnia with an inability to fall asleep or stay asleep, poor appetite, and low mood. She feels less motivated to attend class and submit coursework. She presents for voluntary admission to a local psychiatric hospital after developing thoughts of being better off dead and starting to think of ways to accomplish suicide. She started on bupropion for a provisional diagnosis of major depressive episode, possibility of bipolar II disorder. On the third hospital day, Ms. O's peers in the dayroom note that her eyes roll to the back of her head, she loses consciousness, falls to the floor, and exhibits rhythmic jerking movements.

Is Ms. O's primary problem medical or psychiatric? What factors would be useful to consider in her care? The fact that every living human being has a brain that is connected to their body seems obvious in some ways but may be overlooked in the way health care typically is provided. The aim of this chapter is to elucidate some of the ways in which the mind–body connection is relevant in diagnosis, treatment, and health promotion.

DEFINITIONS AND KEY CONCEPTS

Psychobiology is the study of mental functioning and behavior in relation to other biological processes.

Psychosomatic disorders are conditions of, relating to, concerned with, or involving both mind and body. *Pathophysiology* involves the mind–body connection. In some psychosomatic conditions, an underlying emotional or psychological state (such as anxiety about an upcoming examination) is associated with a physical symptom (such as gastrointestinal distress). In other psychosomatic conditions, an underlying physical or medical symptom (such as antibody production associated with an autoimmune condition) is associated with a behavioral presentation (such as psychotic or manic symptoms). Psychosomatic disorders illustrate the relationship between the mind and body.

The *biopsychosocial approach* integrates the biological, psychological, and social aspects of a disease state, recognizing a multifactorial etiology in contrast to the strictly biomedical aspects of disease.

Consultation-liaison psychiatry is the branch of psychiatry that, in consultation with patients and providing liaison and support to their health care team, aims to help people suffering from a combination of mental and physical symptoms, conditions, disorders, and illnesses.

A *functional disorder* is a condition affecting physiological or psychological functions but not yet determined to have an underlying medical or organic etiology.

INTRODUCTION

The mind and body are interconnected. Physical ailments can produce psychological symptoms. Mental health can affect physical health. As uncontroversial as these sentences may seem, and as much evidence there is that supports a link between mind and body, recognizing the underlying cause can be challenging (Balon, 2006). Given the fact that as many as 25%–30% of the population lives with mental illness in any year (and the proportion of individuals presenting for primary care and/or hospitalization have higher rates of mental illness), it is important to be aware of the likely comorbidities and/or contributions of mental illness to patients' presentations (Matheson et al., 2014). At times, the health care system seems to be set up to treat mind and body as completely separate entities, and patients with so-called "functional disorders," such as fibromyalgia, migraine, and others, may be left feeling invalidated by health care providers who are unable to find a treatable underlying medical illness. Considering the patient as a whole, including situations in which the patient may be experiencing behavioral manifestations of a medical or surgery problem, can improve diagnostic accuracy, timeliness of treatment, and patient satisfaction.

KEY POINT

Consultation–liaison psychiatry, sometimes called psychosomatic medicine, is the branch of psychiatry that focuses on the care of patients experiencing a combination of mental and physical illnesses by consulting with them and liaising with other members of their care team.

The idea of a mind–body connection dates back at least as far as to philosopher Rene Descartes, who seated the soul in the pineal gland. Adolf Meyer, the first professor of psychiatry and chair of the first psychiatric department in the United States at Johns Hopkins University in the early 1900s, championed the role of psychiatry in medical practice. Meyer's brand of psychobiology is considered "the direct predecessor to present-day practices of consultation-liaison psychiatry" (Karl & Holland, 2013). Though terminology has evolved, changed, and reverted over the years, psychosomatic medicine is the practice of mind–body, holistic care for patients who live and function in a biopsychosociocultural context.

Evidence shows that patients with comorbid medical and psychiatric illness experience worse health outcomes and higher costs, particularly in the inpatient setting (Kathol et al., 2015). Over the years, health care systems have implemented various strategies utilizing psychosomatic medicine approaches to improve the situation. Traditional consultation-liaison psychiatry services, proactive or universal psychiatric consultation, and medical complexity intervention units (combined medicine–psychiatry services) incorporate psychosomatic approaches (Jansen et al., 2020). The mind–body connection and alternative explanations for symptom constellations can improve the care of patients in any medical setting, and fully integrating behavioral health in patient-centered medical homes is an evidence-based strategy to improve patient experience and population health, while lowering health care costs (Kathol et al., 2014).

Decades of evidence document an association between mental and physical health; the direction of association is unclear, as are optimal screening and treatment strategies, and prognosis from the underlying medical illness may actually be worse in the presence of depression. Associations are documented between coronary artery disease and depression (Jiang et al., 2002; Khan et al., 2020), stroke and depression (Hackett & Pickles, 2014), and diabetes mellitus and depression (Buchberger et al., 2016). Promoted by the finding of the "broken heart syndrome," or takotsubo cardiomyopathy, researchers have demonstrated evidence that mental stress can induce abnormal left ventricular wall motion in a similar way as physical stress (Jiang, 2015). Cancer, both in itself and because of the diagnosis, can contribute to mood, cognitive, and behavioral changes; its presence can worsen quality of life, and there is some suggestion that psychiatric symptoms also portend worse cancer prognosis (Zahid et al., 2019). Autoimmune disease can be associated with a wide variety of behavioral and affective changes, and individuals who exhibit psychiatric reactions to traumatic stress show a higher risk of developing autoimmune disorders (Song et al., 2018).

QUICK POINT

While in the U.S. psychosomatic medicine is considered a subspecialty of psychiatry and neurology, in some European countries, it is considered a subspecialty of internal medicine.

A variety of endocrine disorders, including hyper- and hypothyroidism, adrenal excess and adrenal insufficiency, parathyroid hormone excess, pheochromocytoma, and others, have predictable and direct correlates with behavioral health manifestations. Less directly evident, but still associated, are other medical and psychiatric illnesses with likely multifactorial and multidirectional effects. A patient with kidney impairment may be depressed or, if the dysfunction is advanced and associated with uremia, confused.

It is beyond the scope of this chapter to provide an exhaustive list depicting the interplay between medical–surgical and psychiatric–behavioral symptoms and signs. See Table 35.1 for a partial listing of psychosomatic medicines one might encounter on clinical clerkships.

TABLE 35.1 Some Medical Conditions and Potential Behavioral Presentations or Manifestations*

	Medical condition	Behavioral presentation
Internal medicine and family medicine	• Thyroid storm • Cushing's disease • Lupus cerebritis • Corticosteroid psychosis or mania • Uncontrolled diabetes • Metabolic syndrome • Paraneoplastic limbic encephalitis • Any number of or combination of medical problems, including infection, ischemia, vasculitis, thiamine deficiency, brain metastases, hyper- or hyponatremia or calcemia, medications, drugs, and withdrawal	• Psychosis, mania, and agitation • Psychosis • Mania and psychosis • Psychosis and mania • Depression • Risk of atypical antipsychotic • Paranoia and mood swings • Delirium or "altered mental status"
Surgery	• Postoperative Ws—wound infection, atelectasis, urinary tract infection, etc. • Trauma (motor vehicle collision and gunshot wound)	• Delirium or "altered mental status" • Substance intoxication and withdrawal
Obstetrics and gynecology	• Peripartum hormone shifts and lack of sleep • Autoimmune encephalitis (NMDA/teratoma) • Paraneoplastic limbic encephalitis (ovarian cancer) • Postoperative infection, malignancy, and urinary tract infection	• Postpartum depression and psychosis • Paranoia and mood swings • Paranoia and mood swings • Delirium or "altered mental status"
Pediatrics	• Diabetic ketoacidosis (e.g., cerebral edema, fluid shifts, and sodium balance disorders) • Frontal lobe lesions • Chronic medical illness	Delirium or "altered mental status" • Inattentiveness and agitation • Chronic illness syndrome (difficulty trusting, fear of caregivers, difficulty forming relationships, and adolescent rebellion) • Posttraumatic stress disorder
Neurology	• Poststroke • Stroke-like presentation • Autoimmune encephalitis • Nonconvulsive status epilepticus • Nutritional (B12, B1) deficiency, neurosyphilis, subdural hematoma, vascular disease, and neurodegenerative disorders, such as CJD and Hashimoto's encephalopathy	• Depression • Differential includes conversion • Mania and psychosis • Catatonia • Dementia (impaired cognition)

(*continues*)

TABLE 35.1 *(Continued)*

	Medical condition	Behavioral presentation
Psychiatry	• Important to be vigilant for medical causes of psychiatric presentations and to assess "medical clearance" for what actually was checked (and what should be): ◦ *AMS*—urinary tract infection, nutritional deficiency, sodium or calcium imbalance, thyroid disorder, and exacerbation of underlying medical illness ◦ *Mania or psychosis*—hyperthyroidism, cortisol excess, neurosarcoidosis, lupus cerebritis, and exogenous androgens or steroids ◦ *Depression*—hypothyroidism, hyperthyroidism, adrenal insufficiency, malignancy, and poststroke. ◦ *Delirium*—any number of medical problems ◦ *Dementia*—nutritional (B12 or B1) deficiency, neurosyphilis, subdural hematoma, vascular disease, neurodegenerative disorders, such as CJD and Hashimoto's encephalopathy	

**This is not intended to be an exhaustive list. Any time a patient presents with behavioral symptoms, it is important to consider whether an underlying medical or surgical etiology might be present and ensure adequate attention to assess for those possibilities.*

THE PSYCHOSOMATIC APPROACH

KEY POINT

The psychosomatic approach to patient care recognizes the connection between the mind and body; this connection is bidirectional.

Psychosomatic approaches to care have been increasingly popular over the past two decades, and the American Board of Psychiatry and Neurology (ABPN) recognized psychosomatic medicine as a specialty in 2003 (Worley et al., 2009). In collaboration with the APA and Academy of Psychosomatic Medicine (now the Academy of Consultation-Liaison Psychiatry [ACLP]), the ABPN defined core components of the practice of the specialty. The scope of practice applies to any patients with psychopathology in general medical settings (e.g., inpatient, outpatient, medical, surgical, and obstetrical). The work involves gathering essential information from reviewing patient medical records; interviewing patients; gathering collateral information from other health care professionals, family members, and caregivers; and paying particular attention to a variety of relevant factors. The consultation-liaison or psychosomatic physician obtains a detailed chief complaint and relevant history with a goal of recognizing the patient's adjustment to illness, relationships with caregivers, response to hospitalizations, and response to specific interventions.

The psychosomatic approach also considers signs and symptoms of intoxication or withdrawal, drug–drug interactions, implications and causes of treatment nonadherence, and issues of polypharmacy or overmedication as well as the course of medical illness, response to interventions, prognosis, functional status, and any associated or resultant physical disabilities. Examination includes physical as well as mental status examination, including with relevant structured bedside cognitive assessment tools and the psychosomatic or consultation-liaison physician may need to assess issues as complex as a patient's decisional capacity or as seemingly mundane as how to improve the relationship between the patient and the health care team (Worley et al., 2009).

The psychosomatic or consultation-liaison physician may need to recommend a plan for diagnostic evaluation as well as implement comprehensive medical-psychiatric treatment plans to include biological, psychological, and sociocultural domains. In providing care to patients in medical settings, the psychosomatic provider is in a position to recognize stressors patients undergoing medical treatment experience. They also are in a position to provide expert consultation regarding use of strategies to decrease patient agitation (ranging from 1:1 sitters to medications to physical restraints) and may also be called on to implement interventions ranging from psychotherapeutic to medication to electroconvulsive therapies for comorbid psychological and/or psychiatric conditions impacting the patient (Worley et al., 2009). Diagnostic challenges range from recognizing underlying medical pathology in a patient who is purported to be "medically clear" to recognizing somatization illnesses (ranging from conversion disorder to somatization disorder to factitious disorder) and helping support the patient and health care team to recognize and address them.

The wide-ranging specialty of psychosomatics encompasses psychiatry and behavioral neurosciences as well as basic medical illness, appropriate treatment interventions, and special considerations with respect to treatments for psychiatric illness in complicated medical patients. In addition to knowledge of disorders and interactions between medical and psychiatric domains, the expert psychosomatic or consultation-liaison consultant is able to establish rapport with a diverse population, including patients, their families, their caregivers, and their physicians. The consultant also effectively communicates recommendations and considerations (including transference, countertransference, conflictual relationships, and difficult team dynamics) in the care of those patients (Worley et al., 2009).

The mind and body are connected. Application of psychosomatic medicine can be broad and deep. A psychiatric specialty (psychosomatic medicine or consultation-liaison psychiatry) and training programs offering combinations of internal medicine, neurology, pediatrics, and family medicine with psychiatry emphasize the importance of holistic evaluation and treatment, but it behooves all medical providers to be alert for those areas of mind–body overlap to optimally diagnose and treat patients and improve their outcomes.

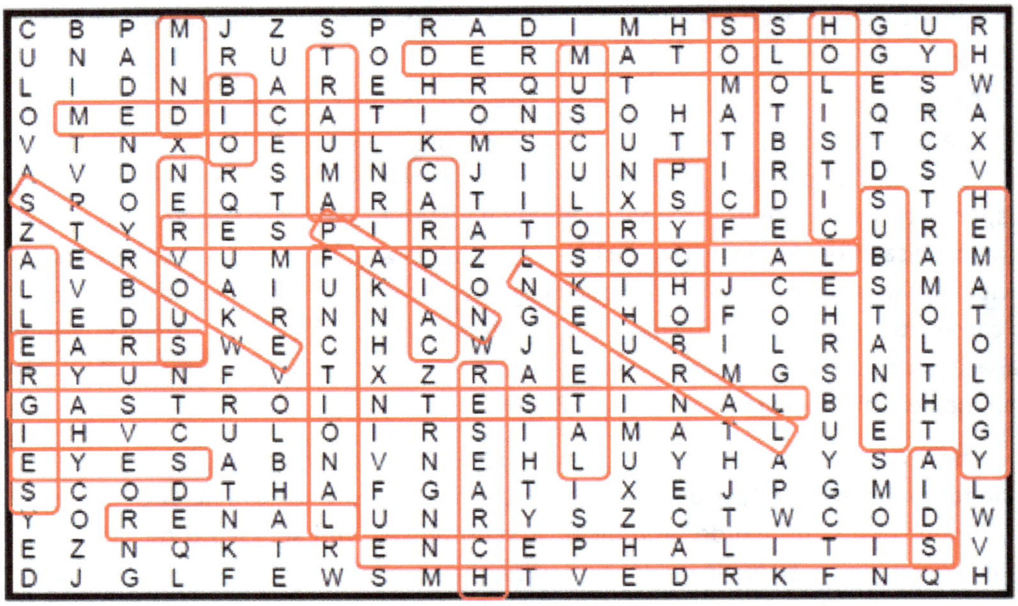

FIGURE 35.1 The psychosomatic approach requires attention to mental health within the various body systems and an understanding of how they overlap.

CASE VIGNETTE

Ms. O, who was started on bupropion for a major depressive episode in the context of multiple life stressors and who has a history of diabetes mellitus, is evaluated in the emergency department after exhibiting seizure-like activity in the dayroom of the psychiatric unit in which she is hospitalized. After obtaining a set of routine labs, including a urine drug screen and a head CT, she is cleared to return to the psychiatric facility, with a provisional diagnosis of orthostatic hypotension, low suspicion for a seizure, and recommendations to discontinue bupropion.

Twenty-four hours after returning to the psychiatric unit, Ms. O develops agitated behavior, disorientation, and confusion. She is brought back to the medical emergency department and is admitted to the combined medicine–psychiatry service. The differential diagnosis for her symptoms is broad. The possibility of actual seizure (related to bupropion, which can lower the seizure threshold or hypoglycemia) needs to be considered. Perhaps, she exhibited syncope (which could be related to orthostatic hypotension related to poor oral intake, vasovagal reaction from stress related to content discussed in the community meeting, or unknown cardiac or neurological underpinnings). Perhaps she was actually having a conversion reaction to the stress of being hospitalized and recalling various life traumas, and this was a psychogenic nonepileptic spell (which is a diagnosis of exclusion). Now that she is encephalopathic, the possibilities of intoxication or withdrawal from psychoactive substances and, depending on vital signs and clinical stability, the possibility of autoimmune encephalitis are worth considering.

EPIDEMIOLOGY

The Epidemiologic Catchment Area (ECA) and National Comorbidity Survey (NCS) were designed toward the end of the last century and were the first efforts to assess baseline rates of mental illness in the United States. A combination of the two studies, with an additional factor for impact on function, reported 1-year prevalence of psychiatric disorders. These range from 12.1%–18.7% for any anxiety disorder, 7.5%–11.1% for any mood disorder (with a 6.4%–10.1% prevalence of major depressive disorder, and approximately 1% for bipolar disorder), greater than 1% for primary psychotic disorder, and an overall 1-year prevalence of 15%–23.4% for any nonsubstance use disorder (Narrow et al., 2002).

For many different categories and types of physical illness, a body of literature exists that evaluates the association with depression, anxiety, psychosis, cognitive changes, and/or other behavioral health manifestations. Historically, the presence of behavioral health symptoms as causative of, associated with, or resulting from medical illness indicates worse prognosis than the medical illness alone. In a retrospective cohort study of veterans with lung cancer, 2.4% of subjects were diagnosed with schizophrenia, which, in turn, was associated with significantly earlier onset of lung cancer diagnosis and a higher risk of death, even after adjustment for confounding factors, including unemployment and homelessness, than cancer-matched controls (Bradford et al., 2016). The presence of mental illness, in 18.9% of a cohort of over 63,000 patients with diabetes mellitus, was associated with worse morbidity and, if the mental illness was substance use disorder or schizophrenia, a higher mortality in type 2 diabetes mellitus (Fernandez de Alba et al., 2020). A cross-sectional study of 174 consecutive pulmonary clinic patients with asthma revealed a 33.3% prevalence of anxiety and 47.7% prevalence of depression (Coban & Aydemir, 2014). In a systematic review with meta-analysis, researchers found that individuals with depression have worse outcomes post-percutaneous coronary intervention than individuals without depression (Patron et al., 2020). Overall, diagnosable psychiatric illness is present in 40% of hospitalized general medical patients and is associated with greater medical cost, longer hospital length of stay, and a higher risk of rehospitalization (Jansen et al., 2018).

QUICK POINT

Whether or not there is a common pathophysiology or causality, the presence of mental illness is associated with worse chronic disease management and worse outcomes. In primary care settings, over 40% of patients have diagnosable and treatable psychiatric illness (Kathol et al., 2014). Up to 40% of hospitalized general medical patients have a diagnosable psychiatric illness, which is associated with greater medical cost, longer hospital length of stay, and a higher risk of rehospitalization (Jansen et al., 2018).

On the other end of the mind–body connection, patients may present for evaluation of seemingly medical symptoms that, after careful review and evaluation, remain unexplained. Patients with somatic symptom disorder rarely present for psychiatric evaluation; rather, they are concerned about the possible medical etiologies and present to primary care, specialists, and, especially, emergency departments (Dunphy et al., 2019). As many as 5%–10% of patients in a general medical clinic setting (more in other settings) may present with somatoform or functional symptoms (Kroenke et al., 2010). Among patients in neurology clinics, as many as 5% have no neurological explanation for their focal symptomatology, and 30% may have their symptoms only partially explained by the underlying neurological disorder (Espay et al., 2018). Diagnoses of exclusion, such as fibromyalgia, chronic headache, irritable bowel syndrome, interstitial cystitis, and dysmenorrhea, are considered somatoform; conversion symptoms, such as psychogenic nonepileptic spells (PNES), are also considered somatoform. As dangerous as failing to recognize and treat a primary medical illness is, failing to recognize somatic symptom disorder can lead to repeated and invasive testing, which can be associated with iatrogenic injury (Dunphy et al., 2019). Additionally, though the descriptor *functional* can infer a certain lack of seriousness to the presenting symptomatology, functional disorders can cause significant impairment in quality of life and status in all domains of life but may be amenable to psychosocial and psychopharmacological treatments (Espay et al., 2018).

NEUROPATHOLOGY

Whether directly or indirectly, many patients find adjustment to medical illness emotionally challenging. Loss of function, loss of control over schedule, loss of usual routines and activities, and direct impacts of physical illness can be challenging for a previously healthy person to accept. Over the long term, the impact of near-death experiences, rebellion that manifests in refusing to take medications, or multiple exacerbations of medical illness requiring hospitalization can take a toll on an individual with chronic illness.

The mind and body are interconnected—in both directions and in many different ways. In a general sense, patients experience medical illness as a "stressor" and may feel psychologically burdened, particularly if they are not able to exert control over the symptoms or their onset. Though the direction of the relationship is not clear, there is an association between psychological distress and overall outcome: The more distressing the patient finds the medical burden to be, the less favorable the overall prognosis may be (Pai et al., 2019). Immune dysregulation (with cytokine production, cell migration, antibody formation, and cytotoxicity) is one way stress can increase vulnerability to disease, mediated by the hypothalamic–pituitary–adrenal (HPA) axis (Levy et al., 2019). In situations of somatic symptom disorder, the presence of a stressor may be unrecognized by the patient, and the symptoms will typically manifest in a somatic way, such as with diarrhea or constipation (irritable bowel syndrome), chronic pain and tension (fibromyalgia), paralysis, or even seizures (conversion disorder).

CLINICAL MANIFESTATIONS

Medical and/or surgical illnesses may present with behavioral disturbances. A classic example is the presentation of an elderly patient with agitation and behavioral disturbances, which turn out to be manifestations of delirium from an underlying urinary tract infection. Less classically considered, but also relevant in light of the possibility of as many as one in four patients presenting without chest pain, is the possibility of acute coronary syndrome presenting as confusion and altered mental status. Though this chapter includes a few specific examples, they are not intended to represent all possible behavioral presentations of or with medical comorbidity. Patients may have physical, psychiatric, or more than one type of illness contributing to an overall presentation. There is no substitute for compassionate, empathic, thorough, and detailed history taking; accurate and detailed physical examination; careful differential diagnosis formation; and rational and adequate diagnostic testing to determine how best to treat an individual patient. Knowledge of diagnostic criteria for psychiatric as well as nonpsychiatric illnesses is important for being able to differentiate. Following are common medical symptoms and conditions that can overlap with psychiatric symptoms.

CLINICAL TIP

Medical and/or surgical illnesses may present with behavioral disturbances. A classic example is the presentation of an elderly patient with agitation and behavioral disturbances, which turn out to be manifestations of delirium from an underlying urinary tract infection.

Heart Disease

Both coronary artery disease and heart failure are associated with depressive symptomatology, an association that persists even after accounting for the physical side effects of medications such as beta blockers and blood pressure-lowering agents (O'Conner et al., 2010; Swenson et al., 2003). Patients with depression experience more significant impairment in functional quality of life than disease-matched patients without depression (Swenson et al., 2003).

Chest Pain

Chest pain, which may occur with or separately from shortness of breath, can occur in the presence of arrhythmia, coronary ischemia, or pulmonary embolism. Associated symptoms, including nausea, shortness of breath, presyncope (feeling lightheaded), and diaphoresis, may occur in ischemic coronary events, which may also present with radiation of pain from the midsternal region up to the jaw or down to one or both arms. Palpitations, or a sensation of the heart beating fast, can be present or absent in patients with atrial fibrillation or other abnormal heart rhythm. Differentiating causes of acute chest pain or palpitations can be challenging when patients present with prominent symptoms of anxiety if the clinician tends to anchor more on the behavioral (i.e., anxiety or panic) than medical (i.e., coronary event, arrhythmia, or pulmonary embolism) side and may ascribe the symptoms to "functional" chest pain instead of "organic" causes. The problem is more challenging in light of the high overlap between panic attack and coronary event symptoms.

The *DSM-5* defines a panic attack as including at least four of the following symptoms: palpitations, sweating, trembling or shaking, shortness of breath or smothering sensation, a feeling of choking, chest pain or discomfort, nausea or abdominal distress, dizziness or lightheadedness, a sense of detachment or unreality, fear of losing control, a fear of dying, paresthesia, and hot flushing. A patient presenting with chest pressure, lightheadedness, sweating, and fear of dying could well be experiencing an acute coronary syndrome, and that patient should undergo appropriate evaluation to exclude an acute coronary event (including careful history taking, such as family history, smoking history, medical history, and prior events) and avoid making assumptions that the symptoms must be psychosomatically mediated. Patients presenting with chest pain should undergo an appropriate evaluation to ensure a coronary or pulmonary cause is not overlooked, and historical details can be very helpful.

Stroke

Stroke results from impaired blood flow in the cerebral vasculature and can occur in patients in a variety of age ranges; recently, with the hypercoagulability seen with infections from SARS-CoV-2 (known as COVID-19), patients with seemingly no other risk factors may present with stroke. Embolic strokes can take place in patients with valvular heart disease, infective endocarditis (which is a risk of injected drug use), and atrial fibrillation (the prevalence of which increased with age). Depending on the vascular distribution of the ischemic or thrombotic event, the patient will exhibit focal neurological symptoms.

Ischemic or thrombotic events can take place in patients with cerebrovascular disease (atherosclerosis) and in patients who undergo vasospasm (from primary vasospastic disorders or from substances that are powerful vasoconstrictors, which is the case for some recreational drugs). Ischemic strokes account for about 85% of strokes, whereas hemorrhagic strokes (from intracranial hemorrhage, which can come from vascular anomalies or from trauma) account for most of the remainder (Robinson & Jorge, 2016). In addition to focal neurological symptoms, a variety of neuropsychiatric syndromes can develop in the presence of cerebrovascular disease. Above and beyond patients' grief reaction to illness and loss of function, depression is highly prevalent in the 5-year period following stroke and can lead to significant debility and impaired quality of life (Robinson & Jorge, 2016). Treatment guidelines for post-stroke recovery include attention to depression and treatment with antidepressant medications (Robinson & Jorge, 2016).

Symptoms that are indistinguishable from stroke may occur in patients with conversion disorder, which is associated with an unconscious stressor and manifests in the same manner as stroke but without MRI findings or other abnormalities to confirm vascular impairment (Espay et al., 2018). Elucidating the underlying stressor(s), enlisting the patient in continuity care and follow-up, and implementing psychological and psychiatric interventions may be useful strategies in the care of patients with conversion symptoms.

Cancer

In addition to the difficulty adjusting to the news of a cancer diagnosis and the difficult side effects of chemotherapy, patients with malignancy may experience major depressive symptoms, posttraumatic stress reactions to their diagnosis and/or treatment, panic attacks, and cognitive impairment associated with cancer and chemotherapy (Holland, 2018). Various malignancies produce antibodies that can contribute to antibody-associated encephalitis, which can be indistinguishable from primary psychiatric disorders because the only systemic manifestation may be autonomic instability (Dalmau & Graus, 2018). Such syndromes are rare, but in light of the importance of diagnosing and treating an underlying malignancy, it is important for physicians and physicians in training to be alert to the presence of fluctuating vital signs and to seek clarification and elucidation of any underlying illness. As a diagnostic tool, it is important to recognize that paraneoplastic syndromes (including those impacting behavior and psychiatric symptomatology) are useful in helping to arrive at an earlier diagnosis of (and possibly more effective treatment strategy for) cancer.

Autoimmune Encephalitis

Closely related to paraneoplastic limbic encephalitis, autoimmune encephalitis can come from underlying malignancy or other as-yet-to-be-clarified autoimmune processes. An example of autoimmune encephalitis comes from author Susannah Cahalan (2012), whose book, *Brain on Fire*, was recently used as the basis for a documentary film. After experiencing hallucinations, insomnia, mood swings, and erratic behavior over the course of about a month, Cahalan was hospitalized psychiatrically and treated for bipolar disorder, schizoaffective disorder, and/or substance use disorder before careful inquiry and re-examination revealed an underlying etiology of autoimmune encephalitis associated with NMDA receptor autoantibodies (Cahalan, 2012). In about half of cases, NMDA receptor antibody encephalitis is associated with an ovarian tumor known as a teratoma, and symptoms improve with both immune-mediated therapy and removal of the tumor.

Adrenal Insufficiency

Neurovegetative symptoms of major depressive disorder include low energy, appetite changes (frequently impaired appetite with weight loss), and a general feeling of low motivation. Patients presenting with the classical symptoms of adrenal insufficiency (weakness, fatigue, anorexia, and weight loss) may not be recognized to additionally exhibit abdominal pain, orthostatic hypotension, and salt craving (Nicolaides, 2017). It is important to maintain a broad differential and to be vigilant about abnormalities and unexpected responses to treatment.

DIAGNOSIS

> **CLINICAL TIP**
>
> The term *medical clearance* is used in different ways. Emergency, medical, and surgical teams use the term *medical clearance* to denote their impression that something other than the diagnoses they usually make is responsible for a patient's symptoms. Psychiatry teams use the term to signify the lack of acute medical contributors to the patent's presentation.

Patients may present with behavioral manifestations of illnesses or conditions that are not primarily psychiatric. Emergency, medical, and surgical teams utilize the term *medical clearance* to denote their impression that something other than the diagnoses they usually make is responsible for a patient's symptoms. Psychiatry teams may also use medical clearance to signify the lack of acute medical contributors to the presentation. The term is controversial. It may lead health care providers to assume in error what diagnostic possibilities have been considered and ruled out (Chennapan et al., 2018). It is important to be cognizant of and work to avoid overreliance on anchoring bias. One of many heuristics humans use to expedite decision-making, anchoring bias occurs when preformed assumptions (or anchors) exert influence on the eventual decision; when this anchor is far from the truth of the matter, errors result.

Factors, such as time pressure (e.g., when needing to make a quick decision regarding triage in the emergency department), cognitive load (e.g., the kind of intellectual engagement required in medical decision-making), and uncertainty can increase the anchoring bias (Lieder et al., 2018). What does this mean for diagnostic evaluation and decision-making? When a patient presents to an acute care setting with dysregulated behaviors, or accompanied by law enforcement, health care providers at the first point of contact may anchor on the likelihood of a primary behavioral disturbance, placing the patient on a care plan that emphasizes timely medical clearance to affect appropriate disposition. Subsequent health care providers encountering the patient may also anchor on the importance of addressing the behavioral concerns without carefully considering the important task of thorough history taking (medical and psychiatric), thoughtful generation of a differential diagnosis, and appropriate diagnostic testing to influence medical decision-making (Chennapan et al., 2018).

The strategies physicians and systems use to improve efficiency and enhance patient throughput, including patient care pathways, protocols for medical clearance, and automated order sets, can at times preclude careful consideration of patient-specific factors. Especially when faced with time pressure, complexity, and a sense of certainty, it is important for health care providers to reach outside of the "usual" comfort zone and consider alternative explanations for the behaviors that caused presentation. It is important to undertake careful, detail-oriented confirmation of the history of the present illness with a hypothesis-driven review of systems, casting a broad net for possible medical contributors to the presentation. It is essential to review and verify medications and substances the patient may have consumed. Finally, it is important for the behavioral health care provider to complete a thorough and hypothesis-driven physical examination (not relying on other health care providers' documentation) to ensure adequate assessment of the full picture of the patient's health status.

In primary care settings, over 40% of patients have diagnosable and treatable psychiatric illness (Kathol et al., 2014). Whether there is a common pathophysiology or causality, the presence of mental illness is associated with worse chronic disease management and worse outcomes, ranging from musculoskeletal pain to asthma to diabetes mellitus (Coban & Aydemir, 2014; Buchberger et al., 2016; Fernandez de Alba et al., 2020; Lentz et al., 2019). Though the case for alleviating human suffering through detecting and treating mental illness is strong, there is also a financial argument for detection and effective treatment of mental illness. Data from 41 million patients in the 2012 Medicare database reveal that the 14% of patients in the cohort with diagnosed mental illness accounted for 32% of the medical expenditures (Kathol et al., 2015). An ever-growing body of evidence points to untreated mental illness as a contributor to higher costs, longer lengths of hospital stays, and higher rates of rehospitalizations for inpatients (Jansen et al., 2018) as well as for outpatients (Wammes et al., 2018).

SCREENING FOR MENTAL HEALTH PROBLEMS IN MEDICAL SETTINGS

How should the busy nonpsychiatric clinician identify patients with mental illness? A number of primary care screening strategies have been developed and implemented in various health systems with high uptake of the Patient Health Questionnaire (PHQ-2 and PHQ-9) to identify individuals with symptoms warranting further investigation regarding presence of major depressive disorder (Mitchell et al., 2016). If it is not feasible to screen all of the patients in an outpatient clinical setting, there may be benefits to screening those patients who are doing less well medically and/or not showing up to their follow-up appointments.

Patients with mental illnesses in medical settings can be challenging to manage. They may be more likely to exhibit suboptimal disease management and have high no-show rates to appointments (Boos et al., 2016). Primary care providers who treat patients with mental illnesses estimate their adherence to recommendations and likelihood of appropriately following up as low (Vistorte et al., 2018). Though challenging to engage in treatment, such patients benefit significantly from the care rendered at each patient encounter. They also stand to benefit from mental health screening, management, and referral when needed. This, in turn, may improve treatment outcomes of their medical illnesses.

Busy clinicians in outpatient settings can be frustrated or confused by the lack of clear-cut or consistent options for referring their patients for evaluation in mental health settings (Mitchell et al., 2016). In health systems in which psychiatric treatments are accessible, uniform uptake of the PHQ in primary care settings may be beneficial, though screening for an illness without the ability to refer for treatment can be frustrating at best and may be counterproductive (Mitchell et al., 2016). Creative solutions, including colocation of mental health providers, task-sharing, technology solutions, and medical provider education, can help expand the clinic's ability to identify and treat mental illness in the patients they see (Hoeft et al., 2018).

In scenarios in which patients present with classic symptoms for which an underlying cause is not elucidated, it is important for the health care provider to carefully review the evaluation that has been undertaken, considering possible medical explanations and somatic symptom disorder and other somatoform disorders as diagnoses of exclusion.

TREATMENT

There is no one-size-fits-all treatment algorithm for comorbid medical and psychiatric illness. An empathic, validating, and reassuring approach to patient interactions can be beneficial at all times. The overarching principle is to be vigilant in evaluating patients' histories and symptoms, apply adequate and appropriate diagnostic testing, and avoid premature closure in arriving at treatment plans. It is important to identify and treat medical etiologies that could be contributing to a behavioral presentation; similarly, it is necessary to identify and treat any psychiatric comorbidities that may be affecting medical care.

Patients undergoing evaluation and management of acute medical illness may exhibit stress responses, and they may benefit from supportive psychotherapy, education in relaxation and mindfulness techniques, and education regarding the diagnostic considerations and anticipated treatments. In acute illness settings, patients may experience a loss of sense of control, which may lead to difficulties interacting productively with the medical staff.

In situations of somatoform or conversion symptoms, patients may feel abandoned or deserted by their specialty physicians as the diagnosis is clarified. It can be especially helpful to ensure support and psychoeducation about the etiology; the role of psychotherapy and, possibly, medications; and the importance of follow-ups when discussing functional disorders with patients who suffer from them.

A variety of experiences leading to and during hospital admission can be inherently traumatizing. Near-death experiences, resuscitative efforts, misperceptions during episodes of delirium, extreme physical distress, adverse reactions to medications, and misunderstanding of the care plan can all lead patients with acute or chronic medical problems to develop a mistrust of the health care system and, in severe cases, actual posttraumatic stress reactions to the hospital setting.

The diagnosis of a chronic medical issue at an early age, particularly one associated with pain or painful procedures, can lead to difficulties trusting, poor self-care, and trauma associated with the episodes of care.

MEDICAL CONSIDERATIONS

A variety of medical conditions can present with behavioral manifestations, and it is important to remain vigilant and to undertake a thorough and detailed history while avoiding anchoring bias. When patients' symptoms do not respond as expected to appropriate interventions, or when the time course or duration does not match the usual or expected course, it can be helpful to step back, reassess data, and determine where there may be gaps in information gathering or diagnostic testing.

While convenient and efficient for the majority of patients presenting with primary psychiatric illness, "medical clearance" protocols that include a set of standard labs may create a sense of false security and should be considered as a part of the evaluation, upon which a careful and thorough historian can add hypothesis-driven diagnostic testing.

SUMMARY

A psychosomatic approach to patient care recognizes the connection between the mind and body; this connection is bidirectional. Patients may present with "functional" medical symptoms without any clear underlying medical pathology. At the same time, patients may present with behavioral symptoms that result from a primary medical illness in the absence of primary psychiatric disease. The majority of patients may exhibit psychological responses to medical illness stressors, and a supportive, validating, and empathic approach can help optimize their response to interventions. In broadening the differential diagnosis to include diseases of the body as well as of the mind, a psychosomatic approach can help the clinician arrive at an accurate diagnosis and a comprehensive treatment plan for patients with a variety of illnesses.

CASE VIGNETTE

The combined medicine–psychiatry team caring for Ms. O considered a broad differential diagnosis and set about undertaking a rational series of examinations and investigations to assess for various possibilities. Urinalysis demonstrated a urinary tract infection; sexually transmitted infections, including gonorrhea, chlamydia, syphilis, and HIV, were ruled out; and she was started on antibiotics for urinary tract infection. Blood sugars remained in the range of 100–180 without any episodes of hypoglycemia. She was monitored on cardiac telemetry and had normal cardiac rhythm. The team considered additional factors, including the possibility of seizure. She had a normal prolonged electroencephalogram,

(*continued*)

and she had a normal brain MRI. With this information, and with the presence of normal vital signs, the team assessed the likelihood of autoimmune encephalitis as low but offered lumbar puncture; the patient declined this intervention. During the entire episode of care the team adopted a trauma-informed approach, working to validate the patient's lived experiences of trauma and completed a deeper assessment of her psychiatric diagnoses, which provisionally included complex posttraumatic stress disorder, bipolar II disorder, and borderline personality disorder. The patient was given educational materials on each of these diagnoses as well as proposed treatment strategies, including fluoxetine and cognitive behavioral therapy, and she agreed to start treatment with fluoxetine and follow-up in the outpatient setting with weekly psychotherapy.

RESOURCES

1. Academy of Consultation-Liaison Psychiatry. www.clpsychiatry.org
2. Association of Medicine and Psychiatry. https://assocmedpsych.org

REFERENCES

Academy of Psychosomatic Medicine. (n.d.). *Consultation-liaison psychiatry.* https://www.clpsychiatry.org/about-aclp/whatis-clp/

American Psychiatric Association. (2013). *Diagnostic and statistical manual of mental disorders* (5th ed.).

Balon, R. (2006). Mood, anxiety, and physical illness: Body and mind, or mind and body? *Depression and Anxiety*, 23, 377–387. https://doi:10.1002/da.20217

Boos, E. M., Bittner, M. J., Kramer, M. R. (2016). A profile of patients who fail to keep appointments in a Veterans Affairs primary care clinic. *Wisconsin Medical Journal*, 115(4), 185–191.

Bradford, D. W., Goulet, J., Hunt, M., Cunningham, N. C., & Hoff, R. (2016). A cohort study of mortality in individuals with and without schizophrenia after diagnosis of lung cancer. *Journal of Clinical Psychiatry*, 77(12), e1626-e1630. https://doi.org/10.4088/JCP.15m10281

Breitbart, W. S., & Alici, Y. (2009). Psycho-oncology. *Harvard Review of Psychiatry*, 17, 361–376.

Buchberger, B., Huppertz, H., Krabbe, L., Lux, B., Mattivi, J. T., & Siafarikas, A. (2016). Symptoms of depression and anxiety in youth with type I diabetes: A systematic review and meta-analysis. *Psychoneuroendocrinology*, 70, 70–84. https://doi:10.1016/j.psyneuen.2016.04.019

Cahalan, S. (2012). *Brain on fire: My month of madness*. Simon & Schuster.

Chennapan, K., Mullinax, S., Anderson, E., Landau, M. J., Nordstrom, K., Seupaul, R. A., & Wilson, M. P. (2018). Medical screening of mental health patients in the emergency department: A systematic review. *The Journal of Emergency Medicine*, 55(6), 799–812. https://doi.org/10.1016/j.jemermed.2018.09.014

Coban, H., & Aydemir, Y. (2014). The relationship between allergy and asthma control, quality of life, and emotional status in patients with asthma: A cross-sectional study. Allergy, *Asthma & Clinical Immunology 10*, 67.

Dalmau, J., & Graus, F. (2018). Antibody-mediated encephalitis. *New England Journal of Medicine*, 378, 840–851. https://doi:10.1056/NEJMra1708712

Dunphy, L., Penna, M., & El-Kafsi, J. (2019). Somatic symptom disorder: A diagnostic dilemma. *BMJ Case Reports*, 12, e231550. https://doi.org/10.1136/bcr-2019-231550

Espay, A. J., Aybek, S., Carson, A., Edwards, M. J., Goldstein, L. H., Hallett, M., LaFaver, K., LaFrance, W. C., Lang, A. E., Nicholson, T., Nielsen, G., Reuber, M., Voon, V., Stone, J., & Morgante, F. (2018). Current concepts in diagnosis and treatment of functional neurological disorders. *JAMA Neurology*, 75(9), 1132–1141. https://doi.org/10.1001/jamaneuro.2018.1264

Fernandez de Alba, I. G., Gimeno-Miguel, A., Poblador-Plou, B., Gimeno-Felieu, L. A., Ioakeim-Skoufa, I., Rojo-Martinez, G., Forjaz, M. J., & Prados-Torres, A. (2020). Association between mental health comorbidity and health outcomes in type 2 diabetes mellitus patients. *Nature Research Scientific Reports, 10*, 19583. https://doi.org/10/1038/s41598-020-76546-9

Hackett, M. L., & Pickles, K. (2014). Part I: Frequency of depression after stroke: An updated systematic review and meta-analysis of observational studies. *International Journal of Stroke*, 9(8), 1017–1025. https://doi:10.1111/ijs.12357

Hoeft, T. J., Fortney, J. C., Patel, V., & Unutzer, J. (2018). Task-sharing approaches to improve mental health in rural and other low-resource settings; A systematic review. *The Journal of Rural Health*, 34, 48–62. https://onlinelibrary.wiley.com/doi/epdf/10.1111/jrh.12229

Holland, J. C. (2018). Psycho-oncology: Overview, obstacles, and opportunities. *Psycho-oncology*, 27, 1364–1376. https://doi:10.1002/pon.4692

Jansen, L., van Schijndel, M., van Waarde, J., & van Busschbach, J. (2018). Health-economic outcomes in hospital patients with medical-psychiatric comorbidity: A systematic review and meta-analysis. *PLOS ONE, 13*(3), e0194029. https://doi.org/10.1371/journal.pone.0194029

Jansen, L. A. W., Ellison, A. E., Nguyen, F., Marina, A., Spencer, J. M., Specker, A., Wierdsma, A. I., Kathol, R. G., & van Schlindel, M. A. (2020). Complexity interventions units in the United States: Organization and dispersion. *Psychosomatic Medicine*, *82*, 805–807. https://doi:10.1097/PSY.0000000000000856

Jiang, W., Krishnan, K. R. R., & O'Connor C. M. (2002). Depression and heart disease: Evidence of a link, and its therapeutic implications. *CNS Drugs*, 16(2), 111–127. https://doi:10.2165/00023210-200216020-00004

Jiang, W. (2015). Emotional triggering of cardiac dysfunction: The present and future. *Current Cardiology Reports*, *17*, 91. https://doi.org/10.1007/s11886-015-0635-3

Karl, S. R., & Holland, J. C. (2013). Looking at the roots of psychosomatic medicine: Adolf Meyer. *Psychosomatics*, *43*, 111–114.

Kathol, R. G., deGruy, F., & Rollman, R. L. (2014). Value-based financially sustainable behavioral health components in patient-centered medical homes. *Annals of Family Medicine*, *12*(2), 172–175. https://doi:10.1370/afm.1619

Kathol, R. G., Melek, S. P., Sargent, S., Sasks, L., & Patel, K. K. (2015). Non-traditional mental health and substance use disorder services as a core part of health in CINs and ACOs. In K. Yale, T. Raskauskas, J. M. Bohn, & C. Konschak (Eds.), *Clinical integration: Population health and accountable care* (3rd ed.; pp. 380-425). Convurgent Publishing.

Kathol, R. G., Patel, K., Sacks, L., Sargent, S., & Melek, S. P. (2015). The role of behavioral health services in accountable care organizations. *American Journal of Managed Care*, *21*(2), e95–e98. https://www.ajmc.com/view/the-role-of-behavioral-health-services-in-accountable-care-organizations

Khan, S. A., Shahzad, U., Zarak, M. S., Channa, J., Khan, I., & Ghani, M. O. A. (2020). Association of depression with subclinical coronary atherosclerosis: A systematic review. *Journal of Cardiovascular Translational Research*, *1*(1). https://doi.org/10.1007/s12265-020-09985-4

Kroenke, K., Spitzer, R. L., Williams, J. B.W., & Lowe, B. (2010). The Patient Health Questionnaire somatic, anxiety, and depressive symptom scales: A systematic review. *General Hospital Psychiatry*, 32, 345–359. https://doi.org/10.1016/j.genhosppsych.2010.03.006

Lentz, T. A., Harman, J. S., Marlow, N. M., Beneciuk, J. M., Fillingim, R. B., & George, S. Z. (2019). Factors associated with persistently high-cost health care utilization for musculoskeletal pain. *PLOS One*, *14*(11), e0225125. https://doi.org/10.1371/journal.pone.0225125

Levy, S., Heruti, I., & Avitsur, R. (2019). Physical injury, stress, and health: Protective role of dispositional optimism. *Stress and Health*, *35*, 267. https://doi.org/10.1002/smi.2859

Lieder, F., Griffiths, T. L., Huys, Q. J. M., & Goodman, N. D. (2018). The anchoring bias reflects rational use of cognitive resources. *Psychonomic Bulletin Review*, *25*, 322–249. https://doi:10.3758/s13423-017-1286-8

Matheson, F. I., Smith, K. L. W., Moineddin, R., Dunn, J. R., & Glazier, R. H. (2014). Mental health status and gender as risk factors for onset of physical illness over 10 years. *Journal of Epidemiology and Community Health, 68*, 64–70. https://jech.bmj.com/content/68/1/64

Merriam-Webster. (n.d.b.). *Biopsychosocial*. https://www.merriam-webster.com/medical/biopsychosocial.

Merriam-Webster. (n.d.a.). *Functional*. https://www.merriam-webster.com/dictionary/functional

Merriam-Webster. (n.d.c.). *Psychobiology*. https://www.merriam-webster.com/medical/psychobiology

Merriam-Webster. (n.d.d.). *Psychosomatic*. https://www.merriam-webster.com/medical/psychosomatic

Mitchell, A. J., Yadegarfar, M., Gill, J., & Stubbs, B. (2016). Case finding and screening clinical utility of the Patient Health questionnaire (PHQ-9 and PHQ-2) for depression in primary care: A diagnostic meta-analysis of 40 studies. *British Journal of Psychiatry Open, 2*, 127–138. https://doi.org/10.1192/bjpo.bp.115.001685

Narrow, N. E., Rae, D. S., Robins, L. N., & Regier, D. A. (2002). Revised prevalence estimates of mental disorders in the United States: Using a clinical significance criterion to reconcile 2 surveys' estimates. *Archives of General Psychiatry, 59*, 115–123.

Nicolaides NC, Chrousos GP, Charmandari E. Adrenal Insufficiency. (2017). In: K. R. Feingold, B. Anawalt, A. Boyce et al. (Eds,). *Endotext*. MDText.com https://www.ncbi.nlm.nih.gov/books/NBK279083/

O'Connor, C. M., Jiang, W., Kuchibhatla, M., Silva, S. G., Cuffe, M. S., Callwood, D. D., Zakhary, B., Stough, W. G., Arias, R. M., Rivelli, S. K., & Krishnan, R. (2010). Safety and efficacy of sertraline for depression in patents wit heart failure: Results of the SADHART-CHF (sertraline against depression and heart disease and chronic heart failure) trial. *Journal of the American College of Cardiology, 56*(9), 692–699. https://doi:10.1016/j.jacc.2010.03.068

Pai, H. C., Li, C. C., Tsai, S. M., Pai, Y. C. (2019). Association between illness representation and psychological distress in stroke patients: A systematic review and meta-analysis. *International Journal of Nursing Studies, 94*, 42–50. https://doi.org/10.1016/j.ijnurstu.2019.01.015

Patron, E., Benvenuti, S. M., Ponchia, A., Gentili, C., Bianconi, S., & Palomba, D. (2020). Depression anticipates patients at risk of poor exercise stress test performance after percutaneous coronary angioplasty: A short-term longitudinal study. *General Hospital Psychiatry, 67*, 10–18. https://doi.org/10.1016/j.genhosppsych.2020.08.009

Robinson, R. G., & Jorge, R. (2016). Post-stroke depression: A review. *American Journal of Psychiatry, 173*, 221–231. https://doi.10.1176/appi.ajp.2015.15030363

Song, H., Fang, F., Tomasson, G., Arnberg, F. K., Mataix-Cols, D., Fernandez de la Cruz, L., Almqvist, C., Fall, K., & Valdimarsdottir U. A. (2018). Association of stress-related disorders with subsequent autoimmune disease. *JAMA, 319*(23), 2388–2400. https://doi:10.1001/jama.2018.7028

Swenson, J. R., O'Connor, C. M., Barton, D., Van Zyl, L. T., Swedberg, K., Forman, L. M., Gaffney, M., & Glassman, A. H.. (2003). Influence of depression and effect of treatment with sertraline on quality of life after hospitalization for acute coronary syndrome. *American Journal of Cardiology, 92*, 1271–1276. https://doi.10.1016/j.amjcard.2003.08.006

Vistorte, A. O. R., Ribeiro, W. S., Jaen, D., Jorge, M. R., Evans-Lacko, S., & Mari, J. (2018). Stigmatizing attitudes of primary care professionals towards people with mental disorders: A systematic review. *The International Journal of Psychiatry in Medicine, 53*(4), 317–338. https://doi.org/10.1177/0091217418778620

Wammes, J. J. G., van der Wees, P. J., Tanke, M. A. C., Western, G. P., & Jeurissen, P. P. T. (2018). Systematic review of high-cost patients' characteristics and healthcare utilization. *BMJ Open, 8*, e023113. https://bmjopen.bmj.com/content/bmjopen/8/9/e023113.full.pdf

Worley, L. L. M., Levenson, J. L., Stern, T. A., Epstein, S. A., Rundell, J. R., Crone, C. C., Wise, T. N., Rummans, T. A., Muskin, P. R., Bourgeois, J. A., Saravay, S. M., Pao, M., Alter, C., Steinberg, M., Wulsin, L., Breitbart, W., Fricchione, G. L., Boland, R., Epstein, L. A., & Winstead, D. (2009). Core competencies for fellowship training in psychosomatic medicine: A collaborative effort by the APA Council on Psychosomatic Medicine, the ABPN Psychosomatic Committee, and the Academy of Psychosomatic Medicine. *Psychosomatics, 50*(6), 557–562. https://doi.org/10.1176/appi.psy.50.6.557

Zahid, J. A., Grummedal, O., Madsen, M. T., & Gogenur, I. (2020). Prevention of depression in patients with cancer: A systematic review and meta-analysis of randomized controlled trials. *Journal of Psychiatric Research*, 120, 113–123. https://doi:10.1016/j.jpsychires.2019.10.009

CHAPTER 36

Adverse Childhood Experiences (ACEs) and Resilience[1]

Edore Onigu-Otite, M.D.; Kammarauche Asuzu, M.D., M.H.S.; and Sindhu Idicula, M.D.

> *"I can be changed by what happens to me. But I refuse to be reduced by it."*
>
> — Maya Angelou

OBJECTIVES

After reading this chapter, students will be able to do the following:

- identify common ACEs
- discuss common risk and protective factors for child abuse and neglect
- review the impact of ACEs on the mental and physical health and social outcomes of individuals

THE CASE OF JAYDA

As an intern on call, you get called to the ER to see a 14-year-old girl who ran away from her foster home. The police rescued her from a man operating a sex trafficking ring. This is her third ER visit this year—all due to behavior concerns. Her foster parents, who had begun the adoption process, are now considering returning her to child protective services (CPS).

(*continued*)

1 Readers may also see "Trauma- and Stressor-Related Disorders" (Chapter 18) for related material.

A look into the child's history shows that for the first 5 years of her life Jayda lived with her biological mother, who had substance use problems. Due to the severity of the substance use disorder symptoms, Jayda's mother could not provide the care her young child needed. Jayda's mother regularly abandoned her, leaving her with relatives, friends, and strangers while using drugs. Jayda went for long periods without food, her clothes were dirty and worn, and she gained little weight. Jayda's mother was in and out of jail for recurrent drug-related misdemeanors. She often left without warning for long periods, leaving Jayda with extended family members and friends. Over the years, Jayda was emotionally, physically, and sexually abused. She repeated two school grades due to a lack of attendance. She struggled to learn, got into fights with other kids, was disrespectful to teachers, and had disciplinary problems.

At age 8, she was taken into CPS custody and placed in a stable environment with two elderly doting foster parents. Things calmed down for the next few years. At age 12, she became belligerent, began leaving home without permission, and had an older boyfriend who was a gang leader. Her foster parents, who had started the adoption process, reversed their plan and returned her to CPS. For the next year, Jayda lived in group homes. About a year ago, she moved to her current home, which everyone hoped would end in adoption. She has been there for 9 months so far. The first 6 months went well. Then Jayda's behavior became problematic. She rebelled against the rules, showed up provocatively dressed to school, began to skip classes, and experimented with drugs. She had multiple sexual partners and was treated for a sexually transmitted disease.

In the ER, you took the time to get a more in-depth look at the case, and this provided you with a better understanding of Jayda's needs. With the social worker's help, Jayda and her family got linked to various resources. With support from CPS and related organizations, Jayda and her family received steady treatment over the next 3 years, including trauma-focused CBT; medications for depression, anxiety, sleep, and PTSD; and drug-related counseling. Although her nightmares and flashbacks and cravings for drugs improved, they never entirely went away. With treatment, Jayda learned practical coping skills and strategies to handle them. Jayda, now a young adult, remains compliant with all aspects of her treatment, as advised by her health care providers. She calls psychotherapy her "painfully beautiful personal space." She got a GED and is now enrolled in a community college program with plans to open a small business, support her family, and be an active contributor to her local community.

DEFINITIONS AND KEY CONCEPTS

Adverse childhood experiences (ACEs) are stressful events and experiences occurring before age 18. These include verbal, physical, or sexual abuse and family dysfunction, such as living in a household with a mentally ill or substance-abusing family member, witnessing a parent being treated violently, or the absence of a parent due to separation, divorce, or incarceration (CDC, 2010). An *ACE score* is the number of categories of ACEs an individual experiences.

Physical abuse is nonaccidental physical injury to a child by another individual. *Child sexual abuse* (CSA) is any sexual act involving a child that is intended to provide sexual gratification to another individual. Psychological abuse (emotional abuse) is nonaccidental verbal or symbolic acts by a child's parent or caregiver that result or have reasonable potential to result in significant psychological harm to the child. *Neglect* is any confirmed or suspected egregious act or omission by a child's parent or other caregiver that deprives the child of basic age-appropriate needs and thereby results, or has reasonable potential to result, in physical or psychological harm to the child. This includes educational, medical, physical, or psychological neglect or abandonment. *Child maltreatment* is any act or series of acts of commission or omission by a parent or other caregiver that results in harm, the potential for harm, or threat of harm to a child. *Resilience* is the ability to dynamically adapt successfully within the context of adversity, tragedy, trauma, significant stress, threat, or danger. It refers to the qualities that enable one to adapt and thrive in the face of adversity of any kind (Horn, 2018; Connor & Davidson, 2003).

INTRODUCTION

ACEs constitute a substantial stressor with long-lasting negative effects on the brain and mental and physical health. ACEs have been robustly linked to unfavorable mental and physical health outcomes and are predictive of higher sociodemographic risk.

The original ACE study led by Felitti et al. (1998, 2019) studied the effects of child abuse, neglect, and household dysfunction in adult life (Figure 36.1). This ground-breaking study uncovered a robust association between the extent of exposure to ACEs during childhood and multiple risk factors for many of the leading causes of death in adulthood. In the study, adults who had experienced four or more ACEs categories had a four to 12-fold increased risk for alcohol or drug use disorders, depression, and suicide attempts. They were two to four times more likely to have 50 or more lifetime sexual intercourse partners and sexually transmitted diseases. They also had a 1.4- to 1.6-fold increased risk of developing severe obesity. Moreover, the number of ACE categories had a graded relationship to adult public health problems, including ischemic heart disease, chronic lung disease, cancer, skeletal fractures, and liver disease. Multiple categories of ACEs were associated with multiple health risk factors through life. In essence, the ACE study identified ACEs as a leading preventable cause of major mental illness and a preventable cause for several leading public health concerns (Felitti, 2002).

KEY POINT

The original ACE study led by Felitti et al. (1998) studied the effects of child abuse, neglect, and household dysfunction in adult life (Figure 36.1). This ground-breaking study uncovered a robust association between the extent of exposure to ACEs during childhood and multiple risk factors for many of the leading causes of death in adulthood.

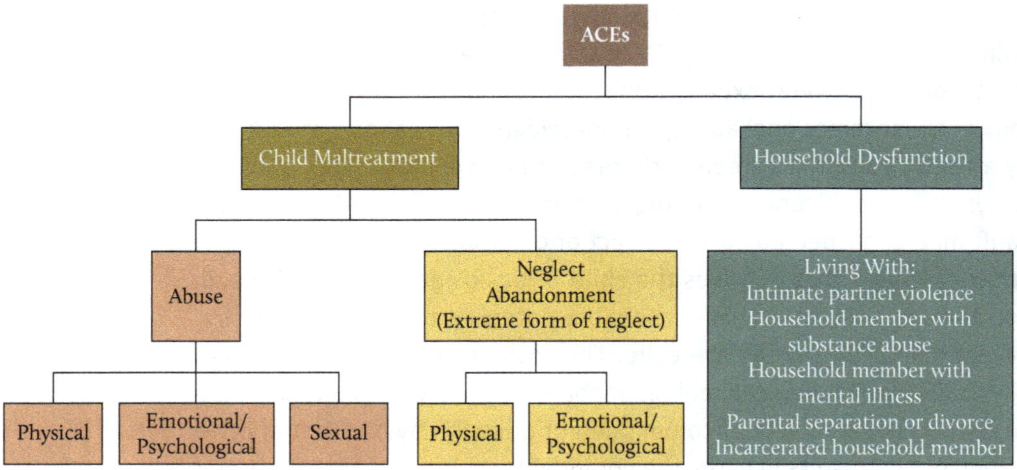

FIGURE 36.1 Categories of ACEs.

Copyright © 2013 by Robert Wood Johnson Foundation. Reprinted with permission.

Since the original ACE study, the ACE research body has expanded, and the original findings are replicated and expanded. The National Survey of Children's Health (NSCH) now assesses nine types of ACEs, including serious economic hardship, alcohol, and substance abuse, mental health problems in the home, domestic violence, parental divorce, loss of parents to death or incarceration, witnessing or experiencing violence in the neighborhood, and social rejection through racial or ethnic discrimination. Consistent with adult studies, child study findings show a linear, dose-response effect of ACEs across a wide range of health and social impacts. ACEs have a lasting negative impact on health, well-being, and opportunity throughout a life span. Increased exposure to ACEs predicts higher sociodemographic risk, including low life potential and premature death by up to 20 years compared to individuals with no ACEs (Figure 36.2). In difficult-to-treat patient cases, where otherwise effective remedies have not been sufficient, it has been suggested that medical practitioners may want to consider the possibility of ACEs (Edwards et al., 2007).

Protective factors against ACEs have been identified, including the presence of at least one safe, stable, and supportive adult and being raised in a stable home and community. Resilience qualities that allow individuals to thrive in the face of adversity buffer against ACEs' harmful effects. Individuals who have and practice resiliency skills may be partly protected against child abuse and neglect's detrimental long-term effects. Preventing ACEs has a pivotal impact on preventing enduring negative consequences. Promoting positive childhood experiences in children within the context of ACEs and delivering interventions that build strengths and resilience in children have been shown to mitigate the impact of ACEs into adulthood (Bethell et al., 2019).

EPIDEMIOLOGY

Nationally representative studies found a high burden of ACEs. Approximately 68% of children 0–17 years old had experienced one or more ACEs. About 60% of adult study participants reported at least one ACE, about 25% reported three or more ACEs, and nearly one in six adults had experienced four or more types of ACEs (Merrick et al., 2018, 2019). Women and several racial and ethnic minority groups were at greater risk of having experienced four or more types of ACEs. In the United States, the risk of having ACEs is higher for Black, Hispanic, and multiracial children compared to White children (Merrick et al., 2018). More ACEs were reported in individuals with less than a high school education, lower incomes, unemployment, and those who identified as gay/lesbian compared to individuals who identified as White, those who completed high school or more education, those in all other income brackets, those who were employed, and those who identified as straight. Emotional abuse was the most prevalent ACE, followed by parental separation or divorce and household substance abuse (Merrick et al., 2018).

The economic and social costs to families, communities, and society are considerable. The CDC estimates that the cost of child maltreatment is a staggering 124 billion annually (Fang et al., 2012). In children, studies showed that three or more ACEs more than quadrupled the risk of experiencing internalizing problems (such as anxiety and depression) and almost quadrupled the risk of experiencing externalizing problems (such as disruptive behaviors) (Clarkson Freeman, 2014). Economic research on human capital indicates significant cost savings potential may occur from implementing effective prevention strategies (Larkin et al., 2014). It has been suggested that a 10% reduction in ACE prevalence could equate to annual savings of three million disability-adjusted life years or $105 billion (Bellis et al., 2019). It is estimated that up to 1.9 million cases of heart disease and 21 million cases of depression could potentially have been avoided by preventing ACEs.

KEY POINT

ACEs have been consistently shown to increase the risk of psychiatric and personality disorders. Both retrospective and prospective studies show a clear association between ACEs and later psychopathology.

ACES AND MENTAL HEALTH

ACEs have consistently been shown to be risks for psychiatric and personality disorders. Both retrospective and prospective studies show a clear association between ACEs and later psychopathology. Both the ACEs themselves and their memory impact the risk of later psychopathology. In children, ACEs are associated with emotional and behavioral problems.

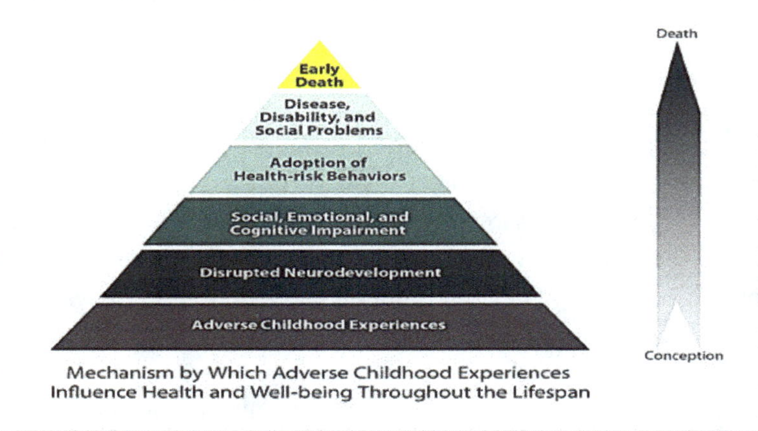

FIGURE 36.2 Impact of ACEs across the life span.

Source: https://www.cdc.gov/violenceprevention/childabuseandneglect/acestudy/ace-graphics.html.

For each additional ACE, there was a 32% increase in the odds of having a problem score on the child behavior checklist (CBCL) and a 21% increase in the odds of having a chronic medical condition. ACEs are a risk factor for many psychiatric disorders that are associated with reduced hippocampal volume, including depression (Anda et al., 2002); PTSD; borderline personality disorder (Zanarini et al., 2000); and dissociative identity disorder/multiple personality disorder (Coons et al., 1994). Childhood maltreatment contributes to the risk of personality disorders, including borderline and antisocial personality disorder (Douglas et al., 2011).

ACEs significantly increase the risk of depression and self-directed violence across the life span. Individuals with four or more types of ACEs are 460% more likely to suffer from depression (Chapman et al., 2004). In the elderly, depression has been significantly correlated with repeated ACEs of all types (Ege et a., 2015). There is a strong association between adult depression and reported CSA (Widom et al., 2007). Some studies found that the only ACE for which a single occurrence was significantly associated with late-life depression was forced sexual intercourse (Ege et al., 2015). Having any ACE increased the risk of attempted suicide two- to five-fold throughout a person's life span (Dube et al., 2001). Individuals with six or more ACEs had over 24.36 times increased odds of attempting suicide (Dube et al., 2001). ACEs are linked to substance use disorders. Each ACE increased the likelihood of early initiation of illicit drug use two- to four-fold. ACEs are associated with alcohol use, nicotine and tobacco use in adulthood, and a higher risk of substance use disorders in the elderly. The association between ACEs and substance use is mediated in part by mood and anxiety disorders, which often precede the onset of drug use (Douglas et al., 2010).

QUICK POINT

Time alone does not heal all wounds. ACEs significantly increase the risk of depression and suicidal behavior across the life span. Individuals with four or more types of ACEs are 460% more likely to suffer from depression (Chapman et al., 2004). In the elderly, depression has been significantly correlated with repeated ACEs of all types (Ege et al., 2015).

Child physical abuse and exposure to domestic violence affects social processing patterns and is associated with later adult intimate partner violence perpetration and victimization. CSA often occurs within the context of other ACEs. Regardless, CSA, alone or within a larger adversity cluster, is associated with a substantially increased risk of subsequent psychopathology. CSA is an established risk factor for adolescent risky sexual behavior. Additional forms of maltreatment elevate the risk, including early sexual initiation and sexual risk behavior, teen pregnancy, prostitution, and the risk for commercial sexual exploitation of children and adults (Seen et al., 2008). Emotional neglect and psychological abuse both have strong relationships with depression. These associations were consistent across ethnic groups.

QUICK POINT

Child physical abuse and exposure to domestic violence affects social processing patterns and is associated with later adult intimate partner violence perpetration and victimization.

CLINICAL TIP

ACEs are linked to substance use disorders. Each ACE increased the likelihood of early initiation of illicit drug use two- to four-fold. ACEs are associated with alcohol use, nicotine and tobacco use in adulthood, and a higher risk of substance use disorders in the elderly. The association between ACEs and substance use is mediated in part by mood and anxiety disorders, which often precede the onset of drug use (Douglas et al., 2010).

ACES, PHYSICAL HEALTH, AND HEALTH SERVICES USAGE

An estimated 19.8% of U.S. children have a chronic medical condition requiring more than routine health and related services. This prevalence increases to 31.6% in children with two or more ACEs (Bethell et al., 2014). ACEs are associated with adult obesity (Williamson et al., 2002), cardiovascular disease (Dong et al., 2004), sleep disturbance (Chapman et al., 2011), diabetes, cancer, sexually transmitted diseases (Hillis et al., 2000), and premature mortality. ACEs are associated with immune function changes and increase the likelihood of hospitalization with a diagnosed autoimmune disease decades into adulthood (Dube et al., 2009). ACEs are linked to negative health behaviors, including lack of treatment compliance. ACEs are linked to increased health service usage. With each additional ACE score, the rate of the number of prescription drugs used increased by 62% (Anda et al., 2008). Adults reporting three or more ACEs were more likely to have significant medical debt with medical expenses exceeding 10% of their household income (Schickedanz et al., 2019).

QUICK POINT

An estimated 19.8% of U.S. children have a chronic medical condition requiring more than routine health and related services. This prevalence increases to 31.6% in children with two or more ACEs (Bethell et al., 2014).

ACES AND SOCIAL OUTCOMES

Children exposed to ACEs are substantially more likely to repeat a grade in school and have shown limited ability to work through challenges (Bethell et al., 2014). Children with multiple ACEs are more likely to live in lower-income homes and have public insurance. An estimated 63.9% of children with both ACEs and emotional disturbances have public insurance (Bethell et al., 2014). In the workforce, ACEs are associated with a higher loss of productivity and lower work performance. An individual with an ACE score of 3 is 2.9 times more likely to have had 14 missed workdays due to mental health issues than individuals with no ACEs.

NEUROPATHOLOGY

The brain is the main body organ responsible for detecting, reacting to, adjusting to, and recovering from stress. Neurobiological studies strongly suggest ACEs are associated with enduring brain dysfunctions that affect physical and mental health throughout the life span (Anda et al., 2006). Specifically, ACEs are associated with changes in the hippocampus, amygdala, prefrontal cortex, and dysregulation of the hypothalamic–pituitary–adrenal (HPA) axis. In individuals with maltreatment history, changes in the brain network affect the relevant processing of trauma-related stimuli and executive control. These changes include decreased grey matter in the prefrontal cortex (responsible for decision-making and self-regulatory skills) and decreased connectivity between the amygdala and ventrolateral prefrontal cortex (involved in the regulation of emotion; Banks et al., 2007; Zannas & West, 2014). An increase in microglia activity (central to the brain's inflammatory response) may contribute to neuroinflammation. ACEs are associated with changes in DNA methylation patterns,both genome wide and in several genes that are associated with anxiety, regulation of the cortisol response, and the SERT serotonin transporter (Zannas & West, 2014). These neurobiological changes, in combination, result in heightened responses to perceived threats and trauma triggers (Bethell et al., 2016). ACEs are associated with shortened telomers and altered gene methylation. Some evidence suggests these changes may be transmitted to offspring (Esteves, 2020).

CLINICAL MANIFESTATIONS

ACEs result in prolonged activation of the stress response. ACEs disrupt neurodevelopment with a resulting impact on the individual's life trajectory (Figure 36.3). Perceived threats can precipitate the body's stress response leading to the activation of the HPA and the sympathetic nervous system, resulting in fear responses, including the fight, flight, or freeze response. The disordered stress response comes on when there is perceived, but perhaps minimal to no real threat, and stays on when the threat is gone or was never present in the first place. This is like a house fire alarm that goes on when there is no fire or when there is perceived fire, such as when the gas stove in the house is on for everyday cooking. The alarm also stays on long after the perceived threat is gone. Psychologically, the individual organizes their awareness to protect themselves from experiencing this distress, leading to psychological avoidance often by employing maladaptive defense mechanisms. Socially, the individual avoids the real or imagined threat, leading to social avoidance. Acute symptoms include behavioral changes, mood and anxiety symptoms, and substance use in some cases. In many cases, responses to

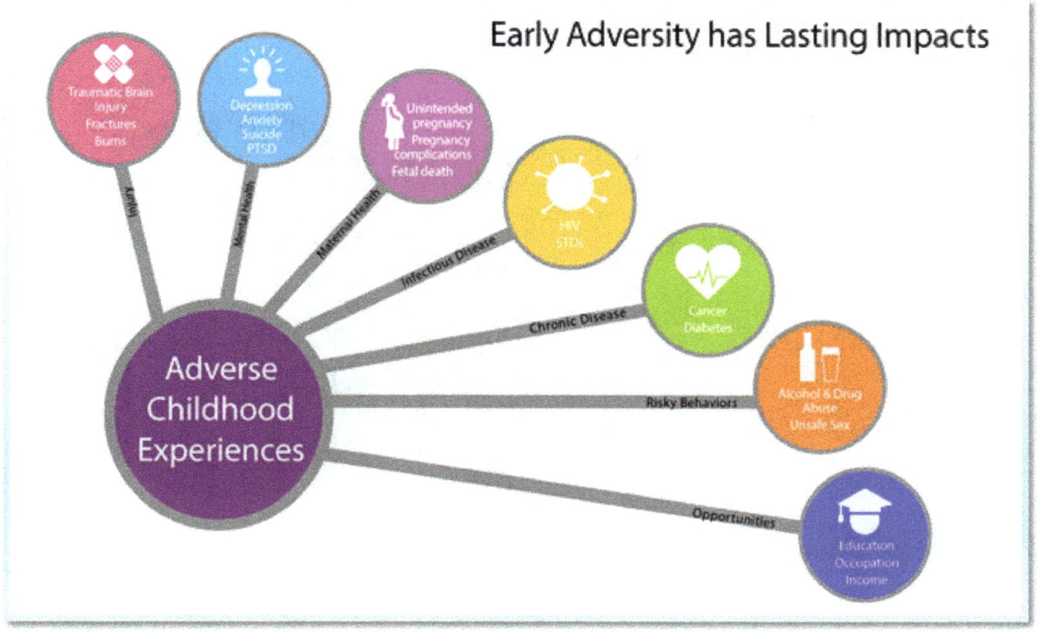

FIGURE 36.3 Early adversity has lasting impacts.

Source: https://www.cdc.gov/violenceprevention/images/acestudy/ACEs-consequences-large.png.

ACEs are more insidious, especially when there are multiple overlapping ACEs. A summary of clinical conditions associated with ACEs is depicted in Figure 36.2 (and more information can be found with the CDC [2013]). Additional clinical information is contained in Chapter 18.

> **CLINICAL TIP**
>
> Individuals with ACEs can experience intense and sometimes unexpected emotions. Emotion coaching at such times can help the individual self-regulate and manage their stress responses.

SCREENING FOR ACES

Qualitative feedback received included highlighting an interest in knowing more about how physicians can identify patients with ACEs. Using the ACE score as a screener may be helpful in clinical practice. To this end, ACE-based screenings and referrals are increasingly being used in pediatric and adult primary care settings (Choi et al., 2019; Gilgoff et al., 2020; Van Neil et al., 2014).

> **CLINICAL TIP**
>
> In the event of ACEs, acute symptoms of a dysregulated stress response include behavioral changes, mood and anxiety symptoms, irritability and aggressive behavior, sleep problems, and substance use in some cases. Responses to ACEs can also be more insidious, especially when there are cumulative, or overlapping ACEs.

TREATMENT

The effects of ACEs can be broad and severe. Optimal treatment includes social, psychological, and biological treatment modalities (Figure 36.4). Treatment includes mitigation of the environment (e.g., removing the child), placement of additional resources for parents, and treatment of household members with mental or substance use disorders. The lingering effects of ACEs experienced in years past can be significant. Treatment often includes trauma-based psychotherapy. Psychotropic medication to address mental

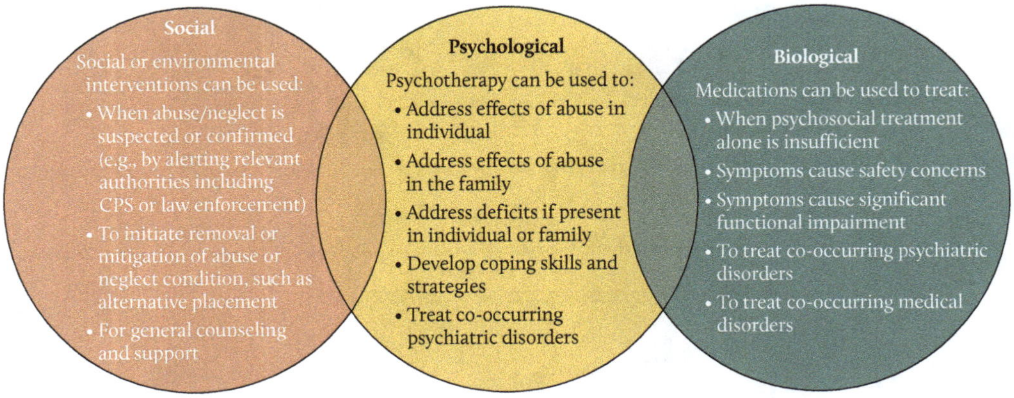

FIGURE 36.4 Modalities for addressing ACEs.

health symptoms can be employed based on the symptom severity and degree of dysfunction.

PROTECTIVE FACTORS

Protective factors are promotive of healthy human development. Research has identified several protective factors against ACEs. The most important protective factor is having a parent available to talk to the child about things that matter to the child and share ideas. The active involvement of a caregiver who has the knowledge, interest, skills, and sensitivity and the supports for the caregiver to work successfully with the child can provide the stable progress the child needs to not only overcome their challenges but to develop a new sense of strength that far outstrips the limitations of their past trauma history. Ideally, such caregivers should be educated on child trauma as well as supported through challenges encountered while parenting the child. Other factors include having over five family meals per week, living in a nonsmoking household, engagement in team sports, growing up in a safe neighborhood, having supportive neighbors, four or more neighborhood amenities, and a well-kept community (Easterlin et al., 2019; Robles et al., 2019).

Prevention programs, such as preschool enrichment and early childhood home visitation programs, have shown success, demonstrating 48–52% reductions in child abuse and neglect rates. Efforts that prevent ACEs can potentially prevent adult chronic conditions, depression, health risk behaviors, and adverse socioeconomic outcomes (Merrick et al., 2019b).

MEMORY TIP

Caregiver skills related to caring for children with trauma, *useful mnemonic*

KISSS
K—Knowledge
I— Interest
S—Skills
S—Sensitivity
S—Supports

(Created by Edore Onigu-Otite)

RESILIENCE

Resilience is the dynamic ability to adapt successfully within the context of adversity, tragedy, trauma, significant stress, or threat. Resilience is the capacity to rebound and successfully adapt in the face of adversity (Connor & Davidson, 2003; Hunt, 2018). Resilience is a factor that mitigates the negative effects of ACEs (Merrick et al., 2019a). In children, in the face of ACEs, resilience often results in more self-efficacy, inner wisdom, and enhanced social or academic competence. Resiliency is an innate capacity; therefore, it can be cultivated in any individual. Identifying and cultivating this in children, including those with ACEs, can significantly impact the child's life trajectory. The concept of resilience promotes hope and optimism—both of which are necessary for overcoming adversity. This also intuitively reduces the sense of hopelessness that can occur in providers working with children with ACEs and helps providers identify and build on assets, while addressing deficits that cause a paradigm shift (Brito & Boller, 2020).

KEY POINT

Resilience is the dynamic ability to adapt successfully within the context of adversity, tragedy, trauma, significant stress, or threat. The concept of resilience promotes hope and optimism—both of which are necessary for overcoming adversity. Resiliency is an innate capacity; therefore, it can be cultivated in any individual.

Several factors impact vulnerability to stress and resilience. These include genetic predisposition, early life experiences, and later life experiences. Vulnerability is increased when the failure to cope with adversity accumulates. Conversely, resilience is increased when successful adaptation occurs in the face of adversity (Daskalakis, 2013). Factors that have been found to be promotive of resilience in children with ACEs include the presence of a supportive adult–child relationship, a sense of self-efficacy, opportunities to practice problem-solving and strengthen self-regulation, and tapping into resources of faith, hope, and related spiritual or cultural traditions. The single most common factor found in children who develop resilience is the stable presence of at least one committed supportive parent, caregiver, or other adult. This includes the adult's consistent availability to respond and provide personalized discussions that help protect the child from developmental disruption and enable the child to positively adapt to the adversity, survive, and, potentially, thrive.

Resilience is not a static construct. It can have a differential impact on the individual at different points in their trajectory and for different ACEs. Protective factors supporting resilience include a stable family environment, supportive family relationships, and personality traits that support social skills (Afifi & Macmillan, 2011). Resiliency skills include self-awareness, attention, flexibility, stability of focus, accepting and letting go physically and mentally, and accessing and sustaining positive emotion. Finding the positive within the adverse experience can facilitate acceptance and shifting forward to thrive. The development and utilization of resiliency skills are results of a combination of biological and psychosocial factors. Children who thrive in the face of misfortune have some biological resistance to adversity and strong relationships with the pivotal adults in their family and community. Children may manifest resilience to one type of adversity but not to others.

PREVENTION OF ACES

> **QUICK POINT**
>
> *"What is predictable is preventable."*
> —Dr. Robert Anda

ACEs are not inevitable, and they can be prevented. Specific strategies for preventing ACEs have been identified (Table 36.1). The Substance and Mental Health Services Administration (SAMHSA) has identified six pillars for trauma-informed care, which represent the guiding principles for providing health care services to individuals with trauma (see Table 18.3 in Chapter 18; CDC, 2018).

TABLE 36.1 Preventing ACEs

Strategy	Approach
Strengthen economic supports to families	• Strengthening household financial security • Family-friendly work policies
Promote social norms that protect against violence and adversity	• Public education campaigns • Legislative approaches to reduce corporal punishment • Bystander approaches • Men and boys as allies in prevention
Ensure a strong start for children	• Early childhood home visitation • High-quality child care • Preschool enrichment with family engagement
Teach skills	• Socioemotional learning • Safe dating and healthy relationship skill programs • Parenting skills and family relationship approaches
Connect youth to caring adults and activities	• Mentoring programs • After-school programs
Intervene to lessen immediate- and long-term harms	• Enhanced primary care • Victim-centered services • Treatment to lessen the harms of ACEs • Treatment to prevent problem behavior and future involvement in violence • Family-centered treatment for substance use disorders

SUMMARY

ACEs exert a considerable toll on mental and physical health, life trajectory, public health, health care dollars, and the broader economy. Reducing risk factors, strengthening protective factors, and developing resilience mitigate the negative impact of ACEs. Improving public health care requires a shift in focus to preventing ACEs, promoting resilience building, and delivering trauma or ACE-informed health care (Garner, 2012; Hughes et al., 2017; Shonkoff, 2016). Increasing comprehensive programs at various levels of society that prevent, detect, and mitigate ACEs' effects should be a target for all.

RESOURCES

1 https://www.nctsn.org/

2 https://developingchild.harvard.edu/resources/toxic-stress-derails-healthy-development/

3 https://www.youtube.com/watch?v=8gm-lNpzU4g

4 https://www.youtube.com/watch?v=fWken5DsJcw

REFERENCES

Afifi, T. O., & Macmillan, H. L. (2011). Resilience following child maltreatment: a review of protective factors. *Canadian Journal of Psychiatry. Revue canadienne de psychiatrie, 56*(5), 266–272.

Anda, R. F., Whitfield, C. L., Felitti, V. J., Chapman, D., Edwards, V. J., Dube, S. R., & Williamson, D. F. (2002). Adverse childhood experiences, alcoholic parents, and later risk of alcoholism and depression. *Psychiatric Services (Washington, D.C.), 53*(8), 1001–1009. https://doi.org/10.1176/appi.ps.53.8.1001

Anda, R. F., Felitti, V. J., Bremner, J. D., Walker, J. D., Whitfield, C., Perry, B. D., Dube, S. R., & Giles, W. H. (2006). The enduring effects of abuse and related adverse experiences in childhood. A convergence of evidence from neurobiology and epidemiology. *European Archives of Psychiatry and Clinical Neuroscience, 256*(3), 174–186. https://doi.org/10.1007/s00406-005-0624-4

Anda, R. F., Brown, D. W., Felitti, V. J., Dube, S. R., & Giles, W. H. (2008). Adverse childhood experiences and prescription drug use in a cohort study of adult HMO patients. *BMC Public Health, 8*, 198. https://doi.org/10.1186/1471-2458-8-198

Banks, S. J., Eddy, K. T., Angstadt, M., Nathan, P. J., & Phan, K. L. (2007). Amygdala-frontal connectivity during emotion regulation. *Social Cognitive and Affective Neuroscience, 2*(4), 303–312. https://doi.org/10.1093/scan/nsm029

Bellis, M. A., Hughes, K., Ford, K., Ramos Rodriguez, G., Sethi, D., & Passmore, J. (2019). Life course health consequences and associated annual costs of adverse childhood experiences across Europe and North America: A systematic review and meta-analysis. *The Lancet. Public Health, 4*(10), e517–e528. https://doi.org/10.1016/S2468-2667(19)30145-8

Bethell, C. D., Newacheck, P., Hawes, E., & Halfon, N. (2014). Adverse childhood experiences: Assessing the impact on health and school engagement and the mitigating role of resilience. *Health Affairs (Project Hope), 33*(12), 2106–2115. https://doi.org/10.1377/hlthaff.2014.0914

Bethell, C., Gombojav, N., Solloway, M., & Wissow, L. (2016). Adverse childhood experiences, resilience and mindfulness-based approaches: Common denominator issues for children with emotional, mental, or behavioral problems. *Child and Adolescent Psychiatric Clinics of North America, 25*(2), 139–156. https://doi.org/10.1016/j.chc.2015.12.001

Bethell, C., Jones, J., Gombojav, N., Linkenbach, J., & Sege, R. (2019). Positive childhood experiences and adult mental and relational health in a statewide sample: Associations across adverse childhood experiences levels. *JAMA pediatrics, 173*(11), e193007. https://doi.org/10.1001/jamapediatrics.2019.3007

Brito, A., & Boller, K. (2020). Changing the pediatric paradigm: Focusing on strengths. *Pediatric Clinics of North America, 67*(2), 247–258. https://doi.org/10.1016/j.pcl.2019.12.010

Centers for Disease Control and Prevention. (2010). Adverse childhood experiences reported by adults—five states, 2009. *MMWR. Morbidity and Mortality Weekly Report, 59*(49), 1609–1613.

Centers for Disease Control and Prevention. (2013). *How do ACEs affect our lives.* https://vetoviolence.cdc.gov/apps/phl/resource_center_infographic.html

Centers for Disease Control and Prevention. (2018). *We can prevent ACEs.*

Chapman, D. P., Whitfield, C. L., Felitti, V. J., Dube, S. R., Edwards, V. J., & Anda, R. F. (2004). Adverse childhood experiences and the risk of depressive disorders in adulthood. *Journal of Affective Disorders, 82*(2), 217–225. https://doi.org/10.1016/j.jad.2003.12.013

Chapman, D. P., Wheaton, A. G., Anda, R. F., Croft, J. B., Edwards, V. J., Liu, Y., Sturgis, S. L., & Perry, G. S. (2011). Adverse childhood experiences and sleep disturbances in adults. *Sleep Medicine, 12*(8), 773–779. https://doi.org/10.1016/j.sleep.2011.03.013

Choi, K. R., McCreary, M., Ford, J. D., Rahmanian Koushkaki, S., Kenan, K. N., & Zima, B. T. (2019). Validation of the Traumatic Events Screening Inventory for ACEs. *Pediatrics, 143*(4), e20182546. https://doi.org/10.1542/peds.2018-2546

Clarkson Freeman, P. A. (2014). Prevalence and relationship between adverse childhood experiences and child behavior among young children. *Infant Mental Health Journal, 35*(6), 544–554.

Connor, K. M., & Davidson, J. R. (2003). Development of a new resilience scale: The Connor–Davidson Resilience Scale (CD-RISC). *Depression and Anxiety, 18*(2), 76–82.

Coons, P. M. (1994). Confirmation of childhood abuse in child and adolescent cases of multiple personality disorder and dissociative disorder not otherwise specified. *The Journal of Nervous and Mental Disease, 182*(8), 461–464.

Daskalakis N. P., Bagot R. C., Parker K. J., Vinkers C. H., & de Kloet E. R. (2013). The three-hit concept of vulnerability and resilience: Toward understanding adaptation to early-life adversity outcome. *Psychoneuroendocrinology, 38*(9), 1858-73. https://www.doi.org/10.1016/j.psyneuen.2013.06.008

Dong, M., Giles, W. H., Felitti, V. J., Dube, S. R., Williams, J. E., Chapman, D. P., & Anda, R. F. (2004). Insights into causal pathways for ischemic heart disease: adverse childhood experiences study. *Circulation, 110*(13), 1761–1766. https://doi.org/10.1161/01.CIR.0000143074.54995.7F

Douglas, K. R., Chan, G., Gelernter, J., Arias, A. J., Anton, R. F., Weiss, R. D., Brady, K., Poling, J., Farrer, L., & Kranzler, H. R. (2010). Adverse childhood events as risk factors for substance dependence: Partial mediation by mood and anxiety disorders. *Addictive Behaviors, 35*(1), 7–13. https://doi.org/10.1016/j.addbeh.2009.07.004

Douglas, K., Chan, G., Gelernter, J., Arias, A. J., Anton, R. F., Poling, J., Farrer, L., & Kranzler, H. R. (2011). 5-HTTLPR as a potential moderator of the effects of adverse childhood experiences on risk of antisocial personality disorder. *Psychiatric Genetics, 21*(5), 240–248. https://doi.org/10.1097/YPG.0b013e3283457c15

Dube, S. R., Anda, R. F., Felitti, V. J., Chapman, D. P., Williamson, D. F., & Giles, W. H. (2001). Childhood abuse, household dysfunction, and the risk of attempted suicide throughout the life span: Findings from the Adverse Childhood Experiences Study. *JAMA, 286*(24), 3089–3096. https://doi.org/10.1001/jama.286.24.3089

Dube, S. R., Fairweather, D., Pearson, W. S., Felitti, V. J., Anda, R. F., & Croft, J. B. (2009). Cumulative childhood stress and autoimmune diseases in adults. *Psychosomatic Medicine, 71*(2), 243–250. https://doi.org/10.1097/PSY.0b013e3181907888

Easterlin, M. C., Chung, P. J., Leng, M., & Dudovitz, R. (2019). Association of team sports participation with long-term mental health outcomes among individuals exposed to adverse childhood experiences. *JAMA Pediatrics, 173*(7), 681–688. https://doi.org/10.1001/jamapediatrics.2019.1212

Edwards, V. J., Anda, R. F., Gu, D., Dube, S. R., & Felitti, V. J. (2007). Adverse childhood experiences and smoking persistence in adults with smoking-related symptoms and illness. *The Permanente Journal*, *11*(2), 5–13. https://doi.org/10.7812/tpp/06-110

Ege, M. A., Messias, E., Thapa, P. B., & Krain, L. P. (2015). Adverse childhood experiences and geriatric depression: Results from the 2010 BRFSS. *The American Journal of Geriatric Psychiatry: Official Journal of the American Association for Geriatric Psychiatry*, *23*(1), 110–114. https://doi.org/10.1016/j.jagp.2014.08.014

Esteves, K. C., Jones, C. W., Wade, M., Callerame, K., Smith, A. K., Theall, K. P., & Drury, S. S. (2020). Adverse childhood experiences: Implications for offspring telomere length and psychopathology. *The American Journal of Psychiatry, 177*(1):47–57. https://doi.org/10.1176/appi.ajp.2019.18030335

Fang, X., Brown, D. S., Florence, C. S., & Mercy, J. A. (2012). The economic burden of child maltreatment in the United States and implications for prevention. *Child Abuse & Neglect*, *36*(2), 156–165. https://doi.org/10.1016/j.chiabu.2011.10.006

Felitti, V. J., Anda, R. F., Nordenberg, D., Williamson, D. F., Spitz, A. M., Edwards, V., Koss, M. P., & Marks, J. S. (1998). Relationship of childhood abuse and household dysfunction to many of the leading causes of death in adults: The Adverse Childhood Experiences (ACE) Study. *American Journal of Preventive Medicine*, *14*(4), 245–258. https://doi.org/10.1016/s0749-3797(98)00017-8

Felitti, V. J., Anda, R. F., Nordenberg, D., Williamson, D. F., Spitz, A. M., Edwards, V., Koss, M. P., & Marks, J. S. (1998). Relationship of childhood abuse and household dysfunction to many of the leading causes of death in adults. The Adverse Childhood Experiences (ACE) study. *American Journal of Preventive Medicine*, *14*(4), 245–258. https://doi.org/10.1016/s0749-3797(98)00017-8

Felitti, V. J., Anda, R. F., Nordenberg, D., Williamson, D. F., Spitz, A. M., Edwards, V., Koss, M. P., & Marks, J. S. (2019). REPRINT OF: Relationship of childhood abuse and household dysfunction to many of the leading causes of death in adults: The Adverse Childhood Experiences (ACE) Study. *American Journal of Preventive Medicine*, *56*(6), 774–786. https://doi.org/10.1016/j.amepre.2019.04.001

Garner, A. S., Shonkoff, J. P., Committee on Psychosocial Aspects of Child and Family Health, Committee on Early Childhood, Adoption, and Dependent Care, & Section on Developmental and Behavioral Pediatrics. (2012). Early childhood adversity, toxic stress, and the role of the pediatrician: Translating developmental science into lifelong health. *Pediatrics*, *129*(1), e224–e231. https://doi.org/10.1542/peds.2011-2662

Gilgoff, R., Singh, L., Koita, K., Gentile, B., & Marques, S. S. (2020). Adverse childhood experiences, outcomes, and interventions. *Pediatric Clinics of North America*, *67*(2), 259–273. https://doi.org/10.1016/j.pcl.2019.12.001

Hillis, S. D., Anda, R. F., Felitti, V. J., Nordenberg, D., & Marchbanks, P. A. (2000). Adverse childhood experiences and sexually transmitted diseases in men and women: A retrospective study. *Pediatrics*, *106*(1), E11. https://doi.org/10.1542/peds.106.1.e11

Horn S. R., Feder A. Understanding resilience and preventing and treating PTSD. (2018). *Harvard Review of Psychiatry, 26*(3), 158–174. https://doi.org/10.1097/HRP.0000000000000194

Hughes, K., Bellis, M. A., Hardcastle, K. A., Sethi, D., Butchart, A., Mikton, C., Jones, L., & Dunne, M. P. (2017). The effect of multiple adverse childhood experiences on health: A systematic review and meta-analysis. *The Lancet. Public Health*, *2*(8), e356–e366. https://doi.org/10.1016/S2468-2667(17)30118-4

Larkin, H., Felitti, V. J., & Anda, R. F. (2014). Social work and adverse childhood experiences research: Implications for practice and health policy. *Social Work in Public Health, 29*(1), 1–16.

Merrick, M. T., Ford, D. C., Ports, K. A., & Guinn, A. S. (2018). Prevalence of adverse childhood experiences from the 2011–2014 behavioral risk factor surveillance system in 23 states. *JAMA Pediatrics, 172*(11), 1038–1044. https://doi.org/10.1001/jamapediatrics.2018.2537

Merrick, J. S., Narayan, A. J., DePasquale, C. E., & Masten, A. S. (2019). Benevolent childhood experiences (BCEs) in homeless parents: A validation and replication study. *Journal of Family Psychology: Journal of the Division of Family Psychology of the American Psychological Association (Division 43)*, *33*(4), 493–498. https://doi.org/10.1037/fam0000521

Merrick, M. T., Ford, D. C., Ports, K. A., Guinn, A. S., Chen, J., Klevens, J., Metzler, M., Jones, C. M., Simon, T. R., Daniel, V. M., Ottley, P., & Mercy, J. A. (2019). Vital signs: Estimated proportion of adult health problems attributable to adverse childhood experiences and implications for prevention - 25 states, 2015-2017. *Morbidity and Mortality Weekly Report*, *68*(44), 999–1005. https://doi.org/10.15585/mmwr.mm6844e1

Onigu-Otite, E., & Idicula, S. (2020). Introducing ACEs (adverse childhood experiences) and resilience to first-year medical students. *MedEdPORTAL*, *16*, 10964.

Onigu-Otite, E. C., and Jamora, M. S. (2017). "Abuse and Neglect." *Johns Hopkins Psychiatry Guide*. www.hopkinsguides.com/hopkins/view/Johns_Hopkins_Psychiatry_Guide/787122/all/Abuse_and_Neglect.

Robles, A., Gjelsvik, A., Hirway, P., Vivier, P. M., & High, P. (2019). Adverse childhood experiences and protective factors with school engagement. *Pediatrics*, *144*(2), e20182945. https://doi.org/10.1542/peds.2018-2945

Schickedanz, A. B., Escarce, J. J., Halfon, N., Sastry, N., & Chung, P. J. (2019). Adverse childhood experiences and household out-of-pocket healthcare costs. *American Journal of Preventive Medicine*, *56*(5), 698–707. https://doi.org/10.1016/j.amepre.2018.11.019

Senn, T. E., Carey, M. P., & Vanable, P. A. (2008). Childhood and adolescent sexual abuse and subsequent sexual risk behavior: Evidence from controlled studies, methodological critique, and suggestions for research. *Clinical Psychology Review*, *28*(5), 711–735

Shonkoff, J.P. (2016). Capitalizing on advances in science to reduce the health consequences of early childhood adversity. *JAMA Pediatrics,*, *170*(10), 1003–1007.

Van Niel, C., Pachter, L. M., Wade, R., Jr, Felitti, V. J., & Stein, M. T. (2014). Adverse events in children: Predictors of adult physical and mental conditions. *Journal of Developmental and Behavioral Pediatrics*, *35*(8), 549–551. https://doi.org/10.1097/DBP.0000000000000102

Widom, C. S., DuMont, K., & Czaja, S. J. (2007). A prospective investigation of major depressive disorder and comorbidity in abused and neglected children grown up. *Archives of General Psychiatry*, *64*(1), 49–56.

Williamson, D. F., Thompson, T. J., Anda, R. F., Dietz, W. H., & Felitti, V. (2002). Body weight and obesity in adults and self-reported abuse in childhood. *International Journal of Obesity and Related Metabolic Disorders: Journal of the International Association for the Study of Obesity*, *26*(8), 1075–1082. https://doi.org/10.1038/sj.ijo.0802038

Zanarini, M. C., Frankenburg, F. R., Reich, D. B., Marino, M. F., Lewis, R. E., Williams, A. A., & Khera, G. S. (2000). Biparental failure in the childhood experiences of borderline patients. *Journal of Personality Disorders*, *14*(3), 264–273. https://doi.org/10.1521/pedi.2000.14.3.264

Zannas, A. S., & West, A. E. (2014). Epigenetics and the regulation of stress vulnerability and resilience. *Neuroscience*, *264*, 157–170.

CHAPTER 37

Social Determinants of Behavioral Health[1]

Olusola Oluwanuga, M.B.B.S.; Malvika Juneja, M.D.; and Harolyn Belcher, M.D., M.H.S.

> *"The essence of global health equity is the idea that something so precious as health might be viewed as a right."*
>
> — Paul Farmer

OBJECTIVES

After completing this chapter, students will be able to do the following:

- define social determinants of health
- describe social determinants of behavioral health
- discuss how social determinants impact the interplay between physical and mental health

CASE VIGNETTE

A 27-year-old male comes into the office for a post-emergency room visit. He was hospitalized recently for diabetic ketoacidosis. He is not sure how you can help him today because "no doctor has been able to cure his diabetes." You notice his low tone and avoidance of eye contact. He does not check his sugars at home and often runs out of insulin mainly because he cannot afford it. He denies using alcohol and tobacco but borrows marijuana from his friend on the weekends to treat his leg pain and get some sleep. When asked about his family history, he informs you that he does not know much about his father, but his mom died of advanced-stage cervical cancer when he and his sister were teenagers. He lives with his grandmother in an apartment, which

(continued)

1 Readers may also see "Diversity and Cultural Psychiatry" (Chapter 42) for related material.

he and his younger sister had moved into after their mother's death. You notice him tear up when he reports that his sister died of an overdose 4 years ago. He does not seem to like the apartment, the neighborhood, and the high school nearby—all of which he blames for his sister's death. He recalls being beaten up outside the same high school while trying to rescue his sister from the people who used to "poison her with drugs." The incident left him with knife injury in his right hip, a limp, chronic pain, and difficulty lifting and walking. Two years after, he was diagnosed with type I diabetes mellitus and started on injectable therapy. Since then, he has tried his best but cannot keep up with his diet recommendations and "the White man's food choices" on the paper that his nurse gave him. He likes to eat the dinner that his grandmother cooks each day, but since she is growing older, he relies on fast food and value meals.

Your questions probe him a bit more, and he reveals that he has been feeling guilty since his sister's death because he could not help her. "What's the point of taking medications? I don't even know what I am living for," he states. He finished 2 years in the local community college but had to stop to get a job to support his grandmother for rent and also because he needed health insurance that could help him with his diabetes medications. He had a girlfriend, but they broke up after his sister's death. You learn that he worked in a pizza place and was almost fired recently after punching an employee who insulted him, addressed him with a derogatory word, and reported him for "injecting stuff" during lunchtime. Because the manager would never believe his side of the story, he stopped using his lunchtime insulin to avoid explanation and confrontation. Since then, he has felt dizzy all the time, but last week, after he got wet in the rain while waiting at the bus stop, he developed a high fever. The next day he was taken to the ER for passing out outside his work.

KEY POINT

The social determinants of health (SDOH) are the conditions in which people are born, grow, live, work, and age. These include a range of factors that influence individuals' or populations' health status. Upstream macroeconomics and policies influence a broader set of political and structural forces that shape the systems in which these behaviors occur.

DEFINITIONS AND KEY CONCEPTS

The social determinants of health (SDOH) are a range of factors that influence individuals' or populations' health status (U.S. Department of Health and Human Services, 2020). Health is determined by complex interactions between social and economic factors, the physical environment, and individual behavior at every stage of life. Upstream macroeconomics and policies influence a broader set of political and structural forces that shape the systems in which these behaviors occur. Inequitable distribution of resources and social hierarchies based on income, gender, and race have emerged as causal factors for health disparities. These factors do not exist in isolation from each other. Instead, they interact together to create a tapestry into which health and life itself are woven.

INTRODUCTION

Human health is largely determined by several social factors, operating from the womb to the tomb, which play a role in determining how long and well an individual will live, the quality of their life, and the societal impact that will be exacted. This chapter aims to focus attention on these elements.

The World Health Organization definition always included social wellbeing in the definition of health. There is an increasing appreciation of the truism that "health is wealth." As the world recognizes the impact of health on economies, the factors influencing health outcomes have assumed significance and infiltrated discussions of policies and structural inequities that have bred these disparities.

KEY POINT

Health and economic inequity undermine human development. The COVID-19 pandemic demonstrated the vast footprint of health on world economics. In multiple ways, it highlighted the impact of SDOHs on pandemic outcomes (Mitchell, 2021; Nagata, 2021; Czeisler, 2020; Mason, 2021).

The COVID-19 pandemic, which shut down the global economy for a substantial part of 2020 and beyond, demonstrated the vast health footprint on world economics. Since it has left an impact on every person in the world in some way or form, its uniquely common preface provides a window through which to view the stark truths of disparity and inequity of provision, access, and services. Simply stated, the poorest amongst us are positioned to have worse health outcomes, and the relationship between poor health and little or no wealth perpetuates in a vicious cycle. This has brought to the fore again the role of the SDOH and the need for a structural transformation in terms of health assets.

Historical Background

The Commission on Determinants of Health (CSDH) was established by the WHO in March 2005. It was a global network of policymakers, researchers, and civil society organizations, brought together by the WHO to support countries and international health partners in addressing the social factors leading to poor health and health inequities (Donkin et al., 2017). The commission aimed to draw governments' and society's attention to the SDOH and the importance of creating better social conditions for health, particularly among the most vulnerable people. The commission delivered its report to the World Health Organization in July 2008, and it subsequently ended its functions. Since then, there have been national initiatives in most parts of the world to adopt a health in all policy (HiAP) approach to governance. This is an acknowledgment of the need to have an intersectoral collaborative approach to health.

MEMORY TIP

Social Determinants Of Health, *useful mnemonic*

SHEEN
S—Social (or community) support system
H—Healthcare access and quality
E—Economic stability
E—Education access and quality
N—Neighborhood / built community

(Created by Edore Onigu-Otite)

QUICK POINT

The approach of public health, policy, and research actions to reduce health disparities coupled with broad local and regional engagement in implementing public health strategies can help reduce disparities. Systemic change also includes medical education (Lewis, 2020; Doobay-Persaud, 2019).

KEY POINT

Social determinants of health generally fall into five domains:

- Economic stability
- Education access and quality
- Health care access and quality
- Neighborhood and built environment
- Social and community context

In the United States, the Healthy People initiative, coordinated by the U.S. Department of Health and Human Services, added SDOHs as a topic area to its agenda in 2010. This effectively recognized the role of social and structural elements in shaping national public health improvement. In addition, in 2011, the National Partnership for Action—the nation's first roadmap for reducing racial and ethnic health disparities—was released by the U.S. Department of Health and Human Services. A dual approach of public health, policy, and research actions directed by federal agencies to reduce health disparities coupled with broad local and regional engagement in implementing public health strategies to reduce disparities are underway (Donkin et al., 2017). These changes have also ushered in a new era in medical education with the ostensible goal of creating pedagogical approaches to discuss health equity and societal systems. The Liaison Committee on Medical Education (LCME) has posted requirements for introducing SDOHs to future physicians for building awareness, attitudes, and competencies for screening for social determinants of health and prescribing solutions to patients. Creating "critical consciousness" came to be viewed as an essential preface to future partnerships between health care and communities in need.

According to the U.S. Department of Health and Human Services (HHS), SDOHs are the conditions in the environments where people are born, live, learn, work, play, worship, and age that affect a wide range of health, functioning, and quality-of-life outcomes and risks.

The HHS's Healthy People 2030 program groups SDOHs into five domains (Figure 37.1):

- Economic stability
- Education access and quality
- Health care access and quality
- Neighborhood and built environment
- Social and community context

Each of these domains represents a cluster of factors that are interconnected. They interact in a complex way to form a web of factors, which, together with personal choices, influence individuals' or populations' health status throughout the life cycle. We will look in detail at these factors and discuss the concept of social determinants of health, particularly mental health, and consider how understanding these concepts plays a role in preventing mental illness and promoting mental health.

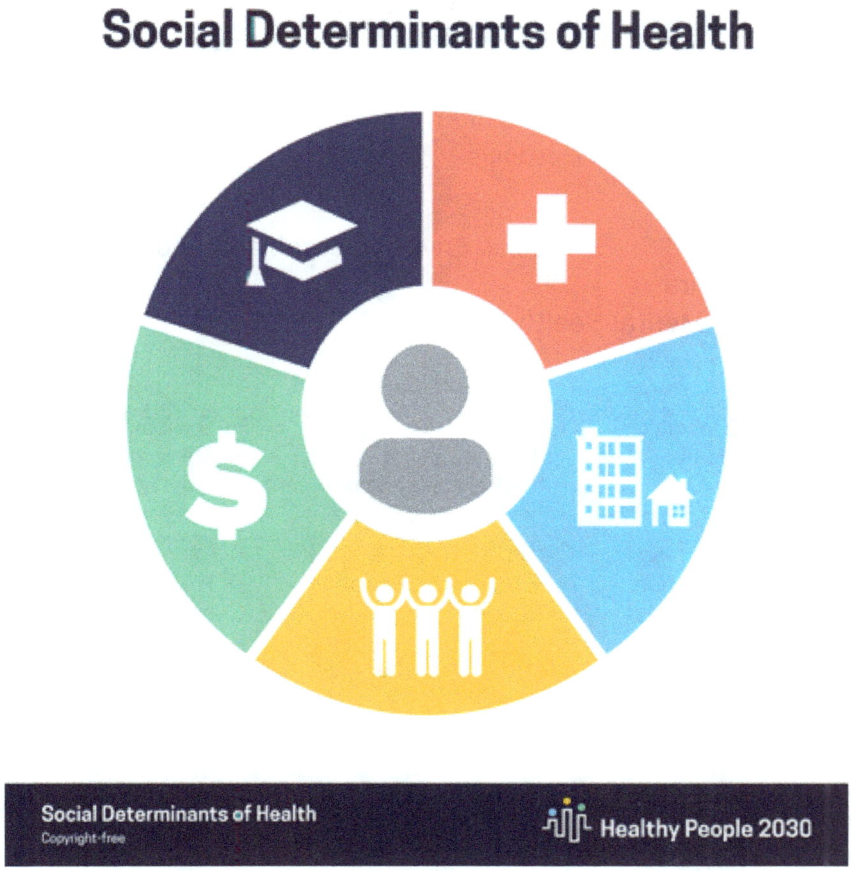

FIGURE 37.1 Social determinants of health.

Source: https://health.gov/healthypeople/objectives-and-data/social-determinants-health.

SOCIAL DETERMINANTS OF BEHAVIORAL HEALTH

Every national body has affirmed the profound impact of SDOHs on mental health and additional downstream issues of substance use, the risk for suicide, and resulting vulnerabilities and disabilities. A national study across many states conducted on 235,067 adults showed that the prevalence of "any depression" was significantly associated with income inequality—the more unequal, the higher the depression prevalence with a correlation coefficient of 43.5 ($p < .001$; Messias, 2011). The association persisted after adjustment for income per capita, percentage with a college degree, and percentage over age 65 (Messias, 2011). Despite the growing evidence that poor and disadvantaged individuals have disproportionately higher mental health issues, it is difficult to distinctly stratify the power and risk of any single SDOH domain. The interlaced issues of social justice, implicit bias, and political climate pose additional challenges in this examination. Scholars find it challenging to articulate discussions about focal elements while discussing

KEY POINT

There is a profound impact of SDOHs on mental health and additional downstream issues of substance use, the risk for suicide, and resulting vulnerabilities and disabilities.

the impact of SDOHs on behavioral health, or vice-versa. One way to approach the review of these determinants could be by dividing this scrutiny into risk factors and protective factors (Table 37.1). Although most of these are interrelated, we will discuss these under the following subheadings.

TABLE 37.1 Social, Environmental, and Economic Determinants of Mental Health

Category	Risk factors	Protective factors
Economic stability	• Poverty • Unemployment • Lack of steady employment • Inadequate childcare • Work stress	• Economic empowerment • Steady employment • Employment programs • Career counseling • High-quality childcare
Education access and quality	• Lack of educational opportunities • Lack of quality education • Lack of school engagement	• Provision of educational opportunities • School and college engagement • School community involvement
Health care access and quality	• Poor nutrition • Lack of access to health care • Lack of, or inadequate, health insurance • Low health literacy	• Adequate nutrition • Access and affordability of health care • Access to preventive health care • Health education
Neighborhood and built environment	• Environmental pollution • Lack of adequate housing • Lack of transportation • Neighborhood disorganization • Easy access to drugs and alcohol • Neighborhood crime and violence • High level of incarceration	• Adequate housing • Adequate transportation • Social cohesion and responsibility • Social tolerance and inclusion • Accessibility of social services • Navigation and utilization of social services
Social and community context	• Social discrimination • Inadequate social support • Urbanization and gentrification • Racial injustice • Ethnic discrimination • War and conflict • Community displacement	• Ethnic minorities integration • Investment in cultural identity • Social tolerance and inclusion • Spirituality and value systems • Social tolerance and inclusion • Community peaceful coexistence

RISK FACTORS

Economic Stability

Economic refers to as the social standing of an individual, family, or group, often measured in terms of income and occupation. . Economic stability depends on factors such as income, housing, food security, cost of living, and affording lifestyle choices, and others. Anxiety, low mood, low self-esteem, and poor sleep could readily occur in the presence of economic instability. Even from conception, economic instability could affect nutrition and antenatal care, putting the developing brain in jeopardy. As of 2020, more than two thirds of Americans were financially vulnerable (Messias, 2011). Thus, it is an important and overarching factor for consideration. Economic stress, including financial hardship and job loss, may worsen mental health and contribute to increases in suicide, substance use, and violence (Galea, 2020; McGinty, 2020; Reeves, 2021).

QUICK POINT

Poverty strikes different demographics differently. In 2018, the poverty rate for two-parent households was only 4.7%. For, single-parent (father-only) households it was 12.7%, and for single-parent (mother-only) households the rate was 24.9%. The poverty rate for people living with a disability, including for mental health, is high, at 25.7%.

Poverty

Poverty is a predisposing factor in mental illness, and mental illness predisposes to poverty (Costello, 2003). It is a vicious cycle of cause and effect. Some studies have found that, with the exception of schizophrenia, poverty is more likely to occur before the onset of mental health disorders (Grohol, 2015). Poverty is associated with several of the other factors mentioned already because it is a common thread through all domains of SDOHs. In addition to the overt risk of stress that poverty inflicts on mental well-being, poverty is also related to reduced access and affordability of mental health resources. Poor and disadvantaged individuals hesitate to seek help, utilize resources, and adhere to therapeutics for mental health conditions.

QUICK POINT

Adults aged 26 or older living below the poverty line were more likely to experience serious mental illness compared to those living at and above the poverty line (7.5% versus 4.1% and 3.1%, respectively; National Surveys on Drug Use and Health, 2016). Adults with mental illness who are living in poverty may face higher health care costs, decreased productivity, and poorer general health (Anakwenze, 2013).

Job Loss, Unemployment, and Lack of Steady Employment

Unemployment, job loss, and lack of steady employment all impact the economics of families and communities, impacting various aspects of health. Having a job positions people to earn an income, provide for their family, have a place in society, and provide a sense of dignity. Employment and the attainment of personal goals positively impact individuals, while loss of employment is known to usher in the risk of isolation, substance use, and violence. Inability to get a job or the loss of a job are associated with anxiety, depression, loss of self-esteem, and even suicide risk. Additionally, loss of employment can significantly set back those individuals who previously had access to mental health treatment and resources through insurance providers. The correlations are not unidimensional, and triggers for mental health issues are tied to employment and sustainability in many ways. For example, a study out of Florida reported that households with an income of less than $20,000 have the highest rate of serious mental disorder, while those with incomes of $75,000 and above, belonging to a higher economic status, have the lowest rates of serious mental illness (Florida Council for Community Mental Health,, 2007.).

Work Stress

Positive stress in the workplace can help drive productivity, but chronic and excessive stress reduces productivity and harms workers' mental health. Microaggressions and explicit discrimination can result in anxiety, depression, burnout, substance use disorders, and a worsening of preexisting mental illness. Mistrust, issues with privacy and fear of loss of employment can further prevent individuals from seeking help for mental health issues.

EDUCATION ACCESS AND QUALITY

Education is a "process and a product" (Hahn, 2015). Education brings exposure and a better understanding of health issues. Ideally, it results in a higher likelihood of prioritizing factors that increase healthy lifestyle behaviors and promote mental health (Hahn, 2015). Like other thematic areas, education does not affect health in isolation but acts in conjunction with other factors. There is an overlap between factors that provide access to good quality education for an individual or community and those that are likely to provide access to good quality health care.

Lack of Education

A lack of education and its attendant consequences of poor health behavior, risky behavior, poor health-seeking, and reduced use of preventive health services are risks for reduced-income generations. People with higher levels of education are more likely to be healthier and live longer. This has led to the emphasis on the need for early childhood education programs, based on strong evidence of the effectiveness in improving educational outcomes associated with long-term health and sufficient evidence of effectiveness of improving social- and health-related outcomes (Community Preventive Services Task Force, 2016).

Low Health Literacy

Education directly affects health literacy. Low health literacy impedes disease identification, engagement in treatment, and treatment outcomes. Early treatment and ongoing medical supervision of mental health depend on sociocultural foundations and literacy about psychiatric disorders and available treatment options. This risk factor is both a risk and a barrier, as low health literacy keeps individuals from seeking timely care and prevents treatment adherence.

HEALTH CARE ACCESS AND QUALITY

Good mental health begins at conception and develops largely in tandem with good physical health. Therefore, access to good quality health care, which comes with prevention, early detection, and intervention, is an important thematic area in determining mental health.

Nutrition and Lifestyle

Nutrition and lifestyle affect the body and the mind. Anxiety, depression, mood disorders, quality of sleep, and poor cognitive functioning have all been linked to poor nutrition. Pathological and physiological changes occur with poor diet and challenge mental and physical state of being. Additionally, food insecurity can change an individual's food choices, paving the way for obesity and chronic diseases.

Behavior Health Equity

Behavioral health equity is the right to access quality health care for all populations, regardless of the individual's race, ethnicity, gender, socioeconomic status, sexual orientation, or geographical location (Substance Abuse and Mental Health Services, 2020; WHO, 2008). With the pandemic, the rapid proliferation of health informatics and digital health innovations has revolutionized health care service delivery. On the other hand, it highlighted the technological divide only made wider by SDOHs. Nevertheless, with appropriate planning and appropriation of resources, this represents a significant opportunity to improve health equity (Brewer, 2020; Vienot, 2019).

NEIGHBORHOOD AND BUILT ENVIRONMENT

The built environment has direct and indirect effects on mental health (Evans, 2003). The zip code of an individual's residence may be an important predictor of their mental health vulnerability. Places of residence have been associated with health inequalities that are becoming more predictive of individuals' health than their genetic codes (Vlahor, 2007; Todman, 2015).

Lack of Housing and Transportation

Lacking basic amenities places people at risk for mental illness. In addition, noise pollution and light pollution experienced in public transportation worsen sleep quality and increase the risk of insomnia. Poor housing, renting accommodation, and homelessness all negatively impact mental health. Depending on related factors, renting and accommodation can be associated with stress and anxiety. They can be a cause of argument and family disharmony, which increases stress and predisposes individuals to mental health problems. Homelessness carries a higher incidence of mental disorders, such as depression, bipolar disorder, schizophrenia, panic attacks, and PTSD. Some members of the homeless population experience psychiatric symptoms, including mood, anxiety, and psychotic symptoms and are at a high risk of substance use disorder and suicidality.

Access to Drugs and Alcohol

Drugs and alcohol are harmful to mental health, often creating a strong cycle of cause and effect. One of the risk factors that increases chances of engaging in drug or alcohol overuse is easier access. Access to these substances is linked to systemic factors, such as poverty, crowded housing, high crime rates, broken school systems, predatory settings, and lawlessness. The midstream effect of domestic instability and additional access to drugs and alcohol from within family systems is another potent driver for adopting risky behaviors. Overall influences of families and neighborhoods were noted as correlating, in many studies, to substance use and mental health disorders. According to a survey of offices in state welfare, the top two issues in their child protection cases were poverty (lower economic status) and parental alcohol and drug use, as claimed in 85% of cases (Substance Abuse and Mental Health Services Administration, 2000).

Neighborhood Social Disorganization

Individuals who live in socially disorganized neighborhoods are more at risk of depression, social withdrawal, dissociative coping, substance use, and PTSD than people who live in environments where crime and violence are less rife. Sidewalks, parks, recreation centers, and neighborhoods are built environments that promote social organization and invite engagement and improved mental wellness (Todman, 2015). A lack of amenities and safety concerns are significant deterrents at an individual level as well as on the community level.

Violence and Crime

Violence is a public health problem in many societies, including in the United States. Violence can be self-perpetuating. Children who grow up in communities with persistent violence are at higher risk of committing violence themselves and at increased risk of delinquency. Both victims and perpetrators have mental health consequences, including depression, anxiety, PTSD, self-harm, and suicide. Violence, both inside and outside the home, impacts the worldview of those involved in it and damages perceptions and societal connections of trust (Pinchevsky, 2012; Coulton, 2007). Exceptionally disproportionate incarceration rates and unprovoked crime in communities of color speak to the significant need for programs that comprehensively heal these communities.

Urbanization

Urbanization has resulted from industrialization and development. Although it comes with economic advantages, a wide range of disorders and deviancies are associated with urbanization (Vlahov, 2007; Srivastava, 2009). Although it comes with economic advantages, a wide range of disorders and deviancies are associated with urbanization. Some of the disorders are severe mental disorders, depression, substance abuse, alcoholism, crime, family disintegration, and alienation. Gentrification is an additional side effect of economic growth and has resulted in destabilizing communities. The resulting state of, or threat of, homelessness has placed undue stress on families, disrupted social ecosystems, and weakened support structures for individuals. An emerging national focus has pointed to the recent rise of environmentally hazardous industries trying to benefit from low land prices in getting placed in close proximity to low-income neighborhoods. Individuals exposed to or working with these substances have presented with a wide range of symptoms, from insomnia to overt psychosis. Thus urbanization, gentrification, and unconstrained industrial growth have in many ways failed disadvantaged groups from direct and indirect risks and created several health disparities, including mental health issues.

SOCIAL AND COMMUNITY CONTEXT

The social context within which a person is placed, their sense of community, available community support, acceptance, and cohesiveness all serve as determinants of their health. This is becoming increasingly relevant as society evolves and individuals ascend in terms of the hierarchy of needs.

Poor Social Capital

Social capital is often seen as the potential of community individuals to work together to create solutions for challenges through networking. A lack of trust and inclusion leads to truncated social networks, weakening discussions of community values, common goals, and mutual obligations. The resulting lowering of social capital causes increased rates of hate crimes and violence and results in mental health issues, including anxiety, paranoia, depression, and insomnia among community members. Social disadvantage may occur because of personal attributes over which the individual may have no control. Factors such as gender, age, race, ethnicity, disability all negatively impact mental health. In general, when human rights are not protected, the socially disadvantaged tend to receive inordinately negative impact on their mental health.

Isolation and Alienation

Isolation and alienation can result in increased stress, anxiety, and cognitive decline. It is hypothesized that alienation is impacted by upstream factors of social injustice and structural forces, including race and gender. These influences force a perpetual focus on survival and predispose individuals to emotions of stress and hopelessness, leading to downstream isolation. Both perceived and explicit, alienation can also create apathy and a loss of desire for personal attainment or social engagement in individuals.

CLINICAL TIP

Negativity arising from discrimination, overt profiling, and implicit and explicit bias based on color, gender, race, weight, social class, political inclination, education, and employment is a substantial structural determinant affecting individuals' mental health and wellness.

Social Discrimination

Social discrimination is a risk factor for depression, PTSD, social avoidance, and suicidality. Negativity arising from discrimination, social rejection by peers, overt profiling, and implicit and explicit bias based on color, gender, race, weight, social class, political inclination, education, and employment is a substantial structural determinant affecting individuals' mental health and wellness. When people experience discrimination or injustice of any kind, it has negative consequences on their mental well-being (Beeri, 2012). Trauma, chronic stress, anxiety, and depression are all associated with racial discrimination. The rise in divisive political and social dialogue in the country and the growth of opinions and expressions on social media are significant factors that shake mood stability and mental wellness. The history of segregation and archaic structural and social justice policies breed fear and trigger mental health issues in marginalized communities.

Deficient Social Support

Individuals with fractured support systems are more prone to developing mental illnesses (Compton, 2015). The bonds of religion, ethnicity, or shared objectives can provide numerous resources and benefits and provide a platform to share frustrations, while providing a safe environment to ask for help. There is a disproportionately higher incidence of mental health disorders among individuals inadequately connected to such systems, including depression, anxiety, insomnia, and PTSD. Among others, vulnerable groups with the highest risk of being negatively impacted by lack of support are post-incarcerated individuals, members of LGBTQ+ groups, those affected by HIV and AIDS, and minimally integrated refugee families. Programs built to support these groups show evidence of this correlation.

War and Conflict

War and conflict often occur, despite diplomatic efforts to prevent them. The mental health consequences of war include anxiety, depression, and PTSD, especially among combat personnel. The long-term and short-term effects on mental health result from grief, loss, and disability accompanying wars and civil unrest. These effects can be debilitating for individuals, families, and societies impacted by wars and community conflict.

Displacement

This social consequence of war, famine, ecological disaster, and other such events is a potent risk factor for mental illness. Displaced people are at greater risk of developing depression, anxiety, PTSD, and psychoses than people living in stable conditions. PTSD is associated with a range of factors, including sociodemographic factors, event exposure characteristics, social support, and personality traits (Neria, 2008). Whether the change is across seas (e.g., immigration or local homelessness), the resultant impact of forced displacements is regarded as a trigger for the development or precipitation of several mental health conditions (Neria, 2008; Grattan, 2011).

QUICK POINT

Social determinants can also act as protective factors to improve mental resilience and improve individuals' chances of staying mentally healthy.

Protective Factors

Social determinants can also act as protective factors to improve mental resilience and improve individuals' chances of staying mentally healthy. These protective factors are listed in Table 37.1

Empowerment

Empowerment refers to uplifting an individual or community by granting autonomy to make choices and access to rights and services. These include freedom of association, access to health services, education, and other services, including economic empowerment. In mental health, empowerment refers specifically to the freedom an individual has to make choices. When people feel that they are part of the decision-making process, they become more engaged, contributing to the development of mental resilience.

CLINICAL TIP

In mental health, empowerment refers specifically to the freedom an individual has to make choices. When people feel that they are part of the decision-making process, they become more engaged, contributing to the development of mental resilience.

Access and Affordability of Health Care

Access is a strong determinant, and communities and individuals who have access to health care options with health insurance are noted to have better health outcomes. Studies show that a person who earns up to $20,000 a year has a one third lower chance of recovering from cocaine abuse than a person that earns more than $70,000 per year (Szalavitz, 2011). Mental health treatments need long-term associations with the health care systems. Along with medical supervision, insured individuals have increased adherence to therapeutics and better utilization of resources.

Ethnic Minorities Integration

Ethnic minorities tend to be disadvantaged, due to a lack of robust support and referral systems. This lack of integration tends to perpetuate the risk factors for poor health. Integration addresses this disadvantage and reduces stigma, a critical factor that prevents minorities from seeking help early for mental health issues. Integration builds communication and pathways to options for ethnic minorities.

QUICK POINT

Ethnic minorities tend to be disadvantaged, due to a lack of robust support and referral systems. This lack of integration tends to perpetuate the risk factors for poor health.

Social Cohesion

Cohesive and collectively poised communities have a chance at better mental health and well-being. Positive interpersonal relationships are based on respect, loyalty, and trust and contribute to resilience and improved mental wellness. Support sharing is foundational for change and allows individuals to adopt best practices even when there is an initial unfamiliarity with the change.

CLINICAL TIP

Individuals end up with better outcomes for both mental and physical health options when their value systems are understood and they are regarded as a microcosm of their communities.

Investment in Cultural Identity

Individuals end up with better outcomes for mental and physical health options when their value systems are understood and they are regarded as a microcosm of their communities. Today, providers are learning to be culturally humble to provide shared medical decisions to manage individuals' mental health issues, keeping their culture and community identity intact. A stronger community identity is protective against the risk of loneliness and isolation. It empowers individuals, provides improved mental well-being and builds mental resilience.

Social Tolerance and Inclusion

Tolerant, adaptable, and inclusive societies do not alienate people dealing with mental health issues. Individuals benefit when they live in a safe and inclusive environment because it gives them a chance to confront their fears and reset responsibility and expectations regarding mental disorders. Lack of inclusiveness creates barriers for those dealing with mental health issues.

Navigation and Utilization of Social Services

Easy navigation of medical systems, improved social services, support, and community networks provide a protective safety net against matters such as domestic violence, child abuse, neglect of the elderly, and others. A strong community network contributes to a sense of safety, which is essential to mental health and well-being. Transparency of cost and care requirements helps promote stronger adherence to medical management of medical disorders. Systems that provide navigators and support services create better outcomes for their members.

Spirituality and Value Systems

Individuals who lean on faith and spirituality have been shown to demonstrate increased resilience and enhanced mental well-being. Overarching spiritual goals usher in emotions of safety and allow individuals to stay positively aligned in their care.

SOCIAL DETERMINANTS OF HEALTH AND THE INTERPLAY BETWEEN PHYSICAL AND MENTAL HEALTH

SDOHs dictate outcomes for both physical and mental health. There is strong evidence that macro-level structural, spiritual, environmental, political, cultural, and economic factors drive proximal measures of community organization and integration; distal measures of individual behaviors; and choices affecting mental and physical health outcomes (Silva, 2016).

Before expanding on equity discussions, we must first acknowledge the interdependability of physical and mental health, as seen in several circumstances (e.g., substance use disorder, cardiovascular disease, diabetes, etc.). The interplay of psychological and psychophysiological mechanisms is so pervasive that the medical field has come to recognize several paradigms in which people with mental conditions end up with worsening physical health and early death. Studies found that in 2000, approximately 245,000 deaths were attributable to low education, 162,000 were due to low social support, 133,000 were due to individual-level poverty, and 119,000 were due to income inequality (Bornstein, 2018). Figure 37.2 depicts major factors impacting human development across the life span.

KEY POINT

The mental health of individuals is shaped by the social, environmental, and economic conditions in which they are born, grow, work, and age. There is strong evidence that macro-level structural, spiritual, environmental, political, cultural, and economic factors drive proximal measures of community organization and integration; distal measures of individual behaviors; and choices affecting mental and physical health outcomes (Silva, 2016).

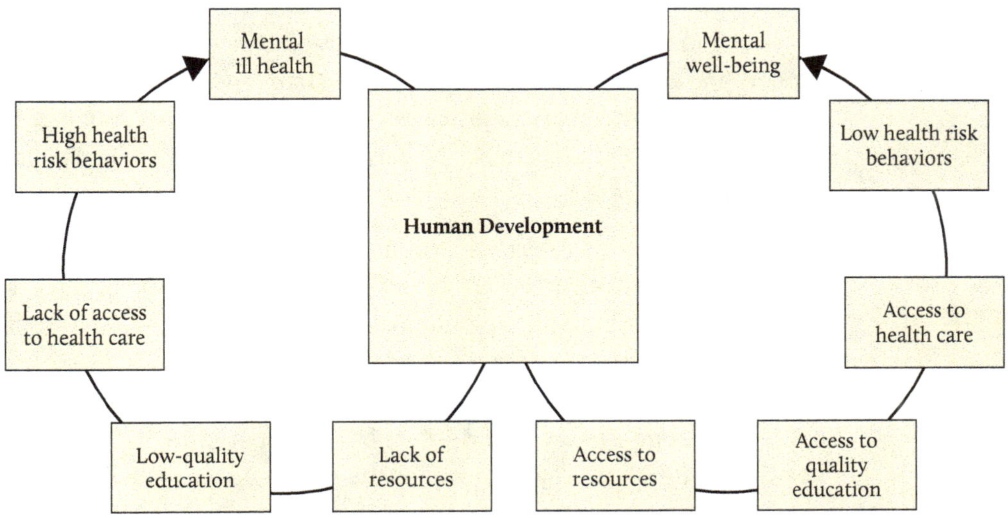

FIGURE 37.2 Social determinants of health, mental well-being, and human development

It is widely understood that the overall quality of physical health and wellness depends on wise choices related to nutrition, exercise, labor, sleep, and social interactions. These choices demand a centered mindset and stable mental health. Individuals with behavioral disorders are often unable to create equilibrium in their lives to support health-oriented decisions. Risky behaviors arising out of dented coping strategies, denial, dependence on alcohol and substance use, preferences for isolation and sedentary habits, unaffordability of low sugar and high-quality foods, and the paranoia toward an already inaccessible health care system together create an intricate cycle of mental and physical disease in these individuals.

Mental health challenges create deficiencies in navigating the health care system, seeking preventive care, demonstrating treatment adherence, and accessing available resources—all of which rely on optimism, social prowess, reliable income, and an overall meaning in life. Suffering from mental disorders, these individuals spiral toward an unending decline in physical health, whereby minimal, reactive, and sporadic interactions with health care cause inadequate chronic disease management, morbidity, and sequelae, leading to the ultimate setting for disability. Therefore, the link between the mind and body is undeniable, such that one cannot be conceived without the other.

Moving the discussion to study the upstream factors that seed these mechanisms and extend the binary associations between physical and mental health, we can concede to the argument that dimensions of both physical and psychological health rely on traditional ecosystems of social support and economic security. Fractured systems and social disadvantage create barriers, shame, hopelessness, and an assumptive outlook of the health care system that perpetuates mistrust, causing a delay in diagnosis and treatment for both.

Race, gender, social class, and poverty continue to play a part in dictating what that environment can offer and, thereby, continue to design end outcomes for both physical and mental health in populations—better for the wealthy and worse for the poor. Economic disparities resulting from cultural imperialism and health disparities resulting from social inequity are perpetuating the cause-and-effect interplay between SDOHs, mental health, and physical health (known as the *spillover phenomenon*).

CLINICAL TIP

An individual's reliance on good physical health to sustain functionality, quality in life, and productivity in society carries a profound reciprocal relationship with their mental well-being as well as their environment.

In effect, an individual's reliance on good physical health to sustain functionality, quality of life, and productivity in society carries a profound reciprocal relationship with their mental wellbeing as well as their environment. Breaking this cycle of mental and physical disease is not feasible without creating a social framework of inclusion, freedom from discrimination, equitable resource distribution, and access to care so that the mind can heal the body, and vice-versa. Today, health care advocates seeking universal improvement in outcomes for physical and mental health demand the promotion of interventions that can make social systems cohesive, invite enduring integration of minorities, reduce food insecurity, create safe green spaces for exercise, provide safe housing, enhance preventive services, offer trauma-informed care, decentralize resources for mental health, offer home-based social support, and elevate consideration of population health in all national policies (Heiman, 2015). Future comprehensive health outcomes will depend on explicit advocacy for transformational restructuring of health care access, social justice reform, nourishment of civic agencies of change, and rejection of all forms of bias.

QUICK POINT

Breaking this cycle of mental and physical disease is not feasible without creating a social framework of inclusion, freedom from discrimination, equitable resource distribution, and access to care so that the mind can heal the body, and vice versa.

SUMMARY

SDOHs involve multiple factors which influence health behaviors, health risk, health access and treatment, and health outcomes. The factors listed above are not exhaustive, but they should set us thinking about the cross-cutting nature of mental health-related matters. Many of these factors do not occur in isolation. Instead, they are often interwoven in a web, creating multilayered vulnerabilities for communities and individuals who are already weakened by social hierarchal disadvantage and challenges of survival. An upsurge of national dialogue in this arena of health care has provided a fresh lens into the role of SDOHs in health disparities and our collective social responsibility to study, frame, dissect and change upstream factors that perpetuate these disparities. Emerging curricula in medical education are preparing health care providers of tomorrow with skills and competencies to lead this change. The undeniable influence of these root causes on mental health and the impact of mental health on the overall growth of individuals, communities, and countries compels an overhaul of mental health policies, resource allocation, and eradication of stigma. Only after that can we realize the dream of equitable health care options for all.

RESOURCES

1 https://health.gov/healthypeople/priority-areas/social-determinants-health

2 https://www.youtube.com/watch?v=zSguDQRjZv0

3 https://www.nami.org/Blogs/NAMI-Blog/August-2020/Ways-We-Can-Address-the-Social-Determinants-of-Mental-Health

REFERENCES

Anakwenze, U., & Zuberi, D. (2013). Mental health and poverty in the inner city. *Health & Social Work, 38*(3), 147–157.

Beeri, A., & Lev-Wiesel, R. (2012) Social rejection by peers: A risk factor for psychological distress. *Child and Adolescent Mental Health, 17*(4)

Brewer, L. C., Fortuna, K. L., Jones, C., Walker, R., Hayes, S. N., Patten, C. A., & Cooper, L. A. (2020). Back to the future: Achieving health equity through health informatics and digital health. *JMIR mHealth and uHealth, 8*(1), e14512. https://doi.org/10.2196/14512

Center for Substance Abuse Treatment. (2000). Substance abuse treatment for persons with child abuse and neglect issues. https://www.ncbi.nlm.nih.gov/books/NBK64904/

Community Preventive Services Task Force. (2016). Recommendation for center-based early childhood education to promote health equity. *Journal of Public Health Management and Practice, 22*(5), E9–E10. https://doi.org/10.1097/PHH.0000000000000354

Compton M. T., Shim R. S. (2015). The social determinants of mental health. *Focus. 13*, 419–25. https://www.doi.org/10.1176/appi.focus.20150017

Costello, E. J. (2003). Relationship between poverty and psychopathology. *JAMA, 290,* 2023-2029

Coulton, C. J., Crampton, D. S., Irwin, M., Spilsbury, J. C., & Korbin, J. E. (2007). How neighborhoods influence child maltreatment: A review of the literature and alternative pathways. *Child Abuse & Neglect, 31*(11–12), 1117-1142.

Czeisler, M. É., Lane, R. I., Petrosky E., Wiley, J. F., Christensen, A., Njai, R., Weaver, M. D., Robbins, R., Facer-Childs, E. R., Barger, L. K., Czeisler, C. A., Howard, M. E., & Rajaratnam, S. M. (2020). Mental health, substance use, and suicidal ideation during the COVID-19 pandemic—United States, June 24–30, 2020. *Morbidity Mortality Weekly Report (MMWR), 69,* 1049–1057. http://dx.doi.org/10.15585/mmwr.mm6932a1external icon

Daniel, H., Bornstein, S. S., & Kane, G. C. (2018). Addressing social determinants to improve patient care and promote health equity: an American College of Physicians position paper. *Annals of Internal Medicine,168*(8), 577–578. https://www.doi.org/10.7326/M17-2441

Donkin, A., Goldblatt, P., Allen, J., Nathanson, V., & Marmot, M. (2017). Global action on the social determinants of health. *BMJ Global Health, 3,* (Supplement 1), e000603. https://doi.org/10.1136/bmjgh-2017-000603

Doobay-Persaud, A., Adler, M. D., & Bartell, T. R., Sheneman, N. E., Martinez, M. D., Mangold, K. A., Smith, P., & Sheehan, K. M.(2019). Teaching the social determinants of health in undergraduate medical education: A scoping review. *Journal of General Internal Medicine, 34*(5), 720–730. https://www.doi.org/10.1007/s11606-019-04876-0

Evans, G. W. (2003). The built environment and mental health. *Journal of Urban Health: Bulletin of the New York Academy of Medicine, 80*(4), 536–555. https://doi.org/10.1093/jurban/jtg063

Grattan, L. M., Roberts, S., Mahan, W. T., Jr, McLaughlin, P. K., Otwell, W. S., & Morris, J. G., Jr. (2011). The early psychological impacts of the Deepwater Horizon oil spill on Florida and Alabama communities. *Environmental Health Perspectives, 119*(6), 838–843

Grohol, J. M. (n.d.). "The Vicious Cycle of Poverty and Mental Health." Psych Central. Accessed June 3, 2015.

Hahn, R. A., & Truman, B. I. (2015). Education improves public health and promotes health equity. *International Journal of Health Services: Planning, Administration, Evaluation, 45*(4), 657–678. https://doi.org/10.1177/0020731415585986

Heiman H. J., & Artiga S. (2015). *Beyond health care: The role of social determinants in promoting health and health equity.* The Henry J. Kaiser Family Foundation.

Holland, K. M., Jones, C., Vivolo-Kantor, A. M., Idaikkadar, N., Zwald, M., Hoots, B., Yard, E., D'Inverno, A., Swedo, E., Chen, M. S., Petrosky, E., Board, A., Martinez, P., Stone, D. M., Law, R., Coletta, M. A., Adjemian, J., Thomas, C., Puddy, R. W., Peacock, G., ... Houry, D. (2021). Trends in US Emergency Department Visits for Mental Health, Overdose, and Violence Outcomes Before and During the COVID-19 Pandemic. *JAMA Psychiatry, 78*(4), 372–379. https://doi.org/10.1001/jamapsychiatry.2020.4402

Lewis, J. H., Lage, O. G., Grant, B. K., Rajasekaran, S. K., Gemeda, M., Like, R. C., Santen, S., & Dekhtyar, M. (2020). *Addressing the social determinants of health in undergraduate medical education curricula: A survey report. Advances in Medical Education and Practice, 11*, 369–377. https://doi.org/10.2147/AMEP.S243827

Mason, M. Welch, S. B., Arunkumar, P., Post, L. A., & Feinglass, J. M. (2021). Opioid overdose deaths before, during, and after an 11-week COVID-19 stay-at-home order—Cook County, Illinois, January 1, 2018—October 6, 2020. *Morbidity Mortality Weekly Report, 70*, 362–363. http://dx.doi.org/10.15585/mmwr.mm7010a3

Mental Illness and Poverty: A Fact Sheet. Florida Council for Community Mental Health (2007)

Messias E., Eaton W. W, & Grooms A. N. (2011). Income inequality and depression prevalence across the United States: An ecological study. *Psychiatric Services (Washington, D.C.), 62*, 710–712

Mitchell, T. O., & Li, L. (2021). State-level data on suicide mortality during COVID-19 quarantine: Early evidence of a disproportionate impact on minorities. *Psychiatry Research, 295*. https://doi.org/10.1016/j.psychres.2020.113629.

Neria Y, Nandi A, Galea S. (2021). Post-traumatic stress disorder following disasters: A systematic review. *Psychological Medicine, 38*(4), 467–480. https://doi.org/10.1017/S0033291707001353

Nagata, J. M., Ganson, K. T., Whittle, H. J., Chu, J., Harris, O. O., Tsai, A. C., Weiser, S. D. (2021). Food insufficiency and mental health in the U.S. during the COVID-19 pandemic. *American Journal of Preventive Medicine*. https://doi.org/10.1016/j.amepre.2020.12.004.

Pinchevsky G. M, Wright E. M. (2012). The impact of neighborhoods on intimate partner violence and victimization. *Trauma Violence Abuse, 13*(2):112–132. https://doi.org/10.1177/152483801244564111

Silva, M., Loureiro, A., & Cardoso, G. (2016). Social determinants of mental health: A review of the evidence *European Journal of Psychiatry, 30*(4).

Srivastava K. (2009). Urbanization and mental health. *Industrrial Psychiatry Journal., 18*(2), 75–76. doi: 10.4103/0972-6748.64028

Substance Abuse and Mental Health Services. (2020). *Behavioral health equity.* https://www.samhsa.gov/behavioral-health-equity. Accessed on October 20, 2021

Substance Abuse and Mental Health Services Administration. (n.d.). *Serious mental illness among adults below the poverty line.* https://www.samhsa.gov/data/sites/default/files/report_2720/Spotlight-2720.html.

Szalavitz, M. *Yes, Addiction Does Discriminate.* (2021). The Fix. https://www.thefix.com/content/economic-inequality-and-addiction8202

Todman L. C., Holliday C. S. (2015). Adverse features of the built environment. In: M. T. Compton, & R. S. Shim (Eds.), *The social determinants of mental health* (pp. 192–212). American Psychiatric Publishing.

U.S. Department of Health and Human Services, Office of Disease Prevention and Health Promotion. (2021). *Healthy people 2030.* https://health.gov/healthypeople/objectives-and-data/social-determinants-health

Veinot, T. C., Ancker, J. S., & Bakken, S. (2019). Health informatics and health equity: Improving our reach and impact. *Journal of the American Medical Informatics Association, 26*(8–9), 689–695. https://doi.org/10.1093/jamia/ocz132

Vlahov, D., Freudenberg, N., Proietti, F., Ompad, D., Quinn, A., Nandi, V., & Galea, S. (2007). Urban as a determinant of health. *Journal of Urban Health: Bulletin of the New York Academy of Medicine, 84*(3 supplement), i16–i26. https://doi.org/10.1007/s11524-007-9169-3

World Health Organization (2008). *Closing the gap in a generation: Health equity through action on the social determinants of health.* Commission on Social Determinants of Health. Geneva, Report reference number: WHO/IER/CSDH/08.1 https://www.who.int/health-topics/social-determinants-of-health#tab=tab_1

CHAPTER 38

Psychiatric Emergencies[1]

Ogboche Andrew Enegela, M.B.B.S., F.W.A.C.P., M.P.H.

and Edore Onigu-Otite, M.D.

"Out of all the things I have lost, I miss my mind the most."

— Mark Twain

OBJECTIVES

After reading this chapter, students will be able to do the following:

- identify common presenting features of psychiatric illness in emergency room settings
- identify common presenting features of psychiatric illness in primary care settings
- identify medical emergencies associated with the use of psychotropic medications
- describe a suicide risk assessment

CASE VIGNETTE

Pedro, a 20-year-old Hispanic-American man, was brought to the emergency room with his older brother, who was concerned about him. Over the past week, Pedro had told his family that he had "no need for food because his energy came from a different world." Five days ago, he stopped sleeping, bathing, and grooming himself. Pedro disclosed he was seeing demons all around him and hearing their voices telling him to kill people or he would be killed. In the last 3 days, he had become increasingly aggressive. This began verbally with his occasionally using curse words. It escalated when his mother reprimanded him for this, and in response, he balled his fists and attempted to strike his mother. Pedro was evaluated by the ER physician, who considered him to have an acute psychotic disorder. A provisional

1 Readers may also see "The Psychiatric Patient Interview" (Chapter 2), "Psychopharmacology" (Chapter 31), "Addiction and Substance Use Disorders" (Chapter 29), and "Prescription Drug Misuse and Abuse: Opioids, Stimulants, Sedative–Hypnotics" (Chapter 30) for related material.

diagnosis of psychosis unspecified was given. While waiting in the emergency room, he became highly irritable and violent toward staff, not responding to verbal attempts to de-escalate his agitation. He was sedated with intravenous lorazepam 2 mg to ensure his and others' safety. Baseline investigations, including a complete blood count, comprehensive metabolic profile, and a urine drug test, were ordered; the results all came back negative, and he was medically cleared for admission. After stabilization in the ER, ensuring the safety of the patient, he was subsequently admitted to the psychiatry ward for further treatment of his psychiatric disorder.

DEFINITIONS AND KEY CONCEPTS

The American Psychiatric Association defines a psychiatric emergency as "an acute disturbance in thought, behavior, mood, or social relationship, which requires immediate intervention as defined by the patient, family, or social unit" (Allen, 2002). Psychiatric emergencies require immediate intervention to prevent the patient or others from imminent danger. Usually, these presentations require intervention when they are recognized to avoid escalation, harm, loss of life or limb, and maintain safety in the ER. *De-escalation* is the intentional reduction of intensity of a conflict or potentially violent situation. De-escalation entails the transfer of a sense of calm into tense situations, using clear, concise, and limit-setting communication. It emphasizes the cultivation of a rapport and a genuine interest in providing help to patients, including for their and others' safety. *Agitation* is a state of anxiety or nervous excitement. This can be conceptualized as vocal and motor behaviors on a continuum of expressions that range from anxiety to aggression. *Neuroleptic malignant syndrome* is a medical urgency or emergency resulting from the cumulative use of dopamine antagonists. *Serotonin syndrome* is a medical urgency or emergency resulting from excessive serotonin caused using incremental serotonergic agents.

INTRODUCTION

Psychiatric emergencies can be challenging and emotionally tasking, even to highly skilled professionals. Professionals should make decisions in the best interests of the patient. Delay in such patient-centered decision-making may result in unwanted mortality, regret on the part of the health workers, and professional liability. This can exert a spiral effect on the patient and those in contact with them. Many families have suffered the anguish of losing a loved one to unrecognized or untreated presentations with psychiatric emergencies. Some of these patient encounters may have been unrecognized due to poor knowledge or attitude from family, onlookers in the community, or staff members unfamiliar with these conditions.

The emergency room (ER) serves as a gateway to the hospital and provides critical access to the health care system for many individuals. The rate of ER visits related to mental health and substance use disorders has increased substantially over the past few decades. The most common mental illness diagnoses in ER settings include depressive disorder, bipolar disorder, schizophrenia, anxiety disorders, and substance use disorders. Suicidality is a common presenting problem in the ER. The percentages of adults having serious thoughts of suicide were higher for past-year alcohol users, past-month binge and heavy alcohol use drinkers, past-year illicit drug users, adults with a past-year substance use disorder (SUD), and adults with a past-year major depressive episode. The number of children presenting in ERs for mental health problems has increased steadily, particularly for self-harm, depression, and behavioral disorders. This proportion increased during the COVID-19 pandemic (Leeb, 2020).

KEY POINT

Professionals should make decisions in the best interests of the patient. Delay in such patient-centered decision-making may result in unwanted mortality, regret on the part of the health workers, and professional liability. This can exert a spiral effect on the patient and those in contact with them.

Psychiatric emergencies are not limited to the ER. Imminent danger, such as suicidal or homicidal ideation and psychotic symptoms, can occur in any medical or mental health setting. Certain psychiatric medication side effects or toxidromes cause urgent medical states, such as serotonin syndrome or neuroleptic malignant syndrome. These are less frequently encountered but equally essential to identify and treat accurately. This chapter seeks to provide insight into psychiatric emergencies, highlighting common presentations, suicidality, differential diagnoses, and treatment options.

KEY POINT

The emergency room (ER) serves as a gateway to the hospital and provides critical access to the health care system for many individuals. Psychiatric emergencies are not limited to the ER. Imminent danger, such as suicidal or homicidal ideation and psychotic symptoms, can occur in any medical or mental health setting. Certain psychiatric medication side effects or toxidromes cause urgent medical states.

COMMON PRESENTING FEATURES OF PSYCHIATRIC ILLNESS IN THE EMERGENCY ROOM

Irritability, Agitation, and Aggression[2]

Irritability, agitation, and aggression are on a spectrum of behavior concerns. Some individuals may be irritable at baseline. Others may shift from being irritable to visibly agitated, then engage in aggressive acts if left without intervention. A few individuals with seemingly no external warning signs may engage in aggressive acts. Yet, it is a clinical skill to identify, assess, and effectively address irritability, agitation, or aggression in emergency settings.

Irritability

Irritability refers to interindividual differences in proneness to anger that may reach a pathological extent (Vidal-Ribas, 2016). This broad definition allows irritability to be viewed as a clinical entity with emotional manifestation. Irritability is a manifestation of mood dysregulation with associated changes in affect. Irritability is a ubiquitous symptom and part of the criteria of many

2 See also Chapter 2, "The Psychiatric Patient Interview."

psychiatric conditions. It is a common presentation in children, teens, adults, and elderly patients who present to the ER. It is prominently recognized in mania and may also result from substance use. Although irritability is not a core diagnostic criterion for depression for adults in the *DSM-5* and *ICD-10*, it is reported in at least one third to half of adults and children with major depression (Balbuena, 2016). Adjusted for baseline psychopathology, irritability is associated with poorer health outcomes and future functional impairment (Vidal-Ribas, 2016). Irritability is a predictor of future mental illness, including depression (OR 1.79), anxiety (OR 1.72), bipolar disorder (OR 1.09), ADHD (OR 1.25), ODD (OR 2.62), substance use disorder (OR 1.11), and conduct disorder (OR 1.04; Vidal, 2016). Irritable depression is also associated with greater severity, lower quality of life, and a history of suicidal attempts, which is itself a criterion for depression (Balbuena, 2016). Therefore, recognizing irritability as a presenting feature of psychiatric illness in the ER is necessary to avoid unsafe discharge of patients who may not reveal their plan to commit suicide.

CLINICAL TIP

Irritability refers proneness to anger. Irritability can be viewed as a clinical entity manifested by mood dysregulation with associated changes in affect. Irritability is a ubiquitous symptom and part of the criteria of many psychiatric conditions. It is a common presentation in children, teens, adults, and elderly patients who present to the ER.

Agitation

Agitation is often seen in the ER and may result in aggressive acts by patients. Agitation can be conceptualized as vocal and motor behaviors on a continuum of expressions that range from anxiety to aggression. Predictors of aggressive behavior include unemployment, young age (< 40 years), a history of violent behavior, and noncompliance to treatment (Sudarsanan, 2004). Other predictors include substance misuse, male gender, low socioeconomic status, extended length of hospitalization, involuntary hospitalization, and specific diagnoses (mania and schizophrenia; Caruso, 2021).

CLINICAL TIP

Agitation can be conceptualized as vocal and motor behaviors on a continuum of expressions that range from anxiety to aggression.

The evaluation of irritable and agitated patients is best carried out nonconfrontationally, aiming for verbal de-escalation. Removal of objects that could inflict injury to self or others is essential in such settings. Psychotropic medication and physical restraint of extremities may be required to ensure patient and staff safety in the ER. Common psychotropic medications used include lorazepam, haloperidol, olanzapine, ziprasidone, which can all be given orally or parenterally. Physically restraining the patient may increase paranoia and agitation, so such physical restraints should be used only when necessary to protect the patient. Chemical restraints are preferred over physical restraints whenever possible. Below are 10 tips for managing the agitated patient.

TEN TIPS FOR MANAGING AN AGITATED PATIENT

> **CLINICAL TIP**
>
> Irritable or agitated patients are often suffering with emotional pain, crisis, or confusion. They may express this via lashing out in words, curt comments, or disrespectful language. Clinical teams have better patient outcomes if they can see beyond the behaviors, identify the needs of the patient, and address them optimally within the circumstances. This is also helpful in building the treatment alliance with the patient and paves the way for better patient outcomes.

Irritable or agitated patients are often suffering from emotional pain, crisis, or confusion. They may express this by lashing out in words, curt comments, or disrespectful language. Clinical teams have better patient outcomes if they can see beyond the behaviors, identify the needs of the patient, and address them optimally within the circumstances. This is also helpful in building the treatment alliance with the patient and paves the way for better patient outcomes. Simple steps that can be taken include:

1. *Prepare for the discussion*—Review the relevant clinical information. This communicates to the patient you care and took the time to find out details of their case.
2. *Take the nonjudgmental stance*—Remember your role is to treat, not to judge. Your goal is simply to get a good patient outcome.
3. *Be respectful*—Use courteous language, tone, and mannerisms. Address the patient by their proper name.
4. *Establish the goal*—Share with them that your goal is to help.
5. *To identify the problem, ask the patient*—Ask the patient what the main problem(s) is/are. If there are multiple problems, you may ask that they specify the top three problems.
6. *Listen*—This communicates respect.
7. *Summarize what the patient said*—This provides direct feedback to them that you heard them correctly.
8. *Validate*—Validate the patient's feelings and wants. Be empathic.
9. *Set expectations and offer choices on the next steps*—Preferably, go for practical solutions. Be realistic. Do not promise or encourage what is not feasible.
10. *Thank the patient*—This provides direct feedback to them that you appreciate them for listening and cooperating with you (if they were able to).

Aggression

Aggression can be defined as behaviors that are intended to hurt or harm oneself, others, or property. As a term, aggression is used to describe behaviors that can potentially cause harm to self, others, or property.

Aggressive acts include self-injurious behavior, assaultive behavior, and violence of any kind. Aggression can be verbal or physical. Verbal aggression can take the form of using harsh words toward another, cursing angrily at a person, suggesting or warning of an intent to harm a person or entity, or making outright threats to inflict harm (e.g., by beating up, killing, maiming, committing acts of arson, or bombing). A terroristic threat is a threat to commit a violent crime to another or others, including to a person, group of persons, place, or entity. Physical aggression ranges from hitting to inflicting wounds (e.g., cuts, scratches, burns, and punches), fighting, threatening, or using a weapon to intimidate, harm, or, ultimately, end life. Hostility refers to irritability, suspiciousness, uncooperativeness, jealousy, or aggression. Several studies have shown a direct link between acts of aggression or cruelty to animals and violence toward humans.

CLINICAL TIP

Aggression can be verbal or physical. Verbal aggression can take the form of using harsh words toward another, cursing angrily at a person, suggesting or warning of an intent to harm a person, or entity, or making outright threats to inflict harm (e.g., by beating up, killing, maiming, committing acts or arson, or bombing).

Psychosis

Psychosis is a symptom rather than a definitive diagnosis, and it is a continuous rather than a categorical phenomenon. It may be a distressing presentation for both patients and family members. At one extreme, patients can be quietly delusional and at risk of self-harm and at the other extreme, patients may be paranoid with poor reality testing posing an extreme and immediate risk to ED staff and other patients. (Peltzer-Jones, 2019). In children, the most common causes of psychosis are anxiety and depression. In addition, brief psychotic phenomena may occur within the context of trauma and trauma reminders. Although psychosis is often a manifestation of an underlying primary mental health disorder, other causes exist. Substance intoxication, withdrawal, and primary brain disorders may have secondary psychotic manifestations (Joyce, 2019). Appropriate management of psychosis is important in the preservation of patient dignity (Zaman, 2017). Verbal de-escalation of psychotic patients may be useful; however, a decision to employ medication may be taken where this is unsuccessful. Short-acting benzodiazepines, including lorazepam and midazolam, and psychotropic medication, such as haloperidol, may resolve the acute disruptive state, allowing evaluation under a controlled setting.

CLINICAL TIP

In children, the most common causes of psychosis are anxiety and depression. In addition, brief psychotic phenomena may occur within context of trauma and trauma reminders.

Suicidality[3]

Suicidality is one of the most frequent reasons for psychiatric presentations to the ER. Over four million presentations with suicidal ideation or attempts occur annually in the United States. The ER is often the first contact setting with patients requiring evaluation for suicidal ideation, and ER staff need to

3 Readers may also see "Suicide" (Chapter 34) for related material.

> **QUICK POINT**
>
> Approximately 10% of all adult ED patients, regardless of chief complaint, have recent suicidal ideation or behaviors, but many will not disclose unless asked (Claassen, 2005; Ilgen, 2009).

> **QUICK POINT**
>
> Performing and adequate suicide risk assessment is fundamental for mental health care in all healthcare settings, including mental health, primary care, and emergency room settings. About 1 in 5 suicide victims had contact with mental health services within a month before their suicide. Leading up to suicide attempts, patients may increase their visits with their PCPs. Contact with primary health care occurred within 1 month of suicide occurs on average in 45% of suicide victims. These contact points with health care professionals provide an opportunity to identify suicide risk factors, conduct a suicide formulation assessment, and intervene effectively.

be adept at assessing suicidal patients (Brucker, 2019). Suicidal patients may convey feelings of worthlessness, guilt, or despair and sometimes articulate in words their wish, intent, or plan to die. Suicidal behaviors can be complex and difficult to predict.

Suicidal patients frequently have presentations with deliberate self-harm and overdoses. Deliberate self-harm, also known as nonsuicidal self-injury (NSSI) may be nonfatal or fatal (Olfson, 2017). However, NSSI increases the risk of completed suicide (Chesin, 2017). Adults treated for deliberate self-harm frequently repeat self-harm in the following year. Although NSSI may range from minor injuries to lacerations requiring suturing, it is essential to keep a record of attendances and note an escalation in the frequency and pattern of injuries. A trend of increasing frequency and severity of injuries may herald the completion of suicide by fatal NSSI. Patients who use violent methods for their initial self-harm have an exceptionally high risk of suicide, particularly right after the initial event, which highlights the importance of careful assessment and close follow-up of this group (Olfson, 2017). Patients with nonfatal NSSI are at higher risk of premature death from multiple causes, including suicide and natural causes, compared to the general population, which is likely related to lifestyle choices (Bergen, 2012; Vuagnat, 2020).

Performing an adequate suicide risk assessment is fundamental for mental health care in all health care settings, including mental health, primary care, and emergency room settings. About one in five suicide victims had contact with mental health services within a month before their suicide. Leading up to suicide attempts, patients may increase their visits with their PCPs. Contact with primary health care occurred within 1 month of suicide occurs on average in 45% of suicide victims (Luoma, 2002; Harmer, 2021). These contact points with health care professionals provide an opportunity to identify suicide risk factors, conduct a suicide formulation assessment, and intervene effectively. Figure 38.1 gives an overview of suicidal thoughts, serious thoughts of suicide, plans, attempts, and completed suicides.

Suicide Risk Assessment and Suicide Risk Formulation

The suicide risk assessment (SRA) focuses on identifying the risk factors for a patient potentially engaging in suicidal acts. It also identifies relevant protective factors that may discourage, prevent, or make it difficult to engage in suicidal acts. This is put together in a suicide risk formulation (SRF). A suicide risk formulation assigns a level of suicide risk that ideally leads to triage and treatment deemed appropriate

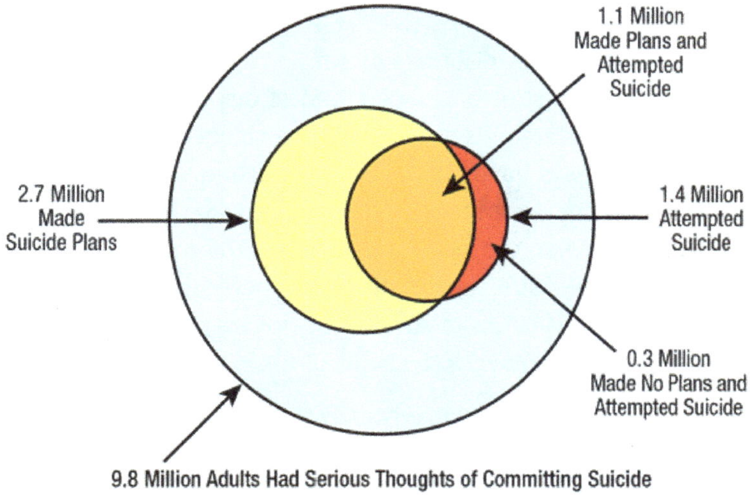

FIGURE 38.1 Suicidal thoughts, plans, and attempts in the past year among adults age 18 or older. Adapted from Substance Abuse and Mental Health Services Administration, 2015.

Source: https://www.samhsa.gov/data/sites/default/files/NSDUH-DR-FFR3-2015/NSDUH-DR-FFR3-2015.htm.

for that level of risk. This includes if a patient is safe, or not safe, to discharge from the ER setting, if additional observation is needed, or if hospitalization is needed to ensure safety.

A limitation in assessing SI is the emphasis laid on the patient's verbal communication of SI. While verbally, a patient may deny SI, their actions in the preceding days or week may suggest the contrary. Examples of behaviors that may suggest a patient may be planning to die of self-inflicted causes include written or electronic messages about things that may happen after their death (such as telling family or friends they are not to blame, that they should carry on with life, or a cause they were involved in), giving away their items, or similar messages. Inquiry on specific methods contemplated for suicide, documentation of plans online or on paper, previous attempts, and injuries sustained are essential components of the history. Standardized evaluation of suicidal patients using validated questionnaires ensures reliable assessment and patient safety. Additional factors for suicide are further discussed in the chapter on suicide.

MEMORY TIP

Suicide Risk Factors to Look for in Psychiatric Emergencies, *useful mnemonic*

SAD HARSH PLANS

S—Suicidal ideation
A—Acute anxiety, agitation, or psychosis
D—Depressed mood

H—Hopelessness
A—Alcohol or substance use intoxication or withdrawal
R—Reliability of others is poor (poor social support)
S—Stressful life event
H—Hospitalization or emergency room visit (recent and for a psychological reason)

P—Plan in consideration, in process, or in place
L—Leaving or withdrawing from family or friends
A—Attempt history
N—New, worsening, or chronic medical illness
S—Story (of family) contains suicide (family history of suicide)

(Created by Edore Onigu-Otite)

Substance Use Disorders and Drug Overdoses[4]

QUICK POINT

Opioids are responsible for over 70% of all overdose deaths in the United States. In 2019, more than 70,000 drug overdose deaths occurred (Mattson, 2021). Provisional data indicates this rose to over 100,000 drug overdose deaths during the 12-month period ending in April 2021 (CDC, 2021). This indicates an almost 30% increase over the same time in the preceding year.

QUICK POINT

While the intensions at the time of overdosing are unclear, as high as 30% of overdose deaths may be suicide attempts (Oquendo, 2018).

The leading substance use disorders presenting in the ER include alcohol-related disorders, substance-induced mental disorders, opioid-related disorders, cocaine-related disorders, and hallucinogen-related disorders. The greatest increases have been substance use in women age 45–64, depression, anxiety or stress reactions in men aged 45–64, and psychosis or bipolar disorders in men and women age 18–44. This increase was largest among the lowest-income communities. The percentage of mental and substance use-related ER visits covered by private insurance decreased, whereas the percentage covered by public insurance (Medicaid) increased.

Drug overdoses can occur with virtually any drug accessible to patients, including psychiatric patients. The rate of overdose-related mortality has risen exponentially (Jalal, 2018). In 2019, more than 70,000 drug overdose deaths occurred in the United States. Opioids are now responsible for over 70% of all overdose deaths in the United States. Prescription opioids, heroin, amphetamine, and fentanyl are agents most frequently associated with drug overdose deaths and represent a changing dynamic in the overdose epidemic in the United States. (Jalal, 2018). While the intentions at the time of overdosing are unclear, as high as 30% of overdose deaths may be suicide attempts (Oquendo, 2018).

A few patients may report an overdose in an attempt to control worsening symptoms, including withdrawal states from substances, hallucinations, or to satisfy cravings that may be seen with opioids or other substances. Mixed overdoses are common, including drugs that may potentiate the effects of others, such as antihistamines and benzodiazepines. Deaths are most frequently due to opioid overdoses. The risk is fourfold higher among patients who use opioids with benzodiazepines compared to those who use opioids alone (Ladapo, 2018). Due to the loss of tolerance, the risk of overdosing from opioids is increased after a period of total or partial abstinence. Naloxone is used for the rapid reversal of opioid-induced cardiorespiratory depression in opioid overdoses. Specific therapy targeted at the drug used in excess can be administered according to best practice guidelines and indications for laboratory testing.

4 Readers may also see "Prescription Drug Abuse: Opioids, Stimulants, and Sedative–Hypnotics" (Chapter 30) for related material.

Alcohol Use Disorder (AUD)[5]

The fifth edition of the *Diagnostic and Statistical Manual of Mental Disorders (DSM-5)*, unlike its predecessors, combines the mental health problems resulting from alcohol use into the entity called alcohol use disorder (AUD). Alcohol use disorder is a mental condition characterized by impairment in the cessation or control of alcohol use, despite adverse consequences relating to health and socioeconomic well-being. AUD encompasses commonly used terms including alcoholism, alcohol dependence, alcohol addiction, and mental health disorder due to alcohol misuse.

Alcohol Intoxication

Alcohol-related illness is the third leading preventable cause of death in the United States. Each year, close to 100,000 people die from alcohol-related causes in the United States (CDC, 2016). The rate of alcohol-related visits to U.S. ERs increased by nearly 50% between 2006 and 2014. This increase was particularly steep among females and drinkers who are middle-aged or older. The rate of visits for acute alcohol consumption increased by 40%, and the rate of visits related to chronic alcohol consumption rose by 58%. In just one decade, the number of people transported to the ER annually for medical emergencies caused or exacerbated by alcohol increased from about three million to five million (White, 2018). Many of these are caused by alcohol intoxication.

QUICK POINT

Alcohol-related illness is the third leading preventable cause of death in the United States. Each year, close to 100,000 people die from alcohol-related causes in the United States. The rate of alcohol-related visits to U.S. emergency departments increased by nearly 50% between 2006 and 2014, especially among females and drinkers who are middle-aged or older (White, 2018).

Alcohol intoxication occurs following consumption of larger volumes of alcohol than can be metabolized by the body, leading to an accumulation in the blood stream and the exertion of its effects on the brain. Intoxicated patients may present to the ER with problems ranging from altercation to fatal motor vehicle accidents (MVAs). Injuries from altercation may vary from blunt to penetrating, although a mixture of different types of injuries is common. Major trauma and death occurring from drunk driving is a preventable, yet tragic, event. Approximately 43% of all fatal motorcycle crashes involve alcohol with more motorcycle-related alcohol ER visits observed in the evening or during the night and by those who did not wear a helmet (Liu, 2021).

In the ER, the management of alcohol intoxication is mainly supportive. This includes serial blood alcohol concentration measurements, protection of the airway, monitoring of vitals, and administration of fluids if needed. Patients with isolated alcohol intoxication typically do not require

5 Readers may also see "Addiction and Substance Use Disorders" (Chapter 29) for related material.

hospitalization, except if there are injuries, comorbid conditions, or the development of signs of moderate to severe withdrawal. Cases of mild withdrawal can be managed as outpatients with the appropriate medications, close supervision, and prompt follow-up.

Alcohol Withdrawal

Alcohol withdrawal is a common presentation of patients with chronic alcohol use. Chronic alcohol use alters the neurochemical homeostasis in the brain, producing a depressant effect. Sudden cessation of alcohol consumption leads to an increase of glutamate-mediated excitatory impulses (Schuckit, 2014).

CLINICAL TIP

Symptoms of alcohol withdrawal include restlessness, sweating, tremors, nausea and vomiting, headache, hallucinations, and tactile abnormalities. Clinical signs may include tachycardia, labile blood pressure fluctuations, elevated body temperature, mydriasis, and tachypnea.

Symptoms of alcohol withdrawal include restlessness, sweating, tremors, nausea and vomiting, headache, hallucinations, and tactile abnormalities. Clinical signs may include tachycardia, labile blood pressure fluctuations, elevated body temperature, mydriasis, and tachypnea (Jesse, 2017). Symptoms manifest as early as 8 hours following abstinence as blood alcohol levels decrease. Although subtle in onset, symptoms progressively increase in severity with time. Without appropriate intervention, deterioration to life-threatening seizures and delirium tremens occur. Delirium tremens is a clinical diagnosis best made according to *DSM-5* diagnostic criteria (Schuckit, 2014; Jesse, 2017).

Standardized assessment for alcohol withdrawal is essential to guide appropriate treatment. The Clinical Institute Withdrawal Assessment (CIWA-Ar) tool for alcohol withdrawal ensures a uniform approach to patients. Although it cannot differentiate between withdrawal and delirium due to other causes, it is nonetheless an extensively used tool in clinical practice (Kattimani, 2013; Sykora, 1989).

KEY POINT

Neuroleptic malignant syndrome (NMS) is caused by unopposed dopamine antagonism. This can occur with cumulative use of dopamine antagonists or abrupt discontinuation of dopamine agonists.

Treatment of alcohol withdrawal entails controlling agitation, fluid and thiamine administration, supportive care to facilitate a functional status, and, importantly, the prevention of seizures. Magnesium, potassium, and phosphorus may be replenished if low. Preconstituted IV bags containing normal saline, thiamine, potassium, magnesium, folic acid, and other vitamins, commonly referred to as a *banana bag*, are helpful in ER settings. Vitamin K may be considered if the prothrombin time is prolonged. Benzodiazepines, which exert their effect through the GABA receptor, are the mainstay of treatment for treating alcohol withdrawal seizures.

EMERGENCIES DUE TO PSYCHOTROPIC DRUGS

Neuroleptic Malignant Syndrome (NsMS)

This is a rare but potentially fatal reaction to antipsychotic medication. It requires a high index of suspicion and immediate treatment to prevent mortality. It may occur as an idiosyncratic drug reaction to the first dose of antipsychotics. However, high doses and rapid dose escalation are key risk factors. NMS appears to be more common in males, but the reasons for this are unclear (Onieb, 2021). Causative agents have central action on the dopaminergic D2 receptors. Both typical and atypical antipsychotics are implicated, although occurrences with atypical agents appear less frequently. Nonantipsychotic agents, including anticonvulsants, antidepressants, and metoclopramide acting on the same receptors, can cause NMS. Abrupt discontinuation of dopamine agonists used for the treatment of Parkinson's disease may also cause NMS (Kuhlwilm, 2020). Drugs associated with NMS are detailed in the table below.

> **MEMORY TIP**
>
> ***Neuroleptic Malignant Syndrome (NMS),*** *useful mnemonic*
>
> **FEVER**
>
> **F**—Fever
> **E**—Encephalopathy
> **V**—Vital sign instability
> **E**—Enzyme elevation—CPK
> **R**—Rigidity
>
> *(Christensen, 2005)*

TABLE 38.1 Medications With Potential for Causing NMS

Medication category	Medication names
Typical antipsychotics	Chlorpromazine, droperidol, fluphenazine, haloperidol, loxapine, molindone, perphenazine, pimozide, thioridazine, thiothixene, trifluoperazine
Atypical antipsychotics	aripiprazole clozapine, lurasidone, olanzapine, paloperidone, quetiapine, risperidone, ziprasidone
Other dopamine antagonists	metoclopramide, prochlorperazine, and promethazine

Symptoms may occur a few hours after the commencement of medication use but may have delayed onset up to a month. The syndrome classically starts with rigidity, although there are a few cases without this symptom (Onieb, 2021). Usually, there is a rapid progression of symptoms with a peak about 3 days following onset (Berman, 2011). Symptoms of NMS are outlined in Table 38.2.

TABLE 38.2 Symptoms of Neuroleptic Malignant Syndrome (NMS)

Category	Symptoms
Major symptoms	• Exposure to dopamine antagonist *or* cessation of dopamine agonist prior to symptom onset • Muscular rigidity • Hyperthermia (100°F or 38°C) • Excessive sweating
Autonomic instability	• Tachycardia or fluctuating heart rate • Hypo- or hypertension or fluctuating blood pressure • Tachypnoea • Excessive salivation • Urinary incontinence
Mental status	• Level of consciousness, qualitative observation: altered or fluctuating consciousness (delirium) • Level of consciousness, quantitative observation: drowsiness, stupor, or coma
Motor symptoms	• Hypertonia (> 25% above baseline or with fluctuation) • Muscle rigidity and akinesia • Tremor, myoclonus, and trismus • Dystonia, dysarthria, and dysphagia
Laboratory findings	• ↑ Leukocytes, ↑ creatinine, ↑ creatinine kinase, and ↑ myoglobin • Hypoxia and metabolic acidosis

Adapted from APA, 2014.

Hyperthermia is often accompanied by tachycardia, flushed dry skin, and labile fluctuations in blood pressure. Hyperthermia is associated with massive rhabdomyolysis and release of intracellular contents, including creatine phosphokinase and calcium, which can accumulate and produce toxic effects on the heart and the kidneys, resulting in serious medical complications from acute renal failure or fatalities from cardiac arrhythmias. Rhabdomyolysis could also trigger the clotting cascade, resulting in disseminated intravascular coagulation (DIC), which can be fatal (Berman, 2011).

Treatment of this syndrome involves cessation of antipsychotic administration or reinstitution of dopaminergic agonists where these were discontinued. Rapid administration of intravenous fluids is required to correct dehydration and prevent tubular damage due to by-products of rhabdomyolysis. External cooling using ice packs and cold blankets may be employed to decrease core body temperature to normal levels. Administration of anticoagulants to prevent deep vein thrombosis may be needed. Although supportive medical therapy is the mainstay of treatment, specific agents may be employed to counteract the features of NMS. Dantrolene and bromocriptine are the main agents employed in the management of NMS. Dantrolene prevents the release of calcium from the sarcoplasmic reticulum and counteracts the tonic skeletal muscle contractions and generation of heat in this condition. Bromocriptine restores depleted dopamine via its agonist effects and is administered orally or via a nasogastric tube

(Vickery, 2018; Berman, 2011). With early recognition and early treatment, the mortality rate is about 10%, and recovery occurs within 2 weeks (Berman, 2011). A delay of at least 2 weeks before recommencement of antipsychotic medication is advocated following NMS. Successful reintroduction of atypical antipsychotics at low doses may be achieved with careful escalation to control psychotic symptoms (Chen, 2018).

Serotonin Syndrome

Serotonin syndrome (SS), also known as serotonin toxicity, is a rare, life-threatening toxidrome due to serotonin excess and characterized by neuromuscular, autonomic, and mental status changes. SS is similar but distinct from NMS in etiology and presentation (Kateon, 2013). SS typically occurs due to the use of two or more medications with serotonergic effects, although it may occur with a single drug taken at therapeutic doses or as an overdose (Gaffney, 2019). SS presentations are more common among adults, but cases among children and adolescents have been described, as the use of serotonergic medications in these age groups has gradually increased (Siqi, 2021). SS can occur when serotonergic drugs are taken with food containing key cytochrome enzyme inhibitors, such as grapefruit juice and caffeine. Supplements containing St. John's wort (*Hypericum perforatum*) may precipitate SS when used in combination with prescribed serotonin agonists. Drugs that can precipitate SS are listed in Table 38.3.

KEY POINT

Serotonin syndrome, also known as serotonin toxicity, is a rare but life-threatening toxidrome due to serotonin excess, characterized by neuromuscular, autonomic, and mental status changes. Serotonin syndrome is similar but distinct from NMS in aetiology and presentation.

TABLE 38.3 Medications Associated With Serotonin Syndrome

Medication category	Medication names
Monoamine oxidase inhibitors	Iproniazid, isocarboxazid, linezolid, moclobemide, nialamide, phenelzine, procarbazine, selegiline, tranylcypromine,
Tricyclic antidepressants (TCAs)	Amitriptyline, clomipramine, imipramine, nortriptyline, tofranil
Selective serotonin reuptake inhibitors (SSRIs)	Citalopram, escitalopram, fluoxetine, fluvoxamine, sertraline, paroxetine,
Serotonin-norepinephrine reuptake inhibitors (SNRIs)	Desvenlafaxine, duloxetine, milnacipran, venlafaxine,
Stimulants	Amphetamines, amphetamine derivatives, cocaine, MDMA (ecstasy)
Serotonin antagonists	Ondansetron, granisetron

Adapted from Kateon, 2013.

Note: Also see Table 31.4: Medications That Have the Potential to Cause or Contribute to the Development of Serotonergic Syndrome (Due to Additive Effect).

MEMORY TIP

Serotonin Syndrome, *useful mnemonic*

SHIVERS

S—Shivering: neuromuscular symptom that is unique to serotonin syndrome

H—Hyperreflexia and myoclonus: seen in mild to moderate cases—most prominent in the lower extremities. This can help differentiate from neuroleptic malignant syndrome, which would present with lead-pipe rigidity.

I— Increased temperature: not always present but usually observed in more severe cases

V—Vital sign abnormalities: tachycardia, tachypnea, and labile blood pressure

E—Encephalopathy: mental status changes, such as agitation, delirium, and confusion

R—Restlessness: common due to excess serotonin activity

S—Sweating: autonomic response to excess serotonin. This symptom can help differentiate from anticholinergic toxicity in which the patients would present with increased temperature but dry to the touch

(Christensen, 2006)

The diagnostic criteria for serotonin syndrome are based on the Sternbach and Hunter criteria for SS, which is simple to apply and useful in clinical settings. The most common clinical features are changes in mental status, restlessness, myoclonus, hyperreflexia, diaphoresis, shivering, and tremor (Sternbach, 1991). Other features of SS include fluctuating blood pressure, vomiting, diarrhea, mydriasis, sweating, restlessness, agitation, and anxiety. The Hunter criteria for diagnosis are outlined in Table 38.4.

Early recognition and prompt treatment of SS are key to preventing mortality. Treatment of SS is supportive with intravenous fluids and external cooling when temperatures are elevated. Severe hypotension can be treated using sympathomimetic agents, including epinephrine, norepinephrine, or phenylephrine. Cyproheptadine has been used in severe cases where supportive measures are likely to be inadequate therapy (Volpi-Abadie, 2013).

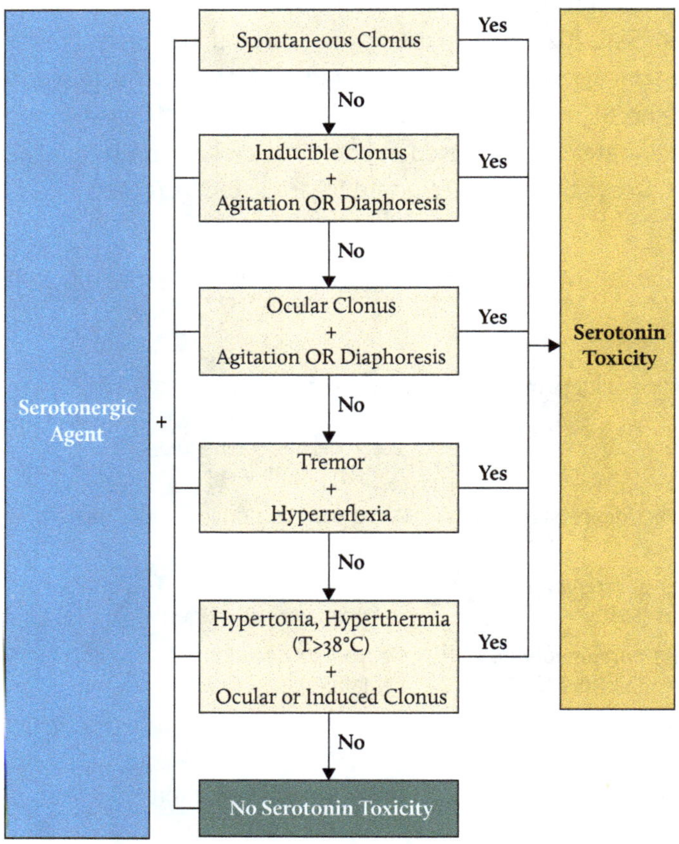

FIGURE 38.2 Hunter criteria for serotonin syndrome. Adapted from Kateon, 2013.

Differentiating NMS and SS may be difficult. Key differentiating factors and similarities are outlined in Table 38.4

TABLE 38.4 Differentiating Neuroleptic Malignant Syndrome and Serotonin Syndrome

Clinical factors	Clinical symptoms and signs	Serotonin syndrome	Neuroleptic malignant syndrome
Precipitating agent(s)		• Cumulative use of serotonergic agents	• Cumulative use of dopamine antagonists • Rapid removal of dopamine agonists
Onset		• Variable • Usually within 24 hours	• Variable • Usually within 72 hours
Similar features	Vital signs	• Blood pressure: hypo- or hypertension or fluctuating blood pressure • Pulse rate: low, high, or fluctuating • Hyperthermia temperature > 38°C/100°F	• BP: hypo- or hypertension or fluctuating blood pressure • Pulse rate: low, high, or fluctuating • Hyperthermia temperature > 38°C/100°F
Overlapping features	Mucosa	• Excessive salivation	• Excessive salivation
	Skin	• Excessive sweating	• Excessive sweating • Pallor
	Muscles	• Hypertonia • (particularly in lower extremities)	• Markedly increased • (lead pipe rigidity in all muscle groups)
Differentiating features	Reflexes	• Hyperreflexia and clonus (spontaneous or inducible)	• Hyporeflexia
	Pupils	• Mydriasis	• Normal
	Bowel sounds	• Hyperactive	• Normal to decreased

Adapted from Kateon, 2013.

MEMORY TIP

Useful mnemonic for items on Hunter's criteria: MOAT-HD.

MOAT-HD

M—Myoclonus (spontaneous, inducible)

O—Ocular clonus (spontaneous, inducible)

A—Agitation

T—Tremor

H—Hyper- (Hyperthermia, Hypertonia, Hyperreflexia)

D—Diaphoresis

CLINICAL TIP

Serotonin syndrome and neuroleptic malignant syndrome have many features in common. While the patient with frequency of movement, the patient with SS is above their baseline. They may appear restless, agitated, and hyperactive, while the patient with NMS is below their baseline. They may be hypo- or akinetic and stiff with lead pipe rigidity and may vocalize less or even seem mute.

KEY POINT

Delirium is an acute state of disturbance in mental state, resulting in altered mental status characterized by changes in consciousness, cognition, perceptual ability, and responsiveness to external stimuli. Delirium is the most common psychiatric disorder in hospitalized patients (Thomas, 2019).

Delirium

Delirium is an acute state of disturbance in mental state resulting in altered mental status characterized by changes in consciousness, cognition, perceptual ability, and responsiveness to external stimuli (Martins, 2012). The acute nature of neurologic dysfunction contrasts this condition with dementia, which runs a chronic course. Delirium is considered a manifestation of acute brain failure with variation in symptom severity. It is the most common psychiatric disorder in hospitalized patients (Thom, 2019). The etiology of delirium could be multifactorial, including psychiatric conditions and medications. Although reversible with early treatment of the cause, delirium may herald a poor prognosis if prolonged and unabating (Oldham, 2018). It is a cause of prolonged hospital stay in the elderly and demands skilled care to ensure a good recovery (Magny, 2018).

Delirium characteristically manifests in different phenotypes, namely hypoactive, hyperactive, and mixed. Hypoactive delirium presents with reduced responsiveness to external stimuli, psychomotor retardation, lethargy, and poor cognition. Hyperactive delirium is characterized by agitation, listlessness, and emotional lability. Mixed delirium is characterized by fluctuating symptoms of both forms earlier described (Thom, 2019). The table below outlines the diagnostic criteria for delirium.

Risk factors for delirium may be categorized into predisposing and precipitating factors. The presence of several predisposing factors indicates a high risk for delirium. Predisposing factors include aging, male sex, preexisting cognitive impairment, alcohol use disorder, and functional disability. Precipitating factors include drugs, acute illness (urinary tract infections, pneumonia), surgery, severe pain, and electrolyte derangements. Anticholinergic agents, tricyclic antidepressants, benzodiazepines, opioids, centrally acting antihistamines, low potency antipsychotics, and alcohol are some common agents that precipitate delirium (Marcantonio, 2017).

MEMORY TIP

Delirium, *useful mnemonic*

DELIRIUM

D— Drugs

E— Electrolyte disturbances

L— Lack of drugs

I— Infections

R— Reduced sensory input

I— Intracranial disorders

U— Urinary and fecal disorders

M—Myocardial and pulmonary disorders

Accurate recognition of delirium in the ER is an important first step in the management of patients. Following its recognition, a thorough evaluation for reversible causes is essential to appropriately treat the condition. Specific treatment is directed at the cause of delirium with supportive measures put in place to maintain functional status and prevent deconditioning of patients. Figures 38.3 and 38.4 outline the specific causes and treatments of delirium.

Drugs

- Alcohol
- Antibiotics (fluoroquinolones)
- Anticholinergics (scopolamine, diphenhydramine, benztropine)
- Anticonvulsants (barbiturates, phenytoin)
- Antihypertensive medication (beta-blockers, methyldopa)
- Antiparkinsonian medication
- Antipsychotics
- Benzodiazepines
- Narcotics
- NSAIDs
- Others: TCAs, lithium

Electrolyte and Metabolic disturbances

- Dehydration
- Hyponatremia/hypernatremia
- Hypoglycemia
- Hypo/hyperthyroid crises
- Hypoxia

Drug withdrawal

- Alcohol
- Narcotics
- Antiparkinsonian medication

Infections

- Pneumonia
- Urinary tract infections
- Sepsis from any other focus

Urinary and fecal disorders

- Constipation/Fecal impaction
- Urinary retention

Myocardial and pulmonary

- Acute decompensated heart failure
- Cardiac surgery
- COPD exacerbation
- Myocardial infarction
- Pulmonary embolism

FIGURE 38.3 Causes of delirium.

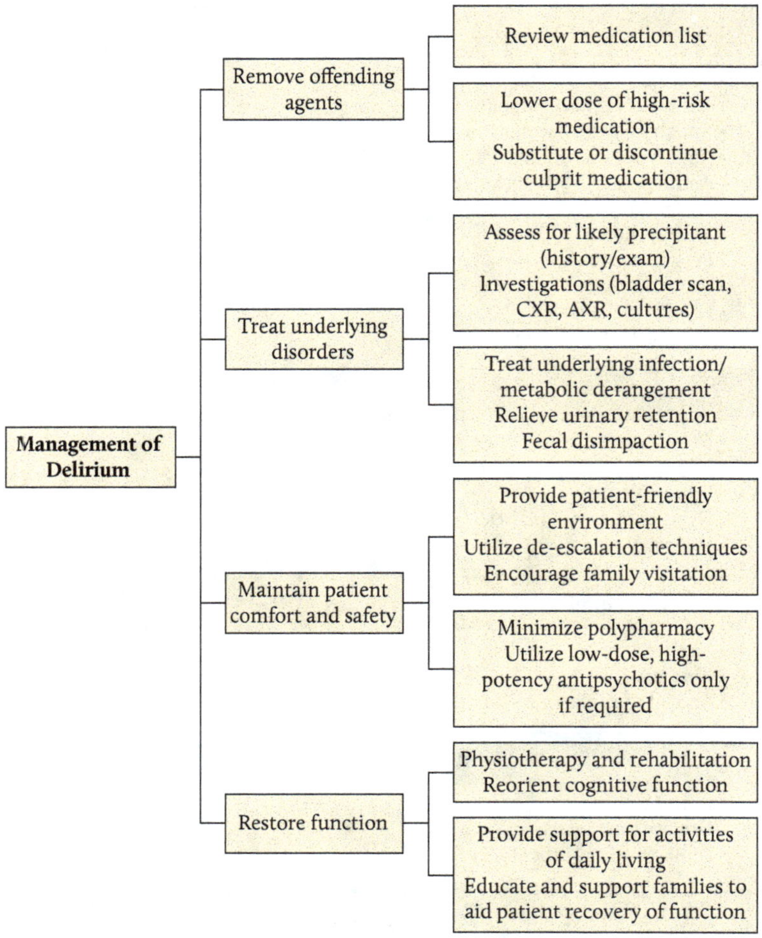

FIGURE 38.4 Management of delirium.

> **KEY POINT**
>
> Psychiatric emergencies are a significant part of emergency care but extends beyond this to medical and psychiatric settings. The spectrum of psychiatric emergencies requires skilled recognition, prompt treatment, and effective interventions to prevent deterioration and loss of life or limb.

SUMMARY

Psychiatric emergencies form a significant part of emergency care. However, the spectrum of psychiatric emergencies is wider and extends beyond the ER settings. Psychiatric emergencies also occur in medical and psychiatric settings. The spectrum of psychiatric emergencies requiring ER care is wide and demands skilled recognition, prompt treatment, and effective interventions to prevent deterioration and loss of life or limb. Compassionate care should be matched with safety precautions for both staff and patients.

RESOURCES

1 https://www.youtube.com/watch?v=wGMPyjWswQQ

2 https://www.acep.org/patient-care/iCar2e/

3 https://www.youtube.com/watch?v=mG4y_JYdFVI

REFERENCES

Adam, A., Faouzi, M., Yersin, B., Bodenmann, P., Daeppen, J. B., & Bertholet, N. (2016). Women and men admitted for alcohol intoxication at an emergency department: alcohol use disorders, substance use and health and social status 7 years later. *Alcohol and Alcoholism, 51*(5), 567–575.

Allen, M. H., Forster, P., Zealberg, J., Currier, G. 2002. *APA task force on psychiatry emergency services*. American Psychiatric Association. https://www.psychiatry.org/File%20Library/Psychiatrists/Directories/Library-and-Archive/task-force-reports/tfr2002_EmergencyCrisis.pdf. Accessed on October 18, 2021.

Antti, M., Anni-Emilia, A., Caroline, S., Tuula, H., Jonna, L., Scott, J. G., Jouko, M & Solja, N. (2021). Age of first alcohol intoxication and psychiatric disorders in young adulthood—A prospective birth cohort study. *Addictive Behaviors, 118*, 106910.

Balbuena, L., Bowen, R., Baetz, M., & Marwaha, S. (2016). Mood instability and irritability as core symptoms of major depression: An exploration using rasch analysis. *Frontiers in Psychiatry, 7*, 174. https://doi.org/10.3389/fpsyt.2016.00174

Bergen, H., Hawton, K., Waters, K., Ness, J., Cooper, J., Steeg, S., & Kapur, N. (2012). Premature death after self-harm: A multicentre cohort study. *The Lancet, 380*(9853), 1568–1574

Berman, B. D. Neuroleptic malignant syndrome: A review for neuro hospitalists. *The Neurohospitalist, 1*(1) (2011): 41–7. https://www.doi.org/10.1177/1941875210386491

Bhatt, M., Perera, S., Zielinski, L., Eisen, R. B., Yeung, S., El-Sheikh, W., DeJesus, J., Rangarajan, S., Sholer, H., Iordan, E., Mackie, P., Islam, S., Dehghan, M., Thabane, L., & Samaan, Z. (2018). Profile of suicide attempts and risk factors among psychiatric patients: A case-control study. *PLoS One, 13*(2), e0192998.

Brucker, K., Duggan, C., Niezer, J., Roseberry, K., Le-Niculescu, H., Niculescu, A. B., & Kline, J. A. (2019). Assessing risk of future suicidality in emergency department patients. *Academic Emergency Medicine: Official Journal of the Society for Academic Emergency Medicine, 26*(4), 376–383. https://doi.org/10.1111/acem.13562

Caruso, R., Antenora, F., Riba, M., Murri, M. B., Biancosino, B., Zerbinati, L., & Grassi, L. (2021). Aggressive behavior and psychiatric inpatients: A narrative review of the literature with a focus on the European experience. *Current Psychiatry Reports, 23*(5), 1–12.

Centers for Disease Control and Prevention. (n.d.). *Alcohol and public health: Alcohol-related disease impact (ardi)*. Centers for Disease Control and Prevention. https://nccd.cdc.gov/DPH_ARDI/Default/

Center for Disease Control and Prevention. (2021). Drug overdose deaths in the U.S. top 100,000 annually. Retrieved February 12, 2022, from https://www.cdc.gov/nchs/pressroom/nchs_press_releases/2021/20211117

Chen, T. R., & Chen, Y. C. (2018). Risperidone-associated neuroleptic malignant syndrome in an inpatient with schizophrenia, with successful rechallenge and 3 year follow-up. *Frontiers in Psychiatry, 9*, 718.

Chesin, M. S., Galfavy, H., Sonmez, C. C., Wong, A., Oquendo, M. A., Mann, J. J., & Stanley, B. (2017). Nonsuicidal self-injury is predictive of suicide attempts among individuals with mood disorders. *Suicide & Life-Threatening Behavior, 47*(5), 567–579. https://doi.org/10.1111/sltb.12331

Christensen, R.C. (2005) Identify neuroleptic malignant syndrome with FEVER. *Current Psychiatry Pearls, 4*(7):102-102

Christensen, R. C. (2006). *Get serotonin syndrome down cold with SHIVERS*. ClinCalc. https://cdn.mdedge.com/files/s3fs-public/Document/September-2017/0502CP_Pearls2.pdf.

Claassen, C. A., & Larkin, G. L. (2005). Occult suicidality in an emergency department population. *The British Journal of Psychiatry: The Journal of Mental Science, 186*, 352–353. https://doi.org/10.1192/bjp.186.4.352

Gaffney, R. R., & Schreibman, I. R. (2015). Serotonin syndrome in a patient on trazodone and duloxetine who received fentanyl following a percutaneous liver biopsy. *Case Reports in Gastroenterology, 9*(2), 132–136.

Hamerle, M., Ghaeni, L., Kowski, A., Weissinger, F., & Holtkamp, M. (2018). Alcohol use and alcohol-related seizures in patients with epilepsy. *Frontiers in Neurology, 9*, 401.

Harmer, B., Lee, S., Duong, T., & Saadabadi, A. (2021). Suicidal ideation. *StatPearls*. StatPearls Publishing.

Hingson, R., Zha, W., & Smyth, D. (2017). Magnitude and trends in heavy episodic drinking, alcohol-impaired driving, and alcohol-related mortality and overdose hospitalizations among emerging adults of college ages 18–24 in the United States, 1998–2014. *Journal of Studies on Alcohol and Drugs, 78*(4), 540–548.

Ilgen, M. A., Walton, M. A., Cunningham, R. M., Barry, K. L., Chermack, S. T., De Chavez, P., & Blow, F. C. (2009). Recent suicidal ideation among patients in an inner-city emergency department. *Suicide & Life-Threatening Behavior, 39*(5), 508–517. https://doi.org/10.1521/suli.2009.39.5.508

Jalal, H., Buchanich, J. M., Roberts, M. S., Balmert, L. C., Zhang, K., & Burke, D. S. (2018). Changing dynamics of the drug overdose epidemic in the United States from 1979 through 2016. *Science, 361*(6408).

Jesse, S., Bråthen, G., Ferrara, M., Keindl, M., Ben-Menachem, E., Tanasescu, R., Brodtkorb, E., Hillbom, M., Leone, M. A., & Ludolph, A. C. (2017). Alcohol withdrawal syndrome: Mechanisms, manifestations, and management. *Acta Neurologica Scandinavica, 135*(1), 4–16. https://doi.org/10.1111/ane.12671

Joyce, E. M. (2018). Organic psychosis: The pathobiology and treatment of delusions. *CNS Neuroscience & Therapeutics, 24*(7), 598–603. https://doi.org/10.1111/cns.12973

Liu, H.-T., Liang, C.-C., Rau, C.-S., Hsu, S.-Y., & Hsieh, C.-H. (2015). Alcohol-related hospitalizations of adult motorcycle riders. *World Journal of Emergency Surgery: WJES, 10*(1), 2. https://doi.org/10.1186/1749-7922-10-2

Luoma, J. B., Martin, C. E., & Pearson, J. L. (2002). Contact with mental health and primary care providers before suicide: A review of the evidence. *The American Journal of Psychiatry, 159*(6), 909–916. https://doi.org/10.1176/appi.ajp.159.6.909

Kateon, H. (2013). Differentiating serotonin syndrome and neuroleptic malignant syndrome. *Mental Health Clinician, 3*(3), 129–133.

Kattimani, S., & Bharadwaj, B. (2013). Clinical management of alcohol withdrawal: A systematic review. *Industrial Psychiatry Journal, 22*(2), 100.

Kuhlwilm, L., Schönfeldt-Lecuona, C., Gahr, M., Connemann, B. J., Keller, F., & Sartorius, A. (2020). The neuroleptic malignant syndrome: A systematic case series analysis focusing on therapy regimes and outcome. *Acta Psychiatrica Scandinavica, 142*(3), 233–241.

Ladapo, J. A., Larochelle, M. R., Chen, A., Villalon, M. M., Vassar, S., Huang, D. Y., & Mafi, J. N. (2018). Physician prescribing of opioids to patients at increased risk of overdose from benzodiazepine use in the United States. *JAMA Psychiatry, 75*(6), 623-630.

Leeb, R. T., Bitsko, R. H., Radhakrishnan, L., Martinez, P., Njai, R., & Holland, K. M. (2020). Mental health-related emergency department visits among children aged < 18 years during the COVID-19 pandemic - United States, January 1–October 17, 2020. *Morbidity and Mortality Weekly Report, 69*(45), 1675–1680. https://doi.org/10.15585/mmwr.mm6945a3

Magny, E., Le Petitcorps, H., Pociumban, M., Bouksani-Kacher, Z., Pautas, É., Belmin, J., Bastuji-Garin, S., & Lafuente-Lafuente, C. (2018). Predisposing and precipitating factors for delirium in community-dwelling older adults admitted to hospital with this condition: A prospective case series. *PLoS One, 13*(2), e0193034.

Martins, S., Fernandes, L. (2012). Delirium in elderly people: A review. *Frontiers in Neurology, 3*(101), 1–12.

Mattson, C. L., Tanz, L. J., Quinn, K., Kariisa, M., Patel, P., Davis, N. L. (2021). Trends and geographic patterns in drug and synthetic opioid overdose deaths—United States, 2013–2019. Morbidity Mortality Weekly Report (MMWR). 70, 202–207.

Oldham, M. A., Flaherty, J. H., & Maldonado, J. R. (2018). Refining delirium: A transtheoretical model of delirium disorder with preliminary neurophysiologic subtypes. *The American Journal of Geriatric Psychiatry, 26*(9), 913–924.

Olfson, M., Wall, M., Wang, S., Crystal, S., Gerhard, T., & Blanco, C. (2017). Suicide following deliberate self-harm. *American Journal of Psychiatry, 174*(8), 765–774.

Oneib, B., & Zaimi, O. (2021). Neuroleptic malignant syndrome: clinical expression, complication, course, and atypical clinical picture. *Middle East Current Psychiatry, 28*(1), 1–6.

Oquendo M. A., & Volkow N. D. (2018). Suicide: A silent contributor to opioid-overdose deaths. *The New England Journal of Medicine, 26;378*(17), 1567–1569. https://doi.org/10.1056/NEJMp1801417

Parsch, C. S., Boonstra, A., Teubner, D., Emmerton, W., McKenny, B., & Ellis, D. Y. (2017). Ketamine reduces the need for intubation in patients with acute severe mental illness and agitation requiring transport to definitive care: An observational study. *Emergency Medicine Australasia, 29*(3), 291–296.

Peltzer-Jones, J., Nordstrom, K., Currier, G., Berlin, J. S., Singh, C., & Schneider, S. (2019). A research agenda for assessment and management of psychosis in emergency department patients. *The Western Journal of Emergency Medicine, 20*(2), 403–408. https://doi.org/10.5811/westjem.2019.1.39263

Richmond, J. S., Berlin, J. S., Fishkind, A. B., Holloman, G. H., Jr, Zeller, S. L., Wilson, M. P., Rifai, M. A., & Ng, A. T. (2012). Verbal de-escalation of the agitated patient: Consensus statement of the American Association for Emergency Psychiatry project beta de-escalation workgroup. *The Western Journal of Emergency Medicine, 13*(1), 17–25. https://doi.org/10.5811/westjem.2011.9.6864

SAMHSA, Center for Behavioral Health Statistics and Quality. (2019). National Survey on Drug Use and Health.

Schuckit, M. A. (2014). Recognition and management of withdrawal delirium (delirium tremens). *New England Journal of Medicine, 371*(22), 2109–2113.

Scotton, W. J., Hill, L. J., Williams, A. C., & Barnes, N. M. (2019). Serotonin syndrome: Pathophysiology, clinical features, management, and potential future directions. *International Journal of Tryptophan Research, 12*. https://doi.org/10.1177/1178646919873925

Siqi Xue, M. D. (2021). Serotonin syncrome in children and adolescents exposed to selective serotonin reuptake inhibitors: A review of literature. *Journal of the Canadian Academy of Child and Adolescent Psychiatry = Journal de l'Academie canadienne de psychiatrie de l'enfant et de l'adolescent, 30*(3), 157

Sternbach H. The serotonin syndrome. (1991). *The American Journal of Psychiatry. 148*(6), 705–13. https://doi.org/10.1176/ajp.148.6.705. PMID: 2035713.

Substance Abuse and Mental Health Services Administration, C. for B. H. S. and Q. (n.d.). *Suicidal thoughts and behavior among adults: Results from the 2015 National Survey on Drug Use and health.* Suicidal Thoughts and Behavior among Adults: Results from the 2015 National Survey on Drug Use and Health. https://www.samhsa.gov/data/sites/default/files/NSDUH-DR-FFR3-2015/NSDUH-DR-FFR3-2015.htm

Sudarsanan, S., Chaudhury, S., Pawar, A. A., Salujha, S. K, & Srivastava, K. (2004). Psychiatric emergencies. Psychiatric Emergencies. *Medical Journal, Armed Forces India.*;60(1):59-62. https://doi.org/10.1016/S0377-1237(04)80162-X

Sullivan, J. T., Sykora, K., Schneiderman, J., Naranjo, C. A., & Sellers, E. M. (1989). Assessment of alcohol withdrawal: The revised clinical institute withdrawal assessment for alcohol scale (CIWA-Ar). *British Journal of Addiction, 84*(11), 1353–1357.

Thom, R. P., Levy-Carrick, N. C., Bui, M., & Silbersweig, D. (2019). Delirium. *American Journal of Psychiatry, 176*(10), 785–793.

Turner, A. H., Nguyen, C. T., Kim, J. J., & McCarron, R. M. (2019). Differentiating serotonin syndrome and neuroleptic malignant syndrome. *Current Psychiatry, 18*, 30–36.

Vickery, P. B., Meadowcraft, L., & Vickery, S. B. (2018). Early detection of an atypical presentation of neuroleptic malignant syndrome: A case report. *The Mental Health Clinician, 7*(3), 137–142. https://doi.org/10.9740/mhc.2017.05.137

Vidal-Ribas, P., Brotman, M. A., Valdivieso, I., Leibenluft, E., & Stringaris, A. (2016). the status of irritability in psychiatry: A conceptual and quantitative review. *Journal of the American Academy of Child and Adolescent Psychiatry, 55*(7), 556–570. https://doi.org/10.1016/j.jaac.2016.04.014

Volpi-Abadie, J., Kaye, A. M., & Kaye, A. D. (2013). Serotonin syndrome. *The Ochsner Journal, 13*(4), 533–540.

Vuagnat, A., Jollant, F., Abbar, M., Hawton, K., & Quantin, C. (2019). Recurrence and mortality 1 year after hospital admission for non-fatal self-harm: A nationwide population-based study. *Epidemiology and Psychiatric Sciences, 29*, e20. https://doi.org/10.1017/S2045796019000039

White, A. M., Slater, M. E., Ng, G., Hingson, R., & Breslow, R. (2018). Trends in alcohol-related emergency department visits in the United States: Results from the nationwide emergency department sample, 2006 to 2014. *Alcoholism, Clinical and Experimental Research, 42*(2), 352–359. https://doi.org/10.1111/acer.13559

Yasin, Y. J., & Banoub, J. A. M. (2018). GBD 2016 Alcohol Collaborators. Alcohol use and burden for 195 countries and territories, 1990–2016: A systematic analysis for the Global Burden of Disease Study 2016. *Lancet, 392*, 1684–735.

Zaman, H., Sampson, S. J., Beck, A., Sharma, T., Clay, F. J., Spyridi, S., Zhao, S., & Gillies, D. (2017). Benzodiazepines for psychosis-induced aggression or agitation. *The Cochrane Database of Systematic Reviews, 2017*(12), CD003079. https://doi.org/10.1002/14651858.CD003079.pub4

CHAPTER 39

Pediatric Mental Health

Sindhu Idicula, M.D. and Betty Del Rio Rodriguez, M.D.

> *"We live in a world in which we need to share responsibility. It's easy to say 'It's not my child, not my community, not my world, not my problem.' Then there are those who see the need and respond. I consider those people my heroes."*
>
> — Fred Rogers

OBJECTIVES

After reading this chapter, students will be able to do the following:

- discuss ways in which the evaluation of adults differs from children and adolescents
- describe the reasons for the necessity for pediatric mental health to be evaluated by both child and adolescent psychiatrists as well as pediatric primary care physicians
- describe common mental health conditions managed in the pediatrician's office

CASE VIGNETTE

Ari comes into your office with his exasperated parents. They note their 8-year-old boy is both sweet and very disruptive. They ask him to do his homework or put his dirty clothes in the hamper and get a frustrated kid who bolts from the room and does what he wants. His teachers note he is a pleasure to teach, he follows the rules well, and maintains a high-A average. His father notes that they have tried a variety of strategies, from giving rewards for good behavior to telling him he is a wonderful child to punishing him with loss of privileges and occasional spankings. He notes, "None of these things work."

As the psychiatrist works with the family, it becomes clear that Ari's well-meaning parents struggle with structure and consistency themselves. As such, Ari functions well within the parameters of the rules within the school environment, but that functioning erodes at home. The conflict lends its way to yelling, and the home is filled with negativity during those times. With the help of some therapy sessions, the psychiatrist is able to help the family think through how to create a structured framework of rules that is sustainable for the family to keep consistent. While Ari's behavior gets worse before it gets better (and the family was warned this might be the case), after several weeks of implementation, Ari is able to follow the rules at home with only occasional temper tantrums.

DEFINITIONS AND KEY CONCEPTS

Pediatric mental health is the emotional, behavioral, and social well-being of a child or adolescent. Pediatric mental health disorders include conditions that change the way a child typically regulates their emotions, behaves, learns, or interacts with other children, adults, or pets. *Consent* is the permission granted by an individual for medical or psychological treatment; for a minor, this would be done by the legal guardian. *Collateral information* is information gathered from other sources, including family members, other providers, schools, and medical records as a supplement to the information gathered from the patient. *Off-label treatment* is the use of medications that do not formally have an FDA indication in that population with that particular disorder, which is more common in pediatric populations where testing lags behind the adult population.

INTRODUCTION

Pediatric mental health conditions can cause significant distress to the patient, their families, and social settings in which the child subsists. Unaddressed in a timely manner or inadequately addressed, they have the potential to seriously affect the trajectory of the individual's life.

The treatment and evaluation of children differ in several key areas from the treatment and evaluation of adults. While the *Diagnostic and Statistical Manual* (*DSM*) remains the same for both populations, there are nuances about development and family relationships that play a much more profound role in the life of a child or adolescent. As such, child and adolescent psychiatrists (CAP) attain specific training to be able to focus on these particular nuances.

While CAPs are well trained at tackling these concerns, there is a worldwide shortage of individuals with this training. There are about

KEY POINT

The treatment and evaluation of children differ in several key areas from the treatment and evaluation of adults. While the *DSM* remains the same for both populations, there are nuances about development and family relationships that play a much more profound role in the life of a child or adolescent.

1.19 CAP per 100,000 youth in high-income countries, while in low- and middle-income countries, the number is less than 0.1 per 100,000 youth (Skokauskas et al., 2019). In the United States, the American Academy of Child and Adolescent Psychiatry estimates that the country needs about 47 child psychiatrists per 100,000 youth. Yet, a study in pediatrics estimates that we have one fourth of that in numbers. Also, the distribution of CAP is weighted toward metropolitan areas, leaving nonmetropolitan counties underserved (McBain et al., 2019).

Given the shortage of CAPs, to have the best chance at treating the vast number of children and adolescents who struggle with mental health disorders, it is vital that this is a joint effort between CAP and pediatricians and others who also do primary care (Foy et al., 2019). Pediatricians and other primary care providers are often the first point of contact for children with mental health conditions within the health care setting. The first part of this chapter highlights some of the key differences in working with pediatric patients to addressing mental health issues, using the American Academy of Child and Adolescent Psychiatry's "Practice Parameters on the Evaluation of Children and Adolescents" as a resource (King, 1997). In the second part, we will discuss pediatric mental health from the pediatrician's perspective.

KEY POINT

Pediatricians and other primary care providers are often the first point of contact for children with mental health conditions within the health care setting.

HOW CHILDREN AND ADOLESCENT EVALUATIONS ARE DIFFERENT FROM ADULT EVALUATIONS

Child and adolescent evaluations differ from adult evaluations in many ways which often more challenging. Firstly, under normal circumstances such evaluations should not occur without first obtaining approval from their parent or legal guardian who may or may not agree with the need for an evaluation. The child's input is generally sort, but the lens through which they view their world, and report their symptoms is often influenced by their level of development. While children may be able to report the nature of symptoms, they may not be accurate in reporting the timing and duration of their problems. This makes clinical evaluations of children and adolescents more elaborate. There are likely to be discrepancies during the process of information gathering. It requires an astute clinician to decipher the information provided by the child, while obtaining additional information from collateral sources including their parents, teachers, and other caregivers involved in the child's life.

Consent

Most adults (with a few exceptions) who come into our consulting rooms or seek an evaluation are able to consent to it. While their visit may be encouraged by someone else (e.g., a frustrated boss or spouse), adults are able to weigh the risks and benefits of going through the evaluation and choose whether this would be in their best interest. This is not the case with children and adolescents. While the age of consent for mental health treatment varies by state (and it is worth your while to become familiar with your local laws), children younger than the age of consent are not seen as able to weigh the risks and benefits able to consent. Their designated grown-up serves that purpose, whether a biological parent or a legally entrusted guardian.

Some situations may present a challenge in properly attaining consent. These may range from a child who presents with a noncustodian grandparent with parents unavailable or a child of divorce, where only one parent is granted medical decision-making power but is not the parent accompanying the child or the medically hospitalized child, whose parent is away from the hospital, and psychiatric consultation is requested by the primary team. Outside of emergent situations, such as risks of harm to self or others, mental health practitioners take consent seriously and try to find many avenues to properly attain it. This may involve setting up practices where consent is clarified when scheduling the appointment, documentation like divorce decrees being reviewed before the appointment, or a request to primary teams that all consults have been discussed with the legal guardian.

Referral and Motivation

Another consideration of children being minors is that typically someone else in their lives is concerned about their mental health struggles. It may be a teacher, or a father, or a pediatrician who may point the family toward care. Some of the people in the child's life may disagree with each other about the problem. For example, a child who presents inattentively in the classroom may have a teacher request an evaluation, whereas the parents may not agree because they see no inattention at home. Here, if the clinician only seeks input from the parents, they may miss the subtle but powerful issues occurring within the classroom. Perhaps the child has a learning disability that may leave them disengaged in the classroom but able to attend at home.

Sources of Information

Gathering collateral information in the context of a child evaluation is vital. Like detective work, child and adolescent psychiatry requires a thorough analysis of the various pieces of the puzzle, both to confirm a story or raise a red flag about an inconsistency that then needs to be pursued. Physicians often reach out to schools to gather data about how a child is performing or contact therapists to find out how a child is progressing in therapy. When appropriate, other family members may share their input. The input of parents is required as well as the input of the child. Often, standard of care involves the use of quantitative instruments, such as standardized scales. For example, a child who comes in with inattention for an initial evaluation may have a standardized scale compiled of information about symptoms of ADHD and comorbidities collected from teachers and parents prior to a solidified diagnosis being made. This may tease out inattention due to a learning disability that expresses inattention solely in the classroom versus inattention as part of ADHD that expresses itself in multiple settings.

STRATEGIES ON CHILD INTERVIEWS

The input of the child may require some creative strategies in the office. Most 6-year-olds will not sit on a couch and share that they have been struggling with sadness and uneasiness about their parents' pending divorce. Children are developing their emotional vocabulary and their narrative skills; they may see things that happen and may not recognize others. Younger children engage in play rather than long conversation as a way to make sense of their worlds. Child psychiatrists often engage with them with toys or crayons, or games. Sitting on the floor with them and playing dolls both allow them to engage in something fun, while sharing whatever they can discuss. It also allows children to tell you the story differently through the play itself. A child who is bullied at school may show those power struggles and fighting through dolls rather than through conversation. A child who worries about his parents' health may draw something telling when asked to draw their family.

ASSESSING WITHIN THE CONTEXT OF DEVELOPMENT

The other piece of the dynamically developing minds and bodies of children is that every evaluation must occur within the context of development. Areas of inquiry include where on the developmental curve a child is, whether they have developed according to age-matched norms, whether development has slowed or reversed, and whether the symptoms are, in reality, a typical developmental pattern of a child their age. For example, temper tantrums are seen as developmentally normal within the context of a 3-year-old—a manifestation of separation individuation and the dilemma a child faces as their ventures on their own. A temper tantrum in an 18-year-old is a whole other scenario; it is developmentally inappropriate and a red flag to keep digging for other issues.

CLINICAL TIP

With children, each evaluation should occur within the context of development.

ASSESSING WITHIN THE CONTEXT OF THE FAMILY

Part of conceptualizing the child's problems includes not solely thinking of the child as an individual but incorporating the dynamic context within which that child lives: the family and other members of that child's life. A child may develop symptoms as a result of their family systems dysfunction—focusing solely on the child could miss the root cause of the symptoms at play, and as a result, the patient may not get better because of an erroneous treatment plan. For example, a child in a family going through a tumultuous divorce may stabilize the family dynamics every time they are ill. As such, the child may unconsciously take on that burden to keep his family intact. Treatment here would focus less on using medications to manage the symptoms the child experiences and finding ways for the family to find a way to stabilize without the child in the sick role.

CLINICAL TIP

A child may develop symptoms because of their family systems dysfunction—focusing solely on the child could miss the root cause of the symptoms at play, and as a result, the patient may not get better because of an erroneous treatment plan.

DISORDERS MAY LOOK DIFFERENT IN PEDIATRIC POPULATIONS

Additionally, presentations may appear differently in children than they do in adults, and becoming familiar with the key features of presentations in children is vital to being able to notice when issues arise. For example, children and adolescents often present with irritability as a key symptom in a major depressive episode, rather than sadness. To miss irritability as a typical presentation of depression may lead a clinician to consider a disorder like bipolar disorder when other criteria may not be suggestive of that. In another example, traumatized children may experience symptoms differently in acute stress disorder and posttraumatic stress disorder (PTSD)—such a subthreshold and nuanced signs may indicate an issue even if a child does not meet full criteria for reexperiencing.

COMORBIDITY IS THE RULE, NOT THE EXCEPTION

With children and adolescents, comorbidity is the rule rather than the exception. For example, in evaluating a child for attention-deficit/hyperactivity disorder (ADHD), a clinician must be sure to consider other disorders that either parade as ADHD or coexist with it. ADHD is highly comorbid with other disorders, such as conduct disorder, oppositional defiant disorder, mood disorders, anxiety disorders, learning disabilities, and intellectual disability (Biederman, 1991). Missing a learning disability or depression may lead to a reductionistic focus on using stimulant medication, which may be dosed higher than needed for the ADHD and that would remain inefficacious at fixing the learning disability or depression.

OFF-LABEL TREATMENT

Treatment using psychopharmacology with children and adolescents frequently involves more use of off-label treatments than with adult work. New medications that come out often get FDA indications for adult uses, but the pediatric indications lag. Physicians start with FDA-approved medications for some disorders and move to off-label medicines if they are inefficacious or not tolerated. There may not be FDA-approved approval for the use of medications for other disorders, so the astute clinician will use the evidence base to consider how off-label approaches may or may not benefit the child.

THERAPEUTIC ALLIANCE

CLINICAL TIP

The therapeutic alliance, also called the working alliance, is a cooperative working relationship between the provider, patient, and their family. The therapeutic alliance is important to develop when working with children and families with mental health concerns.

A vital consideration in the treatment of children and adolescents is that the therapeutic alliance is not just with the child but with the family. While some clinicians may be pulled to empathizing and feeling for a child, or conversely for the parents, it is vital to create an alliance with the child and the family. In periods of conflict, it is crucial to be able to relate to all the players and help each one better understand the perspective of the other. As such, child and adolescent psychiatric work often feel like family psychiatric work, where careful consideration of all the parts of the family is both valuable and necessary. If a parent is struggling with a mental health disorder, their ability to access treatment and become well may have a crucial impact on their child's ability to heal.

CHILD AND ADOLESCENT MENTAL HEALTH IN THE PEDIATRICIAN'S OFFICE

Pediatric primary care providers (PPCP) are the first point of contact for most children and families to access mental health services (Pidano et al., 2020). The PPCP is in an ideal position to screen and treat children with mental health problems (Garner et al., 2011) and help minimize the impact that behavioral and mental health problems can pose for children and adolescents in their development and cognitive and social functioning (Westermair et al., 2018). Special attention should be provided to children faced with adversity early in life, as they are at increased risk of carrying the burden of mental health disorders. Risk factors that increase the likelihood of mental health problems are parents' history of mental health problems, family history of ADHD, exposure to trauma, violence, separation of parents, and poverty (Hardcastle et al., 2020).

Preschool-Aged Children

Young children can be screened for early signs of behavioral and mental health problems during routine well-child check visits, using tools such as the Strength and Difficulties Questionnaire (SDQ), the Ages and Stages Questionnaire-SE (ASQ), and the Pediatric Symptom Checklist (PSC; Hudson, 2016). Positive screening for symptoms of socioemotional and behavioral problems should lead the PPCP to evaluate the child's mental health. Preschool-aged children may present with frequent tantrums, aggression, fighting, hyperactivity, and sleep problems (Egger & Angold, 2006), which could be associated with behavioral or conduct problems, ADHD, or anxiety—the most commonly diagnosed mental health problems at this age (Zaim & Harrison, 2020).

CLINICAL TIP

In the pediatrician's office, young children can, and should, be screened for early signs of behavioral, emotional, and other mental health problems during routine well-child check visits.

Children with severe ADHD are most commonly diagnosed early and usually present with hyperactivity and impulsivity (Danielson et al., 2018; Egger & Angold, 2006). Children with autism, chronic health problems, and some genetic syndromes are at higher risk of having behavioral or mental health problems (Sztein & Lane, 2016). Young children with symptoms of behavioral or mental health problems should receive early intervention with psychoeducation, parenting behavioral therapy, and psychotherapy as the first line of treatment (Sztein & Lane, 2016; Zaim & Harrison, 2020). Children with moderate to severe symptoms, functional impairment, and higher risk factors should be referred to a developmental or mental health specialist.

School-Aged Children

Routine screening at well-child visits can help identify school-aged children at risk for ADHD, conduct problems, anxiety, and depression—the most common mental health diagnoses at this age (CDC, 2020). However, school-aged children usually present to the clinic with school performance problems or somatic symptoms, such as headaches, leg and arm pain, stomach pain, nausea, dizziness, and palpitations (Dillon-Naftolin, 2016; Kutuk et al., 2018; LaVigne et al., 2020).

CLINICAL TIP

Routine screening at well-child visits can help identify school age children at risk for ADHD, conduct problems, anxiety, and depression, which are common mental health diagnoses at this age.

The PPCP can evaluate children with symptoms of ADHD using behavioral rating scales, such as the Vanderbilt or Conners (Hudson, 2016) scales. These scales based on *DSM-5* criteria and the assessment of symptom severity, duration, and level of impairment conducted by the PPCP facilitate making the diagnosis. Other tools, such as the Screen for Childhood Anxiety Related Disorder (SCARED; Birmaher, 1999), are used in children as young as 8 years old to evaluate for anxiety-specific symptoms. These scales are based on *DSM-5* criteria, and the assessment of symptom severity, duration, and level of impairment conducted by the PPCP facilitate making the diagnosis.

ADHD is treated in the PPCP office with medication, behavioral therapy (often provided by a therapist or other mental health providers), or a combination of both (Austerman, 2015; Danielson et al., 2018). Mild anxiety and depression management in the PPCP office start with close monitoring of symptoms and psychoeducation. Behavioral therapy is the first line of treatment for anxiety and depression with mild symptomatology and impairment (Ghandour et al., 2019). Children with moderate to severe impairment should be referred to a mental health specialist for further management.

Adolescents

Adolescents can present to the pediatric office with similar somatic complaints as younger children, but the risk of having a mental health diagnosis increases with age (CDC, 2020; Dalsgaard et al., 2019) and, if left untreated, can lead to persistent mental health problem as adults, decreased educational attainment and economic opportunities, decreased self-esteem, increased risky behaviors and comorbidities, and increased risk of death by suicide (Hardcastle et al., 2020; Kim et al., 2020; Papachristou & Flouri, 2020). The American Academy of Pediatrics recommends routine screening for mental health problems in adolescents starting at the age of 12, as strong evidence shows that early detection can help in getting treatment for adolescents (Cheung et al., 2018). Moreover, depression increases the risk of suicide in adolescents—the second leading cause of death among youth 12–18 years of age in the United States (Guerrero-Ramírez & Cumba-Avilés, 2018; Kim et al., 2020). Adolescents should be screened at the well adolescent and sports physical exam visits using a general psychosocial screener like the PSC-17 to screen for symptoms of attention and externalizing and internalizing symptoms. A significant score in symptoms should trigger the use of specific tools, such as the modified *PHQ-9*, the SCARED, or the GAD-7 (Hudson, 2016). These diagnostic tools can be used when adolescents present with behavioral or mood symptoms as well. The PPCP can integrate them in the evaluation of the severity of symptoms and duration and level of impairment to make a diagnosis. Consideration for comorbidity is important, as having one mental health diagnosis increases the chance of suffering another one (Sztein & Lane, 2016). Mild anxiety and depression can be managed in primary care with close monitoring of symptoms and referral to cognitive behavioral therapy (Dillon-Naftolin, 2016; Ghandour et al., 2019). The PPCP can consider starting medications to treat

CLINICAL TIP

The American Academy of Pediatrics recommends routine screening for mental health problems in adolescents starting at the age of 12 years, as strong evidence shows that early detection can help in getting treatment for adolescents. This is important for suicide prevention, given that suicide is the second leading cause of death in youth.

depression and anxiety, especially when access to psychiatry or mental health services may take some time or is not readily available. Moderate to severe anxiety should be consulted with a mental health specialist.

When to Refer

While primary care providers may manage many mental health disorders, it is also important to recognize situations in which a referral to a child and adolescent psychiatrist is prudent.

TABLE 39.1 Reasons for Referral to a Child and Adolescent Psychiatrist

Reasons for referral	Examples
Urgent or emergent psychiatry evaluation is needed to assess whether hospitalization is required for the safety of the child or others	The presence of suicidal ideation, self-injury, psychosis, aggressive or other out of control behavior, acute symptoms of eating disorder, etc.
Severe symptoms of a psychiatric illness	Severe mental health symptoms or severe functional impairment
Significant functional change or worsening of symptoms	Sudden behavioral change in a previously well-functioning kid or worsening symptoms (e.g., the onset of substance use)
Lack of adequate progress in treatment	Partial response to a course of psychotropic medications or the use of two or more meds; the patient does not get better with intervention in 6 to 8 weeks
Child with significant psychosocial problems needing support and additional treatment modalities, including to address related family or other psychosocial problems	A child with behavioral problems, and caregiver may be impaired or lacking in functioning (e.g., under significant stress, parental conflict or contentious divorce, a parent with mental health or substance use challenges of their own, etc.)
Complex diagnostic issues, including cognitive, psychological, and emotional components that may relate to an organic etiology or complex mental health or legal issues	A history of significant abuse, neglect, abandonment, removal from home, multiple placements, etc.
Patient or family history causing concern for adverse effects from psychotropic medications	A family history of bipolar disorder with concern for flipping child into mania with antidepressant treatment
Preschool children with severe behavior problems	A child under age 5 with severe emotional and behavioral disturbance that may warrant medication
Medically complex children with mental health conditions	A child with chronic medical condition for whom their behavior interferes with the treatment of their medical or mental health conditions

SUMMARY

Mental health disorders are common among children and adolescents and require early identification and intervention. Working with the pediatric population in mental health requires a different skill set and some different ways of conceptualizing care, including issues of consent, alliance, and strategy to collect information. As the prevalence of disorders greatly dwarfs the number of child and adolescent psychiatrists present, both CAP and pediatric mental health providers are needed to provide early interventions for these highly treatable disorders. Working with the pediatric population in mental health requires a different skill set and different ways of conceptualizing care, including consent, alliance, and strategy to collect information.

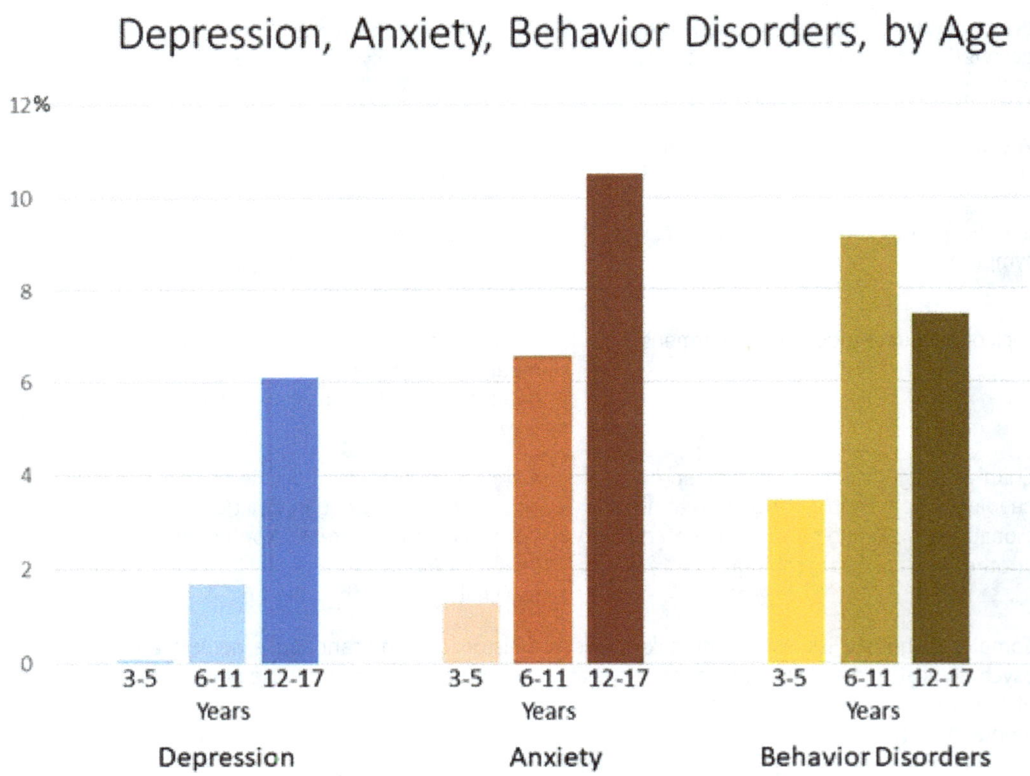

FIGURE 39.1 Common child mental health conditions: depression, anxiety, and behavior disorders by age.

Source: https://www.cdc.gov/childrensmentalhealth/data.html.

RESOURCES

1 Child and Adolescent Mental Health (nih.gov) https://www.nimh.nih.gov/health/topics/child-and-adolescent-mental-health

2 American Academy of Child and Adolescent Psychiatry https://www.aacap.org

3 https://www.cdc.gov/childrensmentalhealth/index.html

4 https://www.aacap.org/AACAP/Resources_for_Primary_Care/CAP_Resources_for_Medical_Student_Educators.aspx

5 Foy JM, Green CM, Earls MF; Committee on Psychosocial Aspects of Child and Family Health, Mental Health Leadership Work Group. (2019). Mental Health Competencies for Pediatric Practice. *Pediatrics*, 144(5):e20192757. doi: 10.1542/peds. 2019-2757.

REFERENCES

American Academy of Child and Adolescent Psychiatry. (n.d.). *When to seek referral or consultation with a CAP*. https://www.aacap.org/AACAP/Member_Resources/Practice_Information/When_to_Seek_Referral_or_Consultation_with_a_CAP.aspx

Austerman, J. (2015). ADHD and behavioral disorders: Assessment, management, and an update from DSM-5. *Cleveland Clinic Journal of Medicine, 82*(11), S2–S7. https://doi.org/10.3949/ccjm.82.s1.01

Biederman, J., Newcorn, J., & Sprich, S. (1991). Comorbidity of attention deficit hyperactivity disorder with conduct, depressive, anxiety, and other disorders. *The American Journal of Psychiatry, 148*(5), 564–577. https://doi.org/10.1176/ajp.148.5.564

Birmaher, B. (1999). *The screen for childhood anxiety related disorders (SCARED)*. https://www.midss.org/content/screen-child-anxiety-related-disorders-scared

CDC. (2020). *Data and statistics on children's mental health*. https://www.cdc.gov/childrensmentalhealth/data.html

Cheung, A. H., Zuckerbrot, R. A., Jensen, P. S., Laraque, D., & Stein, R. E. K. (2018). Guidelines for adolescent depression in primary care (GLAD-PC): Part II: Treatment and ongoing management. *Pediatrics (Evanston), 141*(3), e20174082. https://doi.org/10.1542/peds.2017-4082

Dalsgaard, S., Thorsteinsson, E., Trabjerg, B. B., Schullehner, J., Plana-Ripoll, O., Brikell, I., Wimberley, T., Thygesen, M., Madsen, K. B., Timmerman, A., Schendel, D. McGrath, J. J., Mortesen, P. B., & Pedersen, C. B. (2019). Incidence rates and cumulative incidences of the full spectrum of diagnosed mental disorders in childhood and adolescence. *JAMA Psychiatry, 77*(2), 155–164. https://doi.org/10.1001/jamapsychiatry.2019.3523

Danielson, M. L., Bitsko, R. H., Ghandour, R. M., Holbrook, J. R., Kogan, M. D., & Blumberg, S. J. (2018). Prevalence of parent-reported ADHD diagnosis and associated treatment among U.S. children and adolescents, 2016. *Journal of Clinical Child and Adolescent Psychology: The Official Journal for the Society of Clinical Child and Adolescent Psychology, 47*(2), 199–212. https://doi.org/10.1080/15374416.2017.1417860

Dillon-Naftolin, E. (2016). Identification and treatment of generalized anxiety disorder in children in primary care. *Pediatric Annals, 45*(10), e349–e355. https://doi.org/10.3928/19382359-20160913-01

Egger, H. L., & Angold, A. (2006). Common emotional and behavioral disorders in preschool children: Presentation, nosology, and epidemiology. *Journal of Child Psychology and Psychiatry, 47*(3–4), 313–337. https://doi.org/10.1111/j.1469-7610.2006.01618.x

Foy, J. M., Green, C. M., Earls, M. F., & Committee on Psychosocial Aspects of Child and Family Health, Mental Health Leadership Work Group. (2019). Mental health competencies for pediatric practice. *Pediatrics, 144*(5), e20192757. https://doi.org/10.1542/peds.2019-2757

Garner, A. S., Shonkoff, J. P., Siegel, B. S., Dobbins, M. I., Earls, M. F., McGuinn, L., Pascoe, J., & Wood, D.L. (2011). Early childhood adversity, toxic stress, and the role of the pediatrician: Translating developmental science into lifelong health. *Pediatrics (Evanston), 129*(1), e224–e231. https://doi.org/10.1542/peds.2011-2662

Ghandour, R. M., Sherman, L. J., Vladutiu, C. J., Ali, M. M., Lynch, S. E., Bitsko, R. H., & Blumberg, S. J. (2019). Prevalence and treatment of depression, anxiety, and conduct problems in U.S. children. *The Journal of Pediatrics, 206*, 256–267.e3. https://doi.org/10.1016/j.jpeds.2018.09.021

Guerrero-Ramírez, G., & Cumba-Avilés, E. (2018). Factors associated with suicidal ideation and quality of life in adolescents from Puerto Rico with type 1 diabetes. *Puerto Rico Health Sciences Journal, 37*(1), 19–21. http://search.ebscohost.com/login.aspx?direct=true&db=cmedm&AN=29547680&site=ehost-live

Hardcastle, K., Bellis, M. A., Sharp, C. A., & Hughes, K. (2020). Exploring the health and service utilisation of general practice patients with a history of adverse childhood experiences (ACEs): An observational study using electronic health records. *BMJ Open, 10*(9), e036239. https://doi.org/10.1136/bmjopen-2019-036239

Hudson, D. L. (2016). Quality over quantity: Integrating mental health assessment tools into primary care practice. *Permanente Journal, 20*(3), 15–148. https://doi.org/10.7812/TPP/15-148

Kim, H., Ryu, J. M., & Kim, H. W. (2020). Characteristics and trends of suicide attempt or non-suicidal self-injury in children and adolescents visiting emergency department. *Journal of Korean Medical Science, 35*(33), e276. https://doi.org/10.3346/jkms.2020.35.e276

King, R. A. (1997). Practice parameters for the psychiatric assessment of children and adolescents. *Journal of the American Academy of Child and Adolescent Psychiatry, 36*(10), 4S–20S. https://doi.org/10.1097/00004583-199710001-00002

Kutuk, M. O., Tufan, A. E., Guler, G., Yalin, O. O., Altintas, E., Bag, H. G., Uluduz, D., Toros, F., Aytan, N., Kutuk, O., & Ozge, A. (2018). Migraine and associated comorbidities are three times more frequent in children with ADHD and their mothers. *Brain & Development, 40*(10), 857–864. https://doi.org/10.1016/j.braindev.2018.06.001

LaVigne, T. W., Laake, L. M., & Ibeziako, P. (2020). Somatic symptom and related disorders in pediatric patients: Associations with parent psychiatric and substance use histories. *Clinical Child Psychology and Psychiatry, 25*(4), 932–944. https://doi.org/10.1177/1359104520931579

McBain, R. K., Kofner, A., Stein, B. D., Cantor, J. H., Vogt, W. B., & Yu, H. (2019). Growth and distribution of child psychiatrists in the United States: 2007–2016. *Pediatrics, 144*(6), e20191576. https://doi.org/10.1542/peds.2019-1576

Papachristou, E., & Flouri, E. (2020). Distinct developmental trajectories of internalising and externalising symptoms in childhood: Links with mental health and risky behaviours in early adolescence. *Journal of Affective Disorders, 276*, 1052–1060. https://doi.org/10.1016/j.jad.2020.07.130

Pidano, A. E., Segool, N. K., Delgado, N., Forness, K., Hagen, K., Gurganus, E. A., Honigfeld, L., Hess, C.l Hicks, A., Morgan, C. (2020). Parent perceptions of pediatric primary care providers' mental health–related communication and practices. *Journal of Pediatric Health Care, 34*(5), e49-e58. https://doi.org/10.1016/j.pedhc.2020.04.009

Skokauskas, N., Fung, D., Flaherty, L. T., von Klitzing, K., Pūras, D., Servili, C., Dua, T., Falissard, B., Vostanis, P., Moyano, M. B., Feldman, I., Clark, C., Boričević, V., Patton, G., Leventhal, B., & Guerrero, A. (2019). Shaping the future of child and adolescent psychiatry. *Child and Adolescent Psychiatry and Mental Health, 13*, 19. https://doi.org/10.1186/s13034-019-0279-y

Sztein, D. M., & Lane, W. G. (2016). Examination of the comorbidity of mental illness and somatic conditions in hospitalized children in the United States using the kids' inpatient database, 2009. *Hospital Pediatrics, 6*(3), 126–134. https://doi.org/10.1542/hpeds.2015-0117

Westermair, A. L., Stoll, A. M., Greggersen, W., Kahl, K. G., Hüppe, M., & Schweiger, U. (2018). All unhappy childhoods are unhappy in their own way-differential impact of dimensions of adverse childhood experiences on adult mental health and health behavior. *Frontiers in Psychiatry, 9*, 198. https://doi.org/10.3389/fpsyt.2018.00198

Zaim, N., & Harrison, J. (2020). Pre-school mental health disorders: A review. *International Review of Psychiatry (Abingdon, England), 32*(3), 189–201. https://doi.org/10.1080/09540261.2019.1692793

CHAPTER 40

Geriatric Mental Health[1]

Ajike Ogunsulire-Etumadu, M.D., F.A.C.P., C.H.C.Q.M., PHY-ADV

"Aging is an extraordinary process where you become the person you always should have been."

— David Bowie

OBJECTIVES

After reading this chapter, students will be able to do the following:

- describe the role of the geriatrician as it relates to mental health
- review common mental health conditions seen by geriatricians
- highlight the importance of screening for depression and other mental health conditions in the elderly

CASE VIGNETTE

When it quacks, it is a duck; but when it looks like dementia, it's often not.

Mr. B is a 77-year-old man with several well-controlled chronic medical problems who lives in Florida with his wife in a home they have owned for many years. Mr. B had always prided himself on being independent. He is the head of his family, and his ex-military status makes him regimented and stoic. He does not do well with change. He and his wife have lived in Florida for over 50 years, where they raised their family. His two adult children in California recently told him he needed to move to California to be closer to them, as it would be easier to provide care for them. Of some concern in the preceding years, Mr. B and his wife had suffered from a few falls with consequent multiple emergency department visits and hospitalizations. This had both adult children making multiple trips

(*continued*)

1 Readers may also see "Delirium and Dementia" (Chapter 27) for related material.

from California to Florida. Their adult children lived busy lives and arrived quickly at the decision with little true discussion with their parents.

Mr. B has an age-appropriate memory lapse, but this does not interfere with his day-to-day activities. Over the next 6 months, after he was told what he and his wife needed to do, he began to manifest more memory trouble. He had difficulty remembering the names of his grandchildren and close friends. He could no longer manage his family banking accounts and frequently got lost when shopping for groceries. He lost interest in reading after being an avid reader for many years. He neglected his hygiene and often appeared disheveled and unkempt. He stopped returning calls to his friends and repeatedly turned down invitations to socialize, telling his wife he feared he would not remember friends' names or get lost driving to and from these engagements. Quite alarmed and perplexed at this decline, Mrs. B decided to seek care, convinced that this was slowly worsening dementia. She was sure that her husband would be better served in a specialized memory unit, while she would move into an assisted-living facility (ALF) once they got to California.

At the geriatrician's office, Mr. B was asked about recent events and was administered a geriatric depression scale screening tool. After a thorough physical exam, routine blood work, and a head CT done on account of a history of falls, nothing was found. However, his geriatric depression screen (GDS) was positive for significant depression. He denied having suicidal thoughts but admitted to owning a firearm. His wife was instructed to lock this securely away for safety once she got home.

The cognitive decline, worsening memory loss, poor executive function associated with social withdrawal, and anhedonia symptoms could easily be attributable to dementia. However, given the positive findings on his GDS, a trial of SSRIs and sertraline were started. Within 4 weeks, Mr. B's memory began to improve. He began enjoying reading and speaking with friends again. He now remembered names of familiar places they had visited in the past. Within 12 weeks, he was practically back to his old self. Concurrent psychotherapy revealed deep fears and worries about losing his independence, moving away from friends, and the sense of loss of control he felt, having played no active part in the decision to relocate.

A family meeting with Mr. B and his adult children was done remotely using his psychotherapist's telehealth platform. Mr. B had the opportunity to share his thoughts about the life-adjustment decisions being made. Mr. B voiced his concerns. He worried his opinions would be seen as ingratitude toward his children. His children heard their father and reassured him that his input on decisions for his life were central to the discussion. Mr. B regained his trust and confidence and was no longer anxious and ambivalent about the offered help. He actually started to look forward to the move and the chance to bond with grandchildren, make new friends, renew hobbies, and be cared for safely without feeling like a burden to his children. It became a win–win for everyone.

This case shows how easily psychiatric problems in the elderly can be easily missed or underdiagnosed with a substantial impact on the patient's quality of life. There is a big difference in the cost of health care services between Mr. B going to a memory care facility to be treated for major depressive disorder and living an independent life. Luckily for

Mr. B and his family, he saw a geriatrician who did a thorough workup, including administering a simple in-office geriatric depression screen. One can only imagine the misery he would feel if he were to be wrongly labeled as demented and placed away from family in a memory unit!

DEFINITIONS AND KEY CONCEPTS

A *geriatrician* is a physician who completes a 3-year residency in internal medicine or family medicine and then completes a one- to two-year fellowship in geriatric medicine. It is an American Board of Internal Medicine specialty with board certification status. A geriatrician takes care of patients over 65 years to the end of life, although much younger people are often included, and some consider older than 50 years to be geriatrician-designated worthy. This is more of a reflection of the multiple chronic medical issues often seen in this population.

Why Is a Geriatrician Important in Geriatric Psychiatry?

A geriatrician's training and exposure to ailments and maladies specific to the over 65-year-old (or over 50) population make them good gatekeepers of mental health problems in this unique population. The ability to understand the associations of chronic medical conditions with common symptoms of psychiatric disorders is invaluable. They can detect mental health problems early and know when to refer to a psychiatrist for specialized psychiatric care. They are a vital link in the caregiving loop, which eases the limited geriatric psychiatrists' burden. Most common geriatric psychiatric disorders can be treated and successfully managed by the primary care team or geriatric caregiver.

INTRODUCTION

It is predicted that by 2030 the elderly population, often called seniors, will be twice the size it is today. Sometimes dubbed the "2030 problem," most of the elderly population's growth will be due to the aging of the baby boomers, who will be age 66 to 84, the "young old," and will number 61 million. In addition to the baby boomers, the "oldest old," or those born before 1946, will number nine million.

Looking at these numbers, it becomes evident that health issues, especially those related to mental health in the elderly, need an array of

KEY POINT

It is predicted that by 2030 the elderly population, often called seniors, will be twice the size it is today. Sometimes dubbed the "2030 problem," most of the elderly population's growth will be due to the aging of the baby boomers, who will be aged 66 to 84, the "young old," and will number 61 million.

KEY POINT

Aging is not a disease. From a mental health and economic standpoint, investing in geriatric mental health eases the burden on the aging themselves, their caregivers, and society's burden to fund long-term psychiatric mental health care services.

health care providers to adequately screen, treat, and rehabilitate these older members of society. Adequate health care enables them to age optimally and continue to be valuable members of their communities.

Aging is not a disease. From a mental health and economic standpoint, investing in geriatric mental health eases the burden on the aging themselves, their caregivers, and society's burden to fund long-term psychiatric mental health care services.

Following, we give a brief synopsis on common geriatric psychiatric problems, the association of medical illnesses with geriatric psychiatry symptoms and disorders, how and when to screen to prevent long-term disease burden, diagnoses and treatment options, and when to refer to psychiatry.

SCREENING AND TOOLS AVAILABLE

Screening for ailments, such as late-life depression and behavioral disturbances in dementia, to name a few, can be done using several methods. They should not be used alone, but a clinical diagnostic interview is warranted to see if treatment is indicated or criteria for psychiatric illness are met when a patient tests positive.

COMMON PSYCHIATRIC DISORDERS TREATED BY GERIATRICIANS

Older adults are one of the fastest growing demographics in the United States and other developed countries. As individuals age, they experience and adapt to many changes. This includes cumulative development of medical problems, adjustment to work retirement, death of friends, spouses, siblings, or other family members, and a general contraction of their social circles. In late adult years, brain volume decreases and neurocognitive impairment increases. Neurological conditions such as stroke, dementia, delirium, all increase with impact on mental health symptoms and functioning. For these reasons, mental health is an increasingly important aspect of public health and health worker education.

Depression

Depression in the elderly is common and can present in many forms. Because geriatric patients hardly self-report typical symptoms of feeling blue or depressed, a screen is often the only way to bring out common but easily missed psychiatric problems. Screening for depression should be done be as part of any routine visit for a geriatric patient in the outpatient setting. Screening is either self-reported or performed via an administered questionnaire. Accuracy and specificity have been found to be high and reliable in clinical settings. Geriatric patients' cognitive status should be considered when using and interpreting screening tests for depression (Boyle et al., 2011; Beekman, 1999). Table 40.1 contains commonly used screening tools for depression and tests for cognitive functioning in the elderly (Gallo, 2007).

CLINICAL TIP

Depression in the elderly is common and can present in many forms. Because geriatric patients hardly self-report typical symptoms of feeling blue or depressed, a screen is often the only way to bring out common but easily missed psychiatric problems.

TABLE 40.1 Common Screening Tools Used in Geriatric Mental Health for Depression and Cognitive Functioning

	Name	Utility	Time needed
Depression	Patient Health Questionnaire-2 (PHQ-2)	• Two-item scale • Screens for depressed or anhedonic mood—the core feature of depressive disorders	< 2 mins
	Patient Health Questionnaire-9 (PHQ-99)	• Nine-item scale • Specifically developed for primary care settings and demonstrates ease, validity, and reliability	< 5 mins
	The Geriatric Depression Scale (self-report; GDS)	• Five-item self-report • Two out of five depressive responses suggest depression	
Cognitive functioning	Addenbrooke's Cognitive Examination, Revised (ACE-R)	• Neurocognitive functioning	< 20 mins
	Mini-Cog	• Executive functioning	< 5 mins
	Folstein's Mini-Mental Status Examination (MMSE)	• Neurocognitive functioning	< 10 mins
	Montreal Cognitive Assessment (MOCA)	• Neurocognitive functioning	< 10 mins

Late-Life Depression

Depression is one of the most common psychiatric problems present in the geriatric population. Sadly, depression in the elderly remains underdiagnosed and inadequately treated. Depression is not a normal consequence of aging. Sadness and grief are normal responses to life events in aging, such as grief or bereavement, adjustments to changes in social status upon retirement, and the transition from independent living

> **CLINICAL TIP**
>
> Depression is not a normal consequence of aging. Sadness and grief are normal responses to life events in aging, such as grief or bereavement, adjustments to changes in social status upon retirement, and the transition from independent living to assisted or residential care.

to assisted or residential care. While these changes can be stressors, they do not necessarily cause depression. Accurately diagnosing and treating depression in later life is extremely important, as it affects the quality of life, caregiver burden, and all-cause mortality. Cultural biases include depression being more common in Black persons without spirituality but not a major risk factor in the White population. Older ethnic minorities use mental health services less often than their American counterparts—often maintaining the social taboos and stigmas held in their countries of origin regarding how they are to be diagnosed and subsequently treated. The stigma of a mental health diagnosis still carries across age barriers into the elder community. Hospitalized geriatric patients have a depression rate of over 30%, while patients with stroke, myocardial infarction, or cancer have over 40% risk. Other risk factors for late-life depression include female sex; social isolation; being widowed, divorced, or of separated marital status; lower socioeconomic status; comorbid general medical conditions, uncontrolled pain; insomnia; and functional and cognitive impairment. As many as 50% of nursing home residents manifest depressive disorders symptoms during their first year.

Depressed mood may be the first symptom of several medical conditions that commonly occur in the elderly, including stroke, diabetes, cancer, hypothyroidism, and coronary artery disease. The impact of depression on medical mortality is well documented, increasing mortality post-MI, stroke, and admission to nursing homes in the first year. Depression is a significant risk for suicide in the elderly, who account for about 13% of the U.S. population but 24% of completed suicides. Suicidal behavior in the elderly is a result of the interaction of many factors including mental health symptoms, chronic and debilitating disease conditions, psychological suffering and painful life experiences. Depression and cognitive deficits in several conditions common in late adulthood further increase susceptibility. Acute suicidal ideation requires an urgent psychiatric referral. In the elderly, men have at a higher risk of suicide than women. It is highest in White men over 85, and they have possibly seen a physician in the last month. For this reason, screening for depression is good practice and for firearms in the home is an absolute must once depression is screened for and diagnosed.

> **CLINICAL TIP**
>
> Late-life depression is also associated with an increased risk of developing dementia and may represent a prodrome to dementia or be an independent risk factor. Major depression in the elderly is often associated with cognitive impairment, which develops with mood symptoms or after they have developed.

Late-life depression is also associated with an increased risk of developing dementia and may represent a prodrome to dementia or be an independent risk factor. Major depression in the elderly is often associated with cognitive impairment, which develops with mood symptoms or after they have developed. Antidepressants can resolve the cognitive and mood symptoms, but the risk of conversion to an irreversible dementia syndrome, such as Alzheimer's dementia, remains high. Relapse and chronicity remain high in patients with major depressive disorder in later life.

Vascular or Post-Stroke Depression

Patients with left prefrontal cortex, left hemisphere lesions tend to have more depression and increased severity of symptoms. The risk is highest in the first 2 years after a stroke. Successful treatment of late-life depression depends on addressing comorbid conditions, tailoring pharmacological interventions to each patient, monitoring for effectiveness and side effects, and close follow-up. Serotonin reuptake inhibitors (SSRIs) are the first-line medication treatment with several options in this class. Other medication classes are also available. Apart from medications, other modalities of treatment are also helpful. Psychotherapy, exercise, electroconvulsive therapy (ECT), and bright light therapy, to name a few, are some of the most popular therapies available. The patient's response to treatment can be assessed within 4 weeks, by which time there is often a response if the treatment is effective. Remission, partially or fully, usually occurs within 12 weeks. Multiple failed trials of antidepressants signal the need for psychiatric referral. Suicidal or homicidal ideations or intent signal the need for emergency psychiatry evaluation for possible hospitalization.

Geriatric Bipolar Disorder

Geriatric bipolar disorder (BPD) is characterized by episodes of major depression and mania or hypomania. This group consists of aging BPD patients and those with a first episode generally experienced after 60, although a new presentation after 50 may qualify. Patients typically have a variety of symptoms, ranging from depression to mania. Late-onset mania can often be associated with stroke, dementia, and hyperthyroidism. Some manic episodes can be more symptomatic of confusion, disorientation, distractibility, or irritability, rather than the typical hypomanic mood episodes of the younger BPD patient, and, therefore, are often misdiagnosed as delirium, or vice versa. First-line medications for BPD include lithium, valproate, olanzapine, and quetiapine (Chen, 2011).

Anxiety Disorders in Later Life

Anxiety is commonly associated with pulmonary, cardiovascular, and hyperthyroid disorders. Anxiety symptoms can range from episodic panic to anxiety attacks or nonspecific states of anxiety. They can be worsened by the consumption of common beverages, such as caffeinated drinks. Symptoms can be precipitated or worsened by certain medications, such as

CLINICAL TIP

Anxiety is commonly associated with pulmonary, cardiovascular, and hyperthyroid disorders. Anxiety symptoms can range from episodic panic to anxiety attacks or nonspecific states of anxiety. Symptoms can be precipitated or worsened by certain medications.

theophylline. Related conditions can occur, including obsessive compulsive disorder (OCD), hoarding behaviors, and posttraumatic stress syndrome (PTSD). SSRIs, such as citalopram, sertraline, and escitalopram, are commonly used for treatment. For anxiety, including in the elderly, benzodiazepines, if used, should be prescribed for short periods to control acute symptoms. Various strategies that promote relaxation (e.g., music, aromatherapy, and visual imagery) can be helpful. More formal psychotherapy, such as CBT with cognitive restructuring to identify and respond to stimuli that trigger anxiety, can help develop a range of coping mechanisms to reduce stress and anxiety.

Schizophrenia and Psychotic Disorders

CLINICAL TIP

Late-life psychosis is often associated with neurological conditions, such as stroke, dementia, or Parkinson's disease, as opposed to schizophrenia. Dementia with Lewy bodies is associated with vivid visual hallucinations.

Late-life psychosis is often associated with neurological conditions, such as stroke, dementia, or Parkinson's disease, as opposed to schizophrenia. Dementia with Lewy bodies is associated with vivid visual hallucinations. Conditions manifesting psychotic symptoms should be evaluated for medical causes, including possible delirium, substance use, dementia, stroke, Parkinson's disease, and so on. Acute onset of cognitive decline with the inability to sustain attention and with altered or fluctuating awareness and arousal levels is more likely delirium or possible substance or medication induced. Late-life schizophrenia is considered a new diagnosis after 40 and late after 60 and is often associated with persecutory/paranoid delusions.

Somatic Symptoms and Related Disorder

Somatic symptom complaints are characterized by the seriousness of medical symptoms, persistently high anxiety symptoms, and excessive time and energy spent focusing on somatic symptoms. This is a particularly relevant group in the geriatric population because they are associated with the overuse of medical services; those in this group are usually female and in a lower socioeconomic group. The intent is not to mislead or drive a serious diagnosis, as occurs in malingering, where there is a secondary gain for fictitious symptoms. The symptoms are genuinely perceived as real and are distressing. Acknowledging the concern for symptoms, being empathetic, and scheduling regular visits with the patient are the keys to treatment success. A thorough clinical assessment should be done to exclude the presence of objective disease states.

NEUROPSYCHIATRIC SYMPTOMS OF DEMENTIA

Psychiatry symptoms associated with dementia include agitation, aggression, delusions, hallucinations, paranoia, wandering, depression, apathy, disinhibition, and sleep disturbance. Behavioral disturbances commonly peak in the late afternoon or evening—a phenomenon called *sundowning*. Risk factors for this include poor light exposure and disturbed sleep (Bilwise, 1994). Delusions are also common in Alzheimer's; paranoid beliefs can be distressing to caregivers and patients alike (e.g., family members becoming impostors, unfaithful spouses, etc.; Taylor, 2014).

> **CLINICAL TIP**
>
> Behavioral disturbances commonly peak in the late afternoon or evening—a phenomenon called *sundowning*. Risk factors for this include poor light exposure and disturbed sleep and medical conditions.

Agitation or aggression can arise from various underlying causes in patients with dementia, and identifying the causes is critical to effective management. In some patients, a new infection or medication toxicity can trigger a new behavioral change. Medications that have anticholinergic properties increase risk in dementia patients. In the elderly, these are commonly used to treat sleep disturbance, bladder incontinence, benzodiazepines, and hypnotics or sedatives. Pain is another big risk for neuropsychiatric symptoms in dementia because patients cannot report pain reliably; the screening tool Pain in Advanced Dementia (PAINAD) is a great way to score and assess pain (Chew, 2008).

Agitation in Dementia

Nonpharmacologic strategies include distraction, redirection, and structured routines and providing calm, reassuring responses when patients appear anxious, helping to avert or abort escalation of agitation. Aromatherapy, exercise training, music therapy, touch therapy, and light massage can also be helpful.

While evidence for cholinesterase inhibitors' efficacy is not robust for agitation, they are well tolerated and may have added benefits for cognition and function. The use of SSRI medications, specifically citalopram, has been especially useful in this patient group over 60.

Depression in Dementia

Depression in patients with dementia is often difficult to detect and treat. Cognitive decline is often seen in late-life depression, and cognitive decline is the hallmark of dementia. SSRIs remain the first drug group of choice (Steffens, 2000).

Sleep Disorders in Dementia

Nonpharmacological treatment strategies are preferred. Implementing good sleep hygiene, increasing natural light exposure and activity in the mornings, limiting evening beverages, and eliminating evening alcohol and coffee are all useful measures.

> **QUICK POINT**
>
> Delirium is a clinical syndrome caused by medical conditions, substance intoxication or withdrawal, or medication side effects characterized by a fluctuating disturbance of consciousness with reduced ability to focus, sustain attention, or shift attention. Nearly 30% of hospitalized older medical patients experience delirium.

Wandering and Pacing Behavior

Wandering behaviors can cause safety concerns in elderly patients with dementia. They are some of the most distressing symptoms and most taxing on caregivers, and there is no real way to treat or prevent them. Careful supervision and environmental adjustments can prevent the elderly from getting hurt or lost while wandering. Wandering is often a contributory reason for families and caregivers deciding to place older relatives in nursing homes.

DELIRIUM

Delirium is a clinical syndrome caused by medical conditions, substance intoxication or withdrawal, or medication side effects characterized by a fluctuating disturbance of consciousness with reduced ability to focus, sustain attention, or shift attention. Nearly 30% of hospitalized older medical patients experience delirium. Detecting and treating underlying medical illnesses is an effective way of treating this illness, as is addressing specific hospital issues such as poor sleep, overstimulation by lighting or noise, medication side effects, catheter placements, and unaddressed pain, to name a few. Periodically reviewing and streamlining patients' medication is good clinical practice and one that is essential to prevent and reduce the risk of developing delirium in older patients.

SUMMARY

Psychiatric problems in the elderly are common and often misdiagnosed, underdiagnosed, or totally missed. A geriatrician plays a pivotal role in being a gatekeeper of mental health in the elderly—a patient population where the suspicion for psychiatric issues is often overlooked or missed. The impact on the quality of life and the determinants of overall health and caregivers' outcomes are huge. Both the financial burden from a health care perspective and overall quality of life to the patient and those who care for them can be very burdensome.

RESOURCES

1 Geriatric Psychiatry

2 The State of Mental Health and Aging in America (cdc.gov)

3 Mental health and support as you get older | nidirect

REFERENCES

Beekman, A. T., Copeland, R., & Prince, M. (1999). Review of community prevalence of depression in later life *The British Journal of Psychiatry, 174*(4), 307–311.

Bilwise, D. L. (1994). What is sundowning? *Journal of the American Geriatrics Society, , 42*, 1009.

Boyle, L. L., Richardson, T. M., He, H., Xia, Y., Tu, X., Boustani, M., & Conwell, Y. (2011). How do the PHQ-2, the PHQ-9 perform in aging services clients with cognitive impairment? *International Journal of Geriatric Psychiatry, 26*(9), 952–960. https://doi.org/10.1002/gps.2632

Chen, P., Korobkova, I., Busby, K., & Sajatovic, M. (2011). Late life bipolar disorder: An update. *Aging Health, 7*, 557.

Chew, M. L., Mulsant, B. H., Pollock, B. G., Lehman, M. E., Greenspan, A., Mahmoud, R. A., Kirshner, M. A., Sorisio, D. A., Bies, R. R., & Gharabawi, G. (2008). Anticholinergic activity of 107 medications commonly used by older adults. *Journal of the American Geriatrics Society, 56*(7), 1333–1341. https://doi.org/10.1111/j.1532-5415.2008.01737.x

Gallo, J. J., Bogner, H. R., Morales, K. H., Post, E. P., Lin, J. Y., & Bruce, M. L. (2007). The effect of a primary care practice-based depression intervention on mortality in older adults: A randomized trial. *Annals of Internal Medicine, 146*(10), 689–698. https://doi.org/10.7326/0003-4819-146-10-200705150-00002

Sajatovic, M. (2002). Treatment of bipolar disorder in older adults. *International Journal of Geriatric Psychiatry, 17*, 865.

Steffens, D. C., Skoog, I., Norton, M. C., Hart, A. D., Tschanz, J. T., Plassman, B. L., Wyse, B. W., Welsh-Bohmer, K. A., & Breitner, J. C. (2000). Prevalence of depression and its treatment in an elderly population: The Cache County study. *Archives of General Psychiatry, 57*(6), 601–607. https://doi.org/10.1001/archpsyc.57.6.601

Taylor, W. D. (2014). Clinical practice: Depression in the elderly. *The New England Journal of Medicine, 371*(13), 1228.

Waern, M., Runeson, B. S., Allebeck, P., Beskow, J., Rubenowitz, E., Skoog, I., & Wilhelmsson, K. (2002). Mental disorder in elderly suicides: a case-control study. *The American Journal of Psychiatry, 159*(3), 450–455. https://doi.org/10.1176/appi.ajp.159.3.450

Whooley, M. A., Avins, A. L., Miranda, J., & Browner, W. S. (1997). Case-finding instruments for depression. Two questions are as good as many. *Journal of General Internal Medicine, 12*(7), 439–445. https://doi.org/10.1046/j.1525-1497.1997.00076.x

Wilson, R. S., Barnes, L. L., Mendes de Leon, C. F., Aggarwal, N. T., Schneider, J. S., Bach, J., Pilat, J., Beckett, L. A., Arnold, S. E., Evans, D. A., & Bennett, D. A. (2002). Depressive symptoms, cognitive decline, and risk of AD in older persons. *Neurology, 59*(3), 364–370. https://doi.org/10.1212/wnl.59.3.364

CHAPTER 41

Professional Demeanor and Boundaries With Patients

Elisabeth Netherton, M.D. and Sindhu Idicula, M.D.

> *"I will follow that system of regimen which, according to my ability and judgment, I consider for the benefit of my patients, and abstain from whatever is deleterious and mischievous."*
>
> — Hippocrates

OBJECTIVES

After completing this chapter, students will be able to do the following:

- define boundaries, boundary violation, and boundary boundary-crossing
- list examples of boundary violations and boundary crossings

DEFINITIONS AND KEY CONCEPTS

A *boundary* is a dividing line, a limit of a subject or sphere of activity, or the "edge" of appropriate behavior. A *boundary crossing* is a transient, nonexploitative deviation from the typical practice of medicine. A *boundary violation* is a deviation from typical practice that harms patients.

INTRODUCTION

A boundary is defined as "a dividing line; a limit of a subject or sphere of activity." In clinical practice, we may consider it to be the "edge" of what is appropriate behavior (Gutheil & Gabbard, 1998). Boundaries within interpersonal relationships demarcate where we stop and where someone else begins and help us navigate closeness within relationships, while maintaining our own sense of self, including our bodies, thoughts, feelings, wants, and needs. They help set expectations for the relationship and how we intend to use it.

What Do Boundaries Have to Do With Professional Relationships?

Boundaries define what makes professional relationships "professional." They set expectations for how professional relationships will be conducted and clearly demarcate professional relationships from personal ones. Professional boundaries imply a certain amount of distance, convey respect, and allow for the safety and predictability that is vital for the doctor–patient relationship (Gutheil & Gabbard, 1998).

THE PHYSICIAN–PATIENT RELATIONSHIP

A physician-patient relationship exists when a physician serves a patient's medical needs (AMA, 2021). This is fundamentally a moral activity stemming from the imperative to provide care to patients to relieve symptoms and to alleviate suffering. This relationship is generally based on trust and entered into mutually by the physician and the patient or their surrogate. The physician then has an ethical responsibility to meet these goals while placing the patient's welfare at the center of their dealings (AMA, 2021).

What Is the Role of Boundaries in the Physician–Patient Relationship?

It is sometimes easiest to understand boundaries in contexts in which they become eroded or ineffective. Let's use a case example to see how boundaries can start to shift.

CASE VIGNETTE

Dr. Smith is a psychiatrist taking care of Frank, a young man with depression and severe substance use. Frank is likable, reminding Dr. Smith of his own young-adult son. Frank tries hard and seems to need guidance. Dr. Smith is eager to be helpful to him. Over time, Dr. Smith begins extending his appointments with Frank as they talk about Frank's difficulties. Dr. Smith offers advice from his own life experiences that Frank finds helpful, and they meet more frequently. Dr. Smith hopes the relationship will keep Frank from relapsing on substances. He encourages Frank to call him any time, providing his cell phone number.

(continued)

Frank texts him with increasing frequency. Frank struggles with substance cravings on the weekends, particularly with free time, and Dr. Smith worries about the possibility he might use.

At their next visit, Dr. Smith offers to take Frank with him for his routine Saturday golf game, where they can continue to discuss Frank's future. Soon, Dr. Smith and Frank meet on weekends to play golf together, much as a father and son might. Over time, Frank becomes increasingly uncomfortable sharing more sensitive details of his life with Dr. Smith, worried that he might disappoint or jeopardize their relationship. When he experiences a severe substance relapse, he hides this from Dr. Smith. He feels increasingly depressed but is fearful of disappointing Dr. Smith with his "failure" as a patient. Frank finds that he is no longer able to use this relationship for its original purpose: receiving care for his depression and addiction.

KEY POINT

The physician–patient relationship holds a high level of intimacy—physically, through physical exams, and emotionally, through the discussion of sensitive, private information. Without maintaining proper structure, this relationship can become confusing to patients and physicians alike.

KEY POINT

Boundaries in the physician–patient relationship reinforce that our relationship with our patients within this professional context is one in which we are present for *their* benefit through medical care. While *we* might meet their emotional needs by providing empathic, patient-centered care, they are not there to meet *our* emotional needs.

Physicians carry a fiduciary duty within the physician–patient relationship. Patients give us their trust and rely on us for care, and we, in turn, are ethically bound to act in their best interest. As human beings, we may naturally see our patients as potential new friends, neighbors, or romantic interests but are bound by our fiduciary responsibility to them.

The physician–patient relationship holds a high level of intimacy—physically, through physical exams, and emotionally, through the discussion of sensitive, private information. This can be confusing to patients and physicians alike. The deepening of trust and intimacy over the longitudinal course of the relationship can amplify this confusion (American Medical Association [AMA], 2016).

Boundaries in the physician–patient relationship reinforce that our relationship with our patients within this professional context is one in which we are present for *their* benefit through medical care. While *we* might meet their emotional needs by providing empathic, patient-centered care, they are not there to meet *our* emotional needs. Our only benefit from this relationship is the fee for our professional services and the professional satisfaction of contributing to their health and well-being (AMA, 2016).

In addition to orienting our patients, good boundaries orient us as physicians to the goals of our interactions with our patients. If our goal is to establish a friendship, we might shy away from a difficult conversation or an uncomfortable confrontation, such as ordering a routine urine drug screen or completing a complete physical exam. When this happens, our patients receive suboptimal medical care.

How Do We Set Boundaries in the Physician-Patient Relationship?

Much of our professional boundary setting occurs through nonverbal communication in our professional behavior. We meet at our place of work. We meet during our work hours. We dress in our work clothes, professional attire, or scrubs. We use language that embodies professionalism and respect. Patients call us by our titles, and we refer to them with respect in a manner appropriate to their age and cultural norms. We maintain confidentiality.

Could some of our work happen in another context—for example, in yoga gear at the coffee shop on a first-name basis? With that, our frame is lost. Outside of privacy concerns, now the relationship resembles a friendship and no longer carries the structure and safety our patients need to trust us to care for them.

Physician–patient boundaries also set standards regarding reciprocity. While most relationships have balanced reciprocity, both parties share in an even fashion, the physician–patient relationship does not. We do not use the visits to unload our life struggles, beliefs, or experiences. While this may appear as helpful to empathically connect, doing so can rapidly shut down the availability of relational space for our patients to openly discuss their experiences.

Our relationship exists for our patients' benefit. It is the responsibility of the physician (the professional in the dyad) to hold boundaries for the relationship. Our patients are not expected to know about them, or understand their value, and at times may test them. Can they meet with us after hours or call us by our first name? It is our responsibility to compassionately hold to the frame of our routine clinical practice, emphasizing that the boundaries are necessary to allow us the open and safe space within which to care for their needs.

KEY POINT

Boundary crossings are transient, non-exploitative deviations from our typical practice of medicine—single-event shifts in our typical practice, frequently in response to a specific clinical or emotional need on the part of our patients.

What Happens If Those Boundaries Are Crossed or Violated?

Boundary crossings are transient, nonexploitative deviations from our typical practice of medicine—single-event shifts in our typical practice, frequently in response to a specific clinical or emotional need on the part of our patients. While not fundamentally harmful to our patients, they require thoughtfulness and consideration on the part of physicians to ensure that they do not become repetitive or worsen over time (Gutheil & Gabbard, 1993).

KEY POINT

Boundary violations are deviations from our typical practice that harm our patients; they frequently occur more than once, can worsen over time, and are exploitative in nature.

Boundary violations are deviations from our typical practice that harm our patients; they frequently occur more than once, can worsen over time, and are exploitative in nature. Boundary violations can range from physicians seeking increasing degrees of emotional gratification from their patients to physicians seeking physical or sexual gratification from their patients. Boundary violations do not tend to occur abruptly but as part of a slippery slope of erosion of appropriate professional boundaries over time. These shifts may be slow and result in relationships that markedly differ from routine practice. The case vignette shows one such example, resulting in an emotionally unsafe and emotionally exploitative relationship where good medical care cannot be practiced (Gutheil & Gabbard, 1993).

What Kinds of Situations Lead to Difficulties Holding Boundaries?

Boundary crossings and boundary violations frequently involve issues involving touching patients, gift giving, and personal disclosure from physicians to patients.

Physical touch is inseparable from the work of a physician, due to our use of the physical exam. Outside of this context, great care and careful consideration should be utilized in maintaining good boundaries. Take, for example, a frightened patient being wheeled into surgery reaching out her hand to her physician. Instinctively, we recognize this gesture as an acceptable part of compassionate care. The context helps—the public place, the cultural norms for holding a hand, and the initiation by the patient. In this context, it facilitates, rather than hinders, the physician–patient relationship. Imagine a different scenario in which a male patient who had previously made sexual remarks to a female physician reaches out his hand to hold hers. Here, the boundaries are being tested, and accepting this gesture would *undermine*, rather than enhance, the integrity of the physician–patient relationship. Here, the physician would be wise to reiterate the boundaries of the relationship.

Accepting gifts from patients also deviates from routine clinical practice and is highly contextual. Monetary value may be one key factor, and many institutions hold a cap on monetary value for gifts. However, that is only one component of that decision. Gift giving may signal a need the patient has for the relationship. Patients may give a gift because they feel unworthy of positive regard or feel they won't receive good care without pleasing the physician. They may do it to establish themselves as a "special patient" or because they expect a higher degree of access to their physician. These need to be recognized and, at times, discussed as part of maintaining good boundaries. Some gifts complicate the physician–patient relationship later. Routine practice, such as ordering urine drug screens, declining an inappropriately early refill, or charging a patient a "no-show" fee for failing to cancel adequately, may become complicated or feel more uncomfortable after receiving a gift.

It may feel uncomfortable to decline a gift politely. However, if done properly, it can be conveyed as a sign of caring for the patient. The physician may take the opportunity to emphasize that the relationship is of utmost value to them, and they are concerned that the gift may undermine that. Alternatives include requesting more time to consider whether accepting the gift is in the patient's best interest or sharing the gift with the team, as with gifts of food or flowers.

How Do We Manage Uncertainty With These Boundaries?

Medical training sometimes emphasizes individual knowledge and self-reliance. For these situations, attempting to navigate boundaries alone can be inadvisable. It is important to develop a network of peers and experienced clinicians. Outside observers can frequently offer perspectives that are unavailable from *within* a relationship in which boundaries are being tested, eroded, or broken. One rule of thumb regarding boundary violations may be to reflect on whether we are comfortable seeking consultation. Situations leading to boundary violations are often uncomfortable to seek consultation for. In contrast, those that may include a boundary crossing allow for the physician to openly seek guidance and discuss their actions.

SUMMARY

Boundaries set the expectations for different types of relationships. Professional boundaries are necessary for the safety and predictability of the work of physicians with patients. Transient boundary crossings may happen from time to time, but physicians need to be aware of situations that cross into boundary violations. Consultation with peers or more experienced clinicians may be helpful for recognizing and navigating these situations.

KEY POINT

Boundaries set the expectations for different types of relationships. Professional boundaries are necessary for the safety and predictability of the work of physicians with patients.

RESOURCES

1. Professional Boundaries in Psychiatric Practice. Glen O. Gabbard, Holly Crisp-Han, and Gabrielle S. Hobday. *The Oxford Handbook of Psychiatric Ethics. Edited by John Z. Sadler, K. W. M. Fulford, and Werdie (C.W.) van Staden*

REFERENCES

American Medical Association. (2016). *AMA principles of medical ethics*. Retrieved January 14, 2022, from https://www.ama-assn.org/delivering-care/ama-principles-medical-ethics

American Medical Association. (2021). *Patient-physician relationships*. Ethics of Patient-Physician Relationships. Retrieved January 14, 2022, from https://www.ama-assn.org/delivering-care/ethics/patient-physician-relationships

Gutheil, T. G., & Gabbard, G. O. (1993). The concept of boundaries in clinical practice: Theoretical and risk-management dimensions. *The American Journal of Psychiatry*, *150*(2), 188–196. https://doi.org/10.1176/ajp.150.2.188

Gutheil, T. G., & Gabbard, G. O. (1998). Misuses and misunderstandings of boundary theory in clinical and regulatory settings. *The American Journal of Psychiatry*, *155*(3), 409–414. https://doi.org/10.1176/ajp.155.3.409

CHAPTER 42

Diversity and Cultural Psychiatry[1]

Olusola Oluwanuga, M.B.B.S.; Edore Onigu-Otite, M.D.; and Harolyn Belcher, M.D., M.H.S.

> *"Our ability to reach unity in diversity will be the beauty and the test of our civilization."*
>
> — Mahatma Gandhi

OBJECTIVES

After reading this chapter, learners will be able to:

- define culture, diversity, race, and racism
- discuss the tenets and scope of diversity and cultural psychiatry
- recognize the importance of an individual's culture in the manifestation of their psychopathology
- recognize how diversity impacts mental health assessment and treatment.
- identify several cultural concepts of distress (culture-bound syndromes)

CASE VIGNETTE

Baba is a young adult male who grew up in a foreign country. His parents were affluent in their country, and Baba was considered to be exposed to Western cultures. His dream was to come to America. His parents sent him to the United States to pursue a college education. Baba, an older teen on arrival, found it shocking that the fantasy of America from his country was vastly different from what he saw. He had trouble connecting and making friends. To him, people never said what they thought, and you could never tell what they

---

1 Readers may also see "Social Determinants of Behaviorial Health" (Chapter 37) for related material.

thought because they always kept a straight face. Baba felt his mostly Caucasian and Hispanic teachers did not like him. He felt his African American teachers did not understand him either. He stopped physically going to classes but kept up with the online courses, which his college offered. He could not tell his parents about his struggles because he was the first son, they were pouring a lot of family finances into his education, and he had to succeed. He felt very guilty about this.

Baba had his final exams coming up. So far, academically, he had performed poorly and was on the verge of being asked to withdraw if he did not pass his final exam. Baba stayed up studying, drinking coffee, Monster, and other caffeinated beverages around the clock. He did this for over a month. His sleep schedule was irregular. He slept little and did not leave his room. As was required, on the day of the exam, he went physically to the exam. He sat down to take the exam, and his mind went blank. He starred at the exam questions, unable to comprehend what they said. He thought someone had placed a hex on him from home. They called it *juju* in his native village. He became agitated, began muttering under his breath in the quiet exam hall, then started screaming and bolted for the door. The campus police were called, and Baba was taken to the ER.

In the ER, he was guarded with the doctors. Surprisingly, he seemed more open with the young intern who had a non-American accent. Baba explained the pressures he was under and that he thought he might be depressed. He was afraid he might harm himself he failed the final exam. In reality, he had not taken the exam and knew he was in no state of mind to take the exam. He was calm, listened to the advice of the intern along with the group of doctors. They all recommended he begin treatment for depression. He was treated with an antidepressant, which also improved his sleep at night. His doctors found a therapist with a similar cultural background to his. Baba found it easy to speak with her and looked forward to their sessions. Baba complied with treatment, began to feel better, and, after a while, returned to school. His college professors were happy he was okay and welcomed him back openly. Several of his classmates asked him out. He began to hang out with them and enjoy his college life. He adjusted well, graduated college successfully, and is now raising his family. He was happy he had come to America.

COMMENTARY

Baba had trouble adjusting to the multiple changes, including a new culture, upon coming to the United States. He had less difficulty trusting people of his culture. On the contrary, it was more difficult for him to trust people outside of his culture. He had high expectations from his family and felt the pressure to succeed in his studies, which he knew was expensive to his family. Although he put effort into preparing for his exams, this was a stressor for him. He consumed a lot of caffeine around the clock. Caffeine is a stimulant, and although less common, consumed in large amounts, it can cause psychotic symptoms, including paranoia. Baba was socially withdrawn, experienced anxious and sad mood, and possibly some psychotic symptoms. On the day of the exam, he was likely manifesting symptoms of brain fag. Brain fag is a culture-bound syndrome described in West Africa. Fortunately, in the ER, Baba had health care workers similar to him (i.e., had a non-American accent or similar cultural background), and he was able to be more open, connect, begin, and engage successfully in treatment with a positive outcome.

DEFINITIONS AND KEY CONCEPTS

KEY POINT

Culture refers to shared beliefs, customs, foods, rituals, behaviors, arts, ways of life, and child-rearing practices passed consciously and unconsciously across generations of people and populations. These include, but are not limited to, characteristics such as national origin, language, race, color, disability, ethnicity, gender, age, religion, sexual orientation, gender identity, socioeconomic status, veteran status, and family structures.

KEY POINT

Ethnicity is the grouping of people according to shared attributes including ancestry, history, traditions, and cultural factors such as customs, language, dressing, foods, music, and dance.

Culture refers to shared beliefs, customs, foods, rituals, behaviors, arts, way of life, and child-rearing practices passed consciously and unconsciously across generations of people and populations. These include, but are not limited to, characteristics such as national origin, language, race, color, disability, ethnicity, gender, age, religion, sexual orientation, gender identity, socioeconomic status, veteran status, and family structures. The concept also encompasses differences among people concerning where they are from, where they have lived, and their differences of thought and life experiences (United States Office of Personnel Management, 2011). *Ethnicity is closely associated with culture.* Ethnicity is the grouping of people according to shared attributes, including ancestry, history, traditions, and cultural factors, such as customs, language, dressing, foods, music, and dance. *Diversity* is defined as a collection of individual attributes that help agencies pursue organizational objectives efficiently and effectively (United States Office of Personnel Management, 2011). *Inclusion* is defined as a culture that connects each employee to the organization; encourages collaboration, flexibility, and fairness; and leverages diversity throughout the organization so that all individuals are able to participate and contribute to their full (United States Office of Personnel Management, 2011). It includes the practice or quality of possessing and involving people from various social and ethnic backgrounds, genders, and sexual orientations, which, in turn, helps agencies meet their objectives when conducting their business with clients. Cultural Concepts of Distress (Culture-Bound Syndromes) are a group of syndromes that have been described or tend to manifest in certain cultures or regions of the world. They can be described as a pattern of expression of mental health symptoms or abnormal functioning or behavior that is unique to a specific ethnic or cultural population and does not conform to standard classifications of psychiatric disorders.

Unconscious biases are social stereotypes about certain groups of people that individuals form outside of their own conscious awareness. *Race* is a sociopolitical construct based on external physical characteristics with little to no biological basis. Historically, the origins of the Caucasian, Ethiopian, Mongolian, Red, and Brown "races" date back to supremacy beliefs and the faux science of craniometry in the 1700s (Donovan, 2019). *Racism* is a system that unfairly disadvantages some and advantages others based on physical features. Racism oppresses populations and limits the acknowledgment of the contributions of the oppressed group(s), wasting otherwise valuable human resources (Jones, 2000). *Systemic racism* is a system of structuring opportunity and assigning value based on the social interpretation of how one looks (which is what we call race) that unfairly disadvantages some individuals and communities and unfairly advantages other individuals and communities (Jones, 2000). *Institutionalized racism* is a system that creates differential access to resources, goods, services, and opportunities based on race (Jones, 2000). Institutionalized racism consists of a constellation of structures, policies, practices, norms, and values that collectively result in differential access to goods, services, opportunities offered to society by race. Institutional racism does not require an identifiable perpetrator because it has been institutionalized in laws, customs, and norms (National Academies of Sciences, 2019). Differential access may take the form of loans for housing, quality education, health treatments, or healthy food availability. *Interpersonal racism* is personally mediated racism, which occurs through differential assumptions about others' abilities, motives, and intents by race and differential access or treatment based on these assumptions (National Academies of Sciences, 2019). Examples may include assumptions around health literacy, hasty explanations of medical procedures to select groups of people, failure to attend to or extended time before being attended to within health care systems, and other assumptions. *Internalized racism* occurs when the marginalized group member accepts negative racist stereotypes about their abilities and values (National Academies of Sciences, 2019). Diversity appreciates the differences within and between racial identities. Many individuals are now multiracial, with varied ancestry, histories, cultural affiliations, and exposures. *Racial diversity* is the acknowledgement and celebration of the fascinating differences between racial groups.

KEY POINT

Race is a sociopolitical construct based on external physical characteristics with little to no biological basis. Racism is a system that unfairly disadvantages some and advantages others based on physical features. Diversity appreciates the differences within and between racial identities. Many individuals are now multi-racial, with various combinations of ancestry, histories, cultural affiliations, and exposures. *Racial diversity* is the acknowledgement and celebration of the fascinating differences between racial groups.

INTRODUCTION

Culture and context are often the lenses through which individuals view, identify, and manifest their mental health symptoms. Cultural psychiatry (also known as cross-cultural psychiatry, transcultural psychiatry, or ethnopsychiatry) refers to that aspect of psychiatry that recognizes social and cultural factors in understanding and expressing disease or illness. This branch of psychiatry focuses on psychopathology's social and cultural determinants and the challenges of identifying, treating, and otherwise addressing mental health illness within culturally diverse individuals, subcultures, and groups. On the other hand, culture and context are also lenses through which providers view, identify, and treat mental health symptoms in their patients. Awareness and attention to diversity and contextual clues are effective strategies for reaching optimal patient treatment outcomes.

MEMORY TIP

Both race and ethnicity describe aspects of social group identification. While race refers to a person's external physical characteristics, such as skin tone, hair color, or eye color, ethnicity refers to ancestry and cultural factors. As such, different races may exist within the same ethnic group and different ethnic groups within the same race.

Diversity and inclusion refers to the practice of including and involving people from different social backgrounds, including ethnic, religious,

CLINICAL TIP

Culture and context are often the lenses through which individuals view, identify, and manifest their mental health symptoms. Diversity means understanding and recognizing the uniqueness of each individual, while accepting their differences as is. Health care professionals' appreciation of culture and diversity promotes the knowledge of their clients with impact on health care delivery services and can affect the patient–doctor interaction, engagement, formation, sustenance of the desired therapeutic alliance, and, ultimately, patient outcomes.

KEY POINT

Diversity and inclusion refer to the practice of including and involving people from different social backgrounds, including ethnic, religious, gender, and sexual orientation, in various aspects of the social structure of a community.

gender, and sexual orientation, in various aspects of the social structure of a community. Diversity has become more topical and has even greater relevance with increased migration and globalization. To say we live in a global village is no longer just a cliché; instead, it has become a truism and a living experience for many. Today, personal choices, community structure, and government policies all have, or should have, consideration for diversity to various extents under various circumstances.

Diversity means understanding and recognizing the uniqueness of each individual while accepting their differences as is. Health care professionals' appreciation of diversity promotes the knowledge of their clients with impact on health care delivery services and outcomes. Valuing diversity has even greater relevance for mental health. Matters of diversity are relevant in symptom expression, the understanding and attribution of symptoms, stigma, health-seeking behavior, access to health care, and financing options. All these need to be put into consideration. Sensitivity to diversity can affect the patient–doctor interaction, engagement, formation, and sustenance of the desired therapeutic alliance. Although the most typical considerations for diversity are racial, the shades of diversity have a place in our approach to the social and psychological makeup of patients and provider interactions with them. It is helpful to keep in mind that neither race nor ethnicity is expressed in the human genome. Different responses to diversity are learned and should not be considered inherent, as they are malleable and amenable to change, usually based on new exposure or newly learned behavior.

With increasing diversity in the United States, cultural psychiatry is gaining increasing relevance. *DSM-5* provides an outline of cultural formulation (within the section on emerging measures and models), an upgrade of the one in *DSM-4* (APA, 2013). In addition, there is a glossary of cultural concepts of distress, which seeks to give brief notes about some of the previously termed culture-bound syndromes.

Cultural psychiatry is relevant in clinical practice to help clinicians and researchers diagnose and manage individuals outside the majority culture. Specifically, *DSM-5* calls for a thorough examination of five content areas:

- the cultural identity of the individual
- cultural conceptualizations of distress
- psychosocial stressors and cultural features of vulnerability and resiliency
- cultural characteristics of the relationship between clinician and client
- overall cultural assessment

The *DSM-5* provides the Cultural Formulation Interview (CFI) to make a cultural assessment of the client. The cultural formulations consists of 16 questions that clinicians may use, regardless of their own culture or that of the client.

In the CFI, culture refers explicitly to the following:

- the values, orientations, knowledge, and practices that individuals derive from membership in diverse social groups (e.g., ethnic groups, faith communities, occupational groups, or veteran groups)
- aspects of an individual's background, developmental experiences, and current social contexts may affect their perspectives, such as geographical origin, migration, language, religion, sexual orientation, or race/ethnicity.
- the influence of family, friends, and other community members (the individual's social network) on the individual's illness experience.

The fourth edition of the *Diagnostic and Statistical Manual of Mental Disorders (DSM-4)* used the term "culture-bound syndromes" to describe a group of syndromes that have been described or tend to manifest in certain cultures or regions of the world. This terminology has been changed in the fifth edition of the *DSM* (*DSM-5*), including "cultural concepts of distress."

The updated approach portrays these conditions more accurately for what they are: a group of mental disorders that can manifest in anybody but are characterized by cultural influences on their expression and the individual's experience, That is, although these may be regarded, for example, as anxiety disorders or brief psychotic disorders, they are well recognized in the patients' culture, making them relatable to patients and their families, and thus increasing their relevance to clinical practice.

The recognition of transcultural psychiatry usually results in a more holistic assessment and understanding of patients, especially of minority ethnic or migrant populations, which could result in better outcomes (Tseng, 2006). Each health care worker should have a good understanding of diversity and an appreciation of their blind spots and work progressively toward understanding and appreciating subculture factors and ways to work within this awareness to provide care to culturally diverse clients (Fogel et al., 2020).

CLINICAL TIP

Understanding a person's mental health symptoms and presentations involves an understanding of the culture they identify with and were raised in. This includes a thorough examination of their cultural conceptualizations of distress, psychosocial stressors and cultural features of vulnerability and resiliency, cultural characteristics of the relationship between clinician and client, and overall cultural assessment.

QUICK POINT

The Cultural Formulation Interview (CFI) is used to make a cultural assessment of the client. In the CFI, culture refers explicitly to the following:

- the values, orientations, knowledge, and practices that individuals derive from membership in diverse social groups (e.g., ethnic groups, faith communities, occupational groups, or veteran groups)
- aspects of an individual's background, developmental experiences, and current social contexts may affect their perspectives, such as geographical origin, migration, language, religion, sexual orientation, or race/ethnicity.

- the influence of family, friends, and other community members (the individual's social network) on the individual's illness experience.

QUICK POINT

There are remarkable disparities in access to mental health care in the United States. People of Asian, Latino, and Black ethnicity or descent are 51%, 25%, and 21% less likely to use mental health services, respectively, when compared to White people (Smedley, 2003). The scarcity of mental health providers from historically marginalized populations and culturally congruent mental health practices contributes to mental health disparities.

CLINICAL TIP

Cultural presentation and understanding of mental health symptoms vary across groups. Culture influences how people feel, describe, and report their mental health symptoms. Culture can affect whether a person recognizes their symptoms as a symptom of a mental health condition, their emotional or psychological response to it, how they describe their symptoms, and the degree of the psychological distress it causes.

How Do Culture and Race Affect Mental Health Service Delivery?

There are remarkable disparities in access to mental health care in the United States. People of Asian, Latino, and Black ethnicity or descent are 51%, 25%, and 21% less likely to use mental health services, respectively, when compared to White people (Smedley, 2003). Several factors contribute to these disparities, including stigma, discrimination, lack of coverage, and a shortage of providers, especially those from diverse backgrounds. For example, Black, Latino, and Asian psychologists—combined—account for approximately 13% of the total number of psychologists in the United States (APA, 2016). Only 2% of psychiatrists are Black (McGuire & Miranda, 2008; Milloy, 2020; Turner, 2014). The scarcity of mental health providers from historically marginalized populations and culturally congruent mental health practices contributes to mental health disparities among people of color. Systemic racism has also contributed to decreased access to mental health services for "minoritized" populations. On January 18, 2020, the American Psychiatric Association published an "Apology to Black, Indigenous and People of Color for Its Support of Structural Racism in Psychiatry." The apology acknowledged "our [the American Psychiatric Association's] contributions to the structural racism in our nation and pledged to enact corresponding anti-racist practices. We commit to working together with members and patients in order to achieve the social equality, health equity, and fairness that all human beings deserve. We hope this apology will be a turning point as we strive to make the future of psychiatry more equitable for all" (APA, 2020).

How Do Culture and Race Affect Mental Health Symptom Reporting, Diagnosis, and Treatment?

Cultural presentation and understanding of mental health symptoms vary across groups. Culture influences how people feel, describe, and report their mental health symptoms. Culture can affect whether a person recognizes their symptoms as a symptom of a mental health condition, their emotional or psychological response to it, how they describe their symptoms, and the degree of the psychological distress it causes. Cultural factors also determine the individual's family and community response to their mental health, influencing engagement in treatment and treatment outcomes. Due to stigma, individuals are sometimes left to seek mental health treatment and support alone. In general, the rates of mental illness can be compared across races. However, the impact of mental health symptoms varies across races.

AFRICAN AMERICANS AND MENTAL HEALTH

The African American or Black population is the second-largest racial group in the United States. In combination with other racial populations, the African American population has grown 88.7% since 2010, making up 14.2% (approximately 46.9 million people) of the U.S. population (Jones et al., 2021). The African American population in the United States is a heterogeneous and diverse population consisting of approximately 91% American Descendants of Slavery (ADOS) and 9% Black immigrants. In 2016, the five leading birth countries of Black immigrants in the United States were Jamaica (17.0%), Haiti (15.8%), Nigeria (7.2%), Ethiopia (5.7%), and Trinidad and Tobago (4.5%; Anderson & Lopez, 2018). The history of slavery, institutional and systemic racism, and unethical treatment by the U.S. health care and public health systems has led to health disparities and mistrust of medical institutions among African Americans. Understanding and acknowledging the racial trauma and impact of systems in the United States and countries of origin for the African American population will promote a therapeutic relationship to address mental health concerns. Addressing unconscious bias is a fundamental ongoing process for the mental health provider.

QUICK POINT

The African American or Black population is the second-largest racial group in the United States, making up 14.2% (approximately 46.9 million people) of the U.S. population (Jones et al., 2021). The African American population in the United States is a heterogeneous and diverse population consisting approximately 91% American Descendants of Slavery (ADOS) and 9% Black immigrants. In 2016, the five leading birth countries of Black immigrants in the United States were Jamaica (17.0%), Haiti (15.8%), Nigeria (7.2%), Ethiopia (5.7%), and Trinidad and Tobago (4.5%; Anderson & Lopez, 2018).

Although rates of depression are lower in African-American and Hispanic people than in White people, depression in African American and Hispanic people is likely to be more persistent. African American adults are 20% more likely to report serious psychological distress than White adults. Studies of national representative datasets found the odds of anxiety disorders are 24% lower, mood disorders are 45% lower, and substance use disorders are 32% lower for African American population compared to their European American peers. However, African Americans often experience a disproportionately high burden of disability from mental disorders compared to European Americans (Alvarez et al., 2019). Concerning the place of birth (nativity), African Americans whose parents and survey respondents were not born in the United States had the lowest odds of lifetime mood or substance use disorders. African Americans who were born in the United States and had two parents who immigrated had the highest odds of mood disorder (odds ratio [OR]: 4.16, 95% confidence interval [CI]: 1.27, 13.6) and substance use disorder (OR: 46.53, 95% CI: 9.66, 224.03; Alvarez et al., 2019).

Physician–patient communication differs for African Americans and non-Hispanic Whites. One study found that physicians were 23% more verbally dominant and engaged in 33% less patient-centered communication with African American patients than with White patients (Johnson, 2004).

Studies show that when treating African American patients, clinicians tend to overemphasize the presence and relevance of psychotic symptoms and overlook the existence and relevance of mood symptoms, including depression, compared to acknowledging and placing the same symptoms in patients from other racial or ethnic backgrounds. Perhaps related to this, African Americans are more frequently diagnosed with psychotic disorders and less frequently diagnosed with mood disorders when compared to non-Hispanic Whites with the same symptoms. Differences in how African Americans express symptoms of emotional distress may contribute to misdiagnosis (Bell, 2015). African Americans with mental health conditions, especially schizophrenia, bipolar disorders, and other psychoses, are more likely to be incarcerated than people of other races (U.S. Department of Justice, 2016; Hawthorne, 2012). African American youth are disproportionately overrepresented in the juvenile justice system. Black youth with emotional or behavioral problems conditions are more likely to be directed to the juvenile justice system than to specialty care institutions compared to non-Hispanic White youth (U.S. Department of Justice, 2016).

AMERICAN INDIANS AND ALASKA NATIVE POPULATIONS AND MENTAL HEALTH

QUICK POINT

The American Indian and Alaska Native (AIAN) population includes 574 sovereign tribal nations (National Congress of American Indians, 2020). They are a diverse people with different cultures, languages, and spiritual practices that date back thousands of years before the first Europeans came to America (National Congress of American Indians, 2020). AIAN adults report the highest rates of mental illnesses of any single race identifying group.

In combination with other races, the American Indian and Alaska Native (AIAN) population increased by 160% from 2010 to 2020 (Jones et al., 2021). The 2020 census estimates there are 9.7 million AIAN people alone or in combination in the United States (Jones et al., 2021). There are 574 sovereign tribal nations (National Congress of American Indians, 2020). AIAN populations are diverse people with different cultures, languages, and spiritual practices that date back thousands of years before the first Europeans came to America (National Congress of American Indians, 2020). The U.S. and AIAN history is complex and includes genocide of AIAN peoples, wars, displacement, trauma, oppression, and racism. The consequences of this traumatic history exist today in the mental health and substance abuse disparities of AIAN populations, missing persons, sexual abuse, and poverty.

American Indian and Alaska Native adults report the highest rates of mental illnesses of any single race identifying group. Severe mental illness during the past year was reported in 6.7% of AIAN people compared to 5.2% of overall adults in the United States (Substance Abuse and Mental Health Services Administration, 2020b). Past-year substance use disorder was reported in 10.1% of AIAN compared to the rate of 7.4% among people in the United States age 12 and older (Substance Abuse and Mental Health Services Administration, 2020b). Death rates for suicide are 40% higher for

AIAN females and 20% higher for AIAN males than their European American counterparts (Murphy et al., 2021). Suicide is the second leading cause of death for AIAN people age 10 to 34 (National Center for Injury Prevention and Control, 2021b). AIAN adolescent death rates are 5.2 times higher for females and 2.7 times higher for males than for non-Hispanic European Americans (National Center for Injury Prevention and Control, 2021b). Despite high rates of serious psychological distress and mental illness, AIAN people are 30% less likely to receive mental health services in the past year or prescription medications to treat mental illness (Substance Abuse and Mental Health Services Administration, 2020c, 2020d).

ASIAN-AMERICAN AND PACIFIC ISLANDERS AND MENTAL HEALTH

The Asian American and Pacific Islander (AAPI) population in the United States consists of people from many countries, ethnicities, and cultural identities. There are approximately 22.9 million AAPI living in the United States (U.S. Census Bureau, 2019). The Chinese (except Taiwanese) population was the largest Asian group, followed by Asian Indians (4.6 million), Filipino (4.2 million), Vietnamese (2.2 million), Korean (1.9 million), and Japanese populations (1.5 million; U.S. Census Bureau, 2021).

Many AAPI people have faced trauma due to wars (e.g., survivors of Laos, Cambodia, and Vietnam wars), poverty in their native country and the United States, racism (e.g., historical trauma from colonization of the Hawaiian Islands), and internment (Japanese Americans) in the United States. AAPI populations may be challenged by the privileges of the "model minority" myth that stereotypes AAPI as intelligent by virtue of their race, allowing the complex systems of racism in the United States to persist at the expense of other racial groups (Mental Health America, 2019). Other challenges that AAPI face in the United States include being the "perpetual foreigner" and discrimination due to membership in religious minority groups, such as Buddhism, Confucianism, Hinduism, Islam, Sikhism, or Taoism.

QUICK POINT

The Asian American and Pacific Islander (AAPI) population in the United States consists of people from many countries, ethnicities, and cultural identities. There are approximately 22.9 million AAPI living in the United States (U.S. Census Bureau, 2019). The Chinese (except Taiwanese) population was the largest Asian group, followed by Asian Indians (4.6 million), Filipino (4.2 million), Vietnamese (2.2 million), Korean (1.9 million), and Japanese populations (1.5 million; U.S. Census Bureau, 2021).

AAPI people have the lowest lifetime prevalence of mental disorders (23.5%; Alvarez et al., 2019). According to the 2019 Substance Abuse and Mental Health Services National Survey on Drug Use and Health, 11.7% of AAPI people endorsed having a mental illness or substance in the past year (Substance Abuse and Mental Health Services Administration, 2020a). Opiate use declined significantly from 2018 to 2019 (Substance Abuse and Mental Health Services Administration, 2020a). Marijuana and cocaine use disorder has significantly increased since 2017 for the Asian/NHOPI population age 26 and older (Substance Abuse and Mental Health Services Administration, 2020a). Since 2009, the number of Asian/NHOPI adults age 26–49 who made a suicide plan has significantly increased (Substance Abuse and Mental Health Services Administration, 2020a). Serious mental illness (SMI) among AAPI people has increased since 2014 (Substance Abuse and Mental Health Services Administration, 2020a). Historically, due to lack of insurance, language barriers, stigma, and cultural beliefs, the AAPI population is one of the racial groups least likely to seek mental health services (Mental Health America, 2019; Substance Abuse and Mental Health Services Administration, 2020a).

Nativity differences existed for the odds of mood disorders and substance use disorders in the AAPI population. Respondents to a national survey on mental health and drug use who were born in the United States but neither parent was born in the United States had the highest odds of mood disorders (OR: 3.17, 95% CI: 1.69, 5.95) compared to the AAPI population in which both parents and respondents were born outside of the United States (Alvarez et al., 2019). Respondents who were born in the United States and had one parent who was born in the United States had the highest odds, 11.81% (95% CI: 4.12,33.88), of substance use disorder compared to AAPI respondents with both parents who were born outside of the United States (Alvarez et al., 2019).

EUROPEAN-AMERICANS AND MENTAL HEALTH

QUICK POINT

European-Americans, often referred to as White, constitute the largest racial population (61.6% White alone U.S. census category) in the 2020 US census report (Jones et al., 2021). European-Americans are a diverse population with distinct cultures based on the geographic region in the United States, immigration and nativity status, religious and political affiliation, education and socioeconomic status, and country of family origin.

European-Americans, often referred to as White, constitute the largest racial population (61.6% White alone U.S. census category) in the 2020 U.S. census report (Jones et al., 2021). The White alone racial category decreased 8.6%, while White, in combination with other races, increased 316% over the last decade (Jones et al., 2021). European-Americans are a diverse population with distinct cultures based on the geographic region in the United States, immigration and nativity status, religious and political affiliation, education and socioeconomic status, and country of family origin.

In a nationally representative sample of over 20,000 participants, European Americans had the highest lifetime prevalence (45.6%; Alvarez et al., 2019) of any *Diagnostic and Statistical Manual of Mental Disorders*, fourth edition (APA, 2000) disorder based on the Composite International Diagnostic Interview (*DSM-4*/CIDI) (Kessler & Ustun, 2004). Across any anxiety disorder (26.1%), mood disorder (22.6%), substance use disorder (18.8%), and any disorder (45.6%), European Americans, compared to African

American, Asian, and Latino peers, had the highest lifetime prevalence (Alvarez et al., 2019). Past year substance use disorder among people age 12 and older was higher among non-Hispanic European Americans (7.8%) than the national average of substance use disorders (Substance Abuse and Mental Health Services Administration, 2020b). There was no change in overall reports of past-year substance abuse disorders from 2015 to 2019 for non-Hispanic European Americans (Substance Abuse and Mental Health Services Administration, 2020b). Compared to the national average, the history of past year serious mental illness among adults was higher among non-Hispanic European Americans (5.7%) and lower among other racial groups, including African Americans and AAPI (Substance Abuse and Mental Health Services Administration, 2020b). Odds of mood disorder (OR: 3.00, 95% CI: 1.53, 5.90) and substance use disorder (OR: 3.13, 95% CI: 1.22, 8.06) were highest for European Americans who had one parent and respondent to a national survey on substance use disorder and mental illness who were born in the United States compared to European American respondents who had both parents and were themselves born in another country (Alvarez et al., 2019).

The high rates of mental health disorder among European Americans are essential to recognize, as bias in the United States favoring European Americans may mask early identification of serious mental illness, leading to delays in treatment. Although European Americans have the highest rate of prescription drug use and mental health service use, White adults were the most likely to cite the cost of insurance and belief that services would not help as reasons for not using mental health services compared to other racial groups (Substance Abuse and Mental Health Services Administration, 2015). Understanding the various cultural beliefs and practices among European Americans from different socioeconomic standings, geographic regions, religious backgrounds, and countries of origin is essential for building trust in accepting mental health services.

QUICK POINT

According to the U.S. Census, the Hispanic or Latino population in the United States, which includes people of any race, was 62.1 million in 2020, representing a 23% increase from the 2010 census (Jones et al., 2021). The term Hispanic refers to those whose ancestry comes from a country where Spanish is spoken. In contrast, Latino refers to the country of origin in Latin America (i.e., the Caribbean, Central America, and South America; Fortuna, 2012).

HISPANIC-AMERICANS AND MENTAL HEALTH

Hispanic Americans—or Latinos, Latinas, or Latinx—are a diverse and fast-growing population in the United States. According to the U.S. Census, the Hispanic or Latino population in the United States, which includes people of any race, was 62.1 million in 2020, representing a 23% increase from the 2010 census (Jones et al., 2021). The term *Hispanic* refers to those whose ancestry comes from a country where Spanish is spoken. In contrast, Latino refers to the country of origin in Latin America (i.e., the Caribbean, Central America, and South America; Fortuna, 2012). Not all Latinos speak Spanish.

Latinos are multiracial and multicultural, including indigenous people who speak their native tongues. Mexican Americans (59.9%) represent the largest Hispanic population by country of origin (Statista Research Department, 2020). Historically, there are populations of Mexican-Americans whose descendants "lived in the United States" before the establishment of the modern United States border following the U.S.–Mexican War (1846–1848). Puerto Ricans (9.3%), Cubans (3.9%), Salvadorans (3.7%), and Dominicans (3.4%) are the next most common origins for the U.S. Hispanic population (Statista Research Department, 2020).

Cultural differences, compared to European Americans, include the importance of the extended family as a protective factor (Fortuna, 2012). Respect for parental authority may persist throughout the life span (Fortuna, 2012). Spirituality, collaborative care, and emotional connection may be fundamental components of the mental health therapeutic practice (Fortuna, 2012).

Recent Hispanic immigrants are at risk for traumatic exposures before, during, and after migration. In 2019, suicide was the second leading cause of death for Hispanic youth and young adults age 15 to 34 (National Center for Injury Prevention and Control, 2021a). Approximately 12.2% of Hispanic adults have experienced severe psychological distress during the past year (Office of Minority Health, 2021). Hispanic adults living below the poverty level are over twice as likely to experience severe psychological distress (Office of Minority Health, 2021). Serious mental illness during the past year was reported by 4.9% of the Hispanic adult population (Substance Abuse and Mental Health Services Administration, 2020b). The rate of serious mental illness for Hispanics was similar to the U.S. adult rate of serious mental illness.

The lifetime prevalence of any *DSM-4*/CIDI was lower for Hispanic-American adults (38.3%) than for European American adults (45.6%; Alvarez et al., 2019). The onset of mood disorders occurred later for Hispanic Americans than for Asian, Black, and European Americans (Alvarez et al., 2019). In a national representative sample examining the association between nativity and odds of *DSM-4*/CIDI disorders, the odds of substance use disorders (OR: 6.97, 95% CI 3.01,16.13) were highest for Hispanic respondents who were born in the United States and had one parent born in the United States (Alvarez et al., 2019). Notably, there were no differences in the lifetime odds of having any mood disorder based on nativity (Alvarez et al., 2019).

IMMIGRANTS AND MENTAL HEALTH

The lack of cultural competence of health care providers likely contributes to underdiagnosis and misdiagnosis of mental illness in immigrants. With the development of various cultures and subcultures within society, cultural psychiatry has a broader scope and potential impact than we may think. Understanding an individual's ecosystem or the conditions within which they exist can go a long way in understanding their perspectives of their symptoms and the treatment approaches they may consider. Think of a young man who has developed extremist political ideas and lives within a subculture fed by conspiracy theories or a homeless young female adult who makes a living selling drugs on the streets and whose only contacts are people who use drugs. Although either of these two examples could belong to the ethnic majority, they could still have transcultural issues affecting their mental health and clinical interactions. Another reason for the relevance of these cultural concepts of distress is that many occur amongst the fastest-growing populations in the world. It is important to note that, in the United States, parental and foreign-born child nativity is associated with a lower risk of mental health disorders compared to families in which one or both parents are U.S.- or foreign-born parents with U.S.-born children (Alvarez et al., 2019). There is increasing world trade and migration. With increasing globalization, the possibility of coming across culturally diverse individuals in practice only increases. As stated by Lokko et al. in a perspective contribution in *Academic Psychiatry*, "... the U.S. may have much to learn about how other cultures understand and treat mental illness locally" (Lokko et al., 2016). Psychiatrists participating in global programs that adopt cultural humility and seek to expand their "critical consciousness" can serve as an important link between countries and cultures. They can contribute to the diversification of the mental health workforce, both domestically and abroad (Lokko et al., 2016).

CLINICAL TIP

The lack of cultural competence of health care providers likely contributes to underdiagnosis and misdiagnosis of mental illness in immigrants. With the development of various cultures and subcultures within society, cultural Psychiatry has a broader scope and potential impact than we may think. Understanding an individual's ecosystem or the conditions within which they exist can go a long way in understanding their perspectives of their symptoms and the treatment approaches they may consider.

CLINICAL MANIFESTATIONS OF CULTURAL CONCEPTS OF DISTRESS (CULTURE-BOUND SYNDROMES)

Many cultures around the world believe in causes of mental illness and distress that are not explained by the biopsychosocial model psychiatrists use. This cultural disconnect may be a barrier to accessing mental health care for immigrants and minority populations. The ability to relate these conditions to the culture and recognize them as distressing within the cultural context can help patients and their relatives feel that the condition is understood by the clinician trained in Western medicine. Therefore, the perception of feeling seen and understood can help overcome this barrier to access. For this reason, knowledge of these cultural concepts of distress helps establish a better connection between the health provider and their patients. In this way, a health provider can acquire a mutually acceptable perception of a patient's state of mental and emotional distress.

The clinical manifestations of culture-bound syndromes are diverse. By their very definition, they are described in different ways in various cultures—each with its unique cultural slant. However, they tend to have some features in common, which include the following:

QUICK POINT

There is increasing world trade and migration. With increasing globalization, the possibility of coming across culturally diverse individuals in practice only increases. Many cultures around the world believe in causes of mental illness and distress that are not explained by the biopsychosocial model psychiatrists use. This cultural disconnect may be a barrier to accessing mental health care for immigrants and minority populations.

CLINICAL TIP

Culture bound syndromes are described in different ways in various cultures—each with its unique cultural slant. They often occur without prodromal symptoms and usually include an element of acting out in a manner familiar to the individual's culture. The triggers of the illness may not be readily identified as stressors in Western culture. The patients may need psychological and pharmacological treatments, but they sometimes also improve spontaneously once their distress is recognized and addressed.

- They commonly occur without prodromal symptoms.
- There is usually a particular element of acting out with which the culture is familiar.
- The triggers of the illness may not be readily identified as stressors in the Western culture.
- They often have somatic symptoms related to the gastrointestinal system, the reproductive system, or other physiological functions.
- Patients may need psychological and pharmacological treatments, but they sometimes also improve spontaneously once their distress is recognized and addressed.

The following selected examples of culture-bound syndromes are by no means an exhaustive list. More can be found in *DSM-5* and other reference materials.

Examples of Culture-Bound Syndromes

Different cultures and communities manifest mental health symptoms or distress in different ways. Culture-bound syndromes are often manifested as a combination of psychiatric and somatic symptoms. Below are several examples.

Amok (Rampage)

To run amok describes a sudden bout of murderous madness. Amok is a dissociative condition characterized by a sudden, violent, disorganized rage directed against other objects or persons, sometimes resulting in homicide. It has been described in Southeast Asia and Scandinavian countries, as historically reported by the Viking warriors. It is often associated with sleep deprivation, exhaustion, and amnesia. It can result in retribution for a perceived insult. This behavior can also manifest as a brief psychotic disorder or an acute exacerbation of a chronic psychotic illness. Some parallels have been observed between amok and mass shootings in Western societies, including anger, feelings of prejudice, and paranoid thoughts dominating the internal state of the person experiencing this syndrome. When the weapon of choice switches from a dagger to an automatic gun, the casualties are significantly more significant (Eytan, 2019).

Brain Fag Syndrome (BFS)

According to *DSM-4*, this culture-bound syndrome was common among male high school students and college or university undergraduates in West Africa. This syndrome describes stressor and sleep-related somatic and cognitive complaints; difficulty concentrating and retaining information; and head, eye, and neck pains. BFS could be attributed to be anxiety, the use of psychostimulants and consequent sleep deprivation, or caused by real or perceived excessive pressure to be successful among the young. Treatment for this syndrome can be achieved in mild cases with improved sleep and nutrition, stress management, and relaxation exercises. In more severe cases, counseling, anti-anxiety, and antidepressant medications may be needed (Ayonrinde, 2020; Peltzer et al., 1998).

Dhat Syndrome (DS)

Dhat syndrome (DS) is a condition found in China and other areas in South Asia, including Pakistan, India, Bangladesh, Nepal, and Sri Lanka. The patients, usually young males, report that they suffer from premature ejaculation or impotence and believe that they are losing semen in their urine. Similarly, females complain of excessive vaginal discharge or leucorrhea, also considered a "vital fluid" (Grover et al., 2016). Cognitive behavioral therapy has been found effective in the treatment method of this syndrome. Counseling, antianxiety medications, and antidepressant medications are also effective at treating this syndrome.

Hwabyeong (Fire Illness or Anger Illness)

Hwabyeong has been described among Koreans. A somatization disorder arises when people have difficulty confronting their anger under conditions that they perceive to be unfair. Symptoms of anger illness include palpitations, dry mouth, insomnia, a sad mood, feelings of guilt, and impending doom (Lee et al., 2014). Treatment can take the form of psychotherapy, family therapy, and drug treatment, such as via an antidepressant.

Locura

Locura is translated as "insanity" in the Spanish language. It is primarily seen in the United States and Latin America. It is characterized by severe psychotic symptoms similar to schizophrenia. Locura is thought to be a form of neurosis that develops during times of stress or vulnerability in an individual's life and the accumulation of difficulties or trauma. Symptoms of Locura include agitation, inability to follow rules of social interaction, possible violence, difficulty breathing, hallucination, and other similar symptoms. Antidepressants and antipsychotic medications are potential treatments for Locura.

SUMMARY

Cultural psychiatry makes allowances for an individual's culture and subculture in the recognition, understanding, interpretation, accessing of care, treatment, and response to the treatment of mental health symptoms and disorders. Cultural competence in physicians and mental health workers facilitates accurate diagnosis, which informs effective treatment. With increasing globalization, this is becoming increasingly important in health care delivery. Culture-bound syndromes remind us that culture plays an essential role in the manifestation

KEY POINT

Cultural psychiatry makes allowances for an individual's culture and subculture in the recognition, understanding, interpretation, accessing of care, treatment, and response to the treatment of mental health symptoms and disorders. Cultural competence in physicians and mental health workers facilitates accurate diagnosis, which informs effective treatment. With increasing globalization, this is becoming increasingly important in health care delivery. Culture-bound syndromes remind us that culture plays an essential role in the manifestation and response to the treatment of mental disorders.

and response to the treatment of mental disorders. As globalization increases, there may be a lesser overall impact on the currently known culture-bound syndromes. However, the awareness of the effects of culture and subcultures on mental health and its challenges to health services delivery should enhance culturally competent care and improve patient treatment outcomes (Ventriglio et al., 2016). While race- and language-concordant provider–patient relationships are desirable, mental health care workers should be encouraged to progressively improve all providers' cultural and linguistic competency to optimize patient care and reduce disparities in patient outcomes (Belcher, 2020).

RESOURCES

1 https://www.youtube.com/watch?v=SR3jI6NK0Jw

2 https://www.youtube.com/watch?v=FgNaqfGTysU

3 Correll, C. U. S., B.S; Harsinay, A. (Producer). (2018, August 24, 2018). Culture-Specific Psychiatric Syndromes: A Review. *Medscape Psychiatry.* Retrieved from https://www.medscape.com/viewarticle/901027#vp_2 (Accessed January 28, 2021)

REFERENCES

Alvarez, K., Fillbrunn, M., Green, J. G., Jackson, J. S., Kessler, R. C., McLaughlin, K. A., Sadikova, E., Sampson, N. A., & Alegria, M. (2019). Race/ethnicity, nativity, and lifetime risk of mental disorders in US adults. *Social Psychiatry and Psychiatric Epidemiology, 54*(5), 553–565. https://www.doi.org/10.1007/s00127-018-1644-5

American Psychiatric Association. (2000). *Diagnostic and Statistical Manual of Mental Disorders* (4th ed.).

American Psychiatric Association. (2013). *Diagnostic and statistical manual of mental disorders* (5th ed.).

American Psychiatric Association. (2020). *APA's apology to Black, Indigenous and people of color for its support of structural racism in psychiatry.* https://www.psychiatry.org/newsroom/apa-apology-for-its-support-of-structural-racism-in-psychiatry

American Psychological Association. (2016). *Table 7. Number of active psychologists by race/ethnicity, 2007–2016.* file:///N:/Articles/Healthcare%20Workforce/Psychologist%20race%20ethnicty%202016.pdf

Anderson, M., & Lopez, G. (2018, January 24). *Key facts about Black immigrants in the U.S.* https://www.pewresearch.org/fact-tank/2018/01/24/key-facts-about-black-immigrants-in-the-u-s/

Ayonrinde, O. A. (2020). 'Brain fag': A syndrome associated with 'overstudy' and mental exhaustion in 19th century Britain. *International Review of Psychiatry (Abingdon, England), 32*(5–6), 520–535. https://www.doi.org/10.1080/09540261.2020.1775428

Belcher, H. S., B. (Producer). (2020, Oct 16). Viewpoint: Diversity, equity and inclusion are best for communities – and for health care. *Baltimore Business Journal.* https://www.bizjournals.com/baltimore/news/2020/10/16/viewpoint-diversity-equity-best-for-health-care.html?&https://www.mhaonline.org/?utm_source=Marketing%20Cloud&utm_medium=email&utm_campaign=campaign%20name&utm_content=www.mhaonline.orgutm_source=MarketingCloud&utm_medium=email&utm_campaign=MHA+News+Roundup+%e2%80%93+October+16%2c+2020&utm_content=Viewpoint%3a+Diversity%2c+Equity+and+Inclusion+Are+Best+for+Communities+%e2%80%94+And+for+Health+Care%26nbsp%3b

Bell, C. C., Jackson, W. M., & Bell, B. H. (2015). Misdiagnosis of African-Americans with Psychiatric Issues – Part II. *Journal of the National Medical Association, 107*(3), 35–41. https://doi.org/10.1016/S0027-9684(15)30049-3.

Donovan, J. (2021, April 09). What does "Caucasian" really mean? Retrieved January 6, 2022, from https://science.howstuffworks.com/life/genetic/what-does-caucasian-really-mean.htm

Eytan, A. (2019). From running amok to mass shootings: a psychopathological perspective. *Revue medicale suisse, 15*(663), 1671–1674.

Fogel, A., Nazir, S., Hirapara, K., & Ray, S. (2020). Cultural assessment and treatment of psychiatric patients. *StatPearls*.

Fortuna, L. (2012). Working with Latino/a and Hispanic patients. https://www.psychiatry.org/psychiatrists/cultural-competency/education/best-practice-highlights/working-with-latino-patients

Grover, S., Avasthi, A., Gupta, S., Dan, A., Neogi, R., Behere, P. B., Lakdawala, B., Tripathi, A., Chakraborty, K., Sinha, V., Bhatia, M. S., Patjoshi, A., Rao, T. S., & Rozatkar, A. (2016). Phenomenology and beliefs of patients with Dhat syndrome: A nationwide multicentric study. *The International Journal of Social Psychiatry, 62*(1), 57-66. https://www.doi.org/10.1177/0020764015591857

Hawthorne, W. B., Folsom, D. P., Sommerfeld, D. H., Lanouette, N. M., Lewis, M., Aarons, G. A., Conklin, R. M., Solorzano, E., Lindamer, L. A., & Jeste, D. V. (2012). Incarceration among adults who are in the public mental health system: Rates, risk factors, and short-term outcomes. *Psychiatric Services, 63*(1), 26–32.

Johnson, R. L., Roter, D., Powe, N. R., & Cooper, L. A. (2004). Patient race/ethnicity and quality of patient-physician communication during medical visits. *American Journal of Public Health,* 94(12), 2084–90).

Jones, C. P. (2000). Levels of racism: a theoretic framework and a gardener's tale. *American Journal of Public Health, 90*(8), 1212–1215.

Jones, N., Marks, R., Ramirez, R., & Rios-Vargas, M. (2021). *2020 census illuminates racial and ethnic composition of the country.* https://www.census.gov/library/stories/2021/08/improved-race-ethnicity-measures-reveal-united-states-population-much-more-multiracial.html

Kessler, R. C., & Ustun, T. B. (2004). The World Mental Health (WMH) Survey Initiative version of the World Health Organization (WHO) Composite International Diagnostic Interview (CIDI). *International journal of methods in psychiatric research, 13*(2), 93–121. https://www.doi.org/10.1002/mpr.168

Lee, J., Wachholtz, A., & Choi, K.-H. (2014). A review of the Korean cultural syndrome hwa-byung: Suggestions for theory and intervention. *Asia T'aep'yongyang sangdam yon'gu, 4*(1), 49–49. https://www.doi.org/10.18401/2014.4.1.4

Lokko, H. N., Chen, J. A., Parekh, R. I., & Stern, T. A. (2016). Racial and ethnic Diversity in the US psychiatric workforce: A perspective and recommendations. *Acad Psychiatry, 40*(6), 898–904. https://www.doi.org/10.1007/s40596-016-0591-2

McGuire, T. G., & Miranda, J. (2008). New evidence regarding racial and ethnic disparities in mental health: policy implications. *Health Affairs (Millwood), 27*(2), 393–403. https://www.doi.org/10.1377/hlthaff.27.2.393

Mental Health America. (2019). Asian American/Pacific Islander communities and mental health. *State of Mental Health in America.* https://www.mhanational.org/issues/asian-americanpacific-islander-communities-and-mental-health

Milloy, C. (2020). Black psychiatrists are few. They've never been more needed. *The Washington Post.* https://www.washingtonpost.com/local/black-psychiatrists-are-few-theyve-never-been-more-needed/2020/08/11/7df9eeea-dbeb-11ea-8051-d5f887d73381_story.html

Murphy, S. L., Xu, J., Kochanek, K. D., Arias, E., & Tejada-Vera, B. (2021). *Deaths: Final data for 2018.* National Center for Health Statistics. https://www.cdc.gov/nchs/data/nvsr/nvsr69/nvsr69-13-508.pdf

National Academies of Sciences, E., & Medicine. (2019). In W. Keenan, C. E. Sanchez, E. Kellogg, & S. M. Tracey (Eds.), *Achieving behavioral health equity for children, families, and communities: Proceedings of a workshop.*

National Center for Injury Prevention and Control, C. f. D. C. a. P. (2021a). *10 leading causes of death, United States 2019, all races, Hispanic, both sexes*. https://wisqars.cdc.gov/cgi-bin/broker.exe

National Center for Injury Prevention and Control, C. f. D. C. a. P. (2021b). *10 leading causes of death, United States 2019, Am Indian/AK Native, Non-Hispanic, both sexes*. https://wisqars.cdc.gov/cgi-bin/broker.exe

National Congress of American Indians. (2020). *Tribal Nations and the United States: An introduction*. https://www.ncai.org/tribalnations/introduction/Indian_Country_101_Updated_February_2019.pdf

Office of Minority Health. (2021). *Mental and behavioral health—Hispanics*. https://minorityhealth.hhs.gov/omh/browse.aspx?lvl=4&lvlid=69

Peltzer, K., Cherian, V. I., & Cherian, L. (1998). Brain fag symptoms in rural South African secondary school pupils. *Psychological Reports, 83*(3 Pt 2), 1187–1196. https://www.doi.org/10.2466/pr0.1998.83.3f.1187

Smedley, B., Stith, A., & Nelson, A. R. (2003). In B. D. Smedley, A. Y. Stith, & A. R. Nelson (Eds.), *Unequal treatment: Confronting racial and ethnic disparities in health care.*

Statista Research Department. (2020). *Hispanic population groups in the United States, by country of origin 2019*. https://www.statista.com/statistics/234852/us-hispanic-population/

Substance Abuse and Mental Health Services Administration. (2015). *Racial/ethnic differences in mental health service use among sdults*. (HHS Publication No. SMA-15-4906). Substance Abuse and Mental Health Services Administration. https://www.samhsa.gov/data/sites/default/files/MHServicesUseAmongAdults/MHServicesUseAmongAdults.pdf

Substance Abuse and Mental Health Services Administration. (2020a). *2019 National Survey on drug use and health: Asian/Native Hawaiians and other Pacific Islanders (NHOPI)*. U.S. Department of Health and Human Services. file:///N:/Articles/Mental%20Health_epidemiology/Asian_NHOPI.pdf

Substance Abuse and Mental Health Services Administration. (2020b). *Behavioral health barometer: United States, volume 6: Indicators as measured through the 2019 National Survey on Drug Use and Health and the National Survey of Substance Abuse Treatment Services.*

Substance Abuse and Mental Health Services Administration. (2020c). *Table 8.17B. Received mental health services in past year among persons aged 18 or older, by past year level of mental illness and demographic characteristics: Percentages, 2018 and 2019.* Substance Abuse and Mental Health Services Administration file:///N:/Articles/Mental%20Health_epidemiology/NSDUHDetTabs8-17pe2019.pdf

Substance Abuse and Mental Health Services Administration. (2020d). *Table 8.21B. Received prescription medication as a type of mental health service in past year among persons aged 18 or older, by past year level of mental illness and demographic and socioeconomic characteristics: Percentages, 2018 and 2019.* https://www.samhsa.gov/data/report/2019-nsduh-detailed-tables

Substance Abuse Treatment Services. (HHS Publication No. PEP20-07-02-001). Substance Abuse and Mental Health Services Admininstration https://www.samhsa.gov/data/sites/default/files/reports/rpt32815/National-BH-Barometer_Volume6.pdf

Tseng, W. S. (2006). From peculiar psychiatric disorders through culture-bound syndromes to culture-related specific syndromes. *Transcult Psychiatry, 43*(4), 554–576. https://www.doi.org/10.1177/1363461506070781

Turner, E. A. (2014). *African American mental health: What are the facts?* Retrieved from https://www.psychologytoday.com/us/blog/the-race-good-health/201406/african-american-mental-health-what-are-the-facts

U. S. Census Bureau. (2019). *Annual estimates of the resident population by sex, race, and hispanic origin for the United States: April 1, 2010 to July 1, 2019* (NC-EST2019-SR11H). https://www.census.gov/data/tables/time-series/demo/popest/2010s-national-detail.html

U. S. Census Bureau. (2021). *Asian American and Pacific Islander Heritage Month: May 2021*. https://www.census.gov/newsroom/facts-for-features/2021/asian-american-pacific-islander.html

U.S. Department of Justice. (2016). *Prisoners in 2015*. NCJ 250229 (Bureau of Justice Statistics Bulletin). https://www.bjs.gov/content/pub/pdf/p15.pdf

United States Office of Personnel Management. (2011). *Guidance for agency-specific diversity and inclusion strategic plans*. https://www.opm.gov/policy-data-oversight/diversity-and-inclusion/reports/diagencyspecificstrategicplanguidance.pdf

Vargas, S. M., Huey, S. J., & Miranda, J. (2020). A critical review of current evidence on multiple types of discrimination and mental health. *American Journal of Orthopsychiatry, 90*(3), 374–390. https://www.doi.org/10.1037/ort0000441

Ventriglio, A., Ayonrinde, O., & Bhugra, D. (2016). Relevance of culture-bound syndromes in the 21st century. *Psychiatry and Clinical Neurosciences, 70*(1), 3–6. https://www.doi.org/10.1111/pcn.12359

CHAPTER 43

Research in Psychiatry and Behavioral Sciences

Nidal Moukaddam, M.D., Ph.D.; Edore Onigu-Otite, M.D.; and Asim Shah, M.D.

> *"The art and science of asking questions is the source of all knowledge."*
>
> — Thomas Berger

OBJECTIVES

After reading this chapter, students will be able to do the following:

- review principles of research in psychiatry
- discuss research types and quality of evidence
- summarize drug and device development process

DEFINITIONS AND KEY CONCEPTS

Research is the systematic investigation into and study of materials and associations to establish facts and reach new conclusions. It is a diligent systematic activity aimed at increasing the inventory of knowledge.

KEY POINT

Research is the systematic investigation into and study of materials and associations to establish facts and reach new conclusions. It is a diligent systematic activity aimed at increasing the inventory of knowledge. Research is essential for advancing science.

INTRODUCTION

Research is essential to advance science. In the history of research in psychiatry and behavioral sciences, earlier studies were mainly observational. Some of these studies strongly influenced the understanding of human behavior, such as those on early child development. These studies were conducted at a time when neurobiological factors related to the development of mental illness were not available or in common use. Nevertheless, these studies have their place in psychiatry and behavioral sciences and have led to more sophisticated ways of conducting research in the field.

Human behavior is influenced by biological, psychological, and social factors. This sometimes poses a challenge to conducting studies in behavior and social sciences because the impact of these factors can be difficult to separate. Over time, studies have become progressively more sophisticated and can now include multiple data pieces, including biological markers and neuroimaging in many cases. Consequently, with a growing body of scientific studies, quality research continues to be done, which promotes our understanding and treatment of mental illness.

PRINCIPLES OF RESEARCH METHODOLOGY

In medical education, an emphasis is placed on being able to read and assess research studies and decide whether such studies will affect one's practice and approach to treatment. A medical practitioner also needs to be able to conceptually know how to generate, understand, and report interesting findings. General research principles apply to all academic, scholarly research processes with an emphasis on *experimental designs* in medical disciplines.

KEY POINT

A study hypothesis is an educated guess or prediction that proposes a relationship between two or more variables. This begins with a research question. Posing the right research question and generating the right hypothesis are the foundations of a good study.

In reading a research article or thinking of designing a research project, simple questions underlie the process. A *study hypothesis* is an educated guess or prediction that proposes a relationship between two or more variables. This can be tested through scientific study of the hypothesis. A study hypothesis begins with a research question. Posing the right research question and generating the right hypothesis are the foundations of a good study. Asking the right questions improves your reading through studies as well as designing your own study. If asked in the past tense, the questions can guide the reading or reviewing of a study. On the other hand, if asked in the future tense, the questions can guide study designs. Examples of questions to ask when reading or preparing a study are detailed in Table 43.1.

TABLE 43.1 Study Review or Design Questions

	Reading or reviewing a study	Preparing a study
The question	What was the question asked? What was this study trying to show?	What is the question to be asked? What will the study try to show?
Data collection	What data was collected? How was the data gathered? When was the data gathered? Where was the data gathered? Who were the subjects? Who collected the data? Was the data analyzed correctly?	What data will need to be collected? How will I gather the data? When will I gather the data? Where will I gather the data? Who will the subjects be? Who will collect the data? How can I analyze the data accurately?
Results	Were the results presented objectively—in an unbiased and in a statistically sound manner? Were any major or important findings left out of the conclusion?	How can I present the results objectively—in an unbiased and in a statistically sound manner? How can I capture all important findings?
Conclusion	Was the conclusion presented objectively? Did the study demonstrate the findings it claimed?	How can I present the conclusion objectively? How can I show what I claimed to demonstrate?
Logistics and biases	Who supplied the manpower, access, and analysis, and how was the cost (if applicable) covered?	Who will supply the manpower, access, and analysis, and how will the cost (if applicable) be covered?

More specific human clinical research principles apply when thinking of selecting treatment for patients or understanding whether a new treatment advancing to market is safe and effective. A basic overview of those methodologies is presented in the second half of the chapter.

THE SPECTRUM OF QUALITATIVE TO QUANTITATIVE RESEARCH

Figure 43.1 presents a simplified diagram of research design. Research is either experimental or observational. The terms *quantitative* and *qualitative* are still used and represent the spectrum of the scholarly research process. The gold standard in medical research is the randomized controlled trial (RCT), which is a type of experimental, quantitative trial in which every subject has a control, and the odds of being assigned to either group are randomized. RCTs are the epitome of quantitative research.

Quantitative or experimental research is based on the assumption of a fixed and measurable reality, and inferences are made by analyzing numbers or measurements. Quantitative is not always experimental, but the ability to properly quantify a parameter and the need to have precisely fixed and described setup conditions easily lends itself to modifications and, thus, experimentations.

For experimental research to proceed smoothly, *blinding* and *randomization* are essential to avoid bias in rating or reporting results. A researcher who wants to study a treatment, for instance, might be more likely, in a nonrandomized scenario, to select subjects who could benefit from said treatment. A rater who is blinded to experimental conditions would not know if the subject has received treatment versus placebo and would rate in an unbiased manner.

In circumstances where a field is not ready for experimentation, rigorous analytical observational studies can highlight where further research efforts should be targeted. In this case, the study might lend itself to exploratory data analysis, which looks at all observed data without the imposition of a prior model or hypothesis. Figure 43.1 describes how to select treatments in the absence of gold-standard evidence. Figure 43.2 describes types of analytical observational studies.

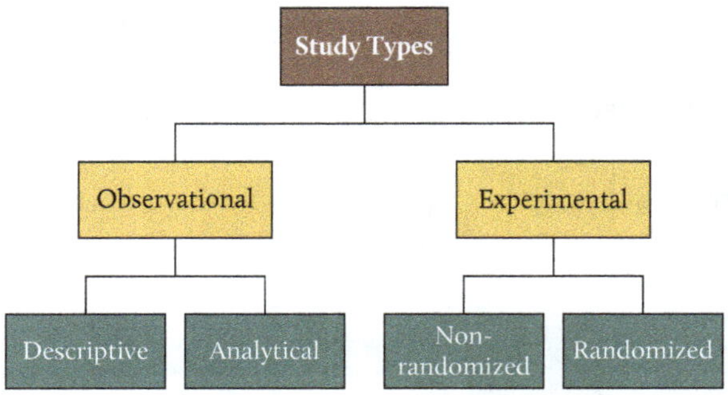

FIGURE 43.1 Types of analytical observational studies.

Cross-sectional studies refer to a snapshot in time with no inherent temporal dimension, highlighting a particular finding within a set of circumstances. Associations are not known, and this type of research is usually the first step preceding experimental manipulations or adjustments, as it serves for hypothesis generation. Case control studies add the element of controls to infer whether exposure could have affected the outcome at hand with the presence or absence of an exposure. Cohort studies, a higher level of observational studies, provide information when experimental studies are not possible, feasible, or ethical. Cohort and other observational studies can be retrospective or prospective and can last decades. A prospective study looks forward; watches for outcomes during the study period, such as the development of a disease; and relates this to other factors, such as suspected risk or protection factor(s). This usually involves taking a group or cohort of subjects and watching them over a long period. A retrospective study looks backward; checks for exposure to suspected risk or protection factors; and relates this to the outcome of interest, such as the development of a disease. Prospective cohort studies have a temporal framework to assess causality and can, therefore, provide the strongest scientific evidence if carefully conducted (Horton, 2011). Twin studies are a powerful example of cohort studies that could not be conducted in a randomized manner; in an examination of 56,396 twin pairs,

Lakhani et al. (2019) tried to distinguish the effects of nature versus nature on medical conditions for 560 phenotypes.

Qualitative research, in contrast to quantitative methodology, is more naturalistic and follows the unfolding of events or outcomes without attempts at control or manipulation from the researcher. Multiple definitions exist with the core features being a variety of methods and data sources (e.g., interviews and in-depth analysis of historical material), an emphasis on understanding motives and motivations, and curiosity toward apparent patterns and behaviors (Aspers & Corte, 2019). Survey data can be longitudinal (panel data) and can rely on assumptions that the explaratory variables are random, fixed, or mixed. Each of these study designs is subject to its own conditions and statistical paradigms.

Observational research, even when producing descriptive results, cannot tell us about associations or causality and cannot exclude systematic or random confounding factors. Some observational qualitative studies include controls, but even then, causality can be inferred, not proven. The scope is meant to be humanistic and discursive, and some think qualitative research is the basis of grounded theories that then sprout proper experimental quantitative research (Corbin & Strauss, 2014). In some cases, qualitative research lags behind until the discovery or adaptation of proper quantitative methods to properly analyze findings. A prime example is deep learning/artificial intelligence methodology that analyzes words used by individuals and can then identify various mental disorders, including depression (Yoo et al., 2020), or identify psychosis based on language prosody (Lucarini et al., 2020). This kind of research would not have been possible a mere decade ago.

Research involving wearables and smartphone apps is another example of a field transitioning from qualitative to quantitative. Digital health, the ability to monitor and track symptoms with digital means, is an area that evolved conceptually first, exploring what can be measured and how this could impact adherence and outcomes. Machine learning methods were then applied, taking digital health to the stage of experimentation by delivering care digitally and predicting responses to selected treatments.

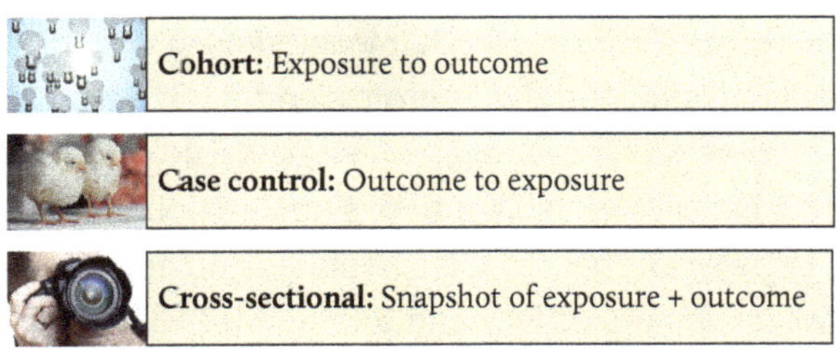

FIGURE 43.2 Types of observational analytical studies.

Copyright © 2015 Depositphotos/peshkov.
Copyright © 2017 Depositphotos/toschevikova.gmail.com.
Copyright © 2012 Depositphotos/Patryk_Kosmider.

CLINICAL RESEARCH

Human research spans comparative and interventional research. Wide-scope mixed methods research can be described as *implementation* research, where a broad range of outcomes can be followed in settings as close to real life as possible in an attempt to understand how to apply research findings in practice and barriers to implementing policies or programs. Human research involves multiple layers of data collection and data management and is also highly regulated in terms of data linkage and sharing between individuals and organizations for purposes of human subject protections, data integrity preservation, and protection from bias. Ethics of data mining and usage of big data in modeling software and artificial intelligence (especially for prediction of behavioral relapses) is a nascent field in biomedical research.

Studies examining whether an intervention or treatment is safe and effective are subject to strict regulations. In interventional research, measures are used to assess whether an intervention or treatment is *safe* and *successful* with studies having primary, secondary, and tertiary outcomes (by order of importance or for exploratory purposes). In randomized controlled trials, primary outcomes are usually the comparison of an intervention group to a placebo group. Subjects are assigned to a placebo or intervention group by chance (random allocation), by cluster (the cluster, rather than the individual, is assigned to intervention or placebo), or in a pragmatic fashion (often by group-level randomization). Multisite trials, involving multiple clinics, sites, or centers, are usually large, sometimes international, and aim to get treatments validated for release into the market. Nuances in study design constitute a whole field and are beyond the scope of this chapter. When a study is designed, outcomes are selected a priori. Associations that were not expected from an experiment are looked at later via post hoc analysis.

QUICK POINT

Clinical trials for pharmaceutical compounds typically follow years of preclinical and basic research. The result of this is a compound that is promising for the treatment of a particular clinical condition.

Clinical trials for pharmaceutical compounds typically follow years of preclinical and basic research (Mochly-Rosen & Grimes, 2014)—the result of which is a compound that is promising for the treatment of a particular clinical condition. Clinical development consists of phases 1 to 3 (Figure 43.3). Phase 1 is typically the first time a new compound is tried in humans. These tend to be small trials that are nonblind and nonrandomized, and they focus on two endpoints: safety and tolerability. Phase 1 trials may also include various dosings of the drug or compound, as the required dose to produce therapeutic effects is not always fully predictable based on allometric scaling from animal data. Other expected results of phase 1 trials include determination of maximum tolerated dosing, safe dosing ranges, CYP and food interactions, and pharmacokinetics.

Phase 2 trials are larger than phase 1 trials and focus on optimizing the conditions (e.g., final dose, route, and regimen) for phase 3 testing. This is also the time to determine what endpoints would be primary and secondary in the phase 3 confirmatory trials. For example, a compound that can work for inattention and for depression may be tested in phase 3 for only one of those as a primary endpoint, as this will shape financial and marketing future steps. Measures of therapeutic effects are added in phase 2, such as biomarkers, imaging, or laboratory datapoints.

QUICK POINT

Clinical development consists of phases 1 to 3 (Figure 43.3). Phase 1 is typically the first time a new compound is tried in humans. These tend to be small, nonblind, and nonrandomized, and they focus on two endpoints: safety and tolerability. Phase 2 trials are focused on optimizing the dosing conditions. Phase 3 trials focus on efficacy within large patient groups and subgroups. Even after FDA approval, post-marketing trials (phase 4) are carried out to ensure continued safety of the drug.

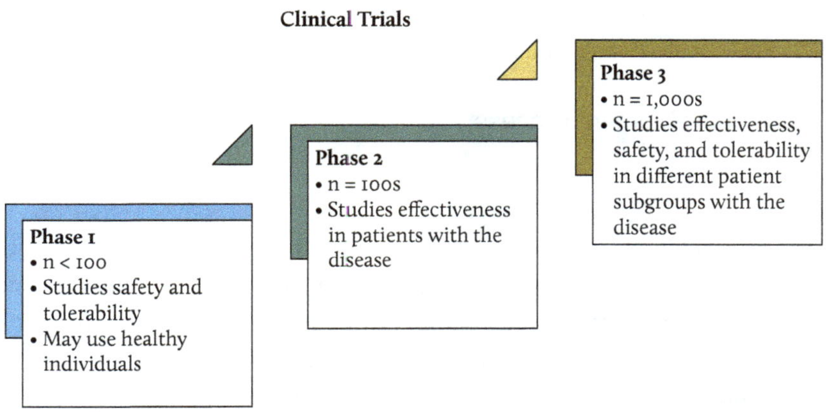

FIGURE 43.3 Phases of a clinical trial.

Phase 3 trials focus on efficacy and have to be large enough to meet Food and Drug Administration (FDA) requirements for safety and efficacy via an approved clinical endpoint with statistical confidence $p < 0.05$. Adverse effects are reported very closely at all trial levels.

Phase 4 (post-marketing) trials are carried out once the drug or device has been approved by the FDA, during the post-market safety monitoring duration. These typically include thousands of volunteers and are very close to real-life conditions in terms of medical comorbidities and polypharmacy use.

KEY POINT

The FDA maintains a thorough process of vetting medications for use in patients. The FDA approves medications for the treatment of specific disorders within the tested doses.

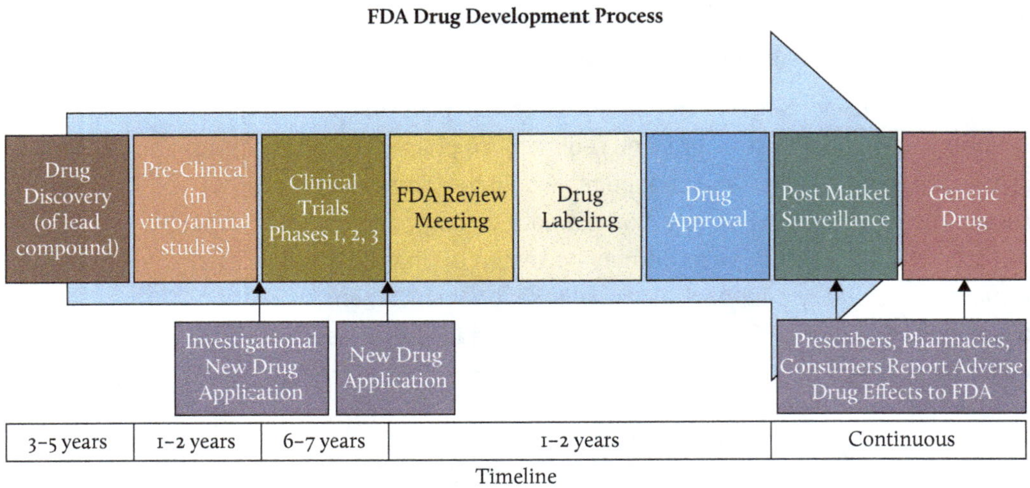

FIGURE 43.4 FDA drug development process.

Funding and Regulatory Oversight

Regulating proper and human conduct of research is essential for protecting human subjects from harm and preventing undue bias in selection, the treatment of subjects, and the reporting of results. Regulatory efforts can be governmental or private in nature and may depend on finding sources for projects. The FDA and institutional review boards (or ethics committees for studies located outside of the United States) seek to ensure that patients are protected. Additionally, regulation of human research seeks to ensure that the risk-to-benefit ratio is acceptable for the proposed clinical studies. Investigational new drug application (IND), including non- and preclinical pharmacology and safety studies; the drug manufacturing and quality assurance (QA) process; and the suggested clinical trial protocol have to be filed with the FDA before clinical trials can begin.

Financial oversight has various levels. First, close scrutiny of individual researchers' conflict of interest ensures adequate reporting of potential conflicts and transparency in the dealings between funders and recipients. This level of transparency is welcome yet slightly at odds with the necessary interface that researchers need to have to promote their work, seek further funding, and seek scalability and commercial applications of their successful discoveries. The second level of scrutiny comes from the funding bodies themselves. In trials funded by the pharmaceutical industry, monitoring on a case-by-case basis is not uncommon, and protocols are rigid and fully manualized. In contrast, governmental research funding, while still requiring a stringent progress report and full compliance with regulatory oversight, leave more flexibility to the research team and provide feedback by renewing or not renewing funding at the end of a set grant period.

TABLE 43.2 Rating Clinical Evidence: Assessment System of the U.S. Preventive Services Task Force

	Quality of evidence
I	Evidence from at least one properly designed randomized controlled trial
II-1	Evidence obtained from well-designed controlled trials without randomization
II-2	Evidence from well-designed cohort or case-control studies, preferably from more than one center or research group
II-3	Evidence from multiple time series with or without the intervention. Important results in uncontrolled experiments (such as the introduction of penicillin treatment in the 1940s) could also be considered as this type of evidence
III	Opinions of respected authorities, based on clinical experience, descriptive studies, or reports of expert committees

SUMMARY

Understanding and designing research is both art and science. It is essential for medical practitioners to have a solid conceptual understanding of research principles to best select treatments for their patients and to be able to keep up with medical literature.

RESOURCES

1 Research Tools - History of Medicine - National Library of Medicine

2 Development and approval process. US Food and Drug Administration

3 Transforming the understanding and treatment of mental illness, National Institute of Mental Health (NIMH)

REFERENCES

Aspers, P., & Corte, U. (2019). What is qualitative in qualitative research. *Qualitative Sociology, 42*(2), 139–160. https://doi.org/10.1007/s11133-019-9413-7

Corbin, J., & Strauss, A. (2014). *Basics of qualitative research: Techniques and procedures for developing grounded theory.* SAGE.

Horton, R. (2011). *Encyclopaedic companion to medical statistics*. Wiley.

Lakhani, C. M., Tierney, B. T., Manrai, A. K., Yang, J., Visscher, P. M., & Patel, C. J. (2019). Repurposing large health insurance claims data to estimate genetic and environmental contributions in 560 phenotypes. *Nature Genetics, 51*(2), 327–334. https://doi.org/10.1038/s41588-018-0313-7

Lucarini, V., Grice, M., Cangemi, F., Zimmermann, J. T., Marchesi, C., Vogeley, K., & Tonna, M. (2020). Speech prosody as a bridge between psychopathology and linguistics: The case of the schizophrenia spectrum. *Front Psychiatry, 11*, 531863. https://doi.org/10.3389/fpsyt.2020.531863

Mochly-Rosen, D., & Grimes, K. (2014). Preparing for the clinic. In D. Mochly-Rosen & K. Grimes (Eds.), *A practical guide to drug development in academia: The SPARK approach* (pp. 79–108). Springer.

Yoo, D. W., Birnbaum, M. L., Van Meter, A. R., Ali, A. F., Arenare, E., Abowd, G. D., & De Choudhury, M. (2020). Designing a clinician-facing tool for using insights from patients' social media activity: Iterative co-design approach. *Journal of Medical Internet Research Mental Health, 7*(8), e16969. https://doi.org/10.2196/16969

INDEX

B

C

D

E

F

G

H

I

J

K

L

M

N

O

P

Q

R

S

T

U

V

W

Y

Z

CPSIA information can be obtained
at www.ICGtesting.com
Printed in the USA
BVHW061301161122
651986BV00002B/3

9 781793 532855